Therapeutic Exercise
Foundations and Techniques
Third Edition

Therapeutic Exercise
Foundations and Techniques
Third Edition

Carolyn Kisner, MS, PT

Assistant Professor
The Ohio State University
School of Allied Medical Professions
Physical Therapy Division
Columbus, Ohio

Lynn Allen Colby, MS, PT

Assistant Professor
The Ohio State University
School of Allied Medical Professions
Physical Therapy Division
Columbus, Ohio

Illustrations by Jerry L. Kisner, MS

F. A. DAVIS COMPANY • PHILADELPHIA

F. A. Davis Company
1915 Arch Street
Philadelphia, PA 19103

Printed in Canada

Last digit indicates print number: 10 9 8 7 6 5 4 3 2 1

Publisher: Jean-François Vilain
Developmental Editor: Crystal McNichol
Production Editor: Roberta Massey
Cover Designer: Steven Ross Morrone

As new scientific information becomes available through basic and clinical research, recommended treatments and drug therapies undergo changes. The authors and publisher have done everything possible to make this book accurate, up to date, and in accord with accepted standards at the time of publication. The authors, editors, and publisher are not responsible for errors or omissions or for consequences from application of the book, and make no warranty, expressed or implied, in regard to the contents of the book. Any practice described in this book should be applied by the reader in accordance with professional standards of care used in regard to the unique circumstances that may apply in each situation. The reader is advised always to check product information (package inserts) for changes and new information regarding dose and contraindications before administering any drug. Caution is especially urged when using new or infrequently ordered drugs.

to Jerry, Craig, & Jodi
CK

to Rick
LC

to our parents, who have been supportive throughout our lives, to our students, who have taught us so much, and to our colleagues, who have been helpful and stimulating in our professional growth
LC and CK

Preface to the Third Edition

Over the past 5 years we have seen many changes in health care delivery. Even though emphasis has always been placed on improving function, the need to document effectiveness of treatment in terms of functional outcome has had a profound impact on the way therapists make decisions for therapeutic intervention. We have attempted to reflect these trends in this edition of *Therapeutic Exercise* while maintaining the original intent and presentation of the text, i.e., to provide a foundation in concepts and techniques upon which an individualized exercise plan can be based. We have also updated information from current research in exercise and postoperative rehabilitation of many orthopedic conditions and have placed greater emphasis on exercises designed to improve stability for functional activities. Illustrations on stabilization and closed-chain exercises have been added to this edition to assist in visualizing application of the techniques. The primary areas of change in the third edition include the following:

- Inclusion in the introductory chapter of the differentiation of the concepts of impairments, disabilities, and handicaps, and emphasis on the importance of measurement of functional outcomes as reflected in the outline for evaluation and assessment.
- Movement of the chapter on aerobic exercise (Chapter 4) from the special section to the first section to emphasize the importance of aerobic conditioning and endurance on exercise training for the overall improvement of functional capacity.
- Development of background information on repetitive trauma syndromes and expanded information on common syndromes in respective extremity and spinal chapters.
- Expansion of concepts and material on functionally related exercises including closed chain, plyometrics, and stabilization training while retaining the need for selective muscle re-education and training through safe and appropriate open-chain exercises.
- Reorganization of each extremity chapter so that, after the brief kinesiology review section, the remaining sections first present a discussion of a common condition followed by the plan for conservative management, then immediately present surgical intervention and plan for postoperative management of the same condition. The final section in each chapter describes and illustrates exercises and progressions that can be used to meet the goals in the treatment plans for the respective joint region. We believe this reorganization will lend greater continuity to the material.

- Reorganization of the spinal chapters so that, following the kinesiology review, approaches for treatment of acute conditions precede treatment of subacute and postural problems. The principles of spinal stabilization training are integrated into the traditional exercises to help the reader recognize the purpose and value of each type of exercise when designing programs for treatment toward functional rehabilitation. Those familiar with the first or second editions of this text will recognize the deletion of the chapter on scoliosis. Pertinent material on this condition has been retained within Chapter 15 on the treatment of spinal problems.
- Revision and expansion of Chapter 17, "Principles of Exercise for the Obstetric Patient" to include trends in prenatal aerobic exercising as supported by recent research and the current statement from The American College of Obstetricians and Gynecologists.
- Updating information in all of the chapters to reflect current research.

Our intent remains to provide the student and clinician with a foundation for designing creative and appropriate therapeutic exercise programs, and we hope that the updated information and reorganization of content in this third edition will continue to serve this purpose.

Preface to the
First Edition

Therapeutic exercise is one of the key tools that a physical therapist uses to restore and improve a patient's musculoskeletal or cardiopulmonary well being. Every therapist needs to have a foundation of knowledge and skills that can be used to manage the majority of patient problems seen. The therapist can then build upon the basic knowledge and progress into specialty areas as interest and patient population dictate. This book has been designed to provide a foundation of appropriate exercise principles and techniques based on current rationale to be used as an instructional tool for the student in the classroom and laboratory setting. It can also be used as a reference for the therapist and other practitioners using exercise in a clinical setting. The scope is inclusive of all basic approaches to exercise including joints, muscles, and other soft tissue and cardiopulmonary conditions. This book does not deal with neuromuscular facilitation techniques because there are many excellent books that specifically address the problems and treatment approaches for the neurologically involved patient. A number of advanced musculoskeletal therapeutic techniques, such as spinal mobilization and manipulation as well as extremity manipulation, have also been excluded from this textbook. We feel a solid foundation in basic skills is necessary prior to learning these advanced skills.

Within this book the reader is directed in the choice of exercise techniques according to the problems presented by the patient and the goals for treatment, not on diagnosis. The book is not a cookbook of exercise routines and protocols for various conditions, because we believe that to learn *how* but not *why* or *when* to apply exercise techniques does not serve the interest of the patient. This book is divided into three major sections to provide a useful foundation in the *how to*, as well as the rationale in the *when* and *why* of therapeutic exercise.

In Part 1, the first chapter begins by drawing together information on a basic approach to evaluation and program development using a simplified problem-solving method and summarizing the typical goals for therapeutic exercise intervention. The remaining four chapters in Part 1 describe the rationale and techniques of therapeutic exercise including range of motion, strengthening procedures, soft tissue stretching, relaxation techniques, and peripheral joint mobilization techniques.

Part 2 presents information on when to apply therapeutic exercise techniques. The section begins with Chapter 6, in which information is presented on soft tissue injury, the repair process, and typical clinical problems. Treatment goals and a general plan of care, based on the clinical problems described, are used to summarize each stage of healing as well as the conditions of rheumatoid arthritis, osteoarthritis, post-fracture management, and surgical management. The goals and plans of care can be used as a foundation for establishing any exercise program and are used as the basis for describing approaches to exercise for each region of the body in the remaining chapters in this section.

The remaining chapters in Part 2 are designed to accomplish three purposes. The first purpose is to provide a review of anatomy, joint mechanics, and muscle function for the region of the body to be treated. This material has been included to help the reader recall important facts that are necessary in designing exercises to restore normal anatomic and biomechanical relationships. The second purpose is to present management approaches in the treatment of joint, soft tissue, and vascular problems common to the region of the body being discussed. The presentation is not comprehensive but is inclusive of enough problems to provide a foundation in treatment approach. The information is not presented as a protocol but rather as a guideline of what to consider for treatment. Patient condition and response to evaluation should be the deciding factors in the choice of techniques. Within each chapter, additional exercise techniques, unique to the region, are described. The third purpose is to include information on the therapeutic exercise management of common surgical procedures. For background information, a brief overview of a variety of surgical procedures is given. Numerous references are provided for in-depth descriptions of surgical procedures if further study is desired. Emphasis is placed on the use of therapeutic exercise in postoperative management by outlining the guidelines, precautions, and progression of the plan of care.

Part 3 includes therapeutic exercise principles and techniques in the specialty areas of chest physical therapy and aerobic exercise. The concluding chapter provides a process for the analysis of physical fitness programs.

We believe the integrated approach used in this book, emphasizing identification of patient problems through skillful evaluation, establishing realistic goals based on the problems, and then deciding on a plan of care to meet the goals, decreases the emphasis on establishing cookbook treatments. This format allows the therapist the challenge of creatively designing an exercise program to best meet the needs of each individual patient. The approach goes beyond the technical doing and allows the therapist to be a thinking contributor to health care.

Acknowledgments

In addition to all those who helped with the previous editions, we wish to thank the following people for their contributions in this revision:

Terri Marble Glenn—for her revision of Chapter 4, "Principles of Aerobic Exercise."

Adam, Mike, and Jodi—for their time, patience, and good humor while posing for the pictures for the third edition, and Carolyn Burnett for again contributing her photographic skills.

The staff at F. A. Davis—Jean-François Vilain, Crystal McNichol, Herb Powell, Jr., Bob Butler, Steve Morrone, and Roberta Massey.

Contributors

Carolyn N. Burnett, MS, PT
Associate Professor Emeritus
Ohio State University
School of Allied Medical Professions
Physical Therapy Division
Columbus, Ohio

Terri M. Glenn, PhD, PT
Lecturer
Ohio State University
School of Allied Medical Professions
Physical Therapy Division
Columbus, Ohio

Cathy J. Konkler, BS, PT
Licking Rehabilitation Services, Inc.
Newark, Ohio

Contents

PART I

General Concepts and Techniques 1

Chapter 1

Introduction to Therapeutic Exercise 3

   I. Approach to Patient Evaluation and Program Development, 4
  II. Goals of Therapeutic Exercise, 13
 III. Summary, 21

Chapter 2

Range of Motion 24

    I. Definitions of Range of Motion Exercises, 25
   II. Indications and Goals for Range of Motion, 25
  III. Limitations of Range of Motion, 26
  IV. Precautions and Contraindications to Range of Motion, 27
   V. Procedures for Applying Range of Motion Techniques, 27
  VI. Techniques for Joint and Muscle ROM Using Anatomic Planes
      of Motion, 28
 VII. Techniques for ROM Using Combined Patterns of Motion, 42
VIII. Techniques of ROM Using Self-Assistance and
      Mechanical Assistance, 43
  IX. Continuous Passive Motion, 52
   X. Range of Motion Through Functional Patterns, 54
  XI. Summary, 54

Chapter 3

Resistance Exercise 56

    I. Definition of Resistance Exercise, 57
   II. Goals and Indications of Resistance Exercise, 57
  III. Precautions for and Contraindications to Resistance Exercise, 59
  IV. Types of Resistance Exercise, 65
   V. Manual Resistance Exercise, 72
  VI. Techniques of Manual Resistance Exercise, 75
 VII. Mechanical Resistance Exercise, 83
VIII. Specific Exercise Regimens, 89
  IX. Use of Equipment With Resistance Exercise, 94
   X. Summary, 107

Chapter 4

Principles of Aerobic Exercise 111

CAROLYN N. BURNETT, MS, PT • TERRI M. GLENN, PhD, PT

    I. Key Terms, 112
    II. Energy Systems, Energy Expenditure, and Efficiency, 115
    III. Physiologic Response to Aerobic Exercise, 118
    IV. Testing as a Basis for Exercise Programs, 120
    V. Determinants of an Exercise Program, 123
    VI. The Exercise Program, 126
    VII. Physiologic Changes That Occur With Training, 129
    VIII. Application of Principles of an Aerobic Conditioning Program for the
       Patient With Coronary Disease, 131
    IX. General Clinical Applications of Aerobic Training, 134
    X. Age Differences, 137
    XI. Summary, 141

Chapter 5

Stretching 143

    I. Definition of Terms Related to Stretching, 144
    II. Properties of Soft Tissue That Affect Elongation, 146
    III. Therapeutic Methods to Elongate Soft Tissues, 155
    IV. Indications and Goals of Stretching, 161
    V. Procedures for Applying Passive Stretching, 161
    VI. Inhibition and Relaxation, 163
    VII. Precautions and Contraindications, 166
    VIII. Techniques of Stretching Using Anatomic Planes of Motion, 167
    IX. Summary, 180

Chapter 6

Peripheral Joint Mobilization 183

    I. Definitions of Joint Mobilization, 184
    II. Basic Concepts of Joint Motion: Arthrokinematics, 185
    III. Indications for Joint Mobilization, 190
    IV. Limitations of Joint Mobilization Techniques, 191
    V. Contraindications and Precautions, 191
    VI. Procedures for Applying Joint Mobilization Techniques, 193
    VII. Peripheral Joint Mobilization Techniques, 199
    VIII. Summary, 232

PART II

Application of Therapeutic Exercise Techniques to Regions
of the Body 235

Chapter 7

Principles of Treating Soft Tissue, Bony, and Postsurgical Problems 237

    I. Soft Tissue Lesions, 238
    II. Stages of Inflammation and Repair: General Descriptions, 240
    III. The Acute Stage: General Treatment Guidelines, 243
    IV. The Subacute Stage: General Treatment Guidelines, 247
    V. The Chronic Stage: General Treatment Guidelines, 250
    VI. Chronic Recurring Pain -- Chronic Inflammation -- General
       Treatment Guidelines, 253
    VII. Rheumatoid Arthritis: General Treatment Guidelines, 257
    VIII. Osteoarthritis: General Treatment Guidelines, 259
    IX. Fractures: General Treatment Guidelines, 261
    X. Surgery, 262
    XI. Summary, 270

Chapter 8
The Shoulder and Shoulder Girdle 273

   I. Review of the Structure and Function of the Shoulder and
      Shoulder Girdle, 274
  II. Joint Problems: Nonoperative Management, 278
  III. Glenohumeral Joint Surgery and Postoperative Management, 287
  IV. Painful Shoulder Syndromes: Repetitive Trauma (Overuse)
      Syndromes, Impingement Syndromes, Shoulder Instabilities, and
      Rotator Cuff Tears, 291
  V. Shoulder Dislocations, 300
  VI. Thoracic Outlet Syndrome, 306
  VII. Reflex Sympathetic Dystrophy, 307
  VIII. Exercise Techniques for Management of Acute and Early Subacute
      Soft Tissue Lesions, 309
  IX. Exercise Techniques for Management of Muscle Strength and
      Flexibility Imbalances in Subacute and Chronic
      Shoulder Problems, 313
  X. Summary, 328

Chapter 9
The Elbow and Forearm Complex 332

   I. Review of the Structure and Function of the Elbow and Forearm, 333
  II. Joint Problems: Nonoperative Management, 336
  III. Joint Surgery and Postoperative Management, 339
  IV. Myositis Ossificans, 342
  V. Overuse Syndromes, Repetitive Trauma Syndromes, 343
  VI. Exercises for Muscle Strength and Flexibility Imbalances, 347
  VII. Summary, 350

Chapter 10
The Wrist and Hand 352

   I. Review of the Structure and Function of the Wrist and Hand, 353
  II. Joint Problems: Nonoperative Management, 358
  III. Joint Surgery and Postoperative Management, 363
  IV. Repetitive Trauma Syndromes/Overuse Syndromes, 372
  V. Traumatic Lesions in the Hand, 374
  VI. Exercises for Muscle Strength or Flexibility Imbalance, 380
  VII. Summary, 384

Chapter 11
The Hip 386

   I. Review of the Structure and Function of the Hip, 387
  II. Joint Problems: Nonoperative Management, 392
  III. Joint Surgery and Postoperative Management, 394
  IV. Fractures of the Proximal Femur and
      Postoperative Management, 399
  V. Overuse Syndromes/Repetitive Trauma Syndromes:
      Nonoperative Management, 401
  VI. Exercises for Muscle Strength or Flexibility Imbalance, 403
  VII. Summary, 415

Chapter 12
The Knee 417

   I. Review of the Structure and Function of the Knee, 417
  II. Joint Problems and Capsular Restrictions:
      Nonoperative Management, 421
  III. Joint Surgery and Postoperative Management, 425
  IV. Patellofemoral Dysfunction: Nonoperative Management, 431

V. Patellofemoral and Extensor Mechanism Surgery and
Postoperative Management, 436
VI. Sprains and Minor Ligamentous Tears, 441
VII. Meniscal Tears, 448
VIII. Exercises for Muscle Strength and Flexibility Imbalances, 453
IX. Summary, 465

Chapter 13
The Ankle and Foot 469

I. Review of the Structure and Function of the Ankle and Foot, 470
II. Joint Problems: Nonoperative Management, 476
III. Joint Surgery and Postoperative Management, 478
IV. Overuse Syndromes/Repetitive Trauma Syndromes, 482
V. Traumatic Soft Tissue Injuries, 484
VI. Exercises for Muscle Strength and Flexibility Imbalances, 488
VII. Summary, 494

Chapter 14
The Spine: Acute Problems 496

I. Review of the Structure and Function of the Spine, 497
II. General Guidelines for Treating Acute Symptoms, 504
III. Intervertebral Disk and Flexion Load Lesions, 506
IV. Facet Joint Lesions in the Spine, 517
V. Muscle and Soft Tissue Lesions: Strains, Tears, and Contusions From
Trauma or Overuse, 521
VI. Selected Conditions, 525
VII. Summary, 528

Chapter 15
The Spine: Subacute, Chronic, and Postural Problems 531

I. The Dynamics of Posture, 532
II. Characteristics and Problems of Common Faulty Postures, 534
III. Procedures to Relieve Pain From Stress and Muscle Tension, 542
IV. Procedures to Increase the Range of Motion of Specific Structures, 545
V. Procedures to Train and Strengthen Muscle Function and to Develop
Endurance for Postural Control (Stabilization Exercises), 551
VI. Procedures to Retrain Kinesthetic and Proprioceptive Awareness for
Posture Correction, 568
VII. Procedures to Teach Management of Posture to Avoid Recurrences
of the Problem, 571
VIII. Summary, 573

Chapter 16
The Spine: Traction Procedures 575

I. Effects of Spinal Traction, 576
II. Definitions and Descriptions of Traction, 578
III. Indications for Spinal Traction, 579
IV. Limitations, Contraindications, and Precautions, 581
V. General Procedures, 582
VI. Cervical Traction Techniques, 583
VII. Lumbar Traction Techniques, 587
VIII. Summary, 590

PART III
Special Areas of Therapeutic Exercise 593

Chapter 17
Principles of Exercise for the Obstetric Patient 595
CATHY J. KONKLER, BS, PT • CAROLYN KISNER, MS, PT

    I. Overview of Pregnancy, Labor, and Delivery, 596
    II. Anatomic and Physiologic Changes of Pregnancy, 598
    III. Pregnancy-Induced Pathology, 602
    IV. Effects of Aerobic Exercise During Pregnancy, 606
    V. Exercise During Pregnancy and Postpartum, 608
    VI. Cesarean Childbirth, 621
    VII. High-Risk Pregnancy, 623
    VIII. Summary, 627

Chapter 18
Management of Vascular Disorders of the Extremities 629

    I. Arterial Disorders, 630
    II. Venous Disorders, 636
    III. Lymphatic Disorders, 640
    IV. Mastectomy, 641
    V. Summary, 647

Chapter 19
Chest Physical Therapy 649

    I. Review of Respiratory Structure and Function, 650
    II. Evaluation in Chest Physical Therapy, 657
    III. Breathing Exercises, 664
    IV. Exercises to Mobilize the Chest, 672
    V. Coughing, 675
    VI. Postural Drainage, 679
    VII. Summary, 687

Chapter 20
Management of Obstructive and Restrictive Pulmonary Conditions 689

    I. Overview of Obstructive Lung Disease, 690
    II. Specific Obstructive Pulmonary Conditions, 691
    III. Overview of Restrictive Lung Disorders, 699
    IV. Specific Restrictive Pulmonary Conditions, 700
    V. Summary, 709

Chapter 21
Critical Analysis of Exercise Programs 711

    I. Designing an Exercise Program: Why Exercise?, 712
    II. Establishing a Baseline by Which Improvement Can
       Be Measured, 712
    III. Establishing Realistic Goals, 718
    IV. Summary, 726

Glossary 727

Index 739

General Concepts and Techniques

Introduction to Therapeutic Exercise

The ultimate goal of any therapeutic exercise program is the achievement of symptom-free movement and function. To effectively administer therapeutic exercise to a patient, the therapist must know the basic principles and effects of exercise on the musculoskeletal, neuromuscular, cardiovascular, and respiratory systems. In addition, the therapist must be able to perform a functional evaluation of the patient and must know the interrelationships of the anatomy and kinesiology of the part, as well as have an understanding of the state of the injury, disease, or surgical procedure and its potential rate of recovery, complications, precautions, and contraindications. Material in this book is presented with the assumption that the reader has had a foundation in human anatomy, physiology, medical kinesiology, and evaluation procedures (including posture evaluation, goniometric measurements, manual and mechanical methods of muscle testing, systematic orthopedic evaluation procedures, and functional outcome testing) and that the reader possesses basic information about the pathology of orthopedic, cardiac, and pulmonary medical conditions.

OBJECTIVES

After studying this chapter, the reader will be able to:

1   Outline a systematic approach to patient evaluation based on critical thinking for the decision-making process of identifying impairments, functional limitations, and disabilities.
2   Identify the sequence of program development based on operationally defined goals, desired functional outcome, and plan of care to meet the goals.
3   Describe basic goals of therapeutic exercise and define related terminology.

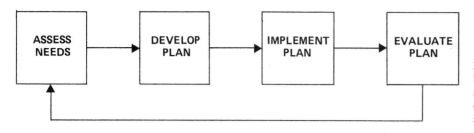

Figure 1–1. Simplified feedback loop depicting a problem-solving approach to patient care. (From Pierson, Burnett, and Kisner,[49] with permission.)

I. Approach to Patient Evaluation and Program Development

Quality patient care involves a problem-solving process whereby the therapist makes effective decisions based on the symptoms, signs, and limitations identified when evaluating and re-evaluating the patient. Simply depicted, it is a feedback loop (Fig. 1–1) and is compatible with models of clinical decision making.[25,26,42,65] A comprehensive evaluation of the patient not only avoids the pitfall of overlooking some important contributing factor and allows for defining the functional limitations of the patient but also influences important decisions regarding the development of the treatment program.[12,42] This section outlines an evaluation process for orthopedic and related problems. The reader is referred to several sources for in-depth study of evaluation procedures and techniques[3,9–11,34,35,41,46,48] and discussion of the role of the physical therapist in diagnosis[12,24,33,42,51,53,65] and functional outcome reporting.[25,26,58]

A. Assess Needs

The first step is to assess the patient's needs. To provide cost-effective quality care in today's health care environment, it is critical to measure needs in terms of the patient's impairments as well as any functional limitations and resulting disabilities or handicaps using objective **outcome measures,** which are clearly defined as measurable activities.[3,6,25] An **impairment** is any loss or abnormality of psychological, physiologic, or anatomic structure or function.[30] It limits or changes an individual's ability to perform a task or activity. **Functional limitation**[24,44] is a limitation from an impairment that is not disabling yet interferes with normal function; **disability** is an inability to undertake normal activities of daily living (ADL); and **handicap** is the social disadvantage resulting from an impairment or disability that prevents or limits the person in his or her occupation, environment, or social setting.[30] (These terms are described in greater detail in the Assessment Section, A.3, of this outline.)

The examination and assessment of the results provide the foundation for establishing a baseline from which outcomes of therapeutic intervention can be measured. The following outline integrates methods for collecting data and identifying the impairments and functional limitations or disabilities of patients with orthopedic difficulties. The discussion of handicaps is beyond the scope of this textbook.

There are many basic examination techniques as well as functional assessment systems.[3,8,9,10,20,34,35,41,48] In recent years, attempts have been made to document the validity and reliability of many of the testing techniques and procedures.[3] There is also a need to validate the tests and procedures in terms of functional outcome. This need for validity has affected the way goals and treatment plans are developed and measured. In addition to assessing patient needs, the needs of the employer and/or caregiver must also be assessed as the findings from the evaluation are interpreted.[25] Although documentation using the SOAP format[16] (subjective/objective/assessment/

plan) is still widespread, some sources describe it as becoming obsolete in preference to functional outcome reporting.[58] The process of obtaining subjective information and objective data to document baseline functional level and subsequent changes is important, no matter which system is used.

1. **Subjective information (the case history)**

   Ask questions so that the patient will:
   a. Describe the onset of the symptoms or mechanism of injury.
      (1) Determine whether symptoms are recent, recurrent, or insidious.
      (2) Determine whether perpetuating circumstances exist.
   b. Describe how the symptoms are perceived.
      (1) Establish the location, type, and nature of the pain or symptoms.
      (2) Determine whether the pain and symptoms fit into a pattern related to segmental reference zones, nerve root patterns, or extrasegmental reference patterns such as dural reference, myofascial pain patterns, peripheral nerve patterns, or circulatory pain.
   c. Describe the behavior of the symptoms through a 24-hour period while carrying out typical daily activities.
      (1) Identify which motions or positions cause or ease the symptoms.
      (2) Determine how severe or how functionally limiting the problem is. The patient describes functional limitations in terms of daily living, work, family, social, and recreational activities.
      (3) Determine how irritable the problem is by how easily the symptoms are evoked and how long they last.
   d. Describe any previous history of the condition. Find out if there has been previous treatment for the problem and the results of the treatment.
   e. Describe related history, such as any medical or surgical intervention.
   f. Briefly describe general health, medications, and x ray or other pertinent studies that have been performed. Identify any medical conditions that may alert you to using special precautions or to contraindications to any testing procedures.

2. **Objective data (the clinical evaluation)**

   Systematically administer tests that will define the **impairment** [the anatomic structure(s) and possible physiologic state] and the **functional limitations** of the patient.
   a. **Inspection**
      Make observations of appearance and basic abilities:
      (1) Use of any adaptive or supportive aids.
      (2) General posture and specific posture or shape of involved body parts such as contour changes, swelling, atrophy, hypertrophy, and asymmetry.
      (3) Appearance of skin, such as scars and discoloration.
      (4) Sitting, stance and gait patterns, general ease of movement, coordination, balance, and ability to disrobe for the evaluation. From this and the results of the diagnostic testing, more detailed tests can be chosen for documentation of functional limitations, disabilities, or handicaps.
   b. **Provocation—selective tension procedures**
      Use the principle of selective tension by administering specific tests in a systematic manner to provoke or re-create the symptoms and thus determine whether the lesion is within an inert structure (joint capsule, ligaments, bursae, fasciae, dura mater, and dural sheaths around nerve roots) or a contractile unit (muscle with its tendons and attachments).[10] Additional joint integrity tests are used to verify problems within the joint.[34] From these tests, it is possible to

identify the forces or stresses reproducing or minimizing the patient's symptoms, the stage of healing, and in many cases, the tissue or tissues causing the
symptoms; that is, identify the impairment(s). From this information it should
be possible to identify a relationship between the stresses to the tissues and the
patient's functional losses. Minimizing and controlling these stresses on the involved tissues form the basis in designing an appropriate therapeutic exercise
program.

(1) Active range of motion (ROM)

The patient is asked to move the body parts related to the symptoms
through their range of motion. From the way the patient moves and the
amount of motion, determine if the patient is able and willing to move the
part. Because both contractile and inert structures are influenced by active
motion, specific problems are not isolated. Anything abnormal in the
movement, any experience of pain, or any changes in sensation are noted.

(2) Passive range of motion

The same movements that the patient performed actively are repeated passively. When the end of the available range is reached, pressure is applied
to get a feel of the resistance of the tissues; the pressure is called **overpressure** and the feel is called **end-feel.** With the muscles relaxed, only
inert structures are being stressed. Note whether any of the tests provoke
the patient's symptoms.

(a) Measure the ROM and compare it with the active ROM. Determine
whether the limitation follows a pattern of restriction typical for that
joint when joint problems exist. (These patterns are described for each
peripheral joint under the respective sections on joint problems in
Chapters 8 through 13.)

(b) Describe the end-feel (the feel the evaluator experiences at the end of
the range when overpressure is applied). Decide whether the feel is
soft (related to compressing or stretching soft tissues), firm (related to
stretching joint capsules and ligaments), or hard (related to a bony
block) or whether there is no end-feel (empty) because the patient will
not allow movement to the end of the available range (related to an
acutely painful condition in which the patient inhibits motion). Decide
whether the end-feel is normal or abnormal for that joint.

Abnormal end-feels include:

—Springy (intra-articular block such as a torn meniscus or articular cartilage)

—Muscle guarding (involuntary muscle contraction in response
to acute pain)

—Muscle spasm (prolonged muscle contraction in response to
circulatory and metabolic changes)

—Muscle spasticity (increased tone and contraction in muscle in
response to central nervous system influences)

—Any end-feel that is different from normal for that joint or at a
different part of the range from normal for the joint being
tested

(c) Determine the stage of pathology by observing when pain is experienced relative to the range of motion. Is the pain or muscle guarding
experienced before the end-feel (acute), concurrent with the end-feel
(subacute), or after application of overpressure (chronic)?

    (d) Determine the *stability* and *mobility* of the joint. Record, using the following grades:

Ankylosed	0
Hypomobile	
Considerable limitation	1
Slight limitation	2
Normal	3
Hypermobile	
Slight increase	4
Considerable increase	5
Unstable	6

    (e) Note whether there is a *painful arc*, which is pain experienced with either active or passive motion somewhere within the ROM. It indicates that some sensitive structure is being pinched during that part of the range of motion. Sometimes pain-sensitive structures are pinched at the end of the range. This is not a painful arc, although such pain should be noted.

(3) Joint integrity (accessory motion) tests

These are passive tests, used to rule out or confirm joint or capsule lesions prior to testing for muscle (contractile) lesions.[27] The tests include:

    (a) Distraction

Separate the joint surfaces and note whether the pain increases or decreases and how easily the bones move apart.

    (b) Compression

Approximate the joint surfaces and note whether the pain increases or decreases. If the pain increases, the compressive force of muscle contraction may also cause increased pain. The source of the pain then is known to be some structure within the joint and not a muscle lesion.

    (c) Gliding

Glide one of the joint surfaces on the other and note the quality and quantity of the joint-play movement (how easily the bones move and whether the joint movement causes pain).

(4) Resisted tests

Resist the related muscles so that they contract isometrically in mid-range to determine whether there is pain or decreased strength in the contractile units. Mid-range isometric contractions are used for minimal movement or stress to the noncontractile structures around the joint. Initially the tests are performed on groups of muscles; then, if a problem is noted, each muscle potentially involved is isolated and tested.

    (a) A strong, yet painful contraction indicates a contractile unit problem (assuming joint problems have been ruled out). Palpate along the entire musculotendinous unit to identify the site of injury.

    (b) A weak and painless contraction may suggest a complete muscle tear, a disused muscle, or a neurologic problem. A muscle tear will have a history of trauma in the region. A disused muscle will usually demonstrate some atrophy and probably not be localized in only one muscle. A neurologic problem will usually have a pattern of sensory loss, as well as weakness in related muscles following a pattern consistent with a nerve root, plexus, or peripheral nerve innervation.

    (c) A weak and painful contraction usually suggests something serious, such as an active lesion, fracture, or inflammation. Relate this to information from the history.

   (d) Document strength with a manual or mechanical muscle test grade.
   (5) Other muscle analysis
      (a) Determine flexibility of two-joint or multijoint muscles.
      (b) Relate imbalances in length and strength between antagonistic muscles.
      (c) Test supporting or stabilizing muscles for strength, coordination, and stabilizing function.

c. Palpation

Palpate, if possible, structures that are incriminated as the source of the problems. Usually palpations are best done after the tests of provocation in order not to increase the irritability of the structures prior to testing. Include:

   (1) Skin and subcutaneous tissue; note temperature, edema, and texture.
   (2) Muscles, tendons, and attachments; note tone, tenderness, trigger points, and contractures.
   (3) Tendon sheaths and bursae; note tenderness, texture, and crepitus.
   (4) Joints; note effusion, tenderness, changes in position or shape, and associated areas such as ligaments.
   (5) Nerves and blood vessels; note presence of neuroma and pulse.

d. Neurologic tests

Any indication of motor weakness or change in sensation directs the evaluator to specific tests to determine nerve, nerve root, or central nervous system involvement. Evaluate:

   (1) Key muscles
      Determine strength and reflexes of muscles related to specific spinal levels and peripheral nerve patterns.
   (2) Motor ability
      Identify any control, balance, or coordination deficits.
   (3) Sensory testing
      Identify changes in perception of temperature, light touch, deep pressure, two-point discrimination, stereognosis, and proprioception and relate loss to peripheral nerve or spinal cord patterns or central nervous system control. If there is a central nervous system impairment, test for body awareness of limbs and trunk, spatial awareness, and perception of vertical alignment.
   (4) Nerve trunk
      Determine whether there is pain on pressure or stretching of the nerve plexus.
   (5) Cranial nerve integrity, if indicated
   (6) Cortical integration and control, if indicated
      Identify abnormal associated reactions, synergies, synkinesis, or postural, righting, and protective reflexes.

e. Additional tests

   (1) Special tests, unique to the specific tissue in each region, are carried out if necessary to confirm or rule out the structures in question.
   (2) Identify the cardiovascular status with measures of endurance or circulatory integrity.
   (3) If indicated, determine respiratory capacity including auscultation, breathing pattern, rate and rhythm of breathing, coughing ability, vital capacity and flow rates, and chest mobility.

(4) Tests performed by physicians or other health personnel may be necessary to identify the source of referred pain patterns and medical disorders.

NOTE: To this point, the outline has addressed a common approach to evaluating orthopedic lesions for the identification of the anatomic structure involved and its stage of inflammation. In addition, testing should be performed to document functional ADL or any activities that restrict job, homemaking, or social and recreational activities.

f. Special tests to document functional limitation, disability, or handicap[3,6,41]
Standardized and consistently measured tests should be used based on the patient's impairment and described limitations. Suggestions include:

(1) Observe gait performance on even and uneven surfaces and with changing directions.

(2) Observe body mechanics and related abilities such as stooping, squatting, kneeling, and bending over.

(3) Observe reaching, pushing, pulling, gripping, and lifting from the floor to various levels.

(4) Observe throwing a ball, running, climbing steps, or rising from a chair.

NOTE: A variety of tests and indices have been developed to document status in ADL, functional independence, level of self-care, and disability ratings. Some have been scrutinized for validity and reliability.[3] Responsibility and care must be taken by the therapist to use standardized tests to develop credibility in documentation of patient care.[59] It is beyond the scope of this text to identify all of the possible tests and their uses.

3. Assessment

Once the subjective and objective data about the patient's tissues and functional abilities (disabilities) are gathered, the information is integrated to determine an overall assessment of the patient and the presenting problems.

a. Identify the diagnosis and impairment.

(1) In the medical model, **diagnosis** is a term used to identify a disease or pathology with characteristic signs and symptoms. Not all physical limitations occur as a result of disease or pathology, yet the term diagnosis is still used to identify the limitation. Diagnosis also refers to the process of making a judgment about the cause or nature of a person's problem.

(2) An **impairment** limits or changes an individual's ability to perform a task or activity. Impairments are identified by the World Health Organization (WHO) in its International Classification of Impairments, Disabilities, and Handicaps (ICIDH) under categories of psychological, physiologic, or anatomic structure.[30] In some instances, an impairment is used as a diagnosis.

(3) Within the field of physical therapy, the role of the physical therapist in identifying impairments and calling them the diagnosis (or physical therapy diagnosis) is being debated and defined.[12,24,33,51,53] The authors of this text believe that the therapist has skills to identify and define physical impairments of the muscloskeletal and neuromuscular systems, and we therefore support the role of the physical therapist in diagnosing structural and functional limitations involving anatomic structures. Currently there is no commonly accepted model encompassing all the possible interpretations and use of the terminology.[45] At the time of this writing it is understood that a

task force has proposed adjustments in the ICIDH to clarify and encompass the definitions and categorization of impairments seen by health professionals that were not identifiable in the original documents.[27] For consistency, although in its evolutionary stages, a generic scheme has been defined by the authors of this text to guide the reader (Table 1–1). In this

TABLE 1–1. Terminology Comparison

World Health Organization's Classification of Impairments, Disabilities, and Handicaps (ICIDH) terminology[30] compared with usage in the physical therapy literature [12,24,33,44,45,51,53] and examples of orthopedic conditions seen by physical therapists.

ICIDH	Suggested Usage	Orthopedic Examples
Disease A pathologic process with a characteristic and identifiable set of signs and symptoms.	**Medical Diagnosis** Related to active pathology from trauma, disease, metabolic imbalance, infection.	Tendinitis, bursitis, rheumatoid arthritis, fracture, surgery, osteoporosis.
Impairment Any loss or abnormality of psychological, physiologic, or anatomic structure or function. It reflects organic dysfunction.	**Diagnostic Categories** Categories of primary dysfunctions identified by the evaluator within the realm of knowledge and practice; may be called an impairment. **Impairments** Related dysfunctions/problems identified by the evaluator associated with the diagnostic category or medical diagnosis.	Overuse syndrome Impingement syndrome Postural syndrome Arthritis/joint restriction Pain at rest, on motion, on repetitive motion, on resistance, on palpation Neurologic symptoms Muscle imbalances Weak muscles Decreased range (muscle/joint) Decreased endurance Poor stability Poor coordination of motion/skill
Disability Any restriction or lack of ability to perform an activity in the manner or within the range considered normal for that individual. Disabilities result from impairments and are categorized as physical, mental, social, and emotional.	**Functional Limitations** Limitations that result from impairments and represent the decreased ability to perform usual roles and daily activities. Interferes with function but is not disabling. Symptoms with specific activities. **Disability** Inability to perform specific activities.	Standing, walking Bending, stooping Kneeling, crouching Lifting, reaching, carrying Driving, cycling Light housework Sports, hobbies Sustained/repetitive activity
Handicap A disadvantage for an individual that limits or prevents fulfillment of a role that is normal for that individual.	**Handicap**	Requires assistance for ADL Unemployable

text, diagnosis encompasses both medical and commonly accepted diagnostic categories, which some references call impairments,[30] primary dysfunctions,[53] or physical therapy diagnoses.[24,51] Use of the term impairments encompasses the problem list, related dysfunctions, or impairments associated with the diagnosis or diagnostic categories.

b. Identify functional limitations or disabilities.

Specifically identify functional limitations or disabilities that are related to the impairments and can be affected by physical therapeutic intervention.[30]

(1) A **disability** "refers to restriction of or inability to perform a normal range of ADL."[24] The World Health Organization identifies physical, mental, social, and emotional disabilities.[30]

(2) Guccione[24] suggests using the category **functional limitations** as described by Nagi[44] to differentiate disabilities that are not truly disabling yet become symptomatic when performing specific activities. The term functional limitations may be more useful than disabilities in these cases because it is more descriptive and less imposing or threatening than disability for many patients with orthopedic injuries. (Heerkens et al[27] propose differentiating disabilities into basic skills and complex skills and suggest using the term abilities rather than disabilities when a positive classification is desired.)

c. Identify any handicaps.

A **handicap** is the social disadvantage that results from the impairment or disability and that prevents or limits the normal role of the person in his or her occupation, environment, or social setting.[30] Most of the conditions addressed in this text do not involve handicaps.

d. Make appropriate referrals.

Identify impairments, limitations, or disabilities beyond or outside the realm of physical therapy and refer to other specialties.

B. Develop Plan

After evaluating and assessing the patient's needs, the next step in the clinical decision-making process is to establish goals and appropriate treatment plan.

1. Factors influencing decisions.[42]

a. The impairments, functional limitations, or disabilities

b. The psychological status, such as the patient's adjustment to the problem, motivation, and personality, as well as ability to understand and learn

c. Socioeconomic support and cultural reactions and expectations

d. Home or alternative care; the physical and emotional environment; family reaction, cooperation, and responsibilities

e. The patient's and employer's vocational plans and goals

f. Ethical considerations and choices

2. Establish goals for expected functional outcome.

a. These are often described as long-term or rehabilitation goals. They are related to how treatment will affect the functional limitations or disability at the conclusion of the therapeutic or rehabilitation program or at the conclusion of one phase of a program. They address whether or not the person will be able to return to work or other defined activity and at what level of participation.

    b. Each goal should be measurable and specific to the conditions or tests used and express the time expected to reach the goal.

3. Identify short-term goals.

    a. These goals are often stated as measurable behavioral objectives affecting the documented impairments.

    b. They usually reflect the component abilities or skills needed to attain the functional outcome such as increasing range, developing proximal stability, increasing endurance, or developing balance.

    c. They progress in difficulty and/or complexity as the patient progresses toward the described functional outcome.

NOTE: Throughout this textbook, lists of treatment goals and plans of care are included. They are written in general terms, not as described here with measurable outcome, tests, and time, because of the global nature of information to which they refer. The therapist should use the lists as guidelines and operationalize the goals for each patient according to his or her condition, desired outcome, and need as described in this section.

4. Develop a plan of care.

    a. Determine what therapeutic approaches will most appropriately meet the goals; consider resources available to the patient's situation.

    b. Select techniques or therapeutic modalities that will fulfill the plan and meet the goals.

    c. Determine what modes of evaluation will be used to document the change reflected in the goals.

    d. Anticipate the length of treatment and plan for discharge; consider any alternate services for treatment.

C. Implement the Plan

1. Once the plan of care is established, use procedures and techniques that will fulfill the plan and meet the goals.
2. Involve the patient (or caregiver) in the management of the impairment(s) both in a home exercise program as well as in the adaptation or modification of the home, work, or recreational environment to minimize or eliminate perpetuating factors contributing to the problem(s).

D. Evaluate the Plan

Frequently evaluate and reassess the effectiveness of the procedures and techniques and modify them or the treatment plan whenever indicated.
1. Compare original data with current data at frequent intervals.
2. Identify goals that have been met, those that need modification, or new goals according to changes in the patient or in his or her lifestyle.

E. Home Program

A home program should be viewed as an extension of the treatment plan of care.
1. Early identification of the patient's home or alternative care setting, family reactions, social and economic capabilities, equipment needed, and vocational plans provide a foundation for anticipating compliance with a home exercise program.

2. If necessary, identify who could and would work with the patient at home.
   a. Involve that person early in the program to make the transition easier.
   b. Teach the person what to do; observe his or her techniques and schedule a follow-up visit to review techniques and answer questions.
3. A home, school, or job visit is advisable in any situation with questions of adaptation or compliance.
4. Motivation and compliance are two situations difficult to control. The following are some suggestions that may influence the patient:
   a. Educate patients about their **impairment** and include them in establishing realistic goals for the management of their problems. This helps them develop ownership of the treatment plan and awareness and participation in the prevention of reinjury or future impairments. Teaching a home program on the day of discharge and expecting understanding and follow-through is unrealistic. The home program should begin at the first treatment and be modified or progressed as patients progress.
   b. Convey the importance of the program with enthusiasm; include open communication and follow-up.
   c. Provide the patient with simple drawings and clearly written instructions of exercises, indicating frequency, duration, number of repetitions, and method of progressing the exercises. Be realistic; provide the least amount of exercises to accomplish the goals. Avoid long, tedious routines.
   d. Work with the patient and family to fit the program into their anticipated daily schedule. It may require that some of the exercises be performed at one time of day and others at another time.
   e. Provide checkpoints for the patient so he or she can see progress or note results of maintenance.
   f. Schedule the patient for re-evaluation at appropriate intervals and revise the program according to the new level of performance. Project a termination date if possible.
5. Maintain a copy of the home program in the patient's records.

II. Goals of Therapeutic Exercise

Following a comprehensive evaluation of the patient and identification of impairments (problems), functional limitations, disabilities, and possible handicaps, the goals of treatment and functional outcomes are developed and the plan of care (treatment plan) is established. In the clinical decision-making process, the therapist must determine the type of therapeutic exercise that can be used to meet the predicted functional outcomes.

The goals of therapeutic exercise include the prevention of dysfunction as well as the development, improvement, restoration, or maintenance of:
—Strength
—Endurance and cardiovascular fitness
—Mobility and flexibility
—Stability
—Relaxation
—Coordination, balance, and functional skills

It is well known that the human body and the individual body systems react, adapt, and develop in response to the forces and stresses placed upon them. Gravity is a constant force that affects the neuromuscular, musculoskeletal, and circulatory systems. Wolff's law states that the skeletal system adapts to the forces placed upon it.[4] In the developing human, gravitational stresses, particularly those that occur in weight-bearing (antigravity) positions, contribute to the growth of the skeletal system.[56] Every normal muscular contraction also places a normal stress on bone and affects its shape and density.[4,56] The neuromuscular and cardiopulmonary systems also adapt as stresses are placed upon them during any movements involved in daily activity.

The absence of normal stresses on the body systems can lead to degeneration, degradation, deformity, or injury. For example, the absence of normal weight bearing, associated with prolonged bed rest, and the absence of normal muscle pull on bone, as seen in flaccid paralysis, will cause osteoporosis and muscle atrophy.[4] Prolonged inactivity will also lead to decreased efficiency of the respiratory and circulatory systems.[4,62] The presence of abnormal stresses, such as the abnormal pull of muscle seen in spastic cerebral palsy, will lead to bone deformity in the immature skeletal system.[56] Repeated and undue stress on the muscular or skeletal systems can cause pain and dysfunction.[4]

In therapeutic exercise, carefully graded stresses and forces are applied to the body systems in a controlled, progressive, and appropriately planned manner to ultimately improve the overall function of the individual to meet the demands of daily living.

To progress the patient through treatment to the desired functional outcome without additional tissue damage, the involved body systems must be progressed through a properly graded program of intervention that addresses the dysfunctions at the level of their loss or limitation. For example, if the functional limitation is the inability to reach overhead, the examination and assessment determine whether the impairments are loss of range, poor strength, poor proximal stability, lack of coordination between antagonists, or poor endurance for repetitive motion. To improve the functional outcome, the component impairments/problems must be addressed through appropriate exercises to the level at which techniques to relearn safe reaching skills can be integrated into the program. The short-term goals will reflect this progression.

An important factor that influences the effectiveness of any therapeutic exercise program is patient education and active involvement in a systematic plan of care. Long-term functional improvements and prevention of future injury will occur only if the patient understands the goals of an exercise plan and incorporates the advice and instructions of the therapist into all aspects of daily living routines.

A. Strength

A major goal that can be achieved through therapeutic exercise is the development, enhancement, or maintenance of strength. Strength is the ability of a muscle or muscle group to produce tension and a resulting force during a maximal effort, either dynamically or statically, in relation to the demands placed upon it.[2,13,18,28]

Throughout the course of normal growth and development, the child and the adult develop normal muscle strength needed for daily activities. Normal strength may refer to adequate, typical, or average strength of a single muscle, of a person, or of a general population group.[35,36] In manual muscle testing, normal is a standard and is defined as the amount or degree of strength of a muscle that allows that muscle to contract against gravity and hold against maximum resistance.[11,35]

As a muscle contracts and develops tension, a force is exerted by that muscle. The amount of force produced depends on a wide variety of biomechanical, physiologic, and neuromuscular factors.

1. Factors that influence the strength of normal muscle

    a. Cross-sectional size of the muscle—the larger the diameter, the greater the strength.[1,2,18,43]

   b. Length-tension relationship of a muscle at the time of contraction—a muscle produces the greatest tension when it is slightly lengthened at the time of contraction.[19,39]

   c. Recruitment of motor units—the greater the number and synchronization of motor units firing, the greater the force output.[2,13,14,17,39,63]

   d. Type of muscle contraction—a muscle produces the most force output when contracting eccentrically (lengthening) against resistance. The muscle produces slightly less force when contracting isometrically (holding) and the least force when contracting concentrically (shortening) against a load.[18,39]

   e. Fiber-type distribution—characteristics of muscle fiber types contribute to a number of contractile properties of muscle such as strength, endurance, power, speed, and resistance to fatigue.[2,52] Type II A and B (fast-twitch) fibers have the ability to generate a great amount of tension but fatigue very quickly. Type I (slow-twitch) fibers develop less tension and do so more slowly than Type II fibers but are more resistant to fatigue.

   f. Energy stores and blood supply—a muscle needs adequate sources of energy (fuel) to contract, generate tension, and resist fatigue.[2,52] The predominant fiber type found in the muscle and the adequacy of blood supply, which transports oxygen and nutrients to muscle, affect the tension-producing capacity of a muscle and its ability to resist fatigue.

   g. Speed of contraction—greater torques are produced at lower speeds, probably because of greater opportunity for recruitment.[7,18,36,39]

   h. Motivation of the patient—a patient must be willing to put forth a maximum effort to generate maximum strength.[18]

2. Changes in the neuromuscular system that lead to increased strength

   a. Hypertrophy*

The strength capacity of a muscle is directly related to the physiologic cross-sectional area of the muscle fiber. The diameter of a muscle fiber is related to muscle bulk. With exercise specifically designed to develop strength, the size of the individual skeletal muscle fibers can be increased. This is called **hypertrophy.** The factors that contribute to hypertrophy are complex but include (1) an increase in the amount of protein in the muscle fiber; (2) an increase in the density of the capillary bed; and (3) biochemical changes in the muscle fiber. When strength in a muscle increases, it has been shown that the type II muscle fibers increase in size and are the primary source of hypertrophy.[2,52]

Although there is only questionable evidence, it has been suggested that the strength of muscle may also be increased with exercise that causes **hyperplasia,** an increase in the *number* of muscle fibers. This increase may be caused by longitudinal fiber splitting.[2,15,22,29] Fiber splitting has been observed in laboratory animals subjected to heavy resistance exercise over a period of time. These findings have been difficult to replicate, and this phenomenon has not yet been observed in normal human beings. The observed fiber splitting may be the result of how the tissue was prepared for analysis rather than biologic changes in the muscle fibers.[52]

   b. Recruitment†

Another important factor that affects a muscle's capacity to increase strength

---

*Refs. 2, 7, 15, 17, 18, 21, 29, 40, 43, 63.
†Refs. 2, 7, 13, 14, 18, 28, 43, 52, 54.

is the recruitment of increased numbers of motor units during exercise. The greater the number of motor units firing, the greater the force output of a muscle. In the early stages of a strength-training program, initial increases in strength are largely due to motor learning that results in neural adaptations such as greater recruitment and synchronization of motor units. It has been shown that strength can be increased without muscle hypertrophy.[7,23,52] Rapid gains in strength in the very early phases of resistance exercise programs are probably the result of recruitment rather than **hypertrophy.**[7,54]

3. Strength changes in noncontractile tissue[60]

In a progressively applied therapeutic exercise program the strength of noncontractile tissue such as bone, tendons, and ligaments can also be improved. As the strength of muscle increases to adapt to increasing demands placed upon it, it appears to also lead to tendon and ligament strength increases at the musculotendinous junction and at the ligament-bone interface. Skeletal tissue also becomes stronger and adapts to increasing demands placed upon it as the result of an exercise program designed to increase strength.

4. Guidelines for developing strength

a. The overload principle

To increase strength, a load that exceeds the metabolic capacity of the muscle must be used during exercise. This will lead to hypertrophy and recruitment and therefore to an increase in strength of the muscle.[28,50]

b. The capacity of a muscle to produce greater tension can be achieved primarily with high-intensity exercise (exercise performed against heavy loads) carried out for a relatively low number of repetitions. In both cases, the muscle must be exercised to the point of fatigue for adaptive increases in strength to occur.[18]

c. Variations in the type and structure of exercise programs, designed to increase strength, will be discussed in Chapter 3.

B. Endurance and Cardiovascular Fitness

Muscular endurance or total-body endurance can also be improved or maintained with therapeutic exercise. Endurance is necessary for performing repeated motor tasks in daily living and carrying on a sustained level of functional activity, such as walking or climbing stairs. Both types of endurance refer to work performed over a prolonged period.

1. Types of endurance

Although they are interrelated, endurance of a single muscle or muscle group and endurance of the total body, particularly as it relates to the cardiovascular and pulmonary systems, will be defined separately.

a. Muscular endurance

The ability of a muscle to contract repeatedly or generate tension, sustain that tension, and resist fatigue over a prolonged period of time. As endurance increases, a muscle will be able to perform a greater number of contractions or hold against a load over an extended period.[7,13,18]

b. General (total) body endurance

The ability of an individual to sustain low-intensity exercise, such as walking, jogging, or climbing, over an extended period.[13,18,31] Endurance exercise, also called aerobic exercise, or conditioning is performed to enhance the cardiovascular or pulmonary fitness of an individual.[7,18,31]

2. **Changes in the muscular, cardiovascular, and pulmonary systems that lead to increased endurance**
   a. Immediate changes during exercise[18]
      (1) Increased blood flow to muscle because of increased demands for oxygen.
      (2) Increased heart rate.
      (3) Increased arterial pressure with heavy exercise. This is due to increased stroke volume, increased cardiac output, increased heart rate, and increased peripheral resistance to blood flow.
      (4) Increased oxygen demand and consumption.
      (5) Increased rate and depth of respiration; secondary muscles of respiration contract to assist the respiration process.
   b. Adaptive (long-term) changes[2,7,18]
      (1) Muscle changes
         The vascularization of the muscle or the density of the capillary bed increases. When a muscle contracts at low intensity for many repetitions to the point of fatigue, aerobic activity occurs in the muscle to provide energy for muscle contraction. Oxygen is necessary for this process to occur. Greater amounts of oxygen can be made available to the muscle as the capillary bed becomes more dense and blood supply to the muscle increases. Adaptive changes in the type I and type IIa muscle fibers are associated with increases in muscular endurance.
      (2) Cardiac and vascular changes[7,18,31]
         (a) Cardiac output and stroke volume increase. This leads to an increase in the efficiency of the working capacity of the heart.
         (b) Resting heart rate decreases. During exercise, of course, the heart rate increases, but as endurance improves, the heart rate returns to a resting level more rapidly after exercise.

         NOTE: Cardiac reserve (the difference between the capacity to do work and the demand for cardiac work) decreases with age and with heart and lung disease. Therefore, the implementation and progression of a conditioning program for the normal young individual versus the patient with cardiopulmonary and circulatory disease will vary greatly (see Chapter 4).

3. **Guidelines for developing endurance**
   a. Muscular endurance[2,7,13,18]
      Active exercise performed repeatedly against a moderate load to the point of fatigue will increase the endurance of a muscle. An increase in muscle endurance will also occur in exercise programs designed to increase strength.
   b. General endurance[2,7,13,18]
      The aerobic capacity of an individual is related to the effective transport of oxygen and maximal oxygen uptake. Exercises that challenge the oxygen transport system will increase endurance, aerobic capacity, and overall cardiopulmonary fitness. Conditioning programs and cardiac rehabilitation programs are designed to meet these goals. These programs often follow these general guidelines:

(1) Exercise is usually directed to large muscle groups, as in walking, running, swimming, and cycling.
(2) Exercise is prolonged and performed for 15 to 45 minutes or more.
(3) The frequency of the exercise varies (every other day, 5 days a week, and so forth), but adequate time for rest is important.
(4) Details of conditioning and aerobic exercises can be found in Chapter 4.

C. Mobility and Flexibility

In addition to strength and endurance, mobility of contractile and noncontractile soft tissues and joints is necessary for the performance of normal functional movements. When an individual with normal neuromuscular control carries out activities of daily living, soft tissues and joints continually elongate and/or shorten, and their appropriate mobility or flexibility is maintained. If normal motion of body parts is restricted in any way, adaptive shortening (tightness) of soft tissues and joints will occur. Disease or trauma to soft tissue and joints, which can cause pain, weakness, or inflammation, can impair mobility. Tightness should be prevented, if possible, but if tightness does occur, mobility exercises may be used to restore the involved structures to their appropriate length.

1. Soft tissue mobility/flexibility

Soft tissue refers to contractile and noncontractile tissues, that is, muscles, connective tissue, and skin. Each will be considered separately.

a. Muscle

Because of the contractile and elastic properties of a muscle, it shortens when stimulated and relaxes after contraction, and it can also be stretched passively. If a muscle is immobile for a period of time, it loses its flexibility and assumes the shortened position in which it has been held. Adaptive shortening of tissue is often referred to as a **contracture.**[38,62]

To restore full flexibility through therapeutic exercise, consideration must be given to the neurophysiologic properties of muscle, such as the function of the muscle spindle and the Golgi tendon organ and to the process of relaxation and the passive elastic properties of muscle. The procedures for lengthening shortened muscles may be done actively or passively.

b. Connective tissue[38,62]

Normal connective tissue is primarily composed of a network of collagen and ground substance. Although it is inert and has no contractile properties, it is somewhat supple and will elongate slowly with a maintained stretch and will adaptively shorten if immobilized.

A denser form of connective tissue is found in scars; it develops when injured soft tissue is immobilized during the healing process. This dense form of connective tissue does not yield to stretch and has no resilient properties.

Prolonged immobilization of soft tissue must be avoided, if possible, to prevent the formation of this dense fibrotic tissue and irreversible contractures. Procedures for maintaining mobility of connective tissue are done passively.

c. Skin

The normal mobility of skin must also be maintained if normal movement is to occur. The suppleness of skin allows it to yield to stretch during active or passive movements of the body.

Skin may develop tightness and cause limitation of motion when scar tissue is formed after severe burns, incisions, or lacerations. Scars do not yield easily to stretch. Early movement, when possible, will minimize tightness from scarring.

2. Joint mobility[34]

For any normal motion to occur, proper joint kinematics are necessary. Adequate capsule laxity is necessary to allow normal roll-sliding to occur between the bony surfaces within the joint.

Any restriction of the capsule or faulty relationship of the joint surfaces will interfere with normal motion. Normal mobility can be restored by either general or specific joint mobilization techniques.

3. Types of mobility exercises

a. Passive stretching

Manual, mechanical, or positional stretch to soft tissues, in which the force is applied opposite to the direction of shortening.

b. Active inhibition

A reflex inhibition and subsequent elongation of muscles, using neurologic principles to reduce tension and lengthen the contractile elements within muscles.[47,61,64]

c. Flexibility exercise

A general term used to describe exercises performed by a person to passively or actively elongate soft tissues without the assistance of a therapist.

d. Joint mobilization

Passive traction and/or gliding movements to joint surfaces that maintain or restore the joint play normally allowed by the capsule, so that the normal roll-glide mechanics can occur as a person moves.

4. Guidelines for developing mobility

Specific procedures, techniques, and precautions for stretching and joint mobilization are discussed in Chapters 5 and 6.

D. Stability

1. General discussion[47,50]

Stability refers to the synergistic coordination of the neuromuscular system to provide a stable base for superimposed functional movements or activities. Stability is usually required in more proximal structures, such as the trunk, hips, and shoulder girdle, for effective positioning and motion of the arms and hands or legs and feet. Stability encompasses adequate mobility for proper placement, adequate strength to hold the position, and adequate endurance and coordination to maintain the position or make adjustments in the position while the distal portion of the kinematic chain is doing the desired activity.

Frequently musculoskeletal dysfunction accompanies weakness in some portion of the kinematic chain, causing inadequate stability and thus jeopardizing some structures by excessive stress.

2. Guidelines for developing stability[47,50]

a. Stabilization exercises are the means by which a patient can learn to control proximal areas of the body and maintain a stable, well-aligned position while carrying out functional activities.

b. An individual can learn to isolate and develop static and dynamic strength in stabilizing muscles. Closed-chain weight-bearing activities using graduated compressive loads stimulate co-contraction in antagonist muscle groups. The term **rhythmic stabilization** is commonly used to describe exercises that are designed to develop stability in proximal muscle joints. Single-plane, controlled motions of the entire segment, with emphasis on proximal stabilizing muscles, are then superimposed.

    c. As control of single-plane movements improves, stabilization exercises are progressed by performing controlled diagonal motions while maintaining proximal stability.

    d. Endurance in stabilizing muscles must be developed with repetitive controlled stresses.

    e. Components of functional activities and finally entire functional activities are practiced using appropriate proximal stabilization.

    f. Additional information on stabilization exercises will be discussed in Chapters 3 and 15.

E. Relaxation

Relaxation refers to a conscious effort to relieve tension in muscles.[37] Through therapeutic exercise an individual can become aware of prolonged muscle tension and can be taught to control or inhibit it.

    Prolonged muscle tension can cause pain, which leads to muscle spasm, which causes more pain. Tension headaches and muscular pain in the region of the cervical spine are often associated with prolonged muscle tension.[37] Patients with severe chronic pulmonary disease often experience tension in the muscles of the upper trunk, which decreases their ability to breathe deeply and efficiently.[37] Pain associated with childbirth may be increased because of increased tension in muscles and the inability of the woman in labor to relax. All of these clinical problems can be diminished by relaxation exercises.

1. Therapeutic basis of relaxation exercises[19,32,37,57]

    a. After an active contraction of skeletal muscle, a reflex relaxation occurs. The stronger the contraction, the greater the subsequent relaxation of that muscle. In addition, as a muscle is contracting, its corresponding antagonistic muscle is inhibited (Sherrington's law of reciprocal innervation).

    b. Conscious thought can also affect tension in muscle. This has been demonstrated in biofeedback and transcendental meditation. Exercise to promote relaxation is based on the therapeutic use of these reflexive and conscious processes, used separately or in combination.

2. Guidelines for promoting relaxation[32,37,57]

    a. The patient is placed in a comfortable position, with all body parts well supported. The patient is taught to progressively contract and relax the musculature.

    b. This process is often coupled with deep-breathing exercise to further promote relaxation. Specific procedures are outlined in Chapters 5 and 15.

F. Coordination, Balance, and Functional Skills[5,37,47,61,64]

1. Definitions and interrelationships

Coordination, balance, and the acquisition of functional skills are all interrelated and are complex aspects of motor control. **Coordination** refers to the ability to use the right muscles at the right time with appropriate sequencing and intensity.[5,47,61,64] Extensive organization within the central nervous system (CNS) is necessary to initiate, guide, and grade patterns of movement. Coordination is the basis of smooth and efficient movement that can occur on a voluntary or involuntary (automatic) level. **Balance** refers to the ability to maintain the center of gravity over the base of support, usually while in an upright position.[47,61] Balance is a dynamic phenomenon that involves a combination of stability and mobility.[47] Balance is necessary to hold a position in space or move in a controlled and coordinated manner. Finally, **functional skills** refer to the varied motor skills necessary to function independently in all aspects of daily living.

Coordination, balance, and functional motor skills[5,47,61] are all dependent upon and affected by the sensory systems, particularly the somatosensory and proprioceptive systems. Coordination and balance must be present if a person is to learn and carry out functional skills. If a patient sustains a musculoskeletal or neuromuscular injury and develops subsequent impairments such as loss of strength, soft tissue immobility, or loss of endurance, then coordination, balance, and functional skills can all be adversely affected, leading to disabilities and handicaps.

2. General principles of exercise to develop coordination, balance, and functional motor skills[5,47,61,64]

The attainment of functional motor skills is dependent upon a background of normal motor control coupled with the ability to learn functional motor tasks. To progress or return a patient to a maximal level of functional activity, therapeutic exercise is coupled with the application of the principles of motor learning. Coordination, balance, and agility training as well as preparatory mobility, stabilization, and strengthening activities are all emphasized to assist the patient in returning to desired functional activities identified by the patient, family, or therapist.

a. Learning or relearning functional motor tasks involves constant repetition of simple to more complex motor activities, use of sensory cues (tactile, visual, or proprioceptive) to enhance motor performance, and removal of sensory cues to enhance problem solving and motor learning.

b. Movements can be initially practiced in simple, anatomic planes of motion and then carried out using combined or diagonal movements.

c. Proximal stability is often emphasized before distal mobility.

d. Simulated and, eventually, specific functional activities, initially simple and then more complex, must be practiced.

e. As the quality of movement improves, so should the speed and timing of movements. Simulated activities should be practiced before returning to optimal functional activities.

NOTE: Isolated exercises to develop strength or endurance should complement or be an integral component of the desired functional tasks.

III. Summary

This chapter has presented a brief outline of an approach to patient program development, using a simplified problem-solving process as the basis for clinical decision making and integrating it with an evaluation and assessment process. It is recommended that the reader have taken a course in evaluation techniques prior to using this book and attempting to choose and administer exercise techniques to patients.

The general goals that can be achieved by the broad scope of therapeutic exercise have also been discussed. Each of these goals has been expanded and is explained in much greater detail in the remaining chapters of this book.

References

1. Allman, FL: Exercises in sports medicine. In Basmajian, JV (ed): Therapeutic Exercise, ed 3. Williams & Wilkins, Baltimore, 1978.
2. Bandy, WD, Lovelace-Chandler, V, and McKitrick-Bandy, B: Adaptation of skeletal muscle to resistance training. Journal of Orthopaedic and Sports Physical Therapy 12:248–255, 1990.
3. Basmajian, J (ed): Physical Rehabilitation Outcome Measures. Canadian Physiotherapy Association in co-operation with Health and Welfare Canada and Canada Communications Group, Toronto, 1994.
4. Browse, NL: The Physiology and Pathology of Bed Rest. Charles C Thomas, Springfield, IL, 1965.
5. Carr, JH, et al: Movement and Science: Foundations for Physical Therapy in Rehabilitation. Aspen Publishers, Rockville, MD 1987.
6. Charnes, AL: Outcomes measurement, intervention versus outcomes. In Cirullo, JA (ed): Orthopaedic Physical Therapy Clinics of North America, Vol. 3. WB Saunders, Philadelphia, 1994, p 147.
7. Ciccone, CD, and Alexander, J: Physiology and therapeutics of exercise. In Goodgold, J (ed): Rehabilitation Medicine, CV Mosby, St Louis, 1988.
8. Clarkson, HM, and Gilewich, GB: Musculoskeletal Assessment: Joint Range of Motion and Manual Muscle Strength. Williams & Wilkins, Baltimore, 1989.
9. Corrigan, B, and Maitland, GD: Practical Orthopaedic Medicine. Butterworth, Boston, 1983.
10. Cyriax, J: Textbook of Orthopaedic Medicine, Vol 1. Diagnosis of Soft Tissue Lesions, ed 8. Bailliere and Tindall, London, 1982.
11. Daniels, L, and Worthingham, C: Muscle Testing: Techniques of Manual Examination, ed 5. WB Saunders, Philadelphia, 1986.
12. Dekker, J, et al: Diagnosis and treatment in physical therapy: An investigation of their relationship. Phys Ther 73:568, 1993.
13. Delateur, BJ: Therapeutic exercise to develop strength and endurance. In Kottke, FJ, Stillwell, GK, and Lehmann, JF (eds): Krusen's Handbook of Physical Medicine and Rehabilitation, ed 3. WB Saunders, Philadelphia, 1982.
14. Delorme, TL, and Watson, AL: Progressive Resistance Exercise. Appleton-Century, New York, 1951.
15. Edgerton, V: Morphology and histochemistry of the soleus muscle from normal and exercised rats. American Journal of Anatomy 127:81, 1970.
16. Feitelberg, S: The Problem Oriented Records System in Physical Therapy. University of Vermont, Burlington, 1975.
17. Fleck, SJ, and Kraemer, WJ: Resistance training: Physiological response and adaptations (Part 2 of 4). The Physician and Sportsmedicine 16:108–124, 1988.
18. Fox, E, and Matthews, D: The Physiological Basis of Physical Education and Athletics, ed 3. Saunders College Publishing, Philadelphia, 1981.
19. Glowitzke, BA, and Milner, M: Understanding the Scientific Basis of Human Movement, ed 2. Williams & Wilkins, Baltimore, 1980.
20. Goldstein, TS: Functional Rehabilitation in Orthopaedics. Aspen Publishers, Gaithersburg, MD, 1995.
21. Gollnick, PD, et al: Muscular enlargement and number of fibers in skeletal muscle of rats. J Appl Physiol 50:936–943, 1981.
22. Gonyea, WJ, Ericson, GC, and Bonde-Petersen, F: Skeletal muscle fiber splitting induced by weightlifting exercise in cats. Acta Physiol Scand 99:105, 1977.
23. Gordon, EE, Kowalski, K, and Fritts, M: Protein changes in quadriceps muscle of rats with repetitive exercises. Arch Phys Med Rehabil 48:296, 1967.
24. Guccione, A: Physical therapy diagnosis and the relationship between impairments and function. Phys Ther 71:449, 1991.
25. Harris, BA: Building documentation using a clinical decision-making model. In Stewart, D, and Abeln, S: Documenting Functional Outcomes in Physical Therapy, Mosby-Yearbook, St Louis, 1993.
26. Harris, BA, and Dyrek, DA: A model of orthopaedic dysfunction for clinical decision making in physical therapy practice. Phys Ther 69:548, 1989.
27. Heerkens, YF, et al: Impairments and disabilities—the difference: Proposal for adjustments of the international classification of impairments, disabilities and handicaps. Phys Ther 74:430, 1994.
28. Hellebrandt, RA, and Houtz, SJ: Mechanisms of muscle training in man: Experimental demonstration of the overload principle. Phys Ther Rev 36:371, 1956.
29. Ho, K, et al: Muscle fiber splitting with weightlifting exercise. Med Sci Sports Exerc 9:65, 1977.
30. International Classification of Impairments, Disabilities and Handicaps: A Manual of Classification Relating to the Consequences of Disease. World Health Organization, Geneva, 1980.
31. Irwin, S, and Tecklin, JS: Cardiopulmonary Physical Therapy. CV Mosby, St Louis, 1985.
32. Jacobson, E: Progressive Relaxation. University of Chicago Press, Chicago, 1938.
33. Jette, AM: Diagnosis and classification by physical therapists: A special communication. Phys Ther 69:967, 1989.
34. Kaltenborn, F: Manual Mobilization of the Extremity Joints: Basic Examination and Treatment Techniques, ed 4. Odas Norlis Bokhandel, Oslo, Norway, 1989.
35. Kendall, FP, et al: Muscles: Testing and Function, ed 4. Williams & Wilkins, Baltimore, 1993.
36. Knutgren, HG: Neuromuscular Mechanisms for Therapeutic and Conditioning Exercise. University Park Press, Baltimore, 1976.
37. Kottke, FJ: Therapeutic exercise to develop neuro-

muscular coordination. In Kottke, FJ, Stillwell, GK, and Lehmann, JF (eds): Krusen's Handbook of Physical Medicine and Rehabilitation, ed 3. WB Saunders, Philadelphia, 1982.

38. Kottke, FJ: Therapeutic exercise to maintain mobility. In Kottke, FJ, Stillwell, GK, and Lehmann, JF (eds): Krusen's Handbook of Physical Medicine and Rehabilitation, ed 3. WB Saunders, Philadelphia, 1982.
39. Lehmkuhl, LD, and Smith, LK: Brunnstrom's Clinical Kinesiology, ed 4. FA Davis Company, Philadelphia, 1983.
40. MacDougall, JD, Sale, DG, Alway, SE, et al: Muscle fiber number in biceps brachii in body builders and control subjects. J Appl Physiol 57:1399–1403, 1984.
41. Magee, D: Orthopedic Physical Assessment, ed 2. WB Saunders, Philadelphia, 1992.
42. Magistro, CM: Clinical decision making in physical therapy: A practitioner's perspective. Phys Ther 69:525, 1989.
43. Moritani, T, and DeVries, HK: Neural factors vs. hypertrophy in the time course of muscle strength gain. Am J Phys Med Rehabil 58:115, 1979.
44. Nagi, SZ: Disability and Rehabilitation. The Ohio State University Press, Columbus, 1969.
45. Nagi, SZ: Disability concepts revisited: implications for prevention. In Pope, AM, and Tarlov, AR (eds): Disability in America. National Academy Press, Washington, DC, 1991.
46. Norkin, CC, and White, DJ: Measurement of Joint Motion: A Guide to Goniometry. FA Davis, Philadelphia, 1985.
47. O'Sullivan, S: Motor control assessment. In O'Sullivan, S, and Schmitz, TJ (eds): Physical Rehabilitation: Assessment and Treatment, ed 3. FA Davis, Philadelphia, 1994.
48. Palmer, ML, and Epler, M: Clinical Assessment Procedures in Physical Therapy. JB Lippincott, Philadelphia, 1990.
49. Pierson, F, Burnett, C, and Kisner, C: A Problem Solving Process. The Ohio State University, Division of Physical Therapy, Columbus, 1986.
50. Prentice, WE: Rehabilitation Techniques in Sports Medicine. Times Mirror/Mosby, St Louis, 1990.
51. Rose, SJ: Physical therapy diagnosis: Role and function. Phys Ther 69:535, 1989.
52. Rose, SJ, and Rothstein, JM: Muscle mutability, part I: General concepts and adaptations to altered patterns of use. Phys Ther 62:1773, 1982.
53. Sahrmann, SA: Diagnosis by the physical therapist: A prerequisite for treatment. Phys Ther 68:1703, 1988.
54. Sanders, MT: Weight training and conditioning. In Sanders, B (ed): Sports Physical Therapy. Appleton & Lange, Norwalk, CT, 1990.
55. Schmitz, TJ: Coordination assessment. In O'Sullivan, S, and Schmitz, TJ (eds): Physical Rehabilitation, ed 3. FA Davis, Philadelphia, 1994.
56. Sharrard, WJW: The hip in cerebral palsy. In Samilson, RL (ed): Orthopedic Aspects of Cerebral Palsy. JB Lippincott, Philadelphia, 1975.
57. Sinclair, JD: Exercise in pulmonary disease. In Basmajian, JV (ed): Therapeutic Exercise, ed 3. Williams & Wilkins, Baltimore, 1978.
58. Swanson, G: Functional outcome report: The next generation in physical therapy reporting. In Stewart, D, and Abeln, S: Documenting Functional Outcomes in Physical Therapy, Mosby-Yearbook, St Louis, 1993.
59. Task Force on Standards for Measurement in Physical Therapy. Standards for tests and measurements in physical therapy practice. Phys Ther 71:589, 1991.
60. Tippett, SR: Closed chain exercise. Orthopedic Physical Therapy Clinics of North America 1:253–267, 1992.
61. Umphried, DA (ed): Neurological Rehabilitation. CV Mosby, St Louis, 1985.
62. Vallbona, C: Bodily responses to immobilization. In Kottke, FJ, Stillwell, GK, and Lehmann, JF (eds): Krusen's Handbook of Physical Medicine and Rehabilitation. WB Saunders, Philadelphia, 1982.
63. Vogel, JA: Introduction to the symposium: Physiological responses and adaptations to resistance exercise. Med Sci Sports Exerc (Suppl)20:131–134, 1988.
64. Voss, DE, Ionta, MK, and Myers, BJ: Proprioceptive Neuromuscular Facilitation, ed 3. Harper & Row, Philadelphia, 1985.
65. Wolf, SL: Clinical Decision Making in Physical Therapy. FA Davis, Philadelphia, 1985.

Range of Motion

Movement of a body segment takes place as muscles or external forces move bones. Bones move with respect to each other at the connecting joints. The structure of the joints, as well as the integrity and flexibility of the soft tissues that pass over the joints, affects the amount of motion that can occur between any two bones. The full motion possible is called the **range of motion (ROM)**. When moving a segment through its range of motion, all structures in the region are affected: muscles, joint surfaces, capsules, ligaments, fasciae, vessels, and nerves. Range of motion activities are most easily described in terms of joint range and muscle range. To describe joint range, terms such as flexion, extension, abduction, adduction, and rotation are used. Ranges of available joint motion are usually measured with a goniometer and recorded in degrees.[2,15,16] Muscle range is related to the functional excursion of muscles.

Functional excursion is the distance that a muscle is capable of shortening after it has been elongated to its maximum.[13] In some cases the functional excursion, or range of a muscle, is directly influenced by the joint it crosses. For example, the range for the brachialis muscle is limited by the range available at the elbow joint. This is true of one-joint muscles (muscles with their proximal and distal attachments on the bones on either side of one joint). For two-joint or multijoint muscles (those muscles that cross over two or more joints), their range goes beyond the limits of any one joint they cross. An example of a two-joint muscle functioning at the elbow is the biceps brachii muscle. If it contracts and moves the elbow into flexion and the forearm into supination while simultaneously moving the shoulder into flexion, it will shorten to a point known as active insufficiency, where it can shorten no more. This is one end of its range. The muscle is lengthened full range by extending the elbow, pronating the forearm, and simultaneously extending the shoulder. When fully elongated it is in a position known as passive insufficiency. Two-joint or multijoint muscles normally function in the mid-portion of their functional excursion, where ideal length-tension relationships exist.[13]

To maintain normal range of motion, the segments must be moved through their available ranges periodically, whether it be the available joint range or muscle range. It is recognized that many factors can lead to decreased ROM, such as systemic, joint, neurologic, or muscular diseases; surgical or traumatic insults; or simply inactivity or immobilization for any reason. Therapeutically, range of motion activities are administered to maintain *existing* joint and soft tissue mobility, which will minimize the effects of contracture formation.[3]

OBJECTIVES

After studying this chapter, the reader will be able to:

1   Describe range of motion and what affects it.
2   Define passive, active, and active-assistive range of motion.
3   Identify indications and goals for passive and active range of motion activities.
4   Identify limitations of passive and active range of motion activities.
5   Identify contraindications to range of motion.
6   Describe procedures for applying range of motion techniques.
7   Apply techniques for joint and muscle range of motion using anatomic planes of motion.
8   Apply techniques for combined range of motion.
9   Apply techniques of range of motion using self-assistance and mechanical assistance including wand, finger ladder, pulley, powder (skate) board, and suspension devices.
10 Describe the benefits and procedures for use of continuous passive motion (CPM) equipment.

I. Definitions of Range of Motion Exercises

A. Passive

Movement within the unrestricted ROM for a segment that is produced entirely by an *external force;* there is no voluntary muscle contraction. The external force may be from gravity, a machine, another individual, or another part of the individual's own body.[5] Passive ROM and passive stretching are not synonymous; see Chapter 5 for definitions and descriptions of passive stretching.

B. Active

Movement within the unrestricted ROM for a segment that is produced by an active contraction of the *muscles* crossing that joint.

C. Active-Assistive

A type of active ROM in which assistance is provided by an outside force, either manually or mechanically, because the prime mover muscles need assistance to complete the motion.

II. Indications and Goals for Range of Motion

A. Passive ROM

1. When a patient is not able to or not supposed to actively move a segment or segments of the body, as when comatose, paralyzed, or on complete bed rest, or when there is an inflammatory reaction and active ROM is painful, controlled **passive ROM** is used to decrease the complications of immobilization in order to:[5]
   a. Maintain joint and soft tissue integrity.
   b. Minimize the effects of the formation of **contractures.**
   c. Maintain mechanical elasticity of muscle.
   d. Assist circulation and vascular dynamics.
   e. Enhance synovial movement for cartilage nutrition and diffusion of materials in the joint.
   f. Decrease or inhibit pain.

g. Assist with the healing process following injury or surgery.

h. Help maintain the patient's awareness of movement.

2. When a therapist is evaluating inert structures (see Chapter 1), passive ROM is used to determine limitations of motion, to determine joint stability, and to determine muscle and other soft tissue elasticity.

3. When a therapist is teaching an active exercise program, passive ROM is used to demonstrate the desired motion.

4. When a therapist is preparing a patient for stretching, passive ROM is often used preceding the passive stretching techniques. Techniques to increase the range of motion when motion is restricted are described in Chapters 5 and 6.

B. Active and Active-Assistive ROM

1. When a patient is able to actively contract the muscles and move a segment either with or without assistance and there are no contraindications, **active ROM** is used to:

   a. Accomplish the same goals of passive ROM with the added benefits that result from muscle contraction.

   b. Maintain physiologic elasticity and contractility of the participating muscles.

   c. Provide sensory feedback from the contracting muscles.

   d. Provide a stimulus for bone and joint tissue integrity.

   e. Increase circulation and prevent thrombus formation.

   f. Develop coordination and motor skills for functional activities.

2. When a patient has weak musculature (poor to fair minus muscle test grade), **active-assistive ROM** is used to provide enough assistance to the muscles in a carefully controlled manner so that the muscle can function at its maximum level and progressively be strengthened.

3. When a patient is placed on an aerobic conditioning program, active-assistive or active ROM can be used to improve cardiovascular and respiratory responses if it is done with multiple repetitions and the results are monitored (see Chapter 4).

C. Special Considerations

1. When a segment of the body is immobilized for a period of time, ROM is used on the regions above and below the immobilized segment to:

   a. Maintain the areas in as normal a condition as possible.

   b. Prepare for new activities, such as walking with crutches.

2. When a patient is on bed rest, ROM is used to avoid the complications of decreased circulation, bone demineralization, and decreased cardiac and respiratory function.

III. Limitations of Range of Motion

A. Limitations of Passive Motion

1. True passive relaxed range of motion may be difficult to obtain when muscle is innervated and the patient is conscious.

2. Passive motion *will not*:

   a. Prevent muscle atrophy.

   b. Increase strength or endurance.

   c. Assist circulation to the extent that active, voluntary muscle contraction does.

B. Limitations of Active ROM

1. For strong muscles, *it will not* maintain or increase strength (see Chapter 3).
2. *It will not* develop skill or coordination except in the movement patterns used.

IV. Precautions and Contraindications to Range of Motion

A. Although both passive and active ROM are contraindicated under any circumstance when motion to a part is disruptive to the healing process, complete immobility leads to adhesion and contracture formation, sluggish circulation, and prolonged recovery time. In light of research by Salter[21] and others,[14] early continuous passive range of motion within a pain-free range has been shown to be beneficial to the healing and early recovery of many soft tissue and joint lesions (see Section IX.A). Historically ROM has been contraindicated immediately following acute tears, fractures, and surgery, but because the benefits of controlled motion have demonstrated decreased pain and an increased rate of recovery, early controlled motion is used as long as the patient's tolerance is monitored. It is imperative that the therapist recognize the value as well as potential abuse of motion and stay within the range, speed, and tolerance of the patient during the acute recovery stage.[5] Additional trauma to the part is contraindicated. Signs of too much or the wrong motion include increased pain and increased inflammation (greater swelling, heat, and redness). (See Chapter 7 for principles of when to use various types of passive and active motion therapeutically.)

B. Usually active ROM of the upper extremities and limited walking near the bed are tolerated as early exercises after myocardial infarction, coronary artery bypass surgery, or percutaneous transluminal coronary angioplasty.[4,7] Careful monitoring of symptoms, perceived exertion, and blood pressure is necessary. If patient response or the condition is life threatening, passive ROM may be carefully initiated to the major joints along with some active ROM to the ankles and feet to avoid venous stasis and thrombus formation. Individualized activities are initiated and progress gradually as the patient tolerates.[4,7]

C. Range of motion is not synonymous with stretching. For precautions and contraindications to passive and active stretching techniques, see Chapters 5 and 6.

V. Procedures for Applying Range of Motion Techniques

A. Based on an evaluation of the patient's impairments and level of function, determine whether passive, active-assistive, or active range of motion will meet the goals.

B. Place the patient in a comfortable position that will allow you to move the segment through the available ROM. Be sure the patient has proper body alignment.

C. Free the region from restrictive clothing, linen, splints, and dressings. Drape the patient as necessary.

D. Position yourself so that proper body mechanics can be used.

E. To control movement, grasp the extremity around the joints. If the joints are painful, modify the grip, still providing support necessary for control.

F. Support areas of poor structural integrity such as a hypermobile joint, recent fracture site, or paralyzed limb segment.

G. Move the segment through its complete pain-free range. Do not force beyond the available range. If you force motion, it becomes a stretching technique. (For principles and techniques of stretching, see Chapter 5.)

H. Perform the motions smoothly and rhythmically, 5 to 10 repetitions. The number of repetitions depends on the objectives of the program and the patient's condition and response to the treatment.

I. If the plan of care includes the use of *passive ROM*:
1. The force for movement is external, being provided by a therapist or mechanical device. When appropriate, a patient may provide the force and be taught to move the part with a normal extremity.
2. No active resistance or assistance is given by the patient's muscles crossing the joint. If so, it becomes an active exercise.
3. The motion is carried out within the free range of motion, that is, the range that is available without forced motion or pain.

J. If the plan of care is the use of *active-assistance or active ROM*:
1. Demonstrate to the patient the motion desired using passive ROM, then ask the patient to perform the motion. Have your hands in position to assist or guide the patient if needed.
2. Assistance is given only as needed for smooth motion. When there is weakness, assistance may be required only at the beginning or end of the ROM.
3. The motion is performed within the available range of motion.

K. ROM techniques may be performed in the
1. Anatomic planes of range of motion (frontal, sagittal, transverse)
2. Muscle range of elongation (antagonistic to the line of pull of the muscle)
3. Combined patterns (combined movements incorporating several planes of motion)
4. Functional patterns (motions used in activities of daily living)

L. Monitor the patient's general condition during and after the procedure. Note any change in vital signs, any change in the warmth and color of the segment, and any change in the range of motion, pain, or quality of movement.

M. Document observable and measurable reactions to the treatment.

N. Modify or progress the treatment as necessary.

VI. Techniques for Joint and Muscle ROM Using Anatomic Planes of Motion

The following descriptions are, for the most part, with the patient in the supine position. Alternate positions for many motions are possible and for some motions are necessary. For efficiency, perform all motions possible in one position, then change the patient's position and perform all appropriate motions in that position, progressing the treatment with minimal turning of the patient. Individual body types or environmental limitations might necessitate variations of the suggested hand placements. Use of good body mechanics by the therapist while applying proper stabilization and motion to the patient to accomplish the goals and avoid injury to weakened structures is the primary consideration.

NOTE: The term "upper or top hand" means the hand of the therapist that is toward the patient's head; "bottom or lower hand" refers to the hand toward the patient's foot. Antagonistic ranges of motion are grouped together for ease of application.

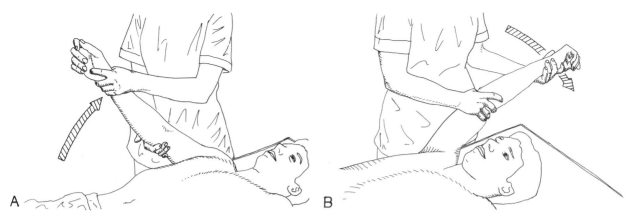

Figure 2–1. Hand placement and positions for (*A*) initiating and (*B*) completing shoulder flexion.

A. Upper Extremity

1. Shoulder: flexion and extension (Fig. 2–1A and B)

HAND PLACEMENT AND MOTION

Grasp the patient's arm under the elbow with your lower hand. With the top hand, cross over and grasp the wrist and palm of the patient's hand. Lift the arm through the available range and return.

NOTE: For normal motion, the scapula should be free to rotate upward as the shoulder flexes. If motion of only the glenohumeral joint is desired, the scapula is stabilized as described in the section on stretching (Chapter 5).

2. Shoulder: extension (hyperextension) (Fig. 2–2)

ALTERNATE POSITIONS

Extension past zero is possible if the patient's shoulder is at the edge of the bed when supine or if the patient is positioned side-lying or prone.

3. Shoulder: abduction and adduction (Fig. 2–3)

HAND PLACEMENT AND MOTION

Use the same hand placement as with flexion, but move the arm out to the side. The elbow may be flexed.

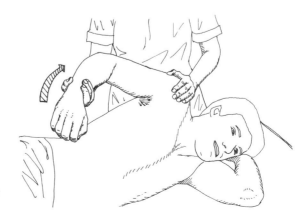

Figure 2–2. Hyperextension of the shoulder with the patient side-lying.

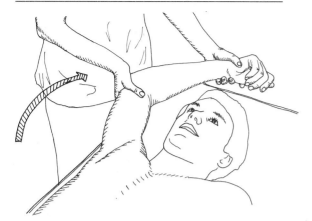

Figure 2–3. Abduction of the shoulder with the elbow flexed.

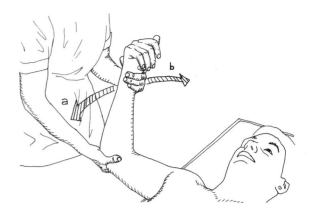

Figure 2–4. Position for initiating (*a*) internal and (*b*) external rotation of the shoulder.

NOTE: To reach full range of abduction, there must be external rotation of the humerus and upward rotation of the scapula.

4. Shoulder: internal (medial) and external (lateral) rotation (Fig. 2–4)

INITIAL POSITION OF THE ARM

If possible, the arm is abducted to 90 degrees, the elbow is flexed to 90 degrees, and the forearm is held in neutral position. Rotation may also be performed with the patient's arm at the side of thorax, but full internal rotation will not be possible.

HAND PLACEMENT AND MOTION

Grasp the hand and the wrist with your index finger between the patient's thumb and index finger. Place your thumb and the rest of your fingers on either side of the patient's wrist, thus stabilizing the wrist. With the other hand, stabilize the elbow. Rotate the humerus by moving the forearm like a spoke on a wheel.

5. Shoulder: horizontal abduction (extension) and adduction (flexion) (Fig. 2–5 A and B)

POSITION OF THE ARM

To reach full horizontal abduction, the shoulder must be at the edge of the table. Begin with the arm either flexed or abducted 90 degrees.

HAND PLACEMENT AND MOTION

Hand placement is the same as with flexion, but the therapist turns his or her body and faces the patient's head as the patient's arm is moved out to the side and then across the body.

6. Scapula: elevation/depression, protraction/retraction, and upward/downward rotation

ALTERNATE POSITIONS

Prone, with the patient's arm at the side (Fig. 2–6), or side-lying, with the patient facing the therapist and the patient's arm draped over the therapist's bottom arm (see Fig. 5–23).

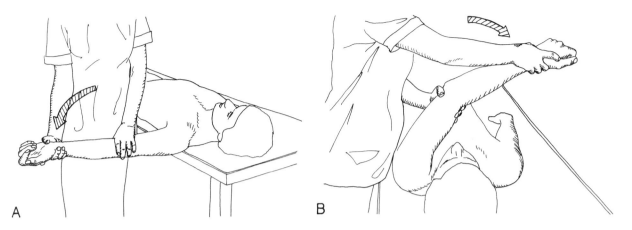

Figure 2–5. Horizontal (*A*) abduction and (*B*) adduction of the shoulder.

HAND PLACEMENT AND MOTION

Cup the top hand over the acromion process, and place the other hand around the inferior angle of the scapula. For elevation, depression, protraction, and retraction, the clavicle also moves as the scapular motions are directed at the acromion process. For rotation, direct the scapular motions at the inferior angle.

7. Elbow: flexion and extension (Fig. 2–7)

HAND PLACEMENT AND MOTION

Hand placement is the same as with shoulder flexion except the motion occurs at the elbow as it is flexed and extended.

NOTE: Control forearm supination and pronation with your fingers around the wrist. Perform elbow flexion and extension with the forearm pronated as well as supinated. The shoulder should not protract when the elbow extends; this disguises the true range.

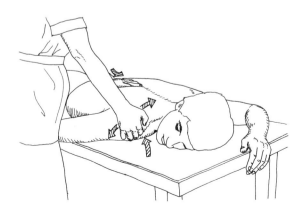

Figure 2–6. Scapular motions with the patient prone.

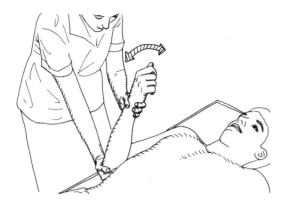

Figure 2–7. Elbow motions with the forearm supinated.

8. **Elongation of two-joint muscles crossing the shoulder and elbow**

   a. Biceps brachii muscle (Fig. 2–8)

      POSITION OF PATIENT

      Supine, with the shoulder at the edge of the treatment table so that the shoulder can be extended past the neutral position.

      HAND PLACEMENT AND MOTION

      First pronate the patient's forearm by grasping around the wrist, and extend the elbow by supporting under the elbow. The shoulder is then extended (hyperextended) until the patient experiences discomfort in the anterior arm region. At this point, full available lengthening of the two-joint muscle is reached.

   b. Long head of the triceps brachii muscle (Fig. 2–9)

      ALTERNATE POSITIONS

      When near-normal range of this muscle is available, the patient must be sitting or standing to reach the full ROM. With marked limitation in muscle range, ROM can be performed in the supine position.

      HAND PLACEMENT AND MOTION

      First, flex the patient's elbow full range with one hand on the distal forearm; then flex the shoulder by lifting up on the humerus with the other hand un-

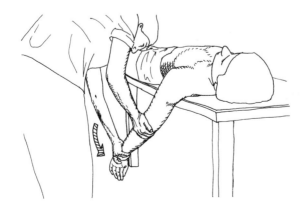

Figure 2–8. End range of motion for the biceps brachii muscle.

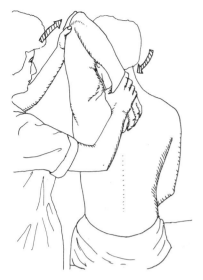

Figure 2–9. End range of motion for the long head of the triceps brachii muscle.

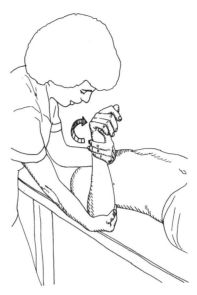

Figure 2–10. Pronation of the forearm.

der the elbow. Full available range is reached when discomfort is experienced in the posterior arm region.

9. Forearm: pronation and supination (Fig. 2–10)

HAND PLACEMENT AND MOTION

Grasp the patient's wrist, supporting the hand with the index finger and placing the thumb and the rest of the fingers on either side of the distal forearm. The motion is a rolling of the radius around the ulna at the distal radius. Stabilize the elbow with the other hand.

ALTERNATE HAND PLACEMENT

Sandwich the patient's distal forearm between the palms of both hands.

NOTE: Pronation and supination should be performed with the elbow both flexed and extended.

   Caution: Do not stress the wrist by twisting the hand; control the pronation and supination motion by moving the radius around the ulna.

10. Wrist: flexion (palmar flexion) and extension (dorsiflexion), radial and ulnar deviation (Fig. 2–11)

HAND PLACEMENT AND MOTION

For all wrist motions, grasp the patient's hand just distal to the joint with one hand, and stabilize the forearm with the other hand.

NOTE: The range of the extrinsic muscles to the fingers will affect the range at the wrist if tension is placed on them. To get full range of the wrist joint, allow the fingers to move freely as you move the wrist.

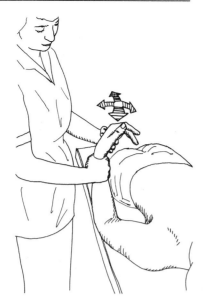

Figure 2–11. ROM at the wrist.

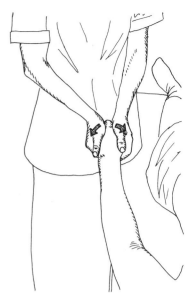

Figure 2–12. ROM to the arch of the hand.

11. Hand: cupping and flattening the arch of the hand at the carpometacarpal and intermetacarpal joints (Fig. 2–12)

HAND PLACEMENT AND MOTION

Face the patient's hand; place the fingers in the palms of the patient's hand and the thumbs on the posterior aspect. Roll the metacarpals to increase the arch, then flatten it.

ALTERNATE HAND PLACEMENT

One hand is placed on the posterior aspect of the patient's hand with the fingers and thumb cupping around the metacarpals.

NOTE: Extension and abduction of the thumb at the carpometacarpal joint are important in maintaining the web space for functional movement of the hand. Isolated flexion-extension and abduction-adduction ROM of this joint should be performed as described in 12.

12. Joints of the thumb and fingers: flexion and extension and abduction and adduction (of the metacarpophalangeal joints of the fingers) (Fig. 2–13A and B)

HAND PLACEMENT AND MOTION

Each joint of the patient's hand can be moved individually by stabilizing the proximal bone with the index finger and thumb of one hand and moving the distal bone with the index finger and thumb of the other hand. Depending on the position of the patient, the forearm and hand can be stabilized on the bed or table or against the therapist's body.

ALTERNATE METHOD

Several joints can be moved simultaneously if proper stabilization is provided. Example: To move all the metacarpophalangeal joints of digits 2 through 5, sta-

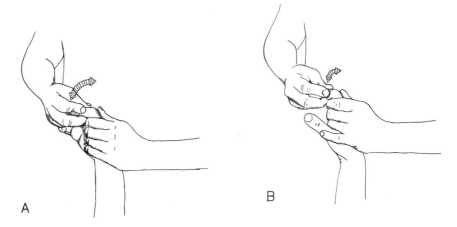

Figure 2–13. ROM to the (*A*) metacarpophalangeal joint of the thumb and (*B*) interphalangeal joint of a finger.

A

B

bilize the metacarpals with one hand and move all the proximal phalanges with the other hand.

NOTE: To accomplish full joint range of motion, do not place tension on the extrinsic muscles going to the fingers. Tension on the muscles can be relieved by altering the wrist position as the fingers are moved.

13. Elongation of extrinsic muscles of the wrist and hand

GENERAL TECHNIQUE

Elongate the muscles over one joint at a time, stabilize that joint, then elongate the muscle over the next joint until the multijoint muscles are at maximum length. To minimize compression of the small joints of the fingers, begin the motion with the distal-most joint.

a. Flexor digitorum profundus and superficialis muscles (Fig. 2–14A)

HAND PLACEMENT AND MOTION

First extend the distal interphalangeal joints, stabilize them, then extend the proximal interphalangeal joints. Hold these joints; then extend the metacarpophalangeal joints.

Stabilize all the finger joints and begin to extend the wrist. When the patient feels discomfort in the forearm, the muscles are fully elongated.

b. Extensor digitorum muscles (Fig. 2–14B)

HAND PLACEMENT AND MOTION

First flex the patient's distal interphalangeal joints and hold them. Next, flex the proximal interphalangeal joints and then the metacarpophalangeal joints. While stabilizing all these joints in the flexed position, begin to flex the wrist until the patient feels discomfort on the dorsum of the hand.

B. Lower Extremity

1. Hip and knee: simultaneous flexion and extension (Fig. 2–15A and B)

HAND PLACEMENT AND MOTION

Support the patient's leg with the fingers of the top hand under the patient's knee and the lower hand under the heel. As the knee flexes full range, swing the fingers to the side of the thigh.

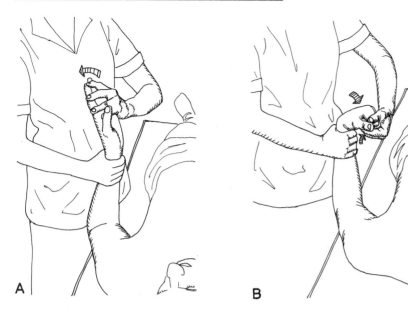

Figure 2–14. End of range for the (A) extrinsic finger flexors and (B) extensors.

NOTE: To reach full range of hip flexion, the knee must also be flexed in order to release tension on the hamstring muscle group. To reach full range of knee flexion, the hip must be flexed in order to release tension on the rectus femoris muscle (see 3).

2. Hip: extension (hyperextension) (Fig. 2–16)

ALTERNATE POSITIONS

Prone or side-lying must be used if the patient has near-normal or normal motion.

HAND PLACEMENT AND MOTION

If the patient is prone, lift the bottom hand under the patient's knee; stabilize the pelvis with the top hand or arm. If the patient is side-lying, bring the bottom hand under the thigh and place the hand on the anterior surface; stabilize the pelvis with the top hand.

NOTE: If the knee is flexed full range, the rectus femoris muscle is placed on a stretch, and full hip range into extension is limited by tension on the muscle (see 3, part b to follow).

3. Elongation of two-joint muscles crossing the hip and knee

a. Hamstring muscle group (Fig. 2–17)

HAND PLACEMENT AND MOTION

Place the lower hand under the patient's heel and the upper hand across the anterior aspect of the patient's knee. Keep the knee in extension as the hip is flexed.

VARIATION

If the hamstrings are so tight as to limit the knee from going into extension, the available range of the muscle is reached simply by extending the knee as far as the muscle allows and not moving the hip.

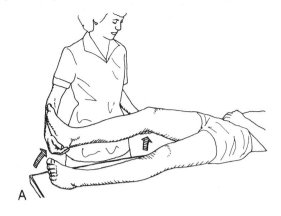

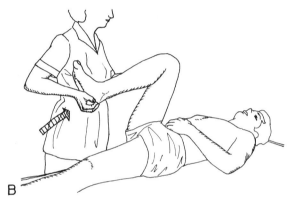

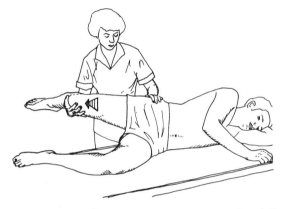

Figure 2–15. (*A*) Initiating and (*B*) completing combined hip and knee flexion.

Figure 2–16. Hand placements to complete full range of hip extension with the patient side-lying.

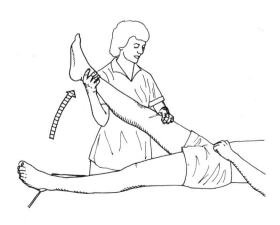

Figure 2–17. ROM to the hamstring muscle group.

ALTERNATE HAND PLACEMENT

If the knee requires support, cradle the patient's leg in your lower arm with your elbow flexed under the calf and your hand across the anterior aspect of the patient's knee. The other hand provides support or stabilization where needed.

b. Rectus femoris muscle

POSITION OF PATIENT AND MOTION

Supine with knees flexed over the edge of the treatment table. Continue to flex the patient's knee until discomfort is experienced in the anterior thigh, which means the full available range is reached.

ALTERNATE POSITION AND MOTION

Prone; flex the patient's knee until discomfort is felt in the anterior thigh (see Fig. 5–18). If the patient has a lot of flexibility, the hip may have to be extended after the knee is flexed full range (similar to Figs. 2–16 and 5–9, except the knee is flexed full range before extending the hip).

4. Hip: abduction and adduction (Fig. 2–18)

HAND PLACEMENT AND MOTION

Support the patient's leg with the upper hand under the knee and the lower hand under the ankle. For full range of adduction, the opposite leg needs to be in a partially abducted position. Keep the patient's hip and knee in extension and neutral to rotation as abduction and adduction are performed.

5. Hip: internal (medial) and external (lateral) rotation

HAND PLACEMENT AND MOTIONS WITH THE HIP AND KNEE EXTENDED

Grasp just proximal to the patient's knee with the top hand and just proximal to the ankle with the bottom hand. Roll the thigh inward and outward.

HAND PLACEMENT AND MOTIONS WITH THE HIP AND KNEE FLEXED (Fig. 2–19)

Flex the patient's hip and knee to 90 degrees; support the knee with the top hand. Cradle the thigh with the bottom arm, and also support the proximal calf with the bottom hand. Rotate the femur by moving the leg like a pendulum. This hand placement provides some support to the knee but still should be used with caution if there is knee instability.

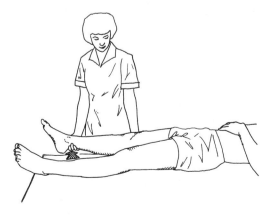

Figure 2–18. Abduction of the hip, maintaining the hip in extension and neutral to rotation.

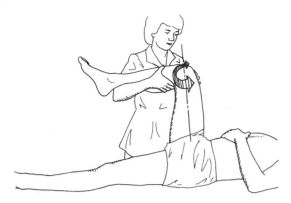

Figure 2–19. Rotation of the hip with the hip positioned in 90 degrees of flexion.

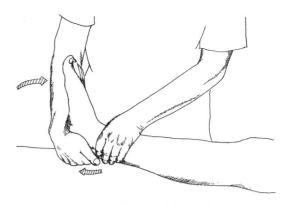

Figure 2–20. Dorsiflexion of the ankle.

6. Ankle: dorsiflexion (Fig. 2–20)

HAND PLACEMENT AND MOTION

Stabilize around the malleoli with the top hand. Cup the patient's heel with the bottom hand and place the forearm along the bottom of the foot. Pull the calcaneus distalward with the thumb and fingers while pushing upward with the forearm.

NOTE: If the knee is flexed, full range of the ankle joint can be obtained. If the knee is extended, the lengthened range of the two-joint gastrocnemius muscle can be obtained, but the gastrocnemius will limit full range of dorsiflexion. Dorsiflexion should be accomplished in both positions of the knee to provide range to both the joint and the muscle.

7. Ankle: plantarflexion

HAND PLACEMENT AND MOTION

Place the top hand on the dorsum of the foot and push it into plantarflexion; the other hand supports the heel.

NOTE: In bed-bound patients the ankle tends to assume a plantarflexed position from the weight of the blankets and pull of gravity, so this motion may not need to be performed.

8. Subtalar (lower ankle) joint: inversion and eversion (Fig. 2–21A and B)

HAND PLACEMENT AND MOTION

Place the thumb medial and the fingers lateral to the joint on either side of the heel; turn the heel inward and outward.

NOTE: Supination of the forefoot may be combined with inversion, and pronation may be combined with eversion.

9. Transverse tarsal joint: supination and pronation (Fig. 2–22)

HAND PLACEMENT AND MOTION

Stabilize the patient's talus and calcaneus with the top hand. With the bottom hand, grasp around the navicular and cuboid. Gently raise and lower the arch.

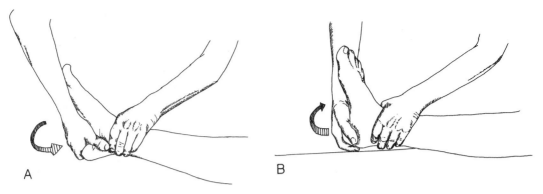

Figure 2–21. End position for (*A*) inversion and (*B*) eversion of the subtalar joint.

10. Joints of the toes: flexion and extension and abduction and adduction (metatarsophalangeal and interphalangeal joints) (Fig. 2–23)

HAND PLACEMENT AND MOTION

With one hand, stabilize the bone proximal to the joint that is to be moved and move the distal bone with the other hand. The technique is the same as with ROM of the fingers.

ALTERNATE METHOD

Several joints of the toes can be moved simultaneously if care is taken not to stress any structure.

C. Cervical Spine

POSITION OF THERAPIST AND HAND PLACEMENT

Standing at the end of the treatment table, securely grasp the patient's head by placing both hands under the occipital region (Fig. 2–24).

1. Flexion (forward-bending)

MOTION

Lift the head as though it were nodding.

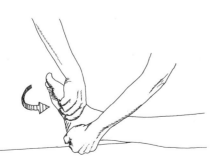

Figure 2–22. End position for supination of the transverse tarsal joint.

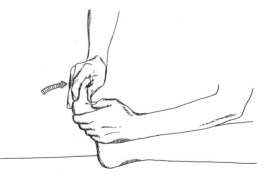

Figure 2–23. Extension of the metatarsophalangeal joint of the large toe.

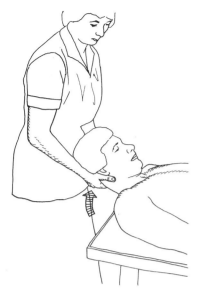

Figure 2–24. Hand placement for cervical motions, illustrating flexion.

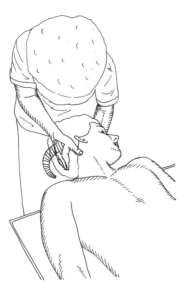

Figure 2–25. Hand placement and end-range for cervical rotation to the left.

2. Extension (backward-bending or hyperextension)

MOTION

Tip the head backward.

NOTE: If the patient is supine, the head must clear the end of the table. The patient may also be prone or sitting.

3. Lateral flexion (side-bending)

MOTION

Maintain the cervical spine neutral to flexion and extension as you direct it into side-bending and approximate the ear toward the shoulder.

4. Rotation (Fig. 2–25)

MOTION

Rotate the head from side to side.

D. Lumbar Spine

1. Flexion (Fig. 2–26)

HAND PLACEMENT AND MOTION

Bring both of the patient's knees to the chest by lifting under the knees (hip and knee flexion). Flexion of the spine occurs as the hips are flexed full range and the pelvis starts to rotate posteriorly. Greater range of flexion can be obtained by lifting under the patient's sacrum with the lower hand.

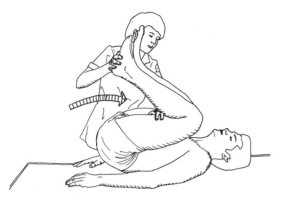

Figure 2–26. Lumbar flexion is achieved by bringing the patient's hips into flexion until the pelvis rotates posteriorly.

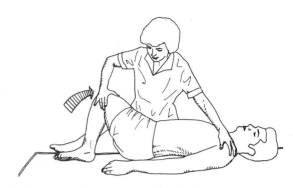

Figure 2–27. Rotation of the lumbar spine results when the thorax is stabilized and the pelvis lifts off the table as far as allowed.

2. Extension

POSITION OF PATIENT
Prone.

HAND PLACEMENT AND MOTION
With hands under the thighs, lift the thighs upward until the pelvis rotates anteriorly and the lumbar spine extends.

3. Rotation (Fig. 2–27)

POSITION OF PATIENT
Hook-lying.

HAND PLACEMENT AND MOTION
Push both of the patient's knees laterally in one direction until the pelvis on the opposite side comes up off the treatment table. Stabilize the patient's thorax with the top hand. Repeat in the opposite direction.

VII. Techniques for ROM Using Combined Patterns of Motion

Effective and efficient ROM can be administered by combining several joint motions that transect several planes. The following examples include portions of patterns similar to the proprioceptive neuromuscular facilitation (PNF) patterns of movement. By using such patterns for passive or active ROM, the goals and program can easily be progressed to facilitation techniques. For explanation and progression of the PNF techniques, the reader is referred to several texts.[24,25] Other patterns can also be developed by the therapist, based on the desired functional outcome.

A. Upper Extremity

1. Position of patient is supine or sitting. Begin with the patient's shoulder extended, abducted, and internally rotated and the forearm pronated. As you flex the patient's shoulder, simultaneously adduct and externally rotate it and supinate the forearm. Then return the arm to the starting position.
2. Begin the same as in 1, except have the shoulder adducted instead of abducted. As you flex the patient's shoulder, simultaneously abduct and externally rotate it and supinate the forearm. Then return the arm to the starting position.

3. The patterns in 1 and 2 can be performed with the elbow flexed or extended, or the elbow can move from one position to the other as the shoulder goes through the ROM.

B. Lower Extremity

1. Position of patient is supine. Begin with the patient's hip extended, abducted, and internally rotated. As you flex the patient's hip, simultaneously adduct and externally rotate it. Then return the lower extremity to the starting position.
2. Begin with the hip extended, adducted, and externally rotated. As you flex the patient's hip, simultaneously abduct and internally rotate it. Then return to the starting position.
3. The patterns in 1 and 2 can be performed with the knee flexed or extended, or the knee can move from one position to the other as the hip goes through the ROM.

VIII. Techniques of ROM Using Self-assistance and Mechanical Assistance

A. Self-Assistance

With cases of unilateral weakness or paralysis, the patient can be taught to use the normal extremity to move the involved extremity through ranges of motion.[23]

1. Arm and forearm

Instruct the patient to reach across the body with the normal extremity and grasp the involved extremity around the wrist, supporting the wrist and hand.

a. Shoulder flexion and extension

The patient lifts the involved extremity over the head and returns it to the side (Fig. 2–28A).

b. Shoulder horizontal abduction and adduction

Beginning with the arm abducted 90 degrees, the patient pulls the extremity across the chest and returns it out to the side (Fig. 2–28B).

c. Shoulder rotation

Beginning with the arm abducted 90 degrees and elbow flexed 90 degrees, the patient rotates the forearm (Fig. 2–29).

d. Elbow flexion and extension

The patient bends the elbow until the hand is near the shoulder and then moves the hand down toward the side of the leg.

e. Pronation and supination of the forearm

Beginning with the forearm resting across the body, the patient rotates the radius around the ulna. Emphasize to the patient not to twist the hand at the wrist joint.

2. Wrist and hand

The patient's normal thumb is moved to the involved hand with the normal fingers along the dorsum of the hand.

a. Wrist flexion and extension and radial and ulnar deviation

The patient moves the wrist in all directions, applying no pressure against the fingers (Fig. 2–30).

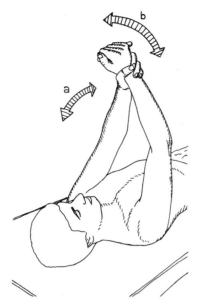

Figure 2–28. Patient giving self-assisted ROM to (*a*) shoulder flexion and extension or (*b*) horizontal abduction and adduction.

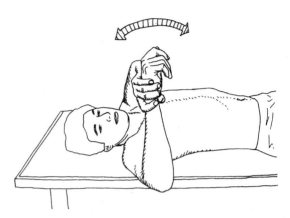

Figure 2–29. Arm position of patient for giving self-assisted ROM to internal and external rotation of shoulder.

b. Finger flexion and extension

The patient uses the normal thumb to extend the involved fingers and cups the normal fingers over the dorsum of the involved fingers to flex them (Fig. 2–31).

c. Thumb flexion with opposition and extension with reposition

The patient cups the normal fingers around the radial border of the thenar eminence of the involved thumb and places the normal thumb along the palmar surface of the involved thumb to extend it (Fig. 2–32). To flex and op-

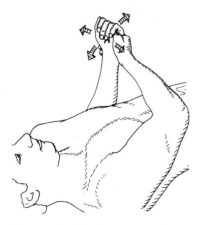

Figure 2–30. Patient applying self-assisted wrist motions.

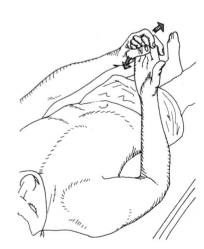

Figure 2–31. Patient applying self-assisted finger flexion and extension.

pose the thumb, the patient cups the normal hand around the dorsal surface of the involved hand and pushes the first metacarpal toward the little finger.

3. Hip and knee

The patient is supine and is instructed to slide the normal foot under the knee of the involved extremity (Fig. 2–33).

a. Hip and knee flexion

Instruct the patient to initiate the motion by lifting up the involved knee with the normal foot. The patient then can grasp the knee with the normal hand and bring the knee up toward the chest.

b. Hip abduction and adduction

Instruct the patient to slide the normal foot from the knee down to the ankle and then move the involved extremity from side to side.

4. Ankle and toes

The patient sits with the involved extremity crossed over the normal one so that the distal leg rests on the normal knee. With the normal hand, the involved ankle can be moved into dorsiflexion and plantarflexion, inversion and eversion, and toe flexion and extension (Fig. 2–34).

B. Wand Exercises

When a patient has voluntary muscle control in an involved upper extremity but needs guidance or motivation to complete the ranges of motion in the shoulder or elbow, a dowel rod (cane, wooden stick, T-bar, or similar object) can be used to provide assistance.

PATIENT POSITION

The choice of position is based on the patient's level of function. Most of the techniques can be performed supine if maximum protection is needed. Sitting or standing requires greater control.

PROCEDURE

Initially, guide the patient through the proper motion for each activity to ensure that he or she does not use substitute motions. The patient grasps the wand with both hands; the normal extremity guides the involved extremity. The patient may be standing, sitting, or supine.

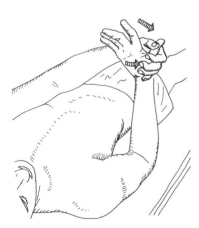

Figure 2–32. Patient applying self-assisted thumb extension.

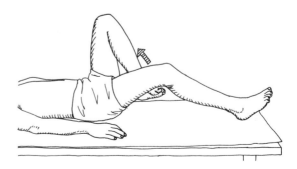

Figure 2–33. Position of patient's foot for initiating self-assisted ROM to the hip.

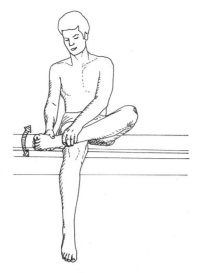

Figure 2–34. Position of patient and hand placement for self-assisted ankle motions.

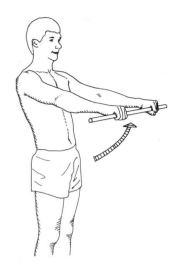

Figure 2–35. Patient using a wand for self-assisted shoulder flexion.

1. Shoulder flexion and return (Fig. 2–35)

The wand is grasped with the hands a shoulder-width apart. The wand is lifted forward and upward through the available range, with the elbows kept in extension if possible. Scapulohumeral motion should be smooth; do not allow scapular elevation or trunk movement.

2. Shoulder horizontal abduction and adduction

The wand is lifted to 90 degrees flexion (same as in Fig. 2–35). Keeping the elbows in extension, the patient pushes and pulls the wand back and forth across the chest through the available range. Do not allow trunk rotation.

3. Shoulder internal and external rotation (Fig. 2–36)

The patient's shoulders are abducted 90 degrees and the elbows flexed 90 degrees. For external rotation, the wand is moved toward the patient's head; for internal rotation, the wand is moved toward the waistline.

ALTERNATE POSITION (see Fig. 8–8)
The patient's arms are at the sides and the elbows are flexed 90 degrees. Rotation of the arms is accomplished by moving the wand from side to side across the trunk while maintaining the elbows at the side. The rotation should occur in the humerus; do not allow elbow flexion and extension.

4. Elbow flexion and extension

The patient's forearms may be pronated or supinated; the hands grasp the wand, a shoulder-width apart. Instruct the patient to flex and extend the elbows.

5. Shoulder hyperextension

The patient may be standing or prone. He or she places the wand behind the buttocks, grasps the wand with hands, a shoulder-width apart, and then lifts the wand backward away from the trunk. The patient should avoid trunk motion.

6. Variations and combinations of movements

For example, the patient begins with the wand behind the buttocks (as in 5) and then moves the wand up the back to achieve scapular winging, shoulder internal rotation, and elbow flexion.

C. Finger Ladder

The finger ladder (or wall climbing) is a device that can provide the patient with objective reinforcement and therefore motivation for performing shoulder range of motion.

Precaution: The patient must be taught the proper motions and not allowed to substitute with trunk side-bending, toe-raising, or shoulder-shrugging.

1. Shoulder flexion

The patient stands, facing the finger ladder an arm's length away, and places the index or middle finger on a step of the ladder. The arm is moved into flexion by climbing with the fingers. The patient steps closer to the ladder as the arm is elevated.

2. Shoulder abduction (Fig. 2–37)

The patient stands sideways, with the affected shoulder toward the ladder an arm's length away. The patient needs to externally rotate the shoulder while abducting the arm.

D. Overhead Pulleys

If properly taught, pulley systems can be effectively used to assist an involved extremity in performing ROM.

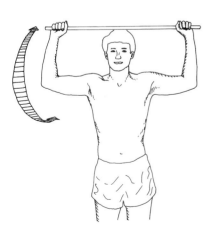

Figure 2–36. Patient using a wand for self-assisted shoulder rotation.

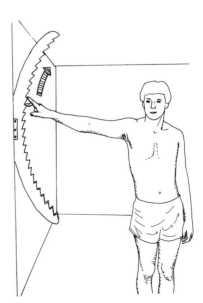

Figure 2–37. Shoulder abduction using a finger ladder.

PULLEY SET-UP

Two pulleys are attached to an overhead bar or to the ceiling approximately shoulder-width apart. A rope is passed over both pulleys, and a handle is attached to each end of the rope. The patient may be sitting, standing, or supine, with the shoulders aligned under the pulleys.

1. Shoulder flexion (Fig. 2–38A) and abduction (Fig. 2–38B)

Instruct the patient to hold one handle in each hand and, with the normal hand, pull the rope and lift the involved extremity either forward (flexion) or out to the side (abduction). The elbow should be kept in extension if possible. The patient should not shrug the shoulder (scapular elevation) or lean the trunk. Guide and instruct the patient so there is smooth motion.

Precaution: Assistive pulley activities for the shoulder are easily misused by the patient, resulting in compression of the humerus against the acromion process. Continual compression will lead to pain and decreased function. Proper patient selection and appropriate instruction can avoid this problem. If a patient cannot learn to use the pulley with proper shoulder mechanics, these exercises should not be performed. With increased pain or decreased mobility, discontinue this activity (see Chapter 8).

2. Shoulder internal and external rotation (Fig. 2–39)

Position the patient with the shoulder abducted 90 degrees and the elbow flexed 90 degrees. Have the arm supported on the back of a chair if the patient is sitting or on the treatment table if the patient is supine. The patient then lifts the forearm with the pulley, causing rotation in the arm.

3. Elbow flexion

With the arm stabilized along the side of the trunk, the patient lifts the forearm and bends the elbow.

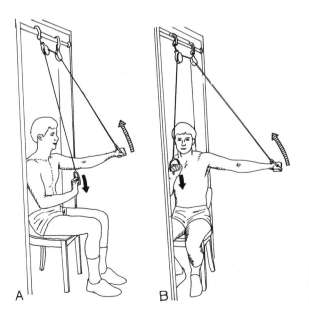

Figure 2–38. (*A*) Shoulder flexion and (*B*) abduction using overhead pulleys to assist the motion.

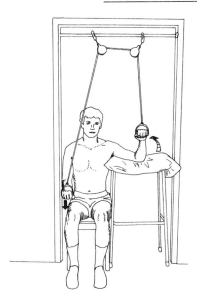

Figure 2–39. Position for shoulder rotation using overhead pulleys to assist the motion.

E. Skate Board; Powder Board

These devices are usually used after surgical procedures to the hip to encourage ROM (see Chapter 11). Proper instructions make them useful, but just telling the patient to move the leg often results in faulty movement or lack of interest.

PROCEDURE

Place the board under the involved extremity. If available, strap a skate to the foot. If no skate is available, place powder or a towel under the extremity to lower the friction of the leg moving on the board.

1. Hip abduction and adduction

POSITION OF PATIENT

The patient is supine. The foot should be pointing upright to keep the hip neutral to rotation. Do not allow the leg to roll outward as the patient moves it from side to side.

2. Hip flexion and extension

POSITION OF PATIENT

The patient is supine. He or she slides the foot up and down the board, allowing the knee to also flex and extend. The hip should not rotate, abduct, or adduct.

ALTERNATE POSITION

The patient is side-lying, with the affected hip up. The board is placed between the legs and supported with pillows if necessary. The skateboard can also be placed on an elevated platform.

Precaution: If side-lying is used after hip surgery, the affected hip must not fall into adduction.

F. Suspension

This technique is used to free a body part from the resistance of friction while it is moving. The part is suspended in a sling attached to a rope that is fixed to an appropriate point above the body segment.[8,9]

1. Two types of suspension

a. Vertical fixation

The point of attachment of the rope is over the center of gravity of the moving segment. The part can then move like a pendulum, describing an arc (Fig. 2–40). Usually the movement is small range, so this type of suspension is primarily used for support.

b. Axial fixation

The point of attachment of all ropes supporting the part is above the axis of the joint to be moved (Fig. 2–41). The part will move on a flat plane, parallel to the floor. This type of fixation allows for maximum movement of a joint.

2. Benefits of suspension for ROM exercises[9]

a. Active participation is required; thus, the patient learns to use the appropriate muscles for the desired movement.

b. Relaxation is promoted through secure support and smooth, rhythmic motion.

c. Little work is required of stabilizing muscles because the part is supported.

d. Modifications can be made to the system to provide grades of exercise resistance.[8–12]

e. After instruction, the patient can often work independently of a therapist.

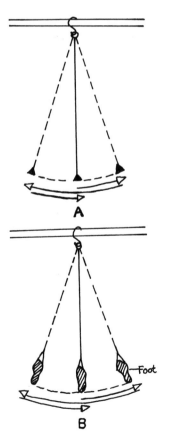

Figure 2–40. Vertical fixation: (*A*) Movement of a pendulum and attachment of the rope over the center of gravity of the extremity results in (*B*) the foot's moving like a pendulum. (Redrawn from Hollis,[8] p 71, with permission.)

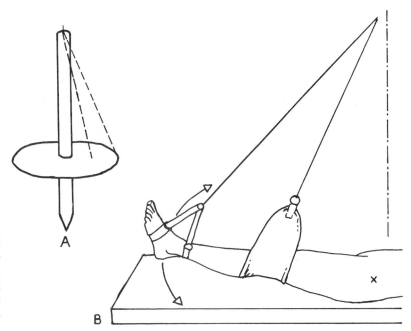

Figure 2–41. Axial fixation: (*A*) A pencil through a circle of paper demonstrates that the paper moves parallel to the floor when the pencil is pivoted. (*B*) Attachment of all ropes above the joint results in the extremity's moving parallel to the floor. (Redrawn from Hollis,[8] p 71, with permission.)

3. **Examples for active ROM using axial fixation suspension**

For extensive descriptions of suspension set-ups, refer to the sources listed in references 8 through 12.
a. Shoulder abduction and adduction with axial fixation (Fig. 2–42)
b. Hip flexion and extension with axial fixation (Fig. 2–43)

G. Reciprocal Exercise Unit

This device can be set up to provide some hip and knee flexion and extension to an involved lower extremity by using the strength of a normal lower extremity. The device is mobile in that it can be attached to a patient's bed, wheelchair, or stan-

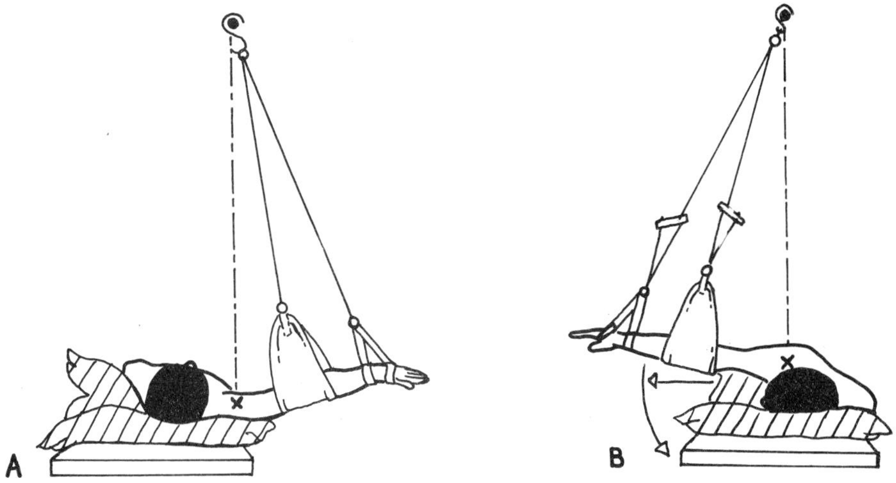

Figure 2–42. Shoulder abduction and adduction in axial fixation (____. ____. axial line) (*A*) supine and (*B*) prone. This position may be used for protraction and retraction of the scapula. (Redrawn from Hollis,[8] p 76, with permission.)

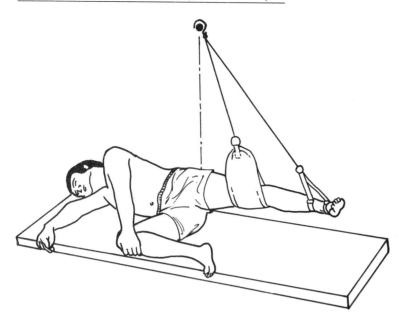

Figure 2–43. Flexion and extension of the hip joint in axial fixation (____. ____. axial line). (Redrawn from Hollis,[8] p 75, with permission.)

dard chair. The circumference of motion as well as excursion of the lower extremities can be adjusted. A reciprocal exercise unit has additional exercise benefits in that it can be used for reciprocal patterning, endurance training, and initiating a strengthening program. (See Chapter 3, Fig. 3–28).

H. Applications

The variety of applications of mechanical devices for assistive ROM is potentially endless, being limited only by the imagination and resources of the therapist. Whenever using equipment, the primary concerns must be:

1. Goals

Does the motion accomplish the goals?

2. Proper mechanics of the moving segment

Is proper stabilization provided and has proper instruction been given to avoid substitute motions?

3. Patient comfort and safety

Are all hazards to the patient from faulty equipment or improper instruction eliminated?

IX. Continuous Passive Motion

Continuous passive motion (CPM), in contrast to intermittent passive motion, is motion that is uninterrupted for extended periods of time.[5] It is usually applied by a mechanical device that moves a desired joint continuously through a controlled range of motion without patient effort for as long as 24 hours a day for 7 or more successive days. The motion is passive so that muscle fatigue does not interfere with the motion. A machine is used because an individual would not be able to apply the controlled motion continuously for the extended periods of time. The treatment technique is based on the research and protocols developed by Robert Salter.[21]

A. Benefits of CPM[5,17-22]

1. CPM is effective in lessening the negative effects of joint immobilization in conditions such as arthritis, contractures, and intra-articular fractures; in decreasing the frequency of postoperative complications; and in improving the recovery rate and range of motion following a variety of surgical procedures.
2. CPM has been shown to:
   a. Prevent development of adhesions and decrease contracture formation.
   b. Decrease postoperative pain.
   c. Enhance nutritional status of the extremity by improving the circulation through the continuous pumping action.
   d. Increase synovial fluid lubrication of the joint.
   e. Decrease joint effusion and wound edema, thus improving wound healing.
   f. Increase the rate of intra-articular cartilage healing and regeneration.
   g. Provide a quicker return of the range of motion.

B. Procedure[1,6,14,21]

NOTE: A variety of protocols have been developed based on individual surgeon's experience. Patient response, surgical procedure, or disease entity may necessitate modifying the range, time, and duration of CPM application.

1. The device may be applied to the involved extremity immediately after surgery while the patient is still under anesthesia or, at least, within 3 days after surgery if bulky dressings prevent early motion.
2. The size and position of the motion arc for the joint is determined. A low arc of 20 to 30 degrees may be used immediately after surgery. The degrees are re-adjusted daily or at an appropriate time interval to progress the patient's range as tolerated.
3. The rate of motion is determined; usually 1 cycle per minute or per 2 minutes is well tolerated.
4. The amount of time on the CPM machine may vary for different protocols: anywhere from continuous for 24 hours to continuous for 1 hour three times a day.[6,14,21] The longer periods of time per day reportedly result in a shorter hospital stay, fewer postoperative complications, and greater range of motion at discharge,[6] although no significant difference was found in a study comparing 5 hours per day with 20 hours per day of CPM.[1]
5. Physical therapy treatments are usually initiated during periods when the patient is not on CPM, including active-assistive or sling exercises.
6. Duration minimum is usually 1 week or when a satisfactory range of motion is reached. A therapeutic exercise program of active exercises is continued until the patient attains appropriate functional goals.

C. Equipment (Fig. 2-44)

Several different companies now manufacture CPM machines. They are designed to be adjustable, easily controlled, versatile, and portable. Some are battery operated to allow the individual to wear the device for up to 8 hours while functioning with daily activities. The batteries are then recharged while the person sleeps. Machines have been developed for just about every peripheral joint.

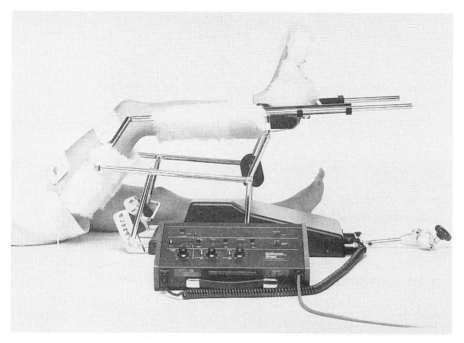

Figure 2–44. CM-100 Continuous Motion Device. (Courtesy of Empi Inc., St. Paul, MN.)

X. Range of Motion Through Functional Patterns

To accomplish motion through functional patterns, first determine what pattern of movement is desired, then move the extremity through that pattern using manual assistance, mechanical assistance if it is appropriate, or self-assistance from the patient. Functional patterning can be beneficial in initiating the teaching of activities of daily living (ADL), as well as in instructing patients with visual impairments in functional activities.

XI. Summary

The benefits, limitations, indications, contraindications, and techniques of both passive and active range of motion exercises have been described. Techniques include manual ROM using anatomic planes and combined patterns, self-assisted ROM, and mechanical assisted ROM.

References

1. Basso, DM, and Knapp, L: Comparison of two continuous passive motion protocols for patients with total knee implants. Phys Ther 67:360, 1987.
2. Clarkson, HM, and Gilewich, GB: Musculoskeletal Assessment: Joint Range of Motion and Manual Muscle Strength. Williams & Wilkins, Baltimore, 1989.
3. Donatelli, R, and Owens-Burckhart, H: Effects of immobilization on the extensibility of periarticular connective tissue. Journal of Orthopaedic and Sports Physical Therapy 3:67, 1981.
4. Fletcher, GF, et al: Exercise Standards: A Statement for Health Professionals. American Heart Association, Dallas, 1991.
5. Frank, C, et al: Physiology and therapeutic value of passive joint motion. Clin Orthop 185:113, 1984.
6. Gose, J: Continuous passive motion in the postoper-

ative treatment of patients with total knee replacement. Phys Ther 67:39, 1987.

7. Guidelines for Exercise Testing and Prescription, ed 4. American College of Sports Medicine, Lea & Febiger, Philadelphia, 1991.

8. Hollis, M: Practical Exercise Therapy. Blackwell Scientific Publications, London, 1976.

9. Johnson, MM, and Bonner, CD: Sling suspension techniques demonstrating the use of a new portable frame. Part I: Introduction, definitions, equipment and advantages. Phys Ther 51:524, 1971.

10. Johnson, MM, and Bonner, CD: Sling suspension techniques demonstrating the use of a new portable frame. Part II: Methods of progression in an exercise program: The upper extremity. Phys Ther 51:1092, 1971.

11. Johnson, MM, and Bonner, CD: Sling suspension techniques demonstrating the use of a new portable frame. Part III: Treatment of motor disabilities: The lower extremity. Phys Ther 51:1288, 1971.

12. Johnson, MM, Ehrenkranz, C, and Bonner, CD: Sling suspension techniques demonstrating the use of a new portable frame. Part IV: Treatment of motor disabilities: Neck and trunk. Phys Ther 58:856, 1973.

13. Lehmkuhl, LD, and Smith, L: Brunnstrom's Clinical Kinesiology, ed 4. FA Davis, Philadelphia, 1983.

14. McCarthy, MR, et al: The clinical use of continuous passive motion in physical therapy. Journal of Orthopaedic and Sports Physical Therapy 15:132, 1992.

15. Norkin, CC, and White, DJ: Measurement of Joint Motion: A Guide to Goniometry, ed 2. FA Davis, Philadelphia, 1994.

16. Palmer, ML, and Epler, M: Clinical Assessment Procedures in Physical Therapy. JB Lippincott, Philadelphia, 1990.

17. Salter, RB, Simmens, DF, and Malcolm, BW: The biological effects of continuous passive motion on the healing of full thickness defects in articular cartilage. J Bone Joint Surg Am 62:1232, 1980.

18. Salter, RB: The prevention of arthritis through the preservation of cartilage. Journal of the Canadian Association of Radiology 31:5, 1981.

19. Salter, RB, Bell, RS, and Keely, FW: The protective effect of continuous passive motion on living cartilage in acute septic arthritis. Clin Orthop 159:223, 1981.

20. Salter, RB: Textbook of Disorders and Injuries of the Musculoskeletal System, ed 2. Williams & Wilkins, Baltimore, 1983.

21. Salter, RB, et al: Clinical application of basic research on continuous passive motion for disorders and injuries of synovial joints. J Orthop Res 1:325, 1984.

22. Stap, LJ, and Woodfin, PM: Continuous passive motion in the treatment of knee flexion contractures: A case report. Phys Ther 66:1720, 1986.

23. Strike Back at Stroke. American Heart Association, New York.

24. Sullivan, PE, Markos, PD: Clinical Decision Making in Therapeutic Exercise. Appleton & Lang, Norwalk, 1995.

25. Voss, DE, Ionta, MK, and Myers, BJ: Proprioceptive Neuromuscular Facilitation, ed 3. Harper & Row, Philadelphia, 1985.

Resistance Exercise

If resistance is applied to a muscle as it contracts, the muscle will adapt and become stronger over time. Adaptive changes can occur in muscle through the use of therapeutic exercise if the metabolic capabilities of the muscle are progressively overloaded. Muscle, which is contractile tissue, becomes stronger as the result of hypertrophy of muscle fibers and an increase in the recruitment of motor units in the muscle.* As the strength of a muscle increases, the cardiovascular response of the muscle improves so that muscular endurance and power also increase.

Many factors, such as disease, disuse, and immobilization, may result in muscle weakness.[74,107] The therapeutic use of resistance in an exercise program, whether applied manually or mechanically, is an integral part of a patient's plan of care when the ultimate goal is to improve strength, endurance, and overall physical function.

When designing a resistance training program, a therapist must always consider the overall level of fitness of the patient, the type of injury or disease, the stage of healing after injury, and, most important, the desired functional outcomes.

OBJECTIVES

After studying this chapter, the reader will be able to:

1 Define resistance exercise.
2 Describe the goals and indications for resistance exercise and differentiate strength, endurance, and power.
3 Explain the precautions and contraindications of resistance exercise.
4 Describe and differentiate between isotonic, isometric, and isokinetic exercise, as well as concentric and eccentric or open-chain and closed-chain exercise.
5 Explain the similarities and differences between manual and mechanical resistance exercise.
6 Explain the principles of application of manual resistance exercise.

*Refs. 6, 11, 31, 32, 40, 62, 63, 80, 87.

7 Describe appropriate techniques of manual resistance exercise using the anatomic planes of motion.

8 Define mechanical resistance exercise.

9 Describe specific regimens of resistance exercise.

10 Discuss the variables found in resistance exercise programs.

11 Identify and explain the use of various types of equipment used in resistance exercise.

I. Definition of Resistance Exercise

Resistance exercise is any form of active exercise in which a dynamic or static muscular contraction is resisted by an outside force.[6,108] The external force may be applied manually or mechanically.

A. Manual Resistance Exercise

Manual resistance exercise is a type of active exercise in which resistance is provided by a therapist or other health professional. Although the amount of resistance cannot be measured quantitatively, this technique is useful in the early stages of an exercise program when the muscle to be strengthened is weak and can overcome only mild to moderate resistance. It is also useful when the range of joint movement needs to be carefully controlled. The amount of resistance given is limited only by the strength of the therapist.

B. Mechanical Resistance Exercise

Mechanical resistance exercise is a form of active exercise in which resistance is applied through the use of equipment or mechanical apparatus. The amount of resistance can be measured quantitatively and progressed over time. It is often used in specific resistance exercise regimens. It is also useful when amounts of resistance greater than the therapist can apply manually are necessary.

II. Goals and Indications of Resistance Exercise

The overall purpose of resistance exercise is to improve function. The specific goals are as follows:

A. Increase Strength

1. Strength refers to the force output of a contracting muscle and is directly related to the amount of tension a contracting muscle can produce.[6,44,49,80,94]
2. To increase the strength of a muscle, the muscle contraction must be loaded or resisted so that increasing levels of tension will develop because of hypertrophy and recruitment of muscle fibers.[73]
3. Strength training has been defined as a muscle or muscle group lifting, lowering, or controlling heavy loads for a relatively low number of repetitions.[6,31,87,108] Resistance training is another term that describes this process. Strength training has been shown to cause selective hypertrophy of type II muscle fibers.[6,80]

B. Increase Muscular Endurance

1. Endurance is the ability to perform low-intensity repetitive exercise over a prolonged period of time.[11,32,68]

2. Muscular endurance is improved by performing exercise against mild resistance (low load) for many repetitions.[68]

3. It has been shown that, in most exercise programs designed to increase strength, muscular endurance also increases.[6,31,80]

4. In certain clinical situations it may be more appropriate to implement a resistance exercise program that will increase a patient's muscular endurance rather than his or her strength. For example, it has been shown that, after many acute or chronic knee injuries, dynamic exercises carried out for a high number of repetitions against light resistance are more comfortable and create less joint irritation than dynamic exercises performed against heavy resistance.[64]

5. Total-body endurance also can be improved with prolonged low-intensity exercise. This will be discussed in detail in Chapter 4.

C. Increase Power

1. Power is also a measure of muscular performance, which is related to strength and speed, and is defined as work per unit of time[43,63,68,93,109] (force $\times$ distance/time). Force times velocity is an equivalent definition.[63,72,88,92,94]

2. The rate at which a muscle contracts and develops force throughout the range of motion and the relationship of speed and force are both factors that affect power.[7,68,71,93,109]

3. Power can be improved by either increasing the work that a muscle must perform in a specified period of time or reducing the amount of time required to produce a given force.[68,84,93,94] Although power is related to strength and speed, speed is the variable that is most often manipulated in power training programs. The greater the intensity of the exercise and the shorter the time period taken to generate a force, the greater the muscular power.

4. Some authors state it is inappropriate to limit the use of the term power to a burst of high-intensity muscle activity. They[32,94] call high-intensity exercise carried out over a short interval of time *anaerobic power* and low-intensity exercise sustained over a long period of time *aerobic power*. (The terms "aerobic power" and "endurance" are often used interchangeably.)

   a. This distinction is made because[32,88,94]:

      (1) Type II (phasic fast-twitch) muscle fibers, which generate a great amount of tension in a short period of time, are geared toward anaerobic metabolic activity and tend to fatigue quickly.

      (2) Type I (tonic, slow-twitch) muscle fibers generate a low level of muscle tension but can sustain the contraction for a long time. These fibers are geared toward aerobic metabolism and are very slow to fatigue.

   b. Muscles are composed of both phasic and tonic fibers.

      (1) Some muscles have a greater distribution of tonic fibers and others have a greater distribution of phasic fibers.

      (2) This leads to differentiation and specialization in muscles. For example, a heavy distribution of type I tonic fibers is found in postural muscles in which low-level, sustained muscle tension constantly holds the body erect against gravity or stabilizes it against repetitive loads.

A high proportion of type II phasic motor units is found in muscles that produce a great burst of tension to enable a person to lift the entire body weight when climbing a flight of stairs; to propel the body forward on crutches; or to lift, push, or pull a heavy load.

5. Resistance exercise programs can be designed to selectively recruit different fiber types in muscles by controlling the intensity, duration, and speed of exercise.

There is no question that strength, endurance, and power are all related and can all be improved with resistance exercises. It is important that the therapist evaluate each clinical situation and design exercise programs that will meet the specific needs of each patient.

III. Precautions for and Contraindications to Resistance Exercise

Although the use of resistance exercise is often the basis of a training program designed to improve a patient's functional capabilities, a therapist must consider a number of precautions and contraindications before implementing and while carrying out a resistance exercise program.

A. Precautions

1. **Cardiovascular precautions**[25,55]

   a. The **Valsalva maneuver,** which is an expiratory effort against a closed glottis, must be avoided during resistance exercise. When a person is exerting a strenuous and prolonged effort, the phenomenon can occur.

   b. Description of the sequence.
      (1) Deep inspiration.
      (2) Closure of the glottis.
      (3) Contraction of abdominal muscles.
      (4) Increase in intrathoracic and intra-abdominal pressures that leads to decreased venous blood flow to the heart. Decreased venous return leads to a decreased cardiac output, which, in turn, causes a temporary drop in arterial blood pressure. This decrease in arterial pressure leads to an increase in the heart rate.
      (5) When the expiratory effort is *released* and expiration occurs, there is a pronounced *increase* in blood pressure up to 200 mm Hg or higher. This is due to rapid venous blood flow into the heart and leads to a forceful contraction of the heart.

   c. Significance in exercise.
      (1) The Valsalva maneuver should be avoided during exercise so that abnormal stress on the cardiovascular system and the abdominal wall can be avoided.
      (2) High-risk patients.
         (a) Patients with a history of cardiovascular problems (cerebrovascular accident, myocardial infarction, or hypertension)
         (b) Geriatric patients
         (c) Patients who have had abdominal surgery or herniation of the abdominal wall

   d. Prevention of the Valsalva maneuver during exercise.[29,55]

(1) Caution the patient about holding his or her breath.

(2) Have the patient exhale when performing a motion.

(3) Ask the patient to count or talk or breathe rhythmically during exercise.

> NOTE: The Valsalva maneuver is most commonly seen when a patient is performing isometric[29] or heavy-resistance exercise.[17] The increase in blood pressure induced by an isometric muscle contraction is proportional to the percentage of maximum voluntary force that is exerted.[106] If a patient exerts maximum effort during dynamic exercise at increasing velocities, the rise in blood pressure appears to be the same at all velocities of movement despite the fact that force output in the muscle decreases.[25] Patients with a history of cardiovascular problems should be monitored closely and may have to avoid isometric or high-effort, dynamic exercises completely.

2. Fatigue

Fatigue is a complex phenomenon that affects functional performance and must be considered in a therapeutic exercise program. Fatigue has a variety of definitions, which are based on the type of fatigue being discussed.

a. **Local muscle fatigue** is the diminished response of a muscle to a repeated stimulus. This is a normal physiologic response of muscle and is characterized by a reduction in the force-producing capacity of the neuromuscular system[26,69] associated with a decrease in the amplitude of the motor unit potentials.[69]

(1) Muscle fatigue can occur during either dynamic or static muscular contractions and whenever high-intensity or low-intensity exercise is performed over a period of time.

(2) The diminished response of the muscle is due to a combination of factors, which include[32,39,99]:

(a) Disturbances in the contractile mechanism of the muscle itself because of a decrease in energy stores, insufficient oxygen, and a build-up of lactic acid.

(b) Inhibitory (protective) influences from the central nervous system

(c) Possibly a decrease in the conduction of impulses at the myoneural junction, particularly in fast-twitch fibers

(3) Muscle fatigue is characterized by a decline in peak torque and is associated with an uncomfortable sensation within the muscle or even pain and spasm. When fatigued, the response of the muscle may be lower or the active range of movement performed by the muscle will be less.[32,69]

b. **General muscular (total-body) fatigue** is the diminished response of a person during prolonged physical activity such as walking or jogging.

(1) General fatigue with prolonged but relatively low-intensity exercise is probably due to[32,39]:

(a) A decrease in blood sugar (glucose) levels

(b) A decrease in glycogen stores in muscle and liver

(c) A depletion of potassium, especially in the elderly patient

(2) This is an important consideration in endurance and conditioning programs and will be discussed further in Chapter 4.

c. Fatigue associated with specific clinical diseases.

(1) Fatigue may occur more rapidly or at predictable intervals in certain diseases associated with neuromuscular or cardiopulmonary dysfunction.

(a) In multiple sclerosis the patient usually awakens rested and functions well in the early morning. By mid-afternoon the patient reaches a peak of fatigue and becomes notably weak. Then by early evening, fatigue diminishes and strength improves.

(b) Patients with cardiac disease, peripheral vascular dysfunction, and pulmonary disease all have deficits that compromise the oxygen transport system. These patients fatigue more rapidly and require a longer period of time for recovery from exercise.

(2) The therapist must be aware of the patterns of fatigue that occur in specific diseases and gear the exercise program accordingly.

3. Recovery from exercise

Adequate time for recovery from fatiguing exercise must be built into every resistance training program. After vigorous exercise, the body must be given time to restore itself to a state that existed prior to the exhaustive exercise.[32,96] Recovery from acute exercise, where the force-producing capacity of muscle returns to 90 to 95% of the pre-exercise capacity, usually takes 3 to 4 minutes, with the most rapid recovery occurring in the first minute.[96]

a. Changes that occur in muscle during recovery.[32]

(1) Energy stores are replenished.

(2) Lactic acid is removed from skeletal muscle and blood in approximately 1 hour after exercise.

(3) Oxygen stores are replenished in muscles.

(4) Glycogen is replaced over several days.

b. It has been shown that if light exercise is performed during the recovery period, recovery from exercise will occur more rapidly than with total rest.[10,32,38]

c. Only if a patient is allowed adequate time to recover from fatigue after each exercise session will long-term physical performance (strength, power, or endurance) improve.

4. Overwork/Overtraining

a. Exercise programs in which heavy resistance is applied or exhaustive training is performed repeatedly must be progressed cautiously to avoid a problem known as overwork or overtraining.[32,106]

b. **Overwork or overtraining** is a phenomenon that actually causes temporary or permanent deterioration of strength as a result of exercise and may occur in normal individuals or in patients with certain neuromuscular diseases. Simply stated, it is not always true that if a little exercise is good, then more exercise must be better.[32,93]

c. Fatigue and overwork are not synonymous terms. Because of the sensation of discomfort that accompanies fatigue in the person with an intact neuromuscular system, overtraining and the resulting muscle weakness usually do not occur. Muscle fiber loss occasionally may occur in a normal individual who trains vigorously but does not have adequate food intake or fat stores to match the increased energy expenditure caused by the exercise. The required energy may be found by the breakdown of body protein in muscle.[106]

d. A progressive deterioration of strength from overwork has been observed clinically in patients with nonprogressive, lower motor neuron disease who participated in vigorous resistance exercise programs.[45]

e. This phenomenon has also been produced in laboratory animals. One study[45,93] demonstrated that, when strenuous exercise was begun soon after a peripheral nerve lesion, the return of functional muscle strength was retarded. It was suggested that this could be due to an excessive protein breakdown in the denervated muscle.

f. Overwork can be avoided if the intensity, duration, and progression of exercise are increased slowly and monitored closely.

g. Careful and periodic re-evaluation of a patient's strength will help the therapist determine whether a patient's strength is improving appropriately as the result of the resistance exercise program.

5. Substitute motions

a. If too much resistance is applied to a contracting muscle during exercise, substitute motions can occur.

b. When muscles are weak because of fatigue, paralysis, or pain, a patient will attempt to carry out the desired movements that those weak muscles normally perform by any means possible.[81] For example, if the deltoid or supraspinatus muscles are weak or abduction of the arm is painful, a patient will elevate the scapula (shrug the shoulder) and laterally flex the trunk to the opposite side. It may appear that the patient is abducting the arm, but in fact he or she is not.

c. To avoid substitute motions in an exercise program, an appropriate amount of resistance and correct stabilization must be applied either manually or with equipment. Specific points of stabilization during resistance exercise are outlined later in this chapter.

6. Osteoporosis

a. **Osteoporosis** is a condition characterized by a reduction of mineralized bone mass that is associated with an imbalance between bone resorption and bone formation.[12,67,107] In addition to the loss of bone mass, there is also a narrowing of the bone shaft and widening of the medullary canal.

b. The changes in bone associated with osteoporosis make the bone unable to withstand normal stresses and highly susceptible to pathologic fracture. A **pathologic fracture** is a fracture of bone already weakened by disease that occurs as the result of very minor stresses to the skeletal system.[12,67] Pathologic fractures most commonly occur in the vertebrae, hips, wrists, and ribs.[12,67]

c. Factors that increase the risk for osteoporosis.

(1) In patients with neuromuscular or musculoskeletal impairments, osteoporosis may develop as the result of prolonged immobilization, bed rest, or inability to bear weight on an extremity.[107]

(a) Patients with flaccid paralysis associated with a spinal cord injury or neuromuscular disease develop bone atrophy rapidly as the result of lack of muscle pull on bone and loss of weight bearing.

(b) Patients with a long history of inflammatory joint disease will develop osteoporosis in the bones near the affected joints. This may be due to prolonged immobilization of affected joints and decreased weight bearing as the result of joint inflammation and pain or long-term systemic steroid therapy.[107]

(2) Although bone loss occurs with normal aging in both men and women, it is most common and severe in postmenopausal white women and seems directly associated with diminishing estrogen secretion.

(3) Nutritional status, specifically lack of dietary intake of calcium, also places a person at risk for developing osteoporosis.

(4) A sedentary lifestyle and lack of regular exercise are also factors associated with the risk of developing osteoporosis.

d. Modifications to exercise programs for patients with osteoporosis.

(1) Emphasis should be placed on endurance exercises or low-intensity strength training. Resistance should be added to a strength-training program very gradually.

(2) Low-impact weight-bearing activities should be incorporated into the exercise program, but explosive twisting movements should be avoided.

7. **Exercise-induced muscle soreness**[13,22,28,34,106,113]

a. **Acute muscle soreness** often develops during or directly after strenuous exercise performed to the point of fatigue.

(1) This response occurs as a muscle becomes fatigued during anaerobic exercise because of lack of adequate blood flow and oxygen (ischemia) and a temporary buildup of metabolites such as lactic acid and potassium in the exercised muscle.[13,24,106]

(2) The muscle pain experienced during intense exercise is transient and subsides quickly after exercise when adequate blood flow and oxygen are restored to the muscle. An appropriate cool-down period of low-intensity exercise can facilitate this process.

b. **Delayed-onset muscle soreness (DOMS)**[13,28,34,36,84,106] after vigorous and unaccustomed exercise or any form of muscular overexertion, muscle tenderness and temporary stiffness may begin to develop at approximately 12 to 24 hours after the completion of exercise. Gradually the DOMS sensation intensifies and usually peaks 24 to 48 hours after exercise. The sensation of tenderness and stiffness in the muscle, which can last as long as 5 to 7 days after exercise, is probably transmitted by unmyelinated group IV afferent neurons, the nerve fibers associated with diffuse muscle pain. Muscle soreness may be felt throughout the muscle belly and at the myotendinous junction.

(1) Although the etiology of DOMS has been investigated for many years, the underlying cause has not yet been determined.

(a) One early theory, the metabolic waste accumulation theory, was reported by Scandinavian researchers who suggested that an accumulation of lactic acid in muscle caused delayed as well as immediate muscle soreness after exercise. This theory has been disproved recently[112] and in earlier studies.[40,43] Studies have shown that it requires only about 1 hour of rest after exercise to exhaustion to remove almost all lactic acid from skeletal muscle and blood.[33,34]

(b) In 1961 deVries[23] proposed the muscle spasm theory as the cause of DOMS. He suggested that a feedback cycle of pain caused by ischemia and buildup of metabolic waste products during exercise led to muscle spasm, which, in turn, caused the DOMS sensation and an on-going reflex pain-spasm cycle that lasted for several days after exercise. The muscle spasm theory has not been supported by subsequent research, which shows no increase in electromyogram (EMG) activity and therefore no evidence of spasm in muscles with delayed soreness.[1,2,106]

(c) Although studies on the specific etiology of DOMS continue, current research seems to suggest that DOMS is linked to some form of contraction-induced microtrauma to muscle fibers and/or connective tissues that results in degeneration and necrosis of these tissues. The necrosis, which is evident for several days after exercise, is accompanied by inflammation and edema.[2,28,35,36,106,113]

(2) Delayed-onset muscle soreness has been frequently reported to be greater after vigorous eccentric exercise than after concentric exercise.[4,35,37,75,76,107] It has been suggested that greater damage to muscle and connective tissue and, therefore, greater DOMS may occur with lengthening contractions than shortening contractions because fewer muscle fibers are contracting during eccentric exercise to control an exercise load, and connective tissues absorb some of the load.[5,17,23,28,101] It is also well established that greater torque can be produced with maximum eccentric muscle contractions than with maximum concentric contractions. Studies suggesting that eccentric exercise is associated with greater DOMS than concentric exercise may not have adequately controlled the intensity or duration of exercise.[30] As the author of one recent study has suggested, differences in the degree of muscle soreness in earlier studies comparing concentric and eccentric exercise may have been the result of differences in the intensity of the muscle contractions rather than the type of muscle contraction.[30] In the recent study, investigators found no differences in the degree of DOMS after concentric and eccentric exercise when these exercises were performed isokinetically with the same levels of intensity (torque production).

(3) Muscle functions, specifically strength and flexibility, are adversely affected during the DOMS time course.

(a) Flexibility and joint range of motion are reduced because of tenderness and stiffness of affected muscles.

(b) There may also be temporary loss of strength that coincides with muscle soreness and may persist several weeks after the DOMS sensation has remitted.[13,41,47,113]

(c) It is questionable whether these temporary limitations are caused directly by the DOMS sensation or by the damage to muscle or connective tissues, resulting in inflammation, edema, disruption of the contractile unit, or neurologic inhibition.

(4) The prevention and/or treatment of DOMS has been only marginally successful.[106] Prevention of delayed-onset muscle soreness at the initiation of an exercise program after a short or long period of inactivity is very difficult. It appears that the only effective method of prevention is several days of previous exercise training. Clinicians believe that the severity of the onset of symptoms may be lessened by *gradually* increasing the intensity and duration of the exercise program, by performing low-intensity warm-up and cool-down exercises, or by gently stretching the muscle to be exercised before and after exercise.[22] Although these techniques are commonly used, little evidence in the literature supports their efficacy in the prevention of DOMS. Effective methods of treatment of the DOMS sensation are continually being sought.[41,47,113] Light, high-speed exercise seems to reduce muscle soreness during the exercise and may hasten permanent relief of

symptoms.[41,106,113] The use of low-frequency, long-pulse-duration trans-cutaneous electrical nerve stimulation (TENS) or thermal agents has also been shown to either decrease[20] or have no effect on the DOMS sensation.[20] Topical salicylate creams, which provide an analgesic effect, have also been shown to reduce the severity of delayed-onset muscle soreness and hasten the relief of symptoms.[47]

B. Contraindications

1. Inflammation

Dynamic resistance exercises are not indicated when a muscle or joint is inflamed or swollen. The use of resistance can lead to increased swelling and more damage to muscles or joints. Low-intensity isometric exercise (muscle setting) can be performed in the presence of inflammation if the activity does not increase pain.

2. Pain

If a patient experiences severe joint or muscle pain during exercise or for more than 24 hours after exercise, the activity should be either entirely eliminated or substantially reduced. A careful evaluation of the cause of pain must be made by the therapist.

IV. Types of Resistance Exercise

Resistance can be applied to either dynamic or static muscle contractions. Resistance exercises can be carried out isotonically (with either concentric or eccentric muscle contractions), isokinetically, and isometrically.[32,36,63,84,92,93] In all cases the ultimate goal is to improve functional performance and capabilities through the development of increased muscular strength, endurance, or power. Before choosing a particular form of exercise, the therapist must consider the concepts of specificity of training and transfer of training.

A. Specificity of Training and Transfer of Training

1. Specificity of training

Specificity of training is a widely accepted assumption, or even principle, that suggests that the adaptive effects of training, such as the improvement of strength, power, and endurance, tend to be highly specific to the training method employed.[32,58,71,84,90,103] Whenever possible, exercises incorporated in a training program should mimic the desired function. For example, if the desired functional activity requires greater muscular endurance than strength, then the intensity and duration of exercises should be geared to improve endurance.[84,90] Specificity of training should also be considered with respect to mode (type) and velocity of exercise as well as patient or limb position during exercise.[9,71,72] For example, if the functional outcome is to be able to ascend and descend stairs, then exercise should be performed eccentrically and concentrically in a closed kinematic chain pattern and progressed to the desired speed and control. It has been suggested that the basis of specificity of training is related to morphologic changes within muscle as well as to motor learning and neural adaptation to the training stimulus.[9,27,51,105]

2. Transfer of training

Carryover of training effects from one variation of exercise to another has also been reported. This phenomenon is called **transfer of training, overflow,** or **cross training.** Transfer of training has been reported to occur on a limited basis with respect to velocity of training, type or mode of exercise, contraction force, and movement pattern.* It has also been suggested that a cross-training effect can occur from an exercised limb to a nonexercised contralateral limb in a resistance training program.[21,50] An example of transfer of training is when eccentric exercise also improves concentric strength and vice versa. A program of exercises designed to develop muscle strength has also been shown to at least moderately improve muscular endurance. Strength training at one speed of exercise has been shown to provide some improvement in strength at higher or lower speeds of exercise. In almost all instances the overflow effects are substantially less than the training effects resulting from specificity of training. Overall, most studies support the importance of designing an exercise program that most closely replicates the desired functional activities. As many variables as possible in the exercise program should match the requirements and demands placed upon a patient during specific functional activities.

B. Isotonic Exercise

Isotonic resistance exercise is a dynamic form of exercise that is carried out against a constant or variable load as a muscle lengthens or shortens through the available range of motion.[32,48,58,84,93] Dynamic strength, muscular endurance, and power can be developed with isotonic exercise.

1. Manual or mechanical resistance

Isotonic exercise can be performed against manual or mechanical resistance, depending on the needs and abilities of the patient. Both manual and mechanical resistance exercises will be discussed extensively in this chapter.

2. Constant versus variable resistance

a. Traditionally isotonic resistance exercise has been performed using a fixed load such as free weights.

b. The term isotonic literally means same or constant tension. But, in fact, when a muscle contracts dynamically against a fixed load (resistance), the tension produced in the muscle varies as it shortens or lengthens through the available range of motion. Maximum muscle tension actually develops at only one point in the range of motion with isotonic exercise performed against a fixed load.[16,32,48,84,93] The weight that is lifted or lowered cannot be greater than the muscle is able to control at the *weakest* point in the ROM.

c. **Variable-resistance exercise**

(1) When isotonic exercise is carried out by using variable-resistance equipment, such as machine weights like the Eagle or Nautilus systems or hydraulic or pneumatic systems, the contracting muscle is subjected to varying amounts of resistance through the range to more effectively load the muscle at multiple points in the range.

(2) When an isotonic muscle contraction is resisted manually, the therapist

---

*Refs. 9, 27, 50, 71, 72, 82, 83, 89, 103.

can vary the resistance appropriately to meet the changing strength capabilities of the muscle throughout the range of motion.[63]

3. Concentric versus eccentric exercise[16,17,63,84]

a. Isotonic resistance exercise can also be performed *concentrically, eccentrically,* or both. That is, resistance can be applied to a muscle as it shortens or lengthens.

b. Most isotonic exercise programs involve a combination of concentric and eccentric exercise, both of which have distinct value, depending on a patient's strength capabilities and functional needs.

c. Although a maximal concentric contraction produces less force than a maximal eccentric contraction, adaptive strength gains after a concentric or eccentric exercise program appear to be similar.[17,27]

d. Greater numbers of motor units must be recruited to control the same load with a concentric contraction as compared with an eccentric contraction, suggesting that concentric exercise has less mechanical efficiency than eccentric exercise.[17,27]

e. As mentioned previously, isotonic strength training performed concentrically appears primarily to improve concentric muscle strength, and eccentric training appears to primarily improve eccentric muscle strength.[3,84,105] Although some research[83] suggests that a limited degree of transfer of training causes eccentric strength gains when concentric training is performed, the majority of the literature suggests that there is little carryover of strength from one mode of exercise to another.

f. The velocity at which concentric or eccentric exercise is performed directly affects the force-generating capacity of the neuromuscular unit.[3,14,27,52,79] At slow velocities, a maximum eccentric contraction generates greater force than a maximum concentric contraction, but as the velocity of exercise increases, concentric contraction forces rapidly decrease and eccentric contraction forces increase slightly and then generally level off or decrease. In a strength-training program, when heavy loads are lifted or lowered, isotonic exercises are usually performed at slow speeds to safely control momentum and minimize the possibility of injury. Additional information on exercise velocity and its impact on concentric and eccentric muscle function is discussed in the section on isokinetic exercise later in this chapter.

g. More extensive information on eccentric exercise as it relates to the application of isotonic and isokinetic training is discussed later in Section IV.D of this chapter.

4. Open kinematic chain versus closed kinematic chain

a. Open-chain exercise[98]

Open-chain exercise refers to movement that occurs in an open kinematic chain, in which the distal segment (the foot or hand) moves freely in space. For example, open-chain movement occurs when the arm lifts or lowers a hand-held weight. Traditionally most manual and mechanical resistance exercise routines have been applied using open-chain exercise. Open-chain exercises can be performed in a dynamic (concentric or eccentric) or static manner. Open-chain exercise may be the only exercise option if weight bearing is contraindicated. But open-chain exercise alone will not adequately prepare a patient for functional weight-bearing activities such as walking, stair climbing, or jumping, which involve muscle action in a closed kinematic chain.

The same muscle functions differently under open-chain and closed-chain conditions. For example, the tibialis posterior functions in an open chain to invert and plantarflex the foot and ankle. In the stance phase of gait, when the foot is planted on the ground in a closed kinematic chain, the tibialis posterior contracts to decelerate the subtalar joint and supinate the foot as well as to externally rotate the lower leg. Therefore, closed-chain exercise must always be considered as an integral aspect of a rehabilitation program.

b. Closed-chain exercise[56,98,104]

Closed-chain exercise refers to movement that occurs in a closed kinematic chain where the body moves over a fixed distal segment. For example, a closed-chain movement occurs in a weight-bearing position when the foot is planted on the ground and muscle action lifts or lowers the body as in stair-climbing or squatting activities. Closed-chain activity occurs in the upper extremities when a person performs a push-up.

Closed-chain exercises are performed in functional postures with some degree of weight bearing and can involve concentric, eccentric, or isometric muscle action. In addition to loading muscles, closed-chain exercises also load bones, joints, and noncontractile soft tissues such as ligaments, tendons, and joint capsules. Because closed-chain activities are done in weight bearing, they stimulate certain mechanoreceptors in and around joints more effectively than open-chain exercises, thereby stimulating muscle co-contraction and adding to joint stability. In addition to improving muscle strength, power, and endurance, closed-chain activities improve stability, balance, coordination, and agility in functional, weight-bearing postures. Obviously, if weight bearing is contraindicated, closed-chain exercise cannot be performed.

Closed-chain activities can be initiated in a rehabilitation program as soon as partial to full weight bearing is permissible. Although closed-chain activities are usually associated with lower extremity function, closed-chain exercises are also important in improving upper extremity function, particularly in developing stability in the shoulder girdle musculature. Sources of resistance applied during closed-chain exercises include manual resistance, mechanical resistance, or simply the weight of the body.

NOTE: Additional guidelines for the application of closed-chain exercises can be found in Section VII.B.7 of this chapter.

C. Isokinetic exercise

Isokinetic exercise is a form of dynamic exercise in which the velocity of muscle shortening or lengthening is controlled by a rate-limiting device that controls (limits) the speed of movement of a body part.[16,48,70,84] The term *isokinetic* refers to movement that occurs at a constant (equal) speed. Muscular force normally used to accelerate a limb is met as resistance.[48,49]

1. Because the velocity of limb movement allowed is constant, the resistance, which the isokinetic exercise unit provides, will vary. For this reason, isokinetic exercise is sometimes referred to as **accommodating resistance exercise.**[16,48,70,71] The resistance met during isokinetic exercise accommodates to the tension-producing capabilities of the muscle and loads the muscle to capacity throughout the range of motion. If the patient is well motivated and is performing with maximum effort, the muscle contracts and works maximally at all points in the range of motion. This may be why several researchers have indicated that isokinetic exercise

programs can strengthen muscles more efficiently than isotonic exercise.[16,48,92,97]

2. When isokinetic exercise units were first developed, only concentric training was possible. Recent advances in technology have led to the development of eccentric isokinetic devices.[3] This allows isokinetic training to occur in either a concentric or eccentric mode depending on the desired functional outcome.

3. Velocity of limb movement is the aspect of exercise that is controlled during isokinetic exercise. Speeds of exercise may range from a slow velocity (15 to 30 degrees per second) to a very fast velocity (over 300 to 400 degrees per second). When concentric isokinetic exercise is performed, the tension-developing capacity of the muscle decreases as the speed of exercise increases. Historically, it has been suggested that, as the speed of an eccentric muscle contraction increases, the force-producing capabilities of the muscle also increase. Investigations that have focused on eccentric isokinetic exercise do not consistently support this concept. In some studies, as the speed of limb movement increased, the force produced also increased, but only up to a point, and then quickly plateaued or decreased. In other instances, the speed of eccentric exercise had little to no effect on the force produced by the contracting muscles.

   Training effects tend to be speed specific. That is, the speed at which strength training occurs tends to be the speed at which strength gains occur. Further discussion on speed-specific isokinetic training can be found later in this chapter.

4. Unlike isotonic exercise, which is usually performed at slow speeds to control momentum and prevent muscle or joint injury, isokinetic exercise can be performed safely at very fast velocities at an appropriate time in a rehabilitation program. During isokinetic exercise the patient need not control the momentum of a rapidly moving weight, which, if uncontrolled, could cause damage to the contracting muscles.

5. Isokinetic exercise has been shown to be an effective means of increasing muscle power and endurance in addition to strength. Isokinetic exercise units allow a patient to safely exercise with a high-intensity effort against a maximal amount of resistance at relatively fast speeds and subsequently improve muscle power. Muscular endurance can also be increased with isokinetic training by performing submaximal muscle contractions for many repetitions at a variety of speeds.

D. Eccentric Exercise

1. As the value of eccentric exercise has become better understood, far more emphasis is being placed on eccentric resistance training in comprehensive rehabilitation programs. As mentioned previously in this chapter, eccentric resistance training may be performed using either isotonic or isokinetic exercises. **Eccentric exercise** is a type of dynamic muscle loading where tension in the muscle develops and physical lengthening of the muscle occurs as an external force is applied to the muscle.[3,17] Eccentric muscle contractions involve negative work and occur in a variety of functional activities such as lowering the body against gravity, descending stairs, or control and deceleration of limb movement during sudden changes of direction or momentum. Eccentric muscle contractions also provide a source of shock absorption during closed-chain functional activities.[3,17,84,89]

2. Some characteristics of eccentric muscle contractions as compared to concentric contractions have been noted in an earlier discussion of isotonic exercise (Section IV.B.3). In addition to an eccentric contraction having greater force-

producing capability than a concentric contraction, an eccentric contraction against a maximum load produces more tension than an isometric contraction. Yet there is little evidence to suggest that adaptive strength gains are any greater at the conclusion of an eccentric training program as compared to either a concentric or isometric training program.[28,32,37,53,54,61,101]

3. It has also been shown that eccentric muscle contractions are more efficient than concentric contractions.[3,5,17,89] That is, fewer motor units must fire to control the same load eccentrically than concentrically; therefore, an individual requires less effort to control a load eccentrically than concentrically. In the early stages of a rehabilitation program, when joint motion is permissible but a muscle is very weak, active eccentric muscle contractions may be easier for a patient to perform than concentric contractions. Initially gravity may be the only source of resistance whereby a patient learns to control the descent or lowering of an involved limb. Later, light mechanical resistance such as a hand-held weight can be added to gradually improve muscle function.

4. In the later stages of rehabilitation the progressive use of eccentric exercises also allows a patient to incorporate very large amounts of resistance into a strength-training program. Because the greatest amount of muscle tension can be generated with an eccentric contraction, the greatest loads can be controlled with eccentric exercise. As a patient begins to return to functional activities, high-speed eccentric exercise against substantial resistance in the form of **stretch-shortening drills** prepares a patient for high-intensity sports or work-related activities that require eccentric muscle control for deceleration or quick changes of direction during movement. (See discussion of stretch-shortening drills in Section VIII.A.5 of this chapter.)

5. Eccentric muscle contractions consume less oxygen and fewer energy stores than concentric muscle contractions against similar loads.[3,5,17,61] When training is performed to improve muscular endurance or aerobic capacity, muscles will demonstrate greater resistance to fatigue, and therefore training effects can be enhanced by emphasizing eccentric activities such as downhill running or high-speed isokinetic eccentric exercise.

6. The issues of specificity of training versus transfer of training with respect to eccentric exercise continue to be debated.[9,27,83,89, 105] As mentioned previously, eccentric isotonic exercise has been shown to be predominantly mode specific. That is, eccentric training primarily increases eccentric strength rather than concentric or isometric strength. Information on specificity of exercise as it applies to the mode and velocity of eccentric isokinetic training is very limited. Isokinetic equipment with an eccentric testing and training mode has been available only for a short period of time. The results of a few recent studies that have investigated specificity versus transfer of training effects with respect to mode or speed of exercise training have generated mixed findings and have been inconclusive.[3]

7. *Precautions for eccentric exercise*
   a. There is potential for excessive stress on the cardiovascular system (i.e., increased heart rate and mean arterial pressure) due to a pressor response when eccentric exercise is performed with maximum effort.[3,17] Therefore, rhythmic breathing techniques during exercise are essential. Caution may also need to be taken in individuals with hypertension and a history of cardiovascular disease or in the elderly population.

b. DOMS has been reported to be more severe and last longer as the result of maximum-effort eccentric exercise as compared to concentric exercise.* An explanation for this may be that greater microtrauma to muscle fibers and connective tissue may occur when a muscle lengthens against resistance than when it shortens. Also, a greater amount of resistance is necessary to overload a muscle performing an eccentric contraction than a concentric contraction, which could lead to greater tissue damage. Therefore, in the early stages of healing following muscle injury, maximum loading during the eccentric phase of exercise should not be done. Light weights, at a submaximal level for concentric exercise, do not stress the muscles during the eccentric phase. Studies that have associated eccentrics with severe DOMS all involved slow-velocity, maximum-effort eccentric exercise. High-velocity isokinetics performed eccentrically may not be as damaging to soft tissues as slow-velocity eccentric exercise, but little research has yet been done in this area.[3,41]

E. Isometric Exercise

Isometric exercise is a static form of exercise that occurs when a muscle contracts without an appreciable change in the length of the muscle or without visible joint motion.[16,49,63] Although there is no physical work done (force × distance), a great amount of tension and force output are produced by the muscle.[63,70] If adaptive changes in muscle, such as increases in strength and endurance, are to occur, isometric contractions should be held against resistance for at least 6 seconds. This allows time for peak tension to develop and for metabolic changes to begin to occur in the muscle with each contraction.[32]

Various forms of isometric exercise and intensities of static muscle contractions are used to meet different goals and functional outcomes at each stage of tissue healing after injury or surgery. Those forms of exercise include muscle-setting exercises, resisted isometric exercises, and stabilization exercises.

1. Muscle-setting exercise

Muscle-setting exercises are low-intensity, isometric exercises performed against little to no resistance. Setting exercises are used to promote muscle relaxation and circulation and to decrease muscle pain and spasm after injury to soft tissues during the acute stage of healing. Muscle setting also maintains mobility between muscle fibers as they heal. Two common examples of muscle setting are to the quadriceps and gluteal muscles. Because muscle setting is not performed against any appreciable resistance, it will not improve muscle strength. Setting exercises can retard muscle atrophy in the very early stages of rehabilitation of a muscle or joint when immobilization is necessary to protect healing structures.[68,84]

2. Resisted isometric exercise

Isometric exercises, performed against manual or mechanical resistance, are used to develop muscle strength when joint movement is painful or inadvisable after injury.

---

*Refs. 3, 13, 16, 17, 28, 34, 37, 61, 75, 76.

a. During isometric training, it is sufficient to use an exercise load (resistance) of 60 to 80 percent of a muscle's force-developing capacity in order to gain strength.[58,69]

b. The length of a muscle at the time of contraction directly affects the amount of tension that a muscle can produce at a specific point in the range of motion.[49,63,66,116] Therefore, the amount of resistance against which a muscle will be able to hold will vary at different points in the range.

c. Because there is no joint movement during isometric exercise, strength will increase only at the joint angle at which the exercise is performed. To develop strength throughout the range of motion, resistance must be applied to static muscle contractions when the joint is in several positions.[32,65]

3. Stabilization exercises

Joint or postural stability can be developed through the application of isometric exercise. **Stability** is achieved by activating co-contraction, that is, the contraction of antagonist muscles that surround proximal joints.[18] Co-contraction is achieved by means of mid-range isometric holding against resistance and in antigravity positions.

a. **Stabilization exercises** are usually performed in weight-bearing postures in a closed kinematic chain.

b. Emphasis is placed on isometrically controlling trunk musculature and proximal muscles of the extremities. A variety of positions are held against manual resistance or against gravity with body weight as the source of resistance.

c. **Rhythmic stabilization** (described in Section VI.C.4 of this chapter) and **dynamic stabilization** exercises (described in Chapters 8, 11, and 15) are forms of isometric exercises designed to develop joint and postural stability.[78,91,100]

4. *Precautions with isometric exercise*

Similar to eccentric exercise, when isometric exercise is performed against resistance, it is associated with a pressor response as a result of the Valsalva maneuver, causing a rapid increase in blood pressure. The magnitude of the response will vary with a patient's age and history. Rhythmic breathing should always be performed during isometric exercise to minimize the pressor response. Isometric exercise, particularly when performed against substantial resistance, may be contraindicated for patients with a history of cardiovascular disease or cerebrovascular accident.

V. Manual Resistance Exercise

A. Definition

Manual resistance exercise is a form of active resistance exercise in which the resistance force is applied by the therapist to either a dynamic or a static muscular contraction.

1. When joint motion is permissible, resistance is usually applied throughout the range of motion as the muscle shortens. Manual resistance may also be applied against a controlled, lengthening contraction or a static contraction of a muscle.

2. Exercise is carried out in the anatomic planes of motion, in diagonal patterns known as proprioceptive neuromuscular facilitation (PNF) techniques,[100,111] or in combined patterns of movement that simulate functional activities.

3. A specific muscle may also be strengthened by resisting the action of that muscle, as described in manual muscle-testing procedures.[15,57]

B. Principles of Applying Manual Resistance Exercise

1. Prior to initiating the exercise

a. Evaluate the patient's range of motion and strength, and identify functional limitations. Manual muscle testing and functional tests will help the therapist establish a qualitative and quantitative baseline level of strength and functional performance against which progress can be measured. It will also help the therapist determine the appropriate amount and type of resistance that should be given in the exercise program.

b. Explain the exercise plan and procedures to the patient.

c. As with ROM exercise (see Chapter 2), place the patient in a comfortable position. Assume a position next to the patient where proper body mechanics can be used. Ensure that the region of the body in which the exercise is to be done is free of restrictive clothing.

d. Demonstrate the desired motion to the patient by passively moving the patient's extremity through the motion.

e. Explain to the patient that he or she must perform the exercise with a maximum but pain-free effort.

f. Ensure that the patient does not hold the breath during the maximum effort to avoid the Valsalva maneuver.[55]

2. During manual resistance exercise

a. Consider the site of application of resistance.

Resistance is usually applied to the distal end of the segment in which the muscle to be strengthened attaches. Distal placement of resistance generates the greatest amount of external torque with the least amount of effort from the therapist. For example, to strengthen the anterior deltoid, resistance is applied to the distal humerus as the patient flexes the shoulder (Fig. 3–1).

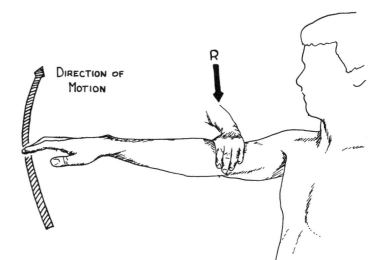

DIRECTION OF MOTION

R

Figure 3–1. Resistance (R) is applied at the distal end of the segment being strengthened and in the direction opposite to the direction of movement of the arm.

(1) The site of application of resistance will vary depending on the strength of the patient and the therapist as well as the stability of the segment.

(2) Resistance may be applied across an intermediate joint if that joint is stable and pain free and if there is adequate muscle strength supporting the joint.

b. Determine the direction of resistance.

Resistance is applied in the direction directly opposite to the desired motion (see Fig. 3–1).

c. Provide stabilization.

To avoid substitute motions when strengthening a specific muscle, appropriate stabilization must be applied by the therapist or with equipment such as splints or belts. Stabilization of a segment is generally applied at the proximal attachment of the muscle to be strengthened. For example, in the case of the biceps brachii muscle, stabilization should occur at the anterior shoulder as elbow flexion is resisted (Fig. 3–2).

d. Apply the appropriate amount of resistance.

Initially, have the patient practice the desired motion against submaximal resistance to get the "feel" of the movement. To increase strength, the optimal response from the patient should be a maximum pain-free effort. In dynamic exercise performed against resistance, the motion should be smooth, not tremulous. The resistance applied should equal the abilities of the muscle at all points in the range of motion. Gradually apply and release resistance so that uncontrolled movements do not occur.

e. Revise the site of application of resistance or decrease the amount of resistance if:

(1) The patient is unable to complete the full range of motion.

(2) The site of application of resistance is painful.

(3) Muscular tremor develops.

(4) Substitute motions occur.

f. Provide appropriate verbal commands.

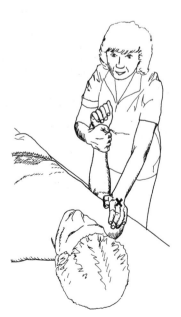

Figure 3–2. Stabilization is applied at the proximal attachment of the muscle being strengthened. In this illustration, the proximal humerus and scapula are stabilized as elbow flexion is resisted.

(1) Give the patient simple verbal commands that are easily understood and do not involve medical terminology or jargon. For example, tell the patient to "Bend and straighten your elbow" rather than "Flex and extend your elbow."

(2) Use different verbal commands to facilitate isometric, concentric, or eccentric contractions.

    (a) To resist an isometric contraction, tell the patient to "Hold" or "Don't let me move you" or "Match my resistance."

    (b) To resist a concentric contraction, tell the patient to "Push" or "Pull."

    (c) To resist an eccentric contraction, tell the patient to "Slowly let go as I push or pull you."

(3) Appropriately coordinate the timing of the verbal commands with the application of manual resistance, particularly when resisting reciprocal movements.

  g. Establish the number of repetitions.

(1) In general, 8 to 10 repetitions of a specific motion will take the patient to a point of muscular fatigue.

(2) Additional repetitions may be carried out after an adequate period of rest is allowed for recovery from fatigue.

VI. Techniques of Manual Resistance Exercise

Consistent with Chapter 2, the majority of exercises described and illustrated in this section are performed with the patient in a *supine position*. Variations in the therapist's position and hand placements may be necessary, depending on the size and strength of the therapist and patient. Alternate positions are described when appropriate or necessary. In all illustrations the direction in which resistance (R) is applied is indicated with a solid arrow.

Opposite motions, such as flexion/extension and abduction/adduction, are often alternately resisted in an exercise program in which strength and balanced neuromuscular control in both an agonist and an antagonist is desired. Resistance to reciprocal movement patterns also enhances a patient's ability to reverse the direction of movement smoothly and quickly, a neuromuscular skill that is necessary in many functional activities. Reversal of direction requires muscular control of both prime movers and stabilizers and combines concentric and eccentric contractions to decrease momentum and make a controlled transition from one direction to the opposite direction of movement.

The manual resistance exercises described in this section are for the upper and lower extremities and are all performed in an open kinematic chain. Additional exercises to increase strength, endurance, and neuromuscular control in the extremities can be found in Chapters 8 through 13. In these chapters many examples and illustrations of resisted eccentric exercises, closed-chain exercises, and exercises in functional movement patterns are included. Resistance exercises for the cervical, thoracic, and lumbar spine are described and illustrated in Chapter 15.

A. The Upper Extremity

1. Flexion of the shoulder (Fig. 3–3)

a. Resistance is applied to the anterior aspect of the distal arm or to the distal portion of the forearm if the elbow is stable and pain free.

b. Stabilization of the scapula and trunk is provided by the treatment table.

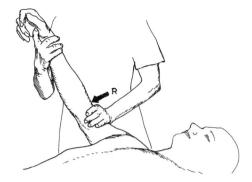

Figure 3–3. Resisted shoulder flexion.

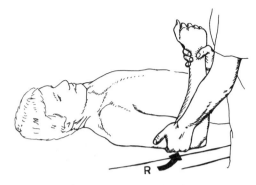

Figure 3–4. Resisted shoulder abduction.

2. **Extension of the shoulder**

   a. Resistance is applied to the posterior aspect of the distal arm or the distal portion of the forearm.
   b. Stabilization of the scapula is provided by the table.

3. **Hyperextension of the shoulder**

   a. The patient may be in the supine position, close to the edge of the table, side-lying, or prone so that hyperextension can occur.
   b. Resistance is applied in the same manner as with extension of the shoulder.
   c. Stabilization is applied to the anterior aspect of the shoulder if the patient is supine. If the patient is side-lying, adequate stabilization must be given to the trunk and scapula. This can usually be done if the therapist places the patient close to the edge of the table and stabilizes the patient with the lower trunk. If the patient is lying prone, manually stabilize the scapula.

4. **Abduction and adduction of the shoulder**

   a. Resistance is applied to the distal portion of the arm with the patient's elbow flexed to 90 degrees. To resist abduction (Fig. 3–4), give resistance to the lateral aspect of the arm; to resist adduction, give resistance to the medial aspect of the arm.
   b. Stabilization (although not pictured in Fig. 3–4) is applied to the superior aspect of the shoulder, if necessary, to prevent the patient from initiating abduction with elevation of the scapula.

5. **Internal and external rotation of the shoulder**

   a. Flex the elbow to 90 degrees and abduct the shoulder to 90 degrees.
   b. Resistance is given to the distal portion of the forearm during internal rotation (Fig. 3–5) and external rotation.
   c. Stabilization is applied at the level of the clavicle during internal rotation. The back and scapula are stabilized by the table during external rotation.

6. **Horizontal abduction and adduction of the shoulder**

   a. Flex the shoulder and elbow to 90 degrees and place the shoulder in neutral rotation.
   b. Resistance is applied to the distal portion of the arm just above the elbow during horizontal adduction and abduction.

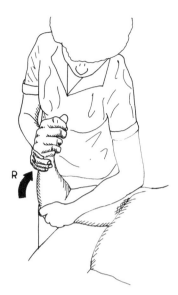

Figure 3–5. Resisted shoulder internal rotation.

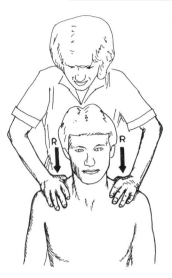

Figure 3–6. Elevation of the shoulders (scapulae), resisted bilaterally.

   c. Stabilization is applied to the anterior aspect of the shoulder during horizontal adduction. The table stabilizes the scapula and trunk during horizontal abduction.

   d. To resist horizontal abduction from 0 to 45 degrees, the patient must be close to the edge of the table while supine or be placed side-lying or prone.

7. Elevation and depression of the scapula

   a. The patient should be in a supine, side-lying, or sitting position.

   b. Resistance is applied along the superior aspect of the shoulder girdle just above the clavicle during scapular elevation (Fig. 3–6 and see Fig. 8–13A).

   c. To resist scapular depression, have the patient attempt to reach down toward the feet and push the hand into the therapist's hand. When the patient has adequate strength, the exercise can be done in a closed kinematic chain by having the patient sit on the edge of a low table and lift the body weight with both hands.

8. Protraction and retraction of the scapula

   a. Resistance is applied to the anterior portion of the shoulder at the head of the humerus to resist protraction and to the posterior aspect of the shoulder to resist retraction.

   b. Resistance may also be applied directly to the scapula if the patient sits or lies on the side facing the therapist. (See Fig. 8–13B.)

   c. Stabilization is applied to the trunk to prevent trunk rotation.

9. Flexion and extension of the elbow

   a. To strengthen the elbow flexors, resistance is applied to the anterior aspect of the distal forearm (Fig. 3–7). The forearm may be positioned in supination, pronation, and neutral to resist individual flexor muscles of the elbow, that is, the brachialis, brachioradialis, and biceps brachii.

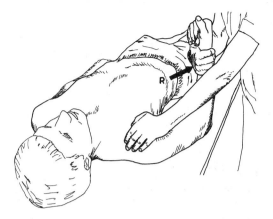

Figure 3–7. Resisted elbow flexion with proximal stabilization.

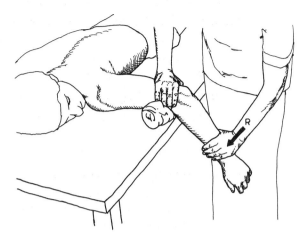

Figure 3–8. Resisted elbow extension.

    b. To strengthen the elbow extensors, place the patient prone (Fig. 3–8) or supine and apply resistance to the distal aspect of the forearm.

    c. Stabilization is applied to the upper portion of the humerus during both motions.

10. Pronation and supination of the forearm (Fig. 3–9)

    a. Resistance is applied to the radius of the distal forearm with the patient's elbow flexed to 90 degrees.

    b. Stabilization may need to be applied to the humerus to prevent motion of the shoulder.

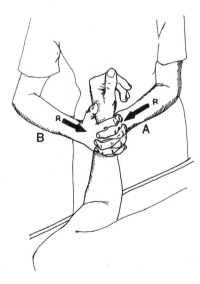

Figure 3–9. (*A*) Resisted pronation. (*B*) Resisted supination of the forearm.

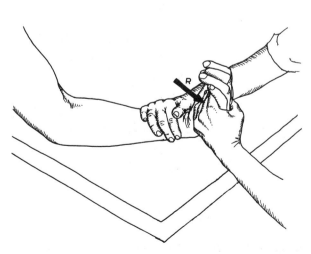

Figure 3–10. Resisted wrist flexion and stabilization of the forearm.

11. Flexion and extension of the wrist (Fig. 3–10)

　　a. Resistance is applied to the volar and dorsal aspects of the hand at the level of the metacarpals to resist flexion and extension, respectively.

　　b. Stabilization is applied to the volar or dorsal aspect of the distal forearm.

12. Radial and ulnar deviation of the wrist

　　a. Resistance is applied to second and fifth metacarpals alternately to resist radial and ulnar deviation.

　　b. Stabilization is applied to the distal forearm.

13. Motions of the fingers (Fig. 3–11) and thumb (Fig. 3–12)

　　a. Resistance is applied just distal to the joint that is moving. Resistance is applied to one joint motion at a time.

　　b. Stabilization should occur at the joints proximal and distal to the joint to be strengthened.

B. The Lower Extremity

1. Flexion of the hip with knee flexion (Fig. 3–13)

　　a. Resistance is applied to the anterior portion of the distal thigh. Simultaneous resistance to knee flexion may be applied at the distal and posterior aspect of the lower leg, just above the ankle.

　　b. Stabilization on the pelvis and lumbar spine is provided by adequate strength of the abdominal muscles.

　　　　Precaution: If, when the opposite hip is extended, the pelvis rotates anteriorly and lordosis in the lumbar spine increases during resisted hip flexion, have the patient flex the opposite hip and knee and plant the foot on the table to protect the low-back region.

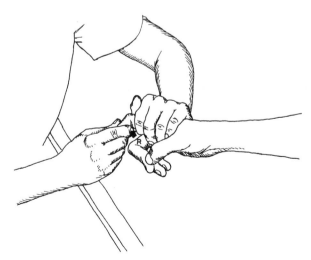

Figure 3–11. Resisted flexion of the proximal interphalangeal (PIP) joint of the index finger with stabilization of the MCP and DIP joints.

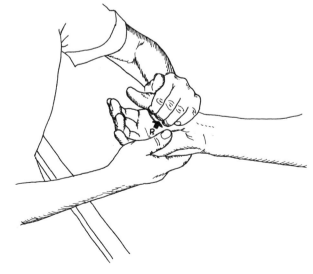

Figure 3–12. Resisted opposition of the thumb.

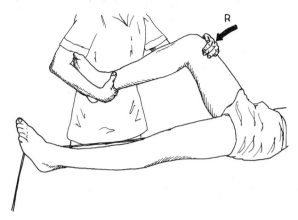

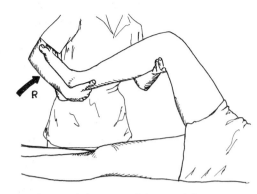

Figure 3–14. Resisted hip and knee extension with hand placement at the popliteal space to prevent hyperextension of the knee.

Figure 3–13. Resisted flexion of the hip with the knee flexed.

2. Extension of the hip (Fig. 3–14)

a. Resistance is applied to the posterior aspect of the distal thigh with one hand and to the inferior and distal aspect of the heel with the other hand.
b. Stabilization of the pelvis and lumbar spine is provided by the table.

3. Hyperextension of the hip (Fig. 3–15)

a. The patient is placed prone.
b. Resistance is given to the posterior aspect of the distal thigh.
c. Stabilization is applied to the posterior aspect of the pelvis to avoid motion of the lumbar spine.

4. Abduction and adduction of the hip (Fig. 3–16)

a. Resistance is applied to the lateral and the medial aspects of the distal thigh to resist abduction and adduction, respectively, or to the lateral and medial

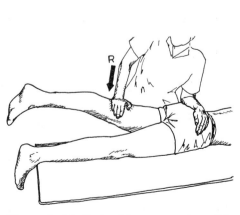

Figure 3–15. Resisted hyperextension of the hip with stabilization of the pelvis.

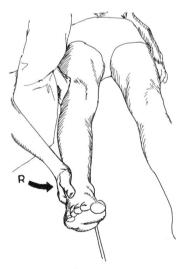

Figure 3–16. Resisted hip abduction.

aspects of the distal leg just above the malleoli if the knee is stable and pain free.

b. Stabilization is applied:

(1) To the pelvis to avoid hip-hiking from substitute action of the quadratus lumborum.

(2) To keep the thigh in neutral position to prevent external rotation of the femur and subsequent substitution by the iliopsoas.

5. Internal and external rotation of the hip

a. With the patient supine and the hip and knee extended:

(1) Resistance is applied to the lateral aspect of the distal thigh to resist external rotation and to the medial aspect of the thigh to resist internal rotation.

(2) Stabilization is applied to the pelvis.

b. With the patient supine and the hip and knee flexed (Fig. 3–17):

(1) Resistance is applied to the medial aspect of the lower leg just above the malleolus during external rotation and to the lateral aspect of the lower leg during internal rotation.

(2) Stabilization is applied to the anterior aspect of the pelvis as the thigh is supported to keep the hip in 90 degrees flexion.

c. With the patient prone, with the hip extended and the knee flexed (Fig. 3–18):

(1) Resistance is applied to the medial and lateral aspects of the lower leg.

(2) Stabilization is given to the pelvis by applying pressure across the buttocks.

6. Flexion of the knee

a. Resistance to knee flexion may be combined with resistance to hip flexion as described earlier with the patient supine.

b. With the patient prone and the hip extended (Fig. 3–19):

(1) Resistance is given to the posterior aspect of the lower leg just above the heel.

(2) Stabilization is given to the posterior pelvis across the buttocks.

c. The patient may also be sitting at the edge of a table with the hips and knees flexed and the trunk supported and stabilized.

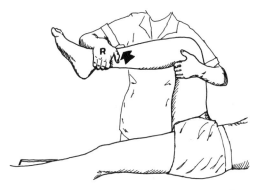

Figure 3–17. Resisted external rotation of the hip with the patient supine.

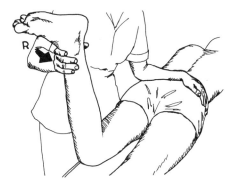

Figure 3–18. Resisted internal rotation of the hip with the patient prone.

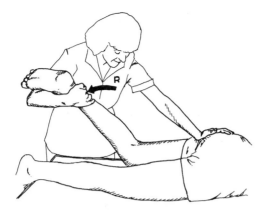

Figure 3–19. Resisted knee flexion with stabilization of the hip.

7. Extension of the knee

a. Resistance is applied to the anterior aspect of the lower leg.

    (1) If the patient is lying supine on a table, the hip must be abducted and the knee flexed so the lower leg is over the side of the table. This position should not be used if the rectus femoris or iliopsoas is tight, because it will cause an anterior tilt of the pelvis and place stress on the low back.

    (2) If the patient is prone, a rolled towel should be placed under the anterior aspect of the distal thigh. This will allow the patella to glide normally during knee extension.

b. Stabilization of the femur and pelvis is necessary.

c. The sitting position is often used for vigorous strengthening of the knee extensors. If this position is used, trunk and back stabilization is necessary for optimum performance.[85]

8. Dorsiflexion and plantarflexion of the ankle

a. Resistance is applied to the dorsum of the foot just above the toes to resist dorsiflexion (Fig. 3–20A) and to the plantar surface of the foot at the metatarsals to resist plantarflexion (Fig. 3–20B).

b. Stabilization is applied to the lower leg.

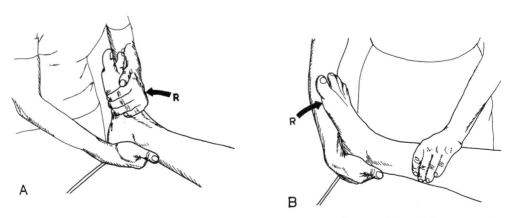

Figure 3–20. (*A*) Resisted dorsiflexion. (*B*) Resisted plantarflexion of the ankle.

9. Inversion and eversion of the ankle

    a. Resistance is applied to the medial aspect of the first metatarsal to resist inversion and to the lateral aspect of the fifth metatarsal to resist eversion.

    b. Stabilization is applied to the lower leg.

10. Flexion and extension of the toes

    a. Resistance is applied to the plantar and dorsal surfaces of the toes as the patient flexes and extends the toes.

    b. Stabilization should occur at the joints above and below the joint that is moving.

C. Additional Modifications of Manual Resistance Exercise

1. The techniques and methods of application of manual resistance exercises described and illustrated can be modified to meet different goals of exercise and individual needs of patients.

2. Although the exercises just described involve manual resistance applied to concentric muscle contractions, manual resistance to eccentric muscle contractions may be equally or more effective for desired functional outcomes.

3. Each exercise described can also be performed isometrically with manual resistance applied at multiple points in the range of motion to improve static muscle strength.

4. As mentioned earlier in this chapter, isometric exercises are often performed to develop co-contraction and stability, particularly in the trunk and in proximal muscle groups of the shoulder girdle and pelvis. A technique known as **rhythmic stabilization**[78,100] is a form of isometric exercise in which manual resistance is applied to one side of a proximal joint and then to the other as the patient holds a closed-chain position to facilitate a simultaneous isometric contraction of muscles on both sides of the joint (see Figs. 8–29A and B). Manual resistance can also be applied alternately to opposite sides of an extremity as a patient holds an isometric muscle contraction in an open kinematic chain (see Fig. 8–30). When using manually resisted isometric techniques to develop stability, manual contacts should be maintained at all times as the isometric contractions are repeated. As a transition is made from one muscle contraction to another, no distinct relaxation phase or joint movement should occur between the opposing contractions.

5. Finally, manual resistance may also be applied in the diagonal patterns of movement as described in proprioceptive neuromuscular facilitation programs.[91,100,111] Application of manual resistance in diagonal planes of movement can strengthen multiple muscle groups simultaneously and may prepare a patient for functional activities more effectively than strengthening activities performed only in the anatomic planes of movement.

VII. Mechanical Resistance Exercise

A. Definition

Mechanical resistance exercise is any form of exercise in which resistance (the exercise load) is applied by the use of some type of equipment. Various terms are used to describe this type of exercise. They include **progressive resistive exer-**

cise (*PRE*),[18,19] *active-resistive training*,[92] *overload training*, and **load-resisting exercise.**[18,19,84,93]

Mechanical resistance exercises are used to increase muscular strength, power, or endurance in rehabilitation or conditioning programs. To improve muscular function, an **overload** must be progressively applied by increasing the resistance or the number of repetitions the exercise is performed. Then, as adaptation to the increased demands occurs, more load must be placed on the muscle or more repetitions must be performed.

Mechanical resistance can be used in place of manual resistance so that a patient can exercise independently or when the strength of the patient becomes greater than the therapist can control.

B. Variables in Mechanical Resistance Exercise Programs

Many variables can be built into a mechanical resistance exercise program. No optimal combination of variables has been determined to be the most effective or most efficient means to improve muscle performance. The necessary components of the desired functional outcomes will dictate which variables are incorporated into the program. Variables may include the intensity of the exercise that is directly related to the exercise load, or how much weight is lifted or lowered; the number of repetitions, or how many times the weight is lifted or lowered; the number of sets or bouts of exercise performed; and the frequency of exercise, or how many times a week the exercise is carried out. Other variables are the type or mode of exercise, the speed at which the exercise is performed, the arc of limb movement, and the position of the patient or limb during exercise.

1. Intensity of exercise and number of repetitions

a. The *intensity* of an exercise program is directly related to the degree to which a muscle or muscle group is loaded, resulting in submaximal or maximal muscle contractions. The goals of the exercise program, the stage of healing of injured tissues, and the patient's current condition and level of fitness must be considered when a therapist determines whether exercise will be carried out against maximal or submaximal muscle loading.

(1) *Submaximal exercise,* whether performed dynamically or statically, is usually indicated when the goal of exercise is to increase muscular endurance or in the early stages of soft tissue healing, when injured tissues must be protected. Submaximal exercise is also appropriate when slow-velocity isokinetic exercise is performed to minimize compressive forces to joints.[16]

(2) Exercise should be performed with maximum intensity in the later stages of rehabilitation when functional levels of strength or power are desired.

Precaution: As the intensity of exercise increases and a patient exerts a maximum or near-maximum effort, cardiovascular risks will substantially increase. A patient needs to be continually reminded to incorporate rhythmic breathing into each repetition of an exercise to minimize these risks.

b. The **exercise load** refers to the amount of resistance imposed on the contracting muscle during exercise. One way to progressively overload a muscle is to gradually increase the amount of resistance used in an exercise program. Generally, in exercise programs that are designed to improve muscular strength, the weight a person lifts, lowers, or holds a specified number of time is progressively increased.[44,84,93]

(1) It is always difficult to determine how much weight a person should use when beginning a resistance exercise program. One early method, devised by DeLorme and Watkins,[18,19] was to determine a **repetition maximum (RM).** A repetition maximum is the greatest amount of weight (load) a muscle can move through the range of motion a specific number of times. DeLorme used 10 RM as a baseline and measurement of the improvement in muscle strength. That is, he determined the greatest amount of weight a subject could move through the range exactly 10 times. Other investigators have recommended a baseline of 6 RM to 15 RM to improve strength.[32,84,92,93]

(2) A repetition maximum is not easy to calculate and is not the most accurate method available today to measure strength before or after a resistance training program. Isokinetic dynamometers and myometers give a more accurate measure of strength. But a repetition maximum is still one way to determine the amount of resistance a person should use to initiate a weight-training program.

(3) In the advanced stages of rehabilitation, another mechanism to determine how much weight can be used to start a resistance training program is based on a percentage of body weight.[84] Percentages vary for different muscle groups. Examples include:

(a) Universal bench press: 30 percent body weight

(b) Universal leg extension: 20 percent body weight

(c) Universal leg extension: 10 to 15 percent body weight

(d) Universal leg press: 50 percent body weight

c. Another variable in a mechanical resistance exercise program is the *number of repetitions* that an exercise is performed against resistance, which is dictated by the intensity of the exercise. If the number of repetitions is progressively increased, the muscle will be continually overloaded and adaptive changes in muscle will occur. Exercise programs that are designed to improve muscle endurance often involve increasing the number of times a person does an exercise without increasing the exercise load.[16,92,93]

d. Training to improve muscular endurance usually involves performing many repetitions of an exercise at a submaximal exercise load. As many as 3 to 5 bouts of 40 to 50 repetitions against light resistance might be used to improve muscular endurance.[84] Endurance training can also be time based. With this type of training, rather than increasing the number of repetitions by a specific amount, the patient simply performs the exercise for a longer period and attempts to complete as many repetitions as possible in that given time.[16]

e. In some programs the amount of resistance and the number of repetitions are both progressively increased to improve strength and endurance. No specific progression of resistance or number of repetitions has been determined to be the most efficient means of improving muscular strength, power, or endurance. As few as 5 to 6 or as many as 15 to 20 repetitions have been recommended.

2. Bouts and frequency of exercise[16,32,62]

a. **Exercise bouts** are the number, or *sets*, performed during each exercise session. Usually several bouts of a specified number of repetitions are carried out, with the patient resting after each bout.

(1) Many combinations of sets and repetitions effectively improve muscular strength and endurance. Strength gains have occurred in programs in which three bouts of 6 RM, two bouts of 12 RM, and six bouts of 3 RM, as well as many other variations, have been used.[32,84,92,93]

(2) Strength gains have even occurred when 1 RM was used.[86] Although 1 RM is not practical in clinical settings, as long as a muscle is progressively overloaded, strength, endurance, or both will increase.

(3) In isokinetic exercise no optimal number of sets of exercise has been determined.[3,16] A set may refer to the number of repetitions performed at each training speed. As with isotonic exercise, the fewer the number of repetitions performed per set, the greater the number of sets in an exercise session.

b. **Exercise frequency** is the number of times an exercise is done within a day or within a week. Most exercise programs are performed every other day or four to five times a week.[32] Adequate time must be allowed for recovery from fatigue if improvement is to occur.

3. Duration of exercise

Exercise duration is the total number of days, weeks, or months during which an exercise program is performed. To significantly increase strength, a program must be at least 6 weeks in duration.[32]

4. Speed of exercise*

a. The speed at which a muscle contracts significantly affects the tension that the muscle produces. As the velocity of muscle shortening increases, the force that the muscle can generate decreases. Electromyogram (EMG) activity and torque decrease as a muscle shortens at faster contractile velocities, because the muscle does not have sufficient time to develop peak tension. As previously mentioned in this chapter, conflicting information exists on force-velocity relationships during eccentric exercise. Some studies suggest that at slow contractile velocities during muscle lengthening against resistance, the force-producing capabilities of the muscle initially increase, but as the contractile velocities continue to increase, force production quickly levels off and then decreases.[3,17,27,89] The initial increase in force production during an eccentric contraction may be a protective response of muscle when it is first overloaded.[14]

b. During isotonic resistance exercise (using free weights or weight-pulley resistance units), only the patient controls the speed of limb movement. Usually isotonic training is performed at slow speeds so that momentum does not become a significant factor during exercise and so that safety for the patient is ensured.

c. *Speed-specific isokinetic training*[†]

(1) Isokinetic exercise devices provide accommodating resistance to limb movement throughout the range of motion at very slow (30 degrees per second) to very fast (500 degrees per second) angular velocities. Al-

---

*Refs. 7, 16, 51, 63, 71, 79, 84, 88, 102, 103, 115.
†Refs. 7, 16, 51, 63, 68, 84, 88, 102, 103, 115.

though the highest speeds available on most isokinetic devices cannot begin to match the very fast velocities (over 1000 degrees per second) of limb movements that occur in some functional activities or sports, isokinetic exercise does provide some foundation for developing dynamic strength and power at rapid speeds of movement.

(2) Numerous studies have investigated how specificity of training relates to the speed of exercise.[27,51,89,95,103] In the early 1970s the concept of specificity of speed of exercise was first introduced by Moffroid et al.[70-72] It was reported that strength gains were the greatest at the training speed and that strength gains, although less substantial, also occurred at speeds other than the training velocities. Although subsequent studies have suggested that physiologic overflow of training effects can occur to a limited degree,[50] the consensus today is that isokinetic exercise should be carried out at velocities consistent with the desired functional activity.[27,51,102] Most functional activities, such as walking or lifting objects, involve medium-to-fast limb movements. Therefore, isokinetic training at medium-to-fast velocities is thought to be the most appropriate preparation for return to functional activities. Isokinetic training that involves exercising at several contractile velocities is called **velocity spectrum rehabilitation** and is discussed later in this chapter.[16,51,84]

5. Mode of exercise

a. The *mode of exercise* refers to the type of muscle contraction, dynamic or static, eccentric or concentric, that occurs during exercise. The types of muscle contractions used in an exercise program are dependent on the type of injury or disease, the stage of tissue healing, the condition of joints and their tolerance for compression or movement, the goals of the exercise program, and ultimately the functional activities to which a patient may want to return.

(1) Consistent with the concept of the specificity of exercise, a therapist will want to choose the mode of resistance exercises to meet the functional needs of a patient. If static strength is required for a specific functional activity, then isometric exercise should be an important aspect of the training program. If dynamic strength is necessary, then concentric or eccentric contractions can be incorporated into the program using isotonic or isokinetic exercise.

(2) In the early stages of a rehabilitation program following a musculoskeletal injury, isometric exercises against progressive resistance may be initiated when a limb is immobilized or when a patient cannot tolerate resisted range of motion.

(3) Eccentric exercise may be indicated when limb movement against resistance is desired but the tension-developing capacity of the muscle is very poor. Initially, eccentric exercise can be performed against manual resistance when joint motion must be carefully controlled. An eccentric muscle contraction may also be more comfortable if a concentric contraction produces pain in the early stages of soft tissue healing.[8]

(4) As a patient progresses, a combination of eccentric and concentric exercise is usually performed because most functional activities require a combination of eccentric and concentric strength or power.

b. The very nature of most mechanical resistance equipment, such as free weights and weight-pulley systems, builds both concentric and eccentric exercise into a training program (see Fig. 3–26).

    (1) When a weight is lifted against gravity, a concentric muscle contraction occurs.

    (2) When a weight is then lowered, an eccentric contraction of the same muscle occurs to control the descent of the weight.

c. Isokinetic exercise can also be performed concentrically and eccentrically with submaximal and then maximal effort for greater resistance.

6. Range of movement—short-arc versus full-arc exercise

Resistance exercises may be done through the entire range of motion (full-arc exercise) or through a limited range **(short-arc exercise).** For example, after surgery for repair of the anterior cruciate ligament, full knee extension against resistance is often contraindicated during early rehabilitation. Therefore, resistance exercises are carried out in only a limited arc of movement to protect the repaired ligament. Gradually, resistance is applied through the complete (full-arc) range of motion to prepare for functional activities.

    Short-arc exercise is also indicated when a patient experiences pain in a portion of the range of motion. For example, if a patient has patellofemoral pain syndrome, bilateral squats from full knee extension to mid-range flexion will strengthen the quadriceps eccentrically and concentrically through a portion of the range. By avoiding squats into full knee flexion there will be fewer compressive forces on the patella that could cause patellofemoral pain.

7. Position of the patient—open-chain versus closed-chain exercise

The position a patient assumes when strengthening a particular muscle group will affect the tension-developing capacity of the muscle, the amount of weight the patient can control, and the carryover of the exercise to functional activities.

a. Resistance exercise can be performed with the distal segment (foot or hand) moving freely in space (open kinematic chain) or with the patient in a weight-bearing position and the distal segment fixed in place or moving while in contact with the ground (closed kinematic chain).

b. The therapist should consider whether strength is necessary in an open or a closed kinematic chain during a specific functional activity and have the patient train accordingly. For example, if the hip and knee extensors are strengthened by having the patient stand and lift the body weight on steps (closed chain), there will be better functional carryover to stair climbing than if the patient strengthens the hip or knee extensors only by lifting or lowering weights with the lower limb moving freely in space (open chain).

c. In open-chain and closed-chain exercises, if the same muscle is exercised with the patient in various positions, the muscle will produce varying amounts of tension because of the relationship between length and tension that exists in muscle. Peak tension develops in a muscle when it is in a slightly lengthened position at the time of contraction.[63,66,116]

d. General guidelines for the progression of open-chain or closed-chain exercises in a resistance training program with respect to the intensity, mode, and speed of the exercise or the number of repetitions and sets performed are similar.

e. Some additional guidelines should be considered when developing closed-chain exercises.

(1) Closed-chain exercises cannot be initiated until weight bearing is permissible. Activities can be modified to initially limit weight bearing and later allow full weight bearing.[56] For example, lower extremity closed-chain activities can be performed in a pool to restrict weight bearing across multiple joints. A patient can perform closed-chain ankle exercise while seated in a chair to limit weight bearing on the involved foot or ankle. An overhead harness system can be used to control (decrease) the percentage of body weight borne on an involved lower extremity so that injured tissues can be protected and the patient can still perform functional, closed-chain activities such as walking or running.

(2) Closed-chain exercises should begin with bilateral weight-bearing activities and progress to unilateral weight-bearing activities.[56]

(3) Closed-chain exercises should first be performed against the resistance of body weight. Later, mechanical resistance can be used to add to body weight.

(4) It is safer and less demanding to begin closed-chain exercises on a stable surface such as the floor before progressing to an unstable surface such as thick foam rubber or a balance board.

(5) In-place weight-bearing activities in which the distal segment is planted as in lateral step-ups should be practiced before closed-chain moving activities such as moving side to side on a slide board.

  f. Ultimately both open-chain and closed-chain activities in various patient positions are incorporated into an exercise program at the intensity, speed, and duration of the desired functional activities.

VIII. Specific Exercise Regimens

Investigators have developed and studied many types of resistance training programs utilizing isotonic, isometric, or isokinetic exercises. The ultimate rationale for the development of each regimen seems to be to design the most effective and efficient method to increase muscular strength, power, or endurance. The optimal intensity of the weight-training program, the optimal number of repetitions and sets, and the optimal frequency of exercise have yet to be determined. Because of the many variations of these parameters found in weight-training regimens, it is difficult to make comparisons or determine which protocol is the best. An overview of several resistance training regimens follows.

A. Isotonic Regimens

1. DeLorme technique[18,19,92]

  a. Originally this technique was called heavy-resistance exercise, but DeLorme later developed the term **progressive resistive exercise (PRE)** to describe his approach to strengthening exercise.

  b. Procedure.

    (1) Determine the 10 RM.

    (2) The patient then carries out

      (a) Ten repetitions at one-half of the 10 RM

      (b) Ten repetitions at three-fourths of the 10 RM

      (c) Ten repetitions at the full 10 RM

    (3) The patient performs all three bouts at each exercise session with a brief rest between bouts.

(4) The approach builds in a warm-up period because the patient initially lifts only one-half and three-fourths of the 10 RM.

(5) The amount of weight is increased weekly as strength increases.

2. The Oxford technique[117]

a. This is the reverse of the three-bout DeLorme system. It was designated to diminish resistance as muscle fatigue develops.

b. Procedure.

  (1) Determine the 10 RM.

  (2) The patient then performs

    (a) Ten repetitions at the full 10 RM

    (b) Ten repetitions at three-fourths of the 10 RM

    (c) Ten repetitions at one-half of the 10 RM

c. This technique attempts to decrease the detrimental effects of fatigue.

d. A general, nonspecific warm-up period of active exercise is advocated prior to beginning the bouts of resistance exercise.

3. Daily adjustable progressive resistance exercise—the DAPRE technique[59,60]

a. The DAPRE technique was developed by Knight to more objectively determine when to increase resistance and how much to increase the resistance in an exercise program.

b. Procedure.

  (1) Determine an initial *working weight* (Knight suggests 6 RM).

  (2) The patient then performs

    Set 1: 10 repetitions of one-half the working weight.

    Set 2: 6 repetitions of three-fourths the working weight.

    Set 3: as many repetitions as possible of the full working weight.

    Set 4: as many repetitions as possible of the *adjusted working weight*. The *adjusted working weight* is based on the number of repetitions of the full working weight performed during set 3.

  (3) The number of repetitions done in set 4 is used to determine the working weight for the next day. Knight points out that the "ideal" maximum number of repetitions (when the patient is asked to perform as many repetitions as possible) is 5 to 7 repetitions.

c. Guidelines for adjustment of the working weight.

Number of Repetitions Performed During Set 3	Adjustment to Working Weight for Set 4	Next Day
0–2	Decrease 5–10 lb and repeat set	Decrease 5–10 lb
3–4	Decrease 0–5 lb	Same weight
5–6	Keep weight the same	Increase 5–10 lb
7–10	Increase 5–10 lb	Increase 5–15 lb
11	Increase 10–15 lb	Increase 10–20 lb

d. The DAPRE system eliminates the arbitrary determination of how much weight should be added in a resistance exercise program on a day-to-day basis.

e. This system can be used with free weights or weight machines.

4. Circuit weight training[92]

Another approach to isotonic resistance exercise is **circuit weight training.** Resistance exercises are carried out in a specific sequence using a variety of exercises for total-body conditioning. Exercises can be done using free weights or weight-training units such as the Universal, Nautilus, or Eagle systems.

a. Exercises could include 8 to 10 RM of
   (1) Bench press
   (2) Leg press
   (3) Situps
   (4) Shoulder press
   (5) Squats
   (6) Curls
b. A rest period (usually 30 seconds to 1 minute) is taken between each bout of exercise.
c. Many examples of circuit weight-training regimens can be found in the athletic training and sports medicine literature.

5. Plyometric training—stretch-shortening drills[42,109,110,114]

a. High-intensity, high-velocity exercises emphasize the development of muscular power and coordination. Quick bursts of force in functional movement patterns are often necessary if a patient is to return to high-demand occupational, recreational, or sports-related activities.
b. **Plyometric training,** often called *stretch-shortening drills*, is an approach to isotonic exercise that combines speed, strength, and functional activities. This form of exercise is appropriate only in the later stages of rehabilitation of young, active individuals who must achieve a high level of physical performance in a specific activity.
c. Plyometrics is defined as a rapid, powerful movement preceded by a preloading countermovement that creates a stretch-shortening cycle in muscle. The eccentric contraction loads and stretches the muscle and is followed by a rapid concentric muscle contraction. For example, a patient stands on a low stool or platform, jumps off the stool, and then quickly jumps back on the stool (see Fig. 12–12). Jumping off the platform and landing on the ground produces an eccentric contraction of the quadriceps as the muscle lengthens. (This is the stretch phase.) To jump back up on the platform, a rapid concentric contraction of the quadriceps occurs. (This is the shortening phase.) Stretch-shortening drills are also used in upper extremity rehabilitation.

   It is thought that the stretch-shortening cycle stimulates the proprioceptors, increases the excitability of the neuromuscular receptors, and improves the reactivity of the neuromuscular system. The term *reactive neuromuscular training* has also been used to describe this approach to exercise.
d. Application and progression of plyometric exercises are as follows:
   (1) Prior to initiation of plyometric training, the patient should have an adequate base of muscle strength and endurance in the muscle to be exercised.
   (2) The plyometric program should be designed with specific functional activities in mind and includes movement patterns in a closed or open kinematic chain that replicate the desired activity.
   (3) All drills should be preceded by adequate warm-up exercises.
   (4) The stretch-shortening activity should be performed as quickly as possible. The rate of stretch of the contracting muscle is more important than

the length of the stretch because velocity of stretch facilitates the mono-synaptic stretch reflex. If a jumping activity is performed, for example, emphasis should be placed on reducing the time on the ground between the eccentric and concentric contractions.

(5) Upper or lower extremity exercises should begin with bilateral stretch-shortening activities and progress to unilateral activities whenever feasible.

(6) Resistance (exercise load) can also be increased to progress the stretch-shortening activity. In the upper extremity, elastic tubing or weighted balls provide additional resistance during the exercises (see Figs. 8–33A and B). In the lower extremity, weights can be added or the height of a platform from which a patient jumps can be cautiously increased.

(7) Finally, the number of repetitions or bouts of exercise performed can also be increased to progressively overload the key muscle groups.

Precaution: Plyometric training should be implemented only in the late stages of rehabilitation with patients who can tolerate high-impact, ballistic forces in an exercise program.

B. Isometric Regimens

1. Brief repetitive isometric exercise[46,64]

a. In the 1950s Hettinger and Muller[46] investigated and advocated isometric exercise as an alternative method of muscle strengthening that they felt was preferable to PRE. Strength gains occurred in 6 weeks when subjects performed a *single* isometric contraction against maximum resistance five to six times per week. Each maximum voluntary contraction was held for 5 to 6 seconds. Although later replications of their study supported and refuted the findings, the most important outcome of the original study was the interest and research on isometric exercise that followed.

b. The brief repetitive isometric exercise (BRIME)[64] regimen was a refinement of the initial research on isometrics. Up to 20 maximum contractions, each held for 6 seconds, were performed daily. A 20-second rest after each contraction as well as rhythmic breathing during the contractions was recommended to prevent increases in blood pressure.

c. This repetitive approach was found to be more effective and maintained the subject's level of motivation better than using a single maximum contraction.

d. Many variations of the BRIME protocol have been studied and shown to be effective for improving static muscle strength.

2. Current use of isometrics in rehabilitation and conditioning

a. These early studies documented that isometric resistance exercise can be an effective means of improving muscle strength if the muscle is repeatedly overloaded.

b. Although isometric exercise can improve muscular endurance, the effect is minimal; dynamic (isotonic and isokinetic) exercises are a more effective means of increasing muscle endurance.

c. **Multiple-angle isometrics** are necessary if the goal of exercise is to improve strength throughout the range of motion. Gains in strength will occur only at or closely adjacent to the training angle.[16,65,84] Physiological overflow occurs only a total of 20 degrees from the training angle (10 degrees in either direction).[58]

(1) Multiple-angle isometrics are initiated when joint motion is permissible

but a resisted dynamic muscle contraction (isotonic or isokinetic) is still uncomfortable or not advisable because of the presence of chronic inflammation. Resistance applied to each point in the ROM should be gradually increased to ensure that the muscle contraction is pain free but that the muscle is progressively overloaded so that strength gains will occur.

(2) Mechanical resistance can be superimposed on multiple-angle isometric muscle contractions by having the patient push against an immovable object or by setting an isokinetic unit at zero degrees per second and having the patient attempt to push or pull with the joint held in various positions.

(3) Resistance should be applied at least every 20 degrees throughout the range.

(4) Although no specific regimen of isometric training has been shown to be most effective, Davies[16] suggests 10 sets of 10 repetitions of 10-second contractions every 10 degrees in the range of motion. (A 10-second contraction may be preferable to a 6-second contraction, as recommended earlier in this chapter to include a 2-second rise time, a 6-second hold time, and a 2-second fall time.)

C. Isokinetic Regimens

1. Velocity spectrum rehabilitation[16,84]

Most isokinetic exercise programs designed to develop strength, endurance, or power involve performing exercises on an isokinetic unit at slow, medium, and fast angular velocities.

NOTE: Most guidelines for velocity spectrum rehabilitation have been directed to concentric isokinetic training. The principles of velocity spectrum training can also be applied to eccentric isokinetic training, but literature documenting guidelines or effectiveness is still scarce.[3]

a. A minimum of three contractile velocities is usually chosen for a training program. A common exercise bout might include training at 60, 120, and 180 degrees per second or 60, 150, and 240 degrees per second. Generally 6 to 10 repetitions are performed at each training velocity with a brief rest after each set. Multiple sets at each velocity may also be performed. No optimal combination of sets and repetitions has been determined.

b. It has been suggested that the effects of training carry over only 15 degrees per second from the training velocity.[16,51] Therefore, some clinicians may choose to set up programs with as many as 8 to 10 training velocities.

c. In the early stages of an isokinetic exercise program, it is useful to begin with submaximal isokinetic exercise in a concentric mode at intermediate and slow speeds so the patient gets the "feel" of the isokinetic equipment and still protects the muscle. As the patient progresses, he or she may exert maximal effort at intermediate speeds. Slow-speed training is usually eliminated when the patient begins to exert maximal effort.

d. During the later stage of a rehabilitation program, it is beneficial to exercise maximally at faster contractile velocities for several reasons.[16,97]

(1) The speed of limb movement during specific functional motor activities, such as walking and running, occurs at fast velocities; therefore, high-speed exercise may better prepare the patient for these activities.

(2) At faster velocities, there are fewer compressive forces on joints.

(3) High-velocity isokinetic training has also been shown to increase muscu-

lar endurance. The muscle is progressively loaded by extending the time the exercise is performed in each session.[68]

e. Finally, specificity of training applies to the velocity at which exercises are done. It is important to choose training speeds that are similar to the speed of movement necessary for a specific functional activity.

2. Eccentric isokinetic training[3,16,52]

Most isokinetic training devices now have an eccentric training mode, but guidelines are limited for eccentric isokinetic exercise programs and how velocity of training should be determined. Most isokinetic protocols and information on speed-specific exercise are based on studies of concentric isokinetic training.

a. Generally, eccentric isokinetic training is introduced in the late stages of rehabilitation. For example, it has been suggested that eccentric isokinetic training should not be initiated after arthroscopic acromioplasty or débridement of the rotator cuff until the patient achieves 80 percent of active shoulder ROM.

b. Eccentric isokinetic training is usually performed at slower speeds than concentric isokinetic training. A range of 60 to 120 degrees per second has been suggested as a safe range for the general population and up to 180 degrees per second for the athlete. Because of the robotic nature of eccentric isokinetic devices, a rapid, unexpected motor-driven movement of the force arm against a limb could injure a patient.

c. To avoid excessive torque production during eccentric isokinetic training, patients are usually instructed to exercise at submaximal levels. In addition, submaximal intensities are suggested to minimize the effects of delayed-onset muscle soreness associated with high-intensity eccentric exercise.

d. Protocols for the use of eccentric isokinetic exercise have been developed and applied to the management of specific diagnoses, primarily in the knee and shoulder. Many protocols suggested by manufacturers of isokinetic products and developed by clinicians have not yet been evaluated or published.

e. The principles of velocity spectrum training are applied to eccentric regimens. Training at four to five slow to medium velocities (60, 90, 120, and 150 degrees per second) with three sets of 20 repetitions at each speed has been suggested.

IX. Use of Equipment With Resistance Exercise

Many types of mechanical apparatus and equipment are available for resistance exercise programs. A simple hand-held weight may adequately meet the needs of a patient carrying out an exercise program at home, whereas a sophisticated isokinetic exercise unit may better suit the needs of another patient.

There are a number of advantages for choosing mechanical resistance over manual resistance in an exercise program. When mechanical equipment is used, the therapist can quantitatively measure a patient's baseline strength prior to initiating the exercise program. The therapist also has an objective measurement of a patient's improvement of strength over time. The patient too can see measurable progress in an exercise program. The level of resistance applied during a given exercise is not limited by the strength of the therapist. The use of equipment also adds variety to an exercise program even in the early stages of rehabilitation when a patient's strength may still be quite limited.

There is an enormous selection of equipment on the market today, specifically for use in resistance training programs. The equipment ranges from simple to complex, small to large, and inexpensive to expensive. The choice of equipment used in a resistance exercise program depends primarily on the individual needs and abilities of the patient carrying out the exercise. The selection of equipment also depends on the availability of the equipment, the cost of purchase of the equipment by a facility or by a patient, and the space requirement for the equipment at home or in a clinical setting.

A. General Principles for the Use of Equipment

To use equipment effectively and safely in a resistance exercise program, the therapist must consider the following:

1. Evaluate the patient's strength, range of motion, joint stability, bone or joint deformities, pain, and integrity of the skin before using the equipment.
2. Determine the most advantageous types of exercise that could be used to improve strength, power, or endurance in the involved muscle groups, and choose the appropriate equipment.
3. Adhere to all safety precautions when applying the equipment.
   a. Be sure all attachments, cuffs, collars, and buckles are securely fastened and adjusted to the individual patient prior to the exercise.
   b. Apply padding for comfort, if necessary, especially over bony prominences.
   c. Stabilize or support appropriate structures to prevent unwanted movement and to prevent undue stress on body parts.
4. When it is appropriate, be certain that the full available range of motion is completed during dynamic exercise without the use of substitute motions.
5. If ROM must be limited to protect healing tissues or to avoid pain, be sure that appropriate range-limiting devices are employed.
6. When the exercise has been completed:
   a. Disengage the equipment and leave it in proper condition for future use.
   b. Never leave broken or potentially hazardous equipment for future use.
7. Observe and re-evaluate the patient to determine how the exercise program was tolerated by the patient. Record observations and objective data as soon as possible.

B. Isotonic Resistance Equipment

1. Free weights

Free weights are graduated weights that are hand held or applied to the upper or lower extremity and include:

a. Barbells
b. Dumbbells (Fig. 3–21)
c. Cuff weights with Velcro closures (Fig. 3–22)
d. Sandbags
e. Weight boots

The variety of free weights available is extensive. The therapist must select equipment for a department that will meet the needs of many patients. Each type of free weight has its advantages and disadvantages. For example, dumbbells, Velcro cuff weights, and sandbags have fixed poundage. Therefore, a series of graduated weights and sizes are necessary to adequately progress a patient as his or her strength increases. On the other hand, barbells and weight boots have interchangeable weights but require time to assemble and adjust to each patient. When strengthening a particular muscle group, a patient will be able to move against less resistance using free weights than when using isotonic machines. Unlike certain weight machines that guide or restrict limb movements,

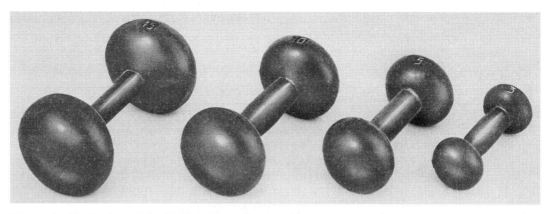

Figure 3–21. Graduated dumbbell weights. (Reprinted by permission of JA Preston Corporation, Clifton, NJ.)

free weights can move in many directions during exercise. The patient must control the plane of motion in which exercise occurs using muscular stabilization, which subsequently decreases the amount of weight the patient can safely control.

2. Elastic resistance devices

    a. Elastic resistance materials and surgical tubing such as Thera-Band and Rehabilitation Xercise Tubing are available in several grades or thicknesses. The thicker the elastic material, the greater the resistance applied to the contracting muscle.

    b. The elastic material can be cut to different lengths and set up so that upper

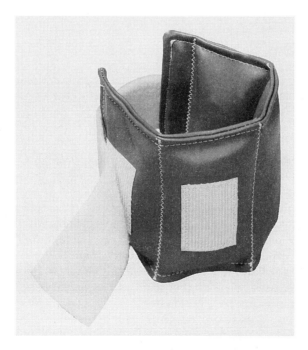

Figure 3–22. The Cuff®, a cuff weight with Velcro closure. (Courtesy of the Dipsters Corporation, Scarsdale, NY. The Cuff® is a trademark of the DIPSTERS Corporation.)

and lower extremity or trunk musculature can be strengthened. (See Figs. 8–24A, 12–10, and 15–20.)

c. One end of the elastic material can be tied to a nylon strap and then attached to a fixed object and the other end held by the patient or looped around the leg or trunk.

d. Elastic resistance can be used with either open-chain or closed-chain exercises. This type of isotonic resistance device is one of the most versatile and widely used forms of resistance during closed-chain activities. (See Figs. 12–11 and 13–4.)

e. The primary disadvantage of elastic resistance is the progressively increasing force caused as the material stretches. The individual may not be able to complete the desired motion because muscles are usually weaker near the end of the range at the point when the resistance is greatest.

3. Pulley systems

Free-standing or wall-mounted pulley systems (with weights or springs) provide either fixed or variable resistance and can be used for upper and lower extremity and trunk strengthening (Fig. 3–23).

a. Permanent or interchangeable weights are available. Permanent weights are usually stacked in 5- to-10-lb increments and can be easily adjusted by changing the placement of a single weight key.

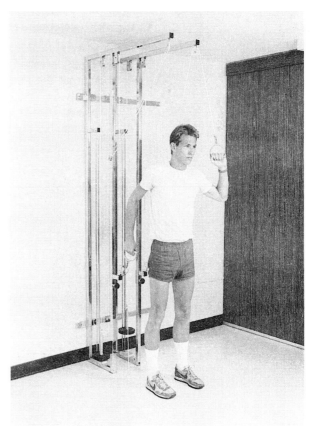

Figure 3–23. The Multi Exercise Pulley Unit can be used to strengthen a variety of muscle groups. (Courtesy of N-K Products Company, Inc., Soquel, CA.)

b. The patient can be set up in many positions, such as sitting in a wheelchair or lying prone on a cart. Many muscle groups may be strengthened by repositioning the patient.

c. Free-standing, multiple-station units, such as the Universal system, allow the patient to exercise multiple muscle groups by moving from one station to another, or they can be used by several patients at a time.

NOTE: When free weights, elastic resistance material, or pulley systems are used as a source of mechanical resistance, strengthening of a muscle often occurs both concentrically and eccentrically. For example, when a patient is holding a weight and strengthening the elbow flexors (Fig. 3–24), the muscle is contracting both concentrically and eccentrically against resistance as the patient lifts and lowers the weight. This needs to be considered when determining the number of repetitions carried out in the exercise program and when evaluating a patient's rate of fatigue and level of delayed muscle soreness.

4. Isotonic torque arm units

a. Exercise equipment such as the N-K Unit (Fig. 3–25) provides constant resistance through either a hydraulic force plate friction mechanism or an interchangeable weight-resistance system.

b. These units are primarily designed to provide resistance to the knee joint but can also be used to strengthen hip and shoulder musculature.[77]

(1) Resisted knee flexion and extension is carried out with the patient sitting or prone.

(2) Resisted hip flexion or extension is carried out with the patient lying or standing.

5. Variable-resistance equipment

a. Some weight-cable equipment systems such as the Eagle (Fig. 3–26) or Nautilus and Universal DVR systems are designed to provide variable resistance throughout the range of motion as a muscle contracts concentrically and eccentrically.

(1) A cam device in the weight-cable system varies the load applied to the contracting muscle, even though the weight selected is constant.

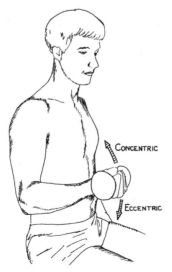

CONCENTRIC

ECCENTRIC

Figure 3–24. Concentric and eccentric strengthening of the elbow flexors occurs as the patient lifts and lowers the weight.

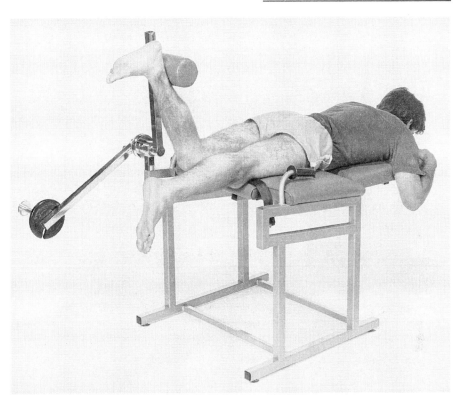

Figure 3–25. N-K Exercise Unit with torque arm and interchangeable weights. (Courtesy of N-K Products Company, Inc., Soquel, CA.)

    (2) In theory, the cam shaft is designed to replicate the torque curve of the muscle being exercised. How effectively this design provides accommodating resistance throughout the range of motion is debatable.

  b. Other variable-resistance units, such as the Hydra-Gym and Keiser Cam II system, use hydraulic or pressurized pneumatic resistance that varies the resistance applied to the muscle through the range of motion.

    (1) Unlike the cam-pulley weight machines that provide resistance to the same muscle group as it contracts concentrically and eccentrically, the hydraulic and pneumatic units provide concentric reciprocal muscle work.

    (2) Hydraulic or pneumatic units also can be used safely at higher velocities than variable-resistance weight-pulley machines.

  c. Many variable-resistance units are designed for exercise of specific muscle groups in the trunk or extremities. For example, a patient may do squats on one machine and leg curls on another machine to strengthen the lower extremities.

  d. The main advantage of variable-resistance equipment over the use of free weights is that the contracting muscle is loaded maximally at multiple points rather than at just one point in the range of motion.

  e. The main disadvantage of variable-resistance equipment is that a great amount of space is needed to set up multiple stations so that many muscle groups can be strengthened.

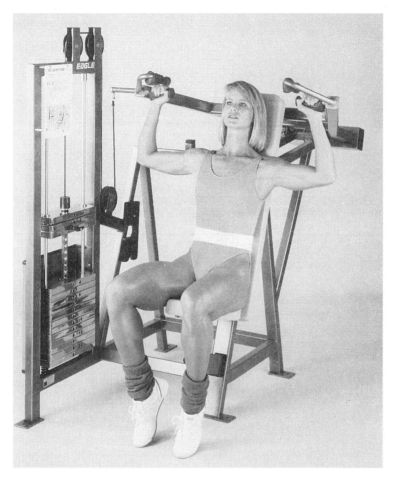

Figure 3–26. The Cybex/Eagle Fitness Systems shoulder press provides variable resistance throughout the range of motion. (Courtesy of Cybex, Division of Lumex, Ronkonkoma, NY.)

6. Exercise bicycle

The stationary exercise bicycle is used to increase lower extremity strength and endurance (Fig. 3–27). Some exercise cycles provide resistance to both the upper and lower extremities. Resistance can be graded with an adjustable friction device. Distance, speed, or duration of exercise can also be monitored.

The exercise bicycle provides resistance to muscles during repetitive, reciprocal movements of the extremities. Passive devices resist only concentric muscle activity as the patient performs either pushing or pulling movements. Motor-driven exercise cycles can be adjusted to provide eccentric as well as concentric resistance. Exercise cycles are particularly appropriate for low-intensity–high-repetition exercises designed to increase muscular or cardiovascular endurance.

7. Resistive reciprocal exercise units

a. A number of resistive exercisers are available and are used for repetitive reciprocal exercise (Fig. 3–28). They are most often used to improve lower extremity endurance, strength, or reciprocal coordination and a person's cardiopulmonary fitness. Many units can also be wall mounted and adapted for upper extremity exercise.

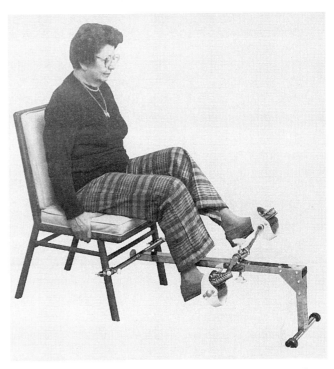

Figure 3–28. The Can-Do® Exerciser, a resistive reciprocal exerciser. (Courtesy of the Dipsters Corporation, Scarsdale, NY. Can-Do® is a trademark of the DIPSTERS Corporation.)

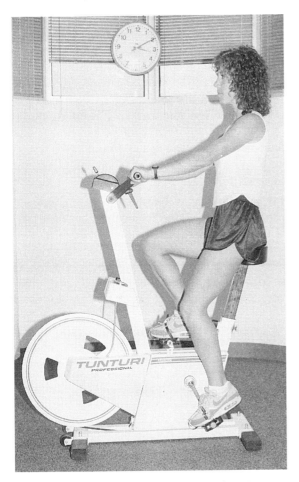

Figure 3–27. Exercise bicycles are used to increase muscular endurance and cardiopulmonary fitness.

    b. A resistance mechanism adjusts to provide light or heavy resistance.

    c. These units are attached to a sturdy straightback chair or wheelchair and are an alternative for patients who cannot safely use a stationary bicycle.

8. Closed-chain resistance devices

Although closed-chain exercises can be performed effectively using only body weight as resistance, several types of isotonic resistance devices from basic to complex and inexpensive to costly can be adapted or have been specifically developed for closed-chain exercises. Some examples include:

    a. Elastic resistance material

    b. Balance boards

        The balance board is used for proprioceptive training in the lower extremities. One example is the BAPS system (Biomechanical Ankle Platform System). (See Fig. 13–7.) Weights can be placed on the board to make the balance activity more challenging.

c. Stepping machines

The StairMaster is an example of a stepping machine that allows the patient to perform stepping movements against adjustable resistance to make the closed-chain activity more difficult.

d. Sliding boards (Fig. 3–29)

The ProFitter consists of a moving platform that slides side to side across an elliptical surface against adjustable resistance. Although it is most often used with the patient standing for lower extremity rehabilitation, it can also provide upper extremity closed-chain resisted movements and trunk stability.

9. Isotonic equipment—points to consider

a. Equipment such as free weights and standard weight-pulley systems that impose a fixed load on a contracting muscle maximally strengthen a muscle at only one point in the range of motion when a patient is in a particular position. The weight that is lifted or lowered through the range of motion can be no greater than what the muscle can control at the *weakest* point in the range. During isotonic exercise performed against constant resistance, a patient will be working maximally at only one small portion of the range of motion.

b. When using free weights, it is possible to vary the point in the range of motion at which the maximum-resistance load is experienced by changing the patient's position with respect to gravity or the direction of the resistance

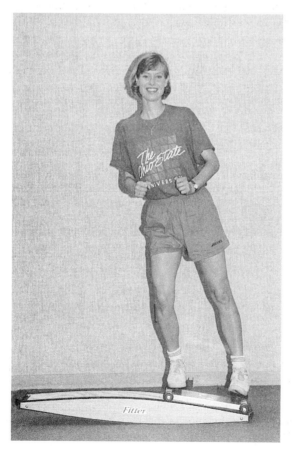

Figure 3–29. The ProFitter provides closed-chain resistance to lower extremity musculature in preparation for functional activities.

load. For example, shoulder flexion may be resisted with the patient standing or supine and holding a weight in the hand.

(1) Patient standing (Fig. 3–30)

Maximum resistance is experienced and maximum torque is produced when the shoulder is at 90 degrees of flexion. Zero torque is produced when the shoulder is at 0 degrees of flexion. Torque again decreases as the patient lifts the weight from 90 to 180 degrees of flexion.

(2) Patient supine (Fig. 3–31)

Maximum resistance is experienced and maximum torque is produced when the shoulder is at 0 degrees of flexion. Zero torque is produced at 90 degrees of shoulder flexion. The shoulder flexors are not active between 90 and 180 degrees of shoulder flexion. Instead, the shoulder extensors must contract eccentrically to control the descent of the arm and weight.

(3) Therefore, the therapist must determine at which portion of the patient's range of movement maximum strength is needed and must choose the optimum in which the exercise should be performed.

c. Standard weight-pulley systems provide maximum resistance when the angle of the pulley is at right angles to the moving bone.

d. With elastic resistance material, the muscle will receive the maximum resistive force when the material is angled 90 degrees to the moving bone. The therapist should determine the range of maximum resistance desired and anchor the elastic material so it is at right angles at that portion of the range. When the material is at an acute angle to the moving bone, there will be less resistance and more joint compressive force.

e. With constant and with most variable resistance equipment, exercises are done slowly to ensure patient safety and minimize momentum and acceleration. One exception is variable-resistance equipment that uses hydraulic or

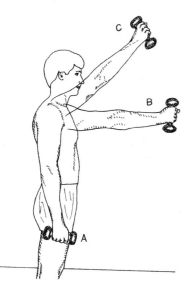

Figure 3–30. When the patient is standing and lifting a weight. (A) Zero torque is produced in the shoulder flexors when the shoulder is at 0 degrees flexion. (B) Maximum torque is produced when the shoulder is at 90 degrees flexion. (C) Torque again decreases as the arm moves from 90 to 180 degrees of shoulder flexion.

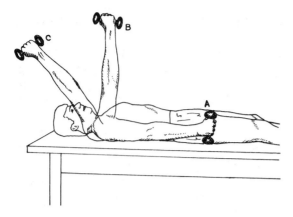

Figure 3–31. When the patient is supine and lifting a weight. (A) Maximum torque is produced at 0 degrees of shoulder flexion. (B) Zero torque is produced at 90 degrees shoulder flexion. (C) The shoulder extensors are active and contract eccentrically against resistance from 90 to 180 degrees shoulder flexion.

pneumatic pressure as a source of resistance. Faster training speeds can be used safely with this type of equipment.

f. Neither constant nor weight-cable isotonic variable resistance equipment can accommodate to a painful arc as a patient moves through the range of motion. Only hydraulic or pneumatic pressure variable-resistance equipment and isokinetic equipment have this capability.

C. Equipment Used with Isometric Exercise

Many pieces of equipment designed for dynamic strengthening exercises can also be modified for use in an isometric strengthening program.

1. When a patient attempts to lift a weight that provides resistance greater than the force the muscle can generate, an isometric contraction occurs.
2. Many of the free weights and weighted pulley systems can be adapted for isometric use.
3. Most isokinetic devices can be set up with the speed set at 0 degrees per second at a variety of joint angles for isometric resistance.
4. Many isometric exercises can be performed against resistance without any equipment. For example, a patient can strengthen the shoulder flexors, abductors, and rotators by pushing the arm against a wall (see Fig. 8–12A, B, and C).

D. Isokinetic Exercise Equipment

Several manufacturers offer isokinetic dynamometers or rate-limiting devices that control the velocity of motion and provide accommodating resistance during dynamic exercise to the extremities or trunk. The equipment provides resistance proportional to the force generated by the person using the machine. The preset rate (degrees per second) cannot be exceeded no matter how vigorously the person pushes against the force arm. Therefore, the muscle contracts to its maximum capacity at all points in the range of motion.

1. Isokinetic training and testing equipment

a. New product lines of isokinetic equipment and improvements in existing equipment are continually being developed. The best source of current information on equipment capabilities are brochures distributed by the manufacturer or product demonstrations at professional meetings.

   b. Some isokinetic exercise systems are designed for both testing and training extremity or trunk musculature. Some examples are the Cybex II+ (Fig. 3–32), the KIN/COM, the Brodex, the Lido, and the Merac. Some systems are designed exclusively for testing or training trunk musculature (Fig. 3–33). Each of these systems has its unique advantages and capabilities.

   c. Other isokinetic units such as the Orthotron II and the Upper Body Exerciser (UBE) (Fig. 3–34) are designed for training only.

   d. Concentric or eccentric resistance exercise can be performed on isokinetic equipment. Some equipment systems have only a concentric mode for exercise, whereas others have both concentric and eccentric modes.

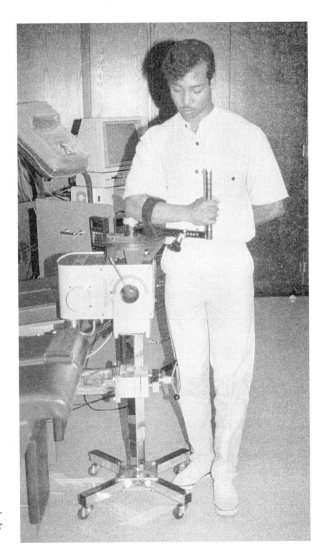

Figure 3–32. The Cybex II +. The isokinetic dynamometer is used for exercise or testing musculature of the extremities.

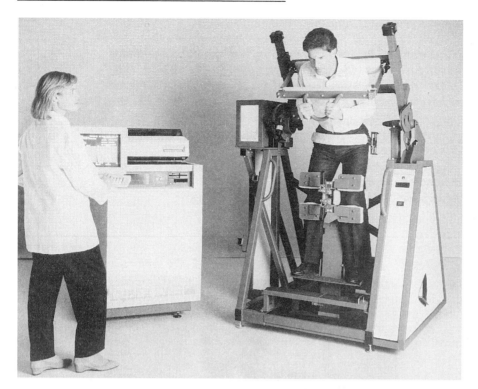

Figure 3–33. Cybex's Back-to-Work Clinic allows assessment and rehabilitation of the back. (Courtesy of Cybex, Division of Lumex, Ronkonkoma, NY.)

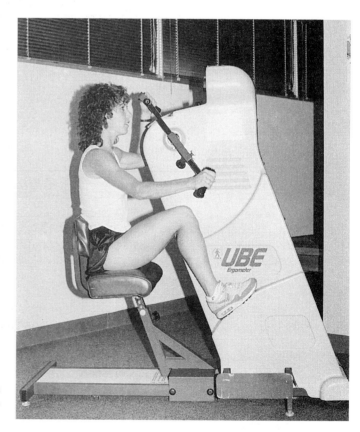

Figure 3–34. The Upper Body Exerciser (UBE) is used for upper extremity strength and endurance training.

e. The range of training and testing velocities available varies from 0 degrees per second to as high as 500 to 1000 degrees per second.

f. Full-arc or short-arc exercise can be performed by controlling the range of movement available with a computer or range-limiting device.

2. Isokinetic equipment—advantages and disadvantages

a. Advantages

(1) Isokinetic equipment can provide maximum resistance at all points in the range of motion as a muscle contracts.

(2) Both high-speed and low-speed training can be done safely and effectively.

(3) The equipment accommodates for a painful arc of motion.

(4) As a patient fatigues, exercise can still continue.

(5) Concentric and eccentric work in the same muscle group can be performed repetitively.

(6) Reciprocal exercise against resistance can be performed, allowing one muscle group to rest while its antagonist contracts. This minimizes muscle ischemia.

(7) Computer-based visual or auditory cues provide feedback to the patient so that submaximal to maximal muscle work can be performed more consistently.

b. Disadvantages

(1) The equipment is large and expensive.

(2) Set-up time and assistance from personnel are necessary if a patient is to exercise multiple muscle groups.

(3) The equipment cannot be used for a home exercise program.

(4) Most units provide only open-chain resistance.

X. Summary

This chapter on resistance exercise has included definitions of manual and mechanical resistance exercise, including isotonic, isometric, and isokinetic exercise. The goals and indications of resistance exercise have been outlined, and the concepts of strength, power, and endurance have been explained. Other factors that must be considered in resistance exercises, such as concentric and eccentric or open-chain and closed-chain muscle activity, have been discussed. Precautions to be considered during resistance exercises have also been summarized. They are fatigue, recovery from exercise, overwork, cardiovascular precautions, muscle soreness, substitute motions, and osteoporosis. Two contraindications—severe pain and acute inflammation—are listed. Principles of manual resistance exercise and techniques for properly applying resistance and stabilization manually during exercise have also been explained.

The use of mechanical resistance exercise has been described, and possible variables in programs have been outlined. These variables include the intensity and mode of exercise; the number of repetitions; bouts, frequency, duration, and speed of exercise; arc of limb motion; and patient position. Resistance training regimens and protocols have been described and compared. Finally, an overview of mechanical equipment and exercise apparatus has been discussed. Advantages and limitations of several pieces of equipment have been explained for use in isotonic, isometric, and isokinetic exercise programs.

References

1. Abraham, WM: Exercise-induced muscle soreness. The Physician and Sportsmedicine 7:57, 1979.
2. Abraham, WM: Factors in delayed muscle soreness. Med Sci Sports Exerc 9:11, 1977.
3. Albert, M: Eccentric Muscle Training in Sports and Orthopedics. Churchill-Livingstone, New York, 1991.
4. Armstrong, RB: Mechanisms of exercise-induced delayed onset muscular soreness: A brief review. Med Sci Sports Exerc 15:529–538, 1984.
5. Asmussen, E: Observations on experimental muscle soreness. Acta Rheumatol Scand 1:109, 1956.
6. Bandy, WD, Lovelace-Chandler, V, and McKitrick-Brandy, B: Adaptation of skeletal muscle to resistance training. Journal of Orthopaedic and Sports Physical Therapy 12:248–255, 1990.
7. Barnes, W: Relationship between motor unit activation to muscular contraction at different contractile velocities. Phys Ther 60:1152, 1980.
8. Bennett, JG, and Stauder, WT: Evaluation and treatment of anterior knee pain using eccentric exercise. Med Sci Sports Exerc 18:526, 1986.
9. Bishop, KN, et al: The effect of eccentric strength training at various speeds on concentric strength of the quadriceps and hamstring muscles. Journal of Orthopaedic and Sports Physical Therapy 13:226–229, 1991.
10. Bonen, A, and Belcastro, AN: Comparison of self-directed recovery methods on lactic acid removal rates. Med Sci Sports Exerc 8:176, 1976.
11. Ciccone, CD, and Alexander, A: Physiology and therapeutics of exercise. In Goodgold, J (ed): Rehabilitation Medicine. CV Mosby, St Louis, 1988.
12. Circulla, JA: Osteoporosis. Clin Man 9:15, 1989.
13. Clarkson, PM, and Tremblay, I: Exercise induced muscle damage, repair and adaptation in humans. J Appl Physiol 65:1–6, 1988.
14. Cress, NM, Peters, KS, and Chandler, JM: Eccentric and concentric force-velocity relationships of the quadriceps femoris muscle. Journal of Orthopaedic and Sports Physical Therapy 16:82–86, 1992.
15. Daniels, L, and Worthingham, C: Muscle Testing: Techniques of Manual Examination, ed 5. WB Saunders, Philadelphia, 1986.
16. Davies, GJ: A Compendium of Isokinetics in Clinical Usage and Rehabilitation Techniques, ed 2. S & S Publishing, La Crosse, WI, 1985.
17. Dean, E: Physiology and therapeutic implications of negative work: A review. Phys Ther 68:233, 1988.
18. Delorme, TL, and Watkins, A: Progressive Resistance Exercise. Appleton-Century, New York, 1951.
19. Delorme, T, and Watkins, A: Technics of progressive resistance exercise. Arch Phys Med Rehabil 29:263, 1948.
20. Denegar, CR, et al: Influence of transcutaneous electrical nerve stimulation on pain, range of motion and serum cortisol concentration in females experiencing delayed onset muscle soreness. Journal of Orthopaedic and Sports Physical Therapy 11:100–103, 1989.
21. DeVine, K: EMG activity recorded from an unexercised muscle during maximum isometric exercise of contralateral agonists and antagonists. Phys Ther 61:898, 1981.
22. DeVries, HA: Electromyographic observations on the effects static stretching has on muscular distress. Research Quarterly 32:468, 1961.
23. Devries, HA: Quantitative electromyographic investigation of the spasm theory of muscle pain. Am J Phys Med Rehabil 45:119, 1966.
24. Dorpat, TL, and Holmes, TH: Mechanisms of skeletal muscle pain and fatigue. Arch Neurol Psychol 74:628, 1955.
25. Douris, PC: Cardiovascular response to velocity-specific isokinetic exercises. Journal of Orthopaedic and Sports Physical Therapy 13:28–32, 1991.
26. Douris, PC: The effect of isokinetic exercise in the relationship between blood lactate and muscle fatigue. Journal of Orthopaedic and Sports Physical Therapy 17:31–35, 1993.
27. Duncan, PW, et al: Mode and speed specificity of eccentric and concentric exercise training. Journal of Orthopaedic and Sports Physical Therapy 11:70–75, 1989.
28. Evans, WJ: Exercise-induced skeletal muscle damage. The Physician and Sportsmedicine 15:89, 1987.
29. Fardy, P: Isometric exercise and the cardiovascular system. The Physician and Sportsmedicine 9:43, 1981.
30. Fitzgerald, GK, et al: Exercise induced muscle soreness after concentric and eccentric isokinetic contractions. Phys Ther 7:505–513, 1991.
31. Fleck, SJ, and Kraemer, WJ: Resistance training: Physiological response and adaptations (Part 2 of 4). The Physician and Sportsmedicine 16:108–124, 1988.
32. Fox, E, and Matthews, D: The Physiological Basis of Physical Education and Athletics, ed 3. Saunders College Publishing, Philadelphia, 1981.
33. Fox, EL, Robinson, S, and Wiegman, D: Metabolic energy sources during continuous and interval running. J Appl Physiol 27:174, 1969.
34. Francis, KT: Delayed muscle soreness: A review. Journal of Orthopaedic and Sports Physical Therapy 5:10, 1983.
35. Franklin, ME, et al: Effect of isokinetic soreness-inducing exercise on blood levels of creatine protein and creatine kinase. Journal of Orthopaedic and Sports Physical Therapy 16:208–214, 1992.
36. Friden, J, Sjostrom, M, and Ekblom B: A morphological study of delayed muscle soreness. Experimentia 37:506, 1981.
37. Friden, J, Sjostrom, M, and Ekblom, B: Myofibrillar damage following intense eccentric exercise in man. Int J Sports Med 4:170, 1983.
38. Gisolti, C, Robinson, S, and Turrell, ES: Effects of aerobic work performed during recovery from exhausting work. J Appl Physiol 21:1767, 1966.
39. Gollnick, P, et al: Glycogen depletion patterns in human skeletal muscle fibers during prolonged work. J Appl Physiol 34:615, 1973.
40. Gordon, EE, Kowalski, K, and Fritts, M: Protein changes in quadriceps muscle of rat with repetitive exercises. Arch Phys Med Rehabil 48:296, 1967.
41. Hasson, S, et al: Therapeutic effect of high speed voluntary muscle contractions on muscle soreness and muscle performance. Journal of Orthopaedic and Sports Physical Therapy 10:499, 1989.

42. Helgeson, K, and Gojdosik, RL: The stretch-shortening cycle of the quadriceps femoris muscle group measured by isokinetic dynamometry. Journal of Orthopaedic and Sports Physical Therapy 17:17–23, 1993.

43. Hellebrandt, FA, and Houtz, SJ: Methods of muscle training: The influence of pacing. Physical Therapy Review 38:319, 1958.

44. Hellebrandt, FA, and Houtz, SJ: Mechanisms of muscle training in man: Experimental demonstration of the overload principle. Physical Therapy Review 36:371, 1956.

45. Herbison, GJ, Jaweed, MM, Ditunno, JF, et al: Effect of overwork during reinnervation of rat muscle. Experimental Neurology 41:1, 1973.

46. Hettinger, T, and Muller, EA: Muskelliestung and Muskeltraining. Arbeitsphysiol 15:111, 1953.

47. Hill, DW, and Richardson, JD: Effectiveness of 10% trolamine salicylate cream on muscular soreness induced by a reproducible program of weight training. Journal of Orthopaedic and Sports Physical Therapy 11:19–23, 1989.

48. Hislop, HJ, and Perrine, J: The isokinetic concept of exercise. Phy Ther 41:114, 1967.

49. Hislop, HJ: Quantitative changes in human muscular strength during isometric exercise. Phys Ther 43:21, 1963.

50. Housh, D, and Housh T: The effects of unilateral velocity-specific concentric strength training. Journal of Orthopaedic and Sports Physical Therapy 17:252–256, 1993.

51. Jenkins, WL, Thackaberry, M, and Killan, C: Speed-specific isokinetic training. Journal of Orthopaedic and Sports Physical Therapy 6:181, 1984.

52. Jenson, K, and DiFabio, RP: Evaluation of eccentric exercise in the treatment of patellar tendonitis. Phys Ther 69:211, 1989.

53. Johnson, BL, et al: A comparison of concentric and eccentric muscle training. Med Sci Sports Exerc 8:35, 1976.

54. Johnson, BL: Eccentric vs. concentric muscle training for strength development. Med Sci Sports Exerc 4:111, 1972.

55. Jones, H: The Valsalva procedure: Its clinical importance to the physical therapist. Phys Ther 45:570, 1965.

56. Kelsey, DD, and Tyson E: A new method of training for the lower extremity using unloading. Journal of Orthopaedic and Sports Physical Therapy 19:218–223, 1994.

57. Kendall, FP, and McCreary, EK: Muscle Testing and Function, ed 3. Williams & Wilkins, Baltimore, 1983.

58. Knapik, JJ, Mawadsley, RH, and Ramos, MU: Angular specificity and test mode specificity of isometric and isokinetic strength training. Journal of Orthopaedic and Sports Physical Therapy 5:58, 1983.

59. Knight, KL: Knee rehabilitation by the daily adjustable progressive resistive exercise technique. Am J Sports Med 7:336, 1979.

60. Knight, KL: Quadriceps strengthening with DAPRE technique: Case studies with neurological implications. Med Sci Sports Exerc 17:636, 1985.

61. Knuttgren, HG: Human performance in high intensity exercise with concentric and eccentric muscle contractions. Int J Sports Med 7:6, 1986.

62. Knuttgren, HG: Neuromuscular Mechanisms for Therapeutic and Conditioning Exercise. University Park Press, Baltimore, 1976.

63. Lehmkuhl, LD, and Smith, LK: Brunnstrom's Clinical Kinesiology, ed 4. FA Davis, Philadelphia, 1983.

64. Liberson, WT: Brief isometric exercise. In Basmajian, JV (ed): Therapeutic Exercise, ed 3. Williams & Wilkins, Baltimore, 1978.

65. Lindh, M: Increase of muscle strength from isometric quadriceps exercise at different knee angles. Scandinavian Journal of Medicine 11:33, 1979.

66. Lunnen, J: Relationship between muscle length, muscle activity and torque of the hamstring muscles. Phys Ther 61:190, 1981.

67. MacKinnon, J: Osteoporosis: A review. Phys Ther 68:1533–1540, 1988.

68. Mangine, R, Heckman, TP, and Eldridge, VL: Improving strength, endurance and power. In Scully, RM, and Barnes, ML (eds): Physical Therapy, JB Lippincott, Philadelphia, 1989.

69. McArdle, WD, Katch, FI, and Katch, VL: Exercise Physiology: Energy, Nutrition and Human Performance. Lea & Febiger, Philadelphia, 1981.

70. Moffroid, M, et al: A study of isokinetic exercise. Phys Ther 49:735, 1969.

71. Moffroid, M, and Whipple, R: Specificity of the speed of exercise. Phys Ther 50:1693, 1970.

72. Moffroid, MT, and Kusick, ET: The power struggle: Definition and evaluation of power of muscular performance. Phys Ther 55:1098, 1975.

73. Mortain, T, and Devries, HA: Neural factors vs. hypertrophy in the time course of muscle strength gain. Am J Phys Med Rehabil 58:115, 1979.

74. Muller, EA: Influence of training and inactivity on muscle strength. Arch Phys Med Rehabil 51:449, 1970.

75. Newman, D: The consequences of eccentric contractions and their relationship to delayed onset muscle pain. Eur J Appl Physiol 57:353–359, 1988.

76. Newman, D, Jones, D, Clarkson, P: Repeated high force eccentric exercise effects on muscle pain and damage. J Appl Physiol 63:1381–1386, 1987.

77. Noland, R, and Kuckhoff, F: Adapted progressive resistance exercise device. Physical Therapy Review 34:333, 1954.

78. O'Sullivan, SB: Strategies to improve motor control and motor learning. In O'Sullivan, SB, and Schmitz, TJ (eds): Physical Rehabilitation: Assessment and Treatment, ed 3. FA Davis, Philadelphia, 1994.

79. Osternig, LR, et al: Influence of torque and limb speed on power production in isokinetic exercise. Am J Phys Med Rehabil 62:163–171, 1983.

80. Pardy W: Strength training. In Basmajian, JV, and Nyberg, R (eds): Rational Manual Therapies, Williams and Wilkins, Baltimore, 1993.

81. Parry, CBW: Vicarious motions (trick movements). In Basmajian, JV (ed): Therapeutic Exercise, ed 3. Williams & Wilkins, Baltimore, 1978.

82. Pavone, E, and Moffat, M: Isometric torque of the quadriceps femoris after concentric, eccentric and isometric exercise training. Arch Phys Med Rehabil 66:168–170, 1985.

83. Petersen, SR, et al: The effects of concentric resistance training and eccentric peak torque and muscle cross-sectional area. Journal of Orthopaedic and Sports Physical Therapy 13:132–137, 1991.

84. Prentice, WE: Rehabilitation Techniques in Sports Medicine. Times Mirror/Mosby, St Louis, 1990.

85. Richard, G, and Currier, D: Back stabilization during knee strengthening exercise. Phys Ther 57:1013, 1977.

86. Rose, DL: Effect of brief maximal exercise on the strength of quadriceps femoris. Arch Phys Med Rehabil 38:157, 1957.

87. Rose, SJ, and Rothstein, JM: Muscle mutability. Part 1. General concepts and adaptations to altered patterns of use. Phys Ther 62:1773–1787, 1982.

88. Rothstein, JM: Muscle biology: Clinical considerations. Phys Ther 62:1823, 1982.

89. Ryan, LM, Magidow, PA, and Duncan, PW: Velocity-specific and mode-specific effects of eccentric isokinetic training of the hamstrings. Journal of Orthopaedic and Sports Physical Therapy 13:33–39, 1991.

90. Sale, DG: Neural adaptation in strength and power training. In Jones, NL, McCartney, N, and McComass, AJ (eds): Human Muscle Power, Human Kinetics, Champaign, IL, 1986.

91. Saliba, VL, Johnson, GS, and Wardlaw, C: Proprioceptive neuromuscular facilitation. In Basmajian, JV, and Nyberg, R (eds): Rational Manual Therapies, Williams and Wilkins, Baltimore, 1993.

92. Sanders, M, and Sanders, B: Mobility: Active-resistive training. In Gould, J, and Davies, G (eds): Orthopedic and Sports Physical Therapy. CV Mosby, St Louis, 1985.

93. Sanders MT: Weight training and conditioning. In Sanders, B (ed): Sports Physical Therapy. Appleton & Lange, Norwalk, CT, 1990.

94. Sapega, AA, and Drillings, G: The definition and assessment of muscular power. Journal of Orthopaedic and Sports Physical Therapy 5:7, 1983.

95. Sherman, WH, et al: Isokinetic strength during rehabilitation following arthrotomy. Athletic Train 16:138, 1981.

96. Sinacore, DR, Bander, BL, and Delitto, A: Recovery from a 1-minute bout of fatiguing exercise: Characteristics, reliability and responsiveness. Phys Ther 74:234–241, 1994.

97. Smith, MJ, and Melton, P: Isokinetic vs. isotonic variable-resistance training. Am J Sports Med 9:275, 1981.

98. Steindler, A: Kinesiology of the Human Body under Normal and Pathological Conditions. Charles C. Thomas, Springfield, IL, 1964.

99. Stephens, JA, and Taylor: Fatigue of maintained voluntary muscle contraction in man. J Physiol (Lond) 220:1, 1972.

100. Sulivan, PE, Markos, PD, and Minor, MAD: An Integrated Approach to Therapeutic Exercise, Reston, Reston, VA, 1982.

101. Talag, TS: Residual muscular soreness as influenced by concentric eccentric and static contractions. Research Quarterly 44:458, 1973.

102. Thomeé, R, et al: Slow or fast isokinetic training after knee ligament surgery. Journal of Orthopaedic and Sports Physical Therapy 8:475, 1988.

103. Timm, KE: Investigation of the physiological overflow effect from speed-specific isokinetic activity. Journal of Orthopaedic and Sports Physical Therapy 9:106, 1987.

104. Tippett, SR: Closed chain exercise. Orthopedic Physical Therapy Clinics of North America 1: 253–267, 1992.

105. Tomberlin, JP, et al: Comparative study of isokinetic eccentric and concentric quadriceps training. Journal of Orthopaedic and Sports Physical Therapy 14: 31–36, 1991.

106. Torg, JS, Welsh, RP, and Shephard, RJ: Current Therapy in Sports Medicine, Vol. 2. B.C. Decker, Toronto, 1990.

107. Vallbona, C: Bodily responses to immobilization. In Kottke, FJ, Stillwell, GK, and Lehmann, JF (eds): Krusen's Handbook of Physical Medicine and Rehabilitation. WB Saunders, Philadelphia, 1982.

108. Vogel, JA: Introduction to the symposium: Physiological responses and adaptations to resistance exercise. Med Sci Sports Exerc (Suppl)20:131–134, 1988.

109. Voight, ML: Stretch strengthening: An introduction to plyometrics. Orthopedic Physical Therapy Clinics of North America, 1:243–252, 1992.

110. Voight, ML, and Draovitch, P: Plyometrics. In Albert, M (ed): Eccentric Muscle Training in Sports and Orthopedics, Churchill-Livingstone, New York, 1991.

111. Voss, DE, Ionta, MK, and Myers, BJ: Proprioceptive Neuromuscular Facility, ed 3. Harper & Row, New York, 1985.

112. Waltrous, B, Armstrong, R, and Schwane, J: The role of lactic acid in delayed onset muscular soreness. Med Sci Sports Exerc 1:380, 1981.

113. Weber, MD, Servedio, F, and Woodall, WR: The effect of three modalities on delayed onset muscle soreness. Journal of Orthopaedic and Sports Physical Therapy 20:236–242, 1994.

114. Wilk, KE, et al: Stretch-shortening drills for the upper extremities: Theory and clinical application. Journal of Orthopaedic and Sports Physical Therapy 17:225–239, 1993.

115. Wilke, DV: The relationship between force and velocity in human muscle. J Physiol 110:249, 1950.

116. Williams, M, and Stutzman, L: Strength variations through the range of joint motion. Physical Therapy Review 39:145, 1959.

117. Zinowieff, AN: Heavy resistance exercise: The Oxford technique. British Journal of Physical Medicine 14:129, 1951.

Principles of
Aerobic Exercise

CAROLYN N. BURNETT, MS, PT • TERRI M. GLENN, PhD, PT

There are numerous sources from which to obtain information on training for endurance in athletes and healthy young people and in individuals with coronary heart disease. But there is little information or emphasis on endurance training and the improvement of fitness in the individual who has other types of chronic disease or disability. This chapter uses information from well-known sources to demonstrate that the physical therapist can use aerobics when working with either healthy individuals or patients with a variety of problems. In addition, some fundamental information about cardiovascular and respiratory parameters in children and the elderly, as well as the young or middle-aged adult, is presented so the physical therapist can be prepared to treat individuals of all ages.

OBJECTIVES

After studying this chapter, the reader will be able to:

1 Define fitness, endurance, conditioning, adaptation, cardiac output, $\dot{V}o_2$ max, a$-\bar{v}O_2$ difference, training stimulus threshold, metabolic equivalent (MET), telemetry, and efficiency.
2 Describe the determination of fitness and/or endurance levels in humans.
3 Discuss the factors influencing the transport of oxygen.
4 Identify the changes that occur with deconditioning and the implications of these changes.
5 Compare the characteristics of the three energy systems.
6 Describe the determination of energy expenditure.
7 Differentiate high-level and low-level activity in terms of energy cost.
8 Differentiate between stress testing and fitness testing.
9 Identify the end points used to determine if $\dot{V}o_2$ max is achieved.
10 List the signs and symptoms that determine cessation of the stress test or the exercise session.
11 Identify the appropriate guidelines for determining the intensity, duration, and frequency of an exercise program.

12 Calculate the maximum heart rate for an individual of a certain age and determine the safest way to calculate the target heart rate for individuals of differing physical capacities, using the maximum heart rate or the heart rate reserve.

13 Discuss the overload principle in endurance training or conditioning.

14 Differentiate between high-level and low-level exercise programs (characteristics, activities, and energy expenditure).

15 Identify some special considerations that should be taken into account when setting up an exercise program.

16 List the cardiovascular and biochemical changes that occur with endurance training and the mechanisms for their occurrence.

17 Compare cardiovascular and respiratory parameters and $\dot{V}o_2$ max in the child, young adult, and aged.

I. Key Terms

A. Fitness

Fitness is a general term used to describe the ability to perform physical work.[1,2] Performing physical work requires cardiorespiratory functioning, muscular strength and endurance, and musculoskeletal flexibility (Fig. 4–1). Optimum body composition is also included when describing fitness.

1. To become physically fit, individuals must participate regularly in some form of physical activity that uses large muscle groups and challenges the cardiorespiratory system. Individuals of all ages can improve their fitness status by participating in activities that include walking, biking, running, and/or training with weights.

2. Fitness levels can be described on a continuum from poor to superior based on energy expenditure during a bout of physical work.[3,11] These ratings are often based on the direct or indirect measurement of the body's maximal oxygen consumption ($\dot{V}o_2$ max).

The US Dept. of Health and Human Services has identified health promotion and disease prevention objectives for Americans for the next century.[26] In the publication *Healthy People 2000*, the following objectives address both cardio-respiratory and musculoskeletal fitness:

Increase to at least 20 percent the proportion of people aged 18 and older and to at least 75 percent the proportion of children and adolescents aged 6 through 17 who engage in vigorous physical activity that promotes the development and maintenance of cardiorespiratory fitness 3 or more days per week for 20 or more minutes per occasion.

Increase to at least 40 percent the proportion of people aged 6 and older who regularly perform physical activities that enhance and maintain muscular strength, muscular endurance and flexibility.

Figure 4–1. Fitness goals for the nation.

a. Oxygen consumption is influenced by age, gender, heredity, inactivity, and disease.

b. Several methods are available to estimate maximal oxygen consumption.

   (1) Cycle ergometer tests include the YMCA Cycle Ergometer Test[15] and the Astrand-Rhyming Test.[4]

   (2) When testing large numbers of subjects, the 3-Min Step Test is often used.[15]

   (3) Distance runs are used when testing active individuals. These include the 1.5-Mile Run[6] and the 12-Min Run.[16]

   (4) Inactive or older individuals can be evaluated using the 1-Mile Walk[16] and the Rockport Fitness Walking Test.[19]

B. Maximal Oxygen Consumption

Maximal oxygen consumption ($\dot{V}o_2$ max) is a measure of the body's capacity to use oxygen.[2,12,21-24] It is usually measured when performing an exercise bout that uses many large muscle groups such as swimming, walking, and running. It is the maximum amount of oxygen consumed per minute when the individual has reached maximal effort. It is usually expressed relative to body weight, as milliliters of oxygen per kilogram of body weight per minute (mL/kg per minute). It is dependent on the transport of oxygen, the oxygen-binding capacity of the blood, cardiac function, oxygen extraction capabilities, and muscular oxidative potential. The $\dot{V}o_2$ can be defined mathematically using the Fick equation.

$$\dot{V}o_2 = \text{cardiac output} \times \text{arteriovenous } O_2 \text{ difference}$$
$$= \dot{Q} \times a - \bar{v}O_2$$
$$\text{Cardiac output } (\dot{Q}) = \text{heart rate} \times \text{stroke volume}$$
$$\text{Arteriovenous } O_2 \text{ difference } (a - \bar{v}O_2) = \text{arterial oxygen} - \text{venous oxygen}$$

C. Endurance

Endurance (a measure of fitness) is the ability to work for prolonged periods of time and the ability to resist fatigue.[21,27,28] It includes muscular endurance and cardiovascular endurance. Muscular endurance refers to the ability of an isolated muscle group to perform repeated contractions over a period of time, whereas cardiovascular endurance refers to the ability to perform large muscle dynamic exercise, such as walking, swimming, and/or biking, for long periods of time.

D. Aerobic Exercise Training (Conditioning)

Aerobic exercise training (conditioning) is an augmentation of the energy capacity of the muscle by means of an exercise program.[21,22,28]

1. Training is dependent on exercise of sufficient intensity, duration, and frequency.

2. Training produces a cardiovascular and/or muscular adaptation and is reflected in an individual's endurance.

3. Training for a particular sport or event is dependent on the *specificity principle*.[27,28] That is, the individual improves in the exercise task used for training and may not improve in other tasks. For example, swimming may enhance one's

performance in swimming events but may not improve one's performance in treadmill running.

E. Adaptation

The cardiovascular system and the muscles used will *adapt* to the training stimulus over time.[21,28] Significant changes can be measured in a minimum of 10 to 12 weeks.

1. **Adaptation** results in increased efficiency of the cardiovascular system and the active muscles. Adaptation represents a variety of neurologic, physical, and biochemical changes within the cardiovascular and muscular systems. Performance increases as a result of these changes.
2. Adaptation is dependent on:
   a. The ability of the organism to change. The person with a low level of fitness will have more potential to improve than the one who has a high level of fitness.
   b. The training stimulus threshold (the stimulus that elicits a training response).
      (1) Training stimulus thresholds are variable.
      (2) The higher the initial level of fitness, the greater the intensity of exercise needed to elicit a significant change.

F. Myocardial Oxygen Consumption

Myocardial oxygen consumption ($m\dot{V}o_2$) is a measure of the oxygen consumed by the myocardial muscle.[12,17,24,28]

1. The need or demand for oxygen is determined by heart rate, systemic blood pressure, myocardial contractility, and afterload. Afterload is determined by the left ventricular wall tension and central aortic pressure. It is the ventricular force required to open the aortic valve at the beginning of systole. Left ventricular wall tension is primarily determined by ventricular size and wall thickness.
2. The ability to supply the myocardium with oxygen is dependent on the arterial oxygen content (blood substrate), hemoglobin oxygen dissociation, and coronary blood flow, which is determined by aortic diastolic pressure, duration of diastole, coronary artery resistance, and collateral circulation.
3. In a healthy individual, a balance between myocardial oxygen supply and demand is maintained during maximal exercise. When the demand for oxygen is greater than the supply, myocardial ischemia results.
4. Since the myocardial muscle extracts 70 to 75 percent of the oxygen from the blood during rest, its main source of supply during exercise is through an increase in coronary blood flow.

G. Deconditioning

Deconditioning occurs with prolonged bed rest, and its effects are frequently seen in the patient who has had an extended illness. Decreases in maximal oxygen consumption, cardiac output (stroke volume), and muscular strength occur very rapidly. These effects are also seen, although possibly to a lesser degree, in the individual who has spent a period of time on bed rest without any accompanying disease process and in the individual who is sedentary because of lifestyle and increasing age (Fig. 4–2).

```
↓ muscle mass
↓ strength
↓ cardiovascular function
↓ total blood volume
↓ plasma volume
↓ heart volume
↓ orthostatic tolerance
↓ exercise tolerance
↓ bone mineral density
```

Figure 4–2. Deconditioning effects associated with bed rest. (Data from American College of Sports Medicine: Resource Manual for Guidelines for Exercise Testing and Prescription, ed 2. Lea & Febiger, Philadelphia, 1993.)

II. Energy Systems, Energy Expenditure, and Efficiency

A. Energy Systems

Energy systems are metabolic systems involving a series of biochemical reactions resulting in the formation of adenosine triphosphate (ATP), carbon dioxide, and water.[21-23] The cell uses the energy produced from the conversion of ATP to adenosine diphosphate (ADP) and phosphate (P) to perform metabolic activities. Muscle cells use this energy for actin-myosin cross-bridge formation when contracting. There are three major energy systems. The intensity and duration of activity determine when and to what extent each metabolic system contributes.

1. The Phosphagen or ATP-PC system

The ATP-PC system (adenosine triphosphate-phosphocreatine) has the following characteristics:
a. Phosphocreatine and ATP are stored in the muscle cell.
b. Phosphocreatine is the chemical fuel source.
c. No oxygen is required.
d. When muscle is rested, the supply of ATP-PC is replenished.
e. The maximal capacity of the system is small (0.7 mol ATP).
f. The maximal power of the system is great (3.7 mol ATP/min).
g. The system provides energy for short, quick bursts of activity.
h. It is the major source of energy during the first 30 seconds of intense exercise.

2. The anaerobic glycolytic system

The anaerobic glycolytic system has the following characteristics:
a. Glycogen (glucose) is the fuel source.
b. No oxygen is required.
c. ATP is resynthesized in the muscle cell.
d. Lactic acid is produced.
e. The maximal capacity of the system is intermediate (1.2 mol ATP).

f. The maximal power of the system is intermediate (1.6 mol ATP/min).

g. The systems provide energy for activity of moderate intensity and short duration.

h. It is the major source of energy from the 30th to 90th second of exercise.

3. The aerobic system

The aerobic system has the following characteristics:

a. Glycogen, fats, and proteins are fuel sources.

b. Oxygen is required.

c. ATP is resynthesized in the mitochondria of the muscle cell. The ability to metabolize oxygen and other substrates is related to the number and concentration of the mitochondria and cells.

d. The maximal capacity of the system is great (90.0 mol ATP).

e. The maximal power of the system is small (1.0 mol ATP/min).

f. The system predominates over the other energy systems after the second minute of exercise.

4. Recruitment of motor units

Recruitment of motor units is dependent on rate of work. Fibers are recruited selectively during exercise.[21,28]

a. Slow-twitch fibers (type I) are characterized by a slow contractile response, are rich in myoglobin and mitochondria, have a high oxidative capacity and a low anaerobic capacity, and are recruited for activities demanding endurance. These fibers are supplied by small neurons with a low threshold of activation and are used preferentially in low-intensity exercise.

b. Fast-twitch fibers (type IIb) are characterized by a fast contractile response, have a low myoglobin content and few mitochondria, have a high glycolytic capacity, and are recruited for activities requiring power.

c. Fast-twitch fibers (type IIa) have characteristics of both type I and type IIb fibers and are recruited for both anaerobic and aerobic activities.

B. Functional Implications[5]

1. Bursts of intense activity (seconds) develop muscle strength and stronger tendons and ligaments. ATP is supplied by the phosphagen system.

2. Intense activity (1 to 2 minutes) repeated after 4 minutes of rest or mild exercise provides anaerobic power. ATP is supplied by the phosphagen and anaerobic glycolytic system.

3. Activity with large muscles, which is less than maximal intensity for 3 to 5 minutes repeated after rest or mild exercise of similar duration, may develop aerobic power and endurance capabilities. ATP is supplied by the phosphagen, anaerobic glycolytic, and aerobic systems.

4. Activity that is of submaximal intensity lasting 30 minutes or more taxes a high percentage of the aerobic system and develops endurance.

C. Energy Expenditure

Energy is expended by individuals engaging in physical activity. Activities can be categorized as light or heavy by determining the energy cost. Most daily activities are light activity and are aerobic because they require little power but occur over prolonged periods.[21,22] Heavy work usually requires energy supplied by both the aerobic and anaerobic systems.

1. Energy expenditure can be determined easily by open-circuit spirometry or telemetry.
   a. *Open-circuit portable spirometry* requires that the individual breathe into and out of a mouthpiece with a valve.[21]
      (1) The expired air passes directly through a gas analyzer that measures volume and analyzes the oxygen and carbon dioxide composition of the expired sample. This occurs automatically on a breath-by-breath basis.
      (2) The energy expenditure is computed from the amount of oxygen consumed.
   b. *Telemetry*, or physiologic radio transmission, allows the individual to move freely. The heart rate of the individual is transmitted to a graphic printout system, producing an electrocardiographic strip.
      (1) Heart rate is linearly related to the work performed.
      (2) Heart rate is therefore linearly related to the amount of oxygen consumed per minute.
2. Energy expended is computed from the amount of oxygen consumed.
   Units used to quantify energy expenditure are kilocalories and METs (Fig. 4–3).
   a. A *kilocalorie* is a measure expressing the energy value of food. It is the amount of heat necessary to raise 1 kilogram (kg) of water 1°C. A kilocalorie (kcal) can be expressed in oxygen equivalents. Five kilocalories equal approximately one liter of oxygen consumed (5 kcal = 1 liter O_2).
   b. A *MET* is defined as the oxygen consumed (milliliters) per kilogram of body weight per minute (mL/kg). It is equal to approximately 3.5 mL/kg per minute.[2]
   c. Activities are classified as light or heavy according to energy expended or oxygen consumed while accomplishing them.[20]
      (1) Light work for the average male (65 kg) requires 2.0 to 4.9 kcal/min, or 6.1 to 15.2 mL O_2/kg per minute, or 1.6 to 3.9 METs. Strolling 1.6 km/h, or 1.0 mph, is considered light work.
      (2) Heavy work for the average male (65 kg) requires 7.5 to 9.9 kcal/min, or 23.0 to 30.6 mL O_2/kg per minute, or 6.0 to 7.9 METs. Jogging 8.0 km/h, or 5.0 mph, is considered heavy work.
      (3) Jogging 8.0 km/h, or 5.0 mph, requires 25 to 28 mL O_2/kg per minute and is considered heavy work. The energy expended is equivalent to 8 to 10 kcal/min, or 7 to 8 METs.
3. The energy expenditure necessary for most industrial jobs requires less than three times the energy expenditure at rest.[21]
4. Energy expenditure of certain physical activities can vary, depending on factors such as skill, pace, and fitness level.[21]

The average individual engaged in normal daily tasks expends 1800 to 3000 kcal per day. Athletes engaged in intense training can use more than 10,000 kcal per day.

Figure 4–3. Daily energy expenditure. (Data from Wilmore, JH, and Costill, DL: Physiology of Sport and Exercise. Human Kinetics, Champaign, IL, 1994.)

D. Efficiency

Efficiency is usually expressed as a percentage[21]:

$$Percent\ efficiency = \frac{useful\ work\ output}{energy\ expended\ or\ work\ input} \times 100$$

1. Work output equals force times distance ($W = F \times D$). It can be expressed in power units or work per unit of time ($P = w/t$).
   a. On a treadmill, work equals the weight of the subject times the vertical distance the subject is raised walking up the incline of the treadmill.
   b. On an ergometer bicycle, work equals the distance (which is the circumference of the flywheel times the number of revolutions) times the bicycle resistance.
2. Work input equals energy expenditure and is expressed as the net oxygen consumption per unit of time.
   a. With aerobic exercise, the resting volume of oxygen used per unit of time ($\dot{V}o_2$ value) is subtracted from the oxygen consumed during 1 minute of the steady state period.
      (1) Steady state is reached within 3 to 4 minutes after exercise has started.
      (2) In the steady state period, $\dot{V}o_2$ remains at a constant (steady) value.
   b. Total net oxygen cost is multiplied by the total time in minutes that the exercise is performed.
3. The higher the net oxygen cost, the lower the efficiency in performing the activity.
4. Efficiency of large muscle activities is usually 20 to 25 percent.

III. Physiologic Response to Aerobic Exercise

The rapid increase in energy requirements during exercise requires equally rapid circulatory adjustments to meet the increased need for oxygen and nutrients to remove the end products of metabolism such as carbon dioxide and lactic acid and to dissipate excess heat. The shift in body metabolism occurs through a coordinated activity of all the systems of body; neuromuscular, respiratory, cardiovascular, metabolic, and hormonal (Fig. 4–4). Oxygen transport and its utilization by the mitochondria of the contracting muscle are dependent on adequate blood flow in conjunction with cellular respiration.[21-25]

Ambient temperature, humidity, and altitude can affect the physiologic responses to acute exercise. Diurnal fluctuations as well as changes associated with a female's menstrual cycle can affect these responses as well. Therefore, researchers control these factors as much as possible when evaluating the response to exercise.

Figure 4–4. Factors affecting the response to acute exercise.

A. Cardiovascular Response to Exercise[12,17,24,25]

1. The exercise pressor response.
   Stimulation of small myelinated and unmyelinated fibers in skeletal muscle involves a sympathetic nervous system (SNS) response. The central pathways are not known.
   a. The SNS response includes a generalized peripheral vasoconstriction and increased myocardial contractility, an increased heart rate, and hypertension. This results in a marked increase and redistribution of the cardiac output.
   b. The degree of the response equals the muscle mass involved and the intensity of the exercise.
2. Cardiac effects.
   a. Frequency of sinoatrial node depolarization increases and heart rate increases; there is a decrease in vagal stimuli as well as an increase in SNS stimulation.
   b. There is an increase in the force development of the myofibers; a direct inotropic response of the SNS increases myocardial contractility.
3. Peripheral effects.
   a. Generalized vasoconstriction occurs that allows blood to be shunted from the nonworking muscles, kidneys, liver, spleen, and splanchnic area to the working muscles.
   b. A locally mediated reduction in resistance in the working muscle arterial vascular bed, independent of the autonomic nervous system, is produced by metabolites such as Mg^{2+}, Ca^{2+}, ADP, and P_{CO_2}.[21]
   c. The veins of the working as well as the nonworking muscles remain constricted.
   d. A *net* reduction in total peripheral resistance results.
4. The cardiac output increases because of the
   a. Increase in myocardial contractility
   b. Increase in heart rate
   c. Increase in the blood flow through the working muscle
   d. Increase in the constriction of the capacitance vessels on the venous side of the circulation in both the working and nonworking muscles, raising the peripheral venous pressure
   e. Net reduction in the total peripheral resistance
5. The increase in the systolic blood pressure is the result of the augmented cardiac output.

B. Respiratory Response to Exercise[21-23]

1. Respiratory changes occur rapidly with an increased gas exchange by the first or second breath. During exercise there is a decrease in venous O_2 saturation, an increase in P_{CO_2} and H^+, an increase in body temperature, increased epinephrine, and an increased stimulation of receptors of the joints and muscles; any of these factors, alone or in combination, may stimulate the respiratory system. Baroreceptor reflexes, protective reflexes, pain, emotion, and voluntary control of respiration may also contribute to the increase in respiration.
2. Minute ventilation increases as respiratory frequency and tidal volume increase.
3. Alveolar ventilation, occurring with the diffusion of gases across the capillary-alveolar membrane, increases 10-fold to 20-fold in heavy exercise to supply the additional oxygen needed and excrete the excess carbon dioxide produced.

C. Responses Providing Additional Oxygen to Muscle

1. The increased blood flow to the working muscle previously discussed provides additional oxygen.
2. There is also extraction of more oxygen from each liter of blood. There are several changes that allow for this.
   a. A decrease of the local tissue P_{O_2} occurs because of the use of more oxygen by the working muscle. As the partial pressure of oxygen decreases, the unloading of oxygen from hemoglobin is facilitated.
   b. The production of more carbon dioxide causes the tissue to become acidotic (the hydrogen ion concentration increases) and the temperature of the tissue to increase. Both situations increase the amount of oxygen released from hemoglobin at any given partial pressure.
   c. The increase of red blood cell 2,3-diphosphoglycerate (DPG) produced by glycolysis during exercise also contributes to the enhanced release of oxygen.
3. Factors determining how much of the oxygen is consumed are:
   a. Vascularity of the muscles
   b. Fiber distribution
   c. Number of mitochondria
   d. Oxidative mitochondrial enzymes present in the fibers
      The oxidative capacity of the muscle is reflected in the $a-\bar{v}O_2$ difference, which is the difference between the oxygen content of arterial and venous blood.

IV. Testing as a Basis for Exercise Programs

Testing for physical fitness of healthy individuals should be distinct from graded exercise testing of convalescing patients, individuals with symptoms of coronary heart disease, or individuals who are age 35 years or older but asymptomatic.[1,2] Regardless of the type of testing, the level of performance is based on the submaximal or maximal oxygen uptake ($\dot{V}O_2$ max) or the symptom-limited oxygen uptake. The capacity of the individual to transport and utilize oxygen is reflected in the oxygen uptake. Readers are referred to the American College of Sports Medicine: *Guidelines for Exercise Testing and Prescription*, ed 4 (Lea & Febiger, Philadelphia, 1991), and the American College of Sports Medicine: *Resource Manual for Guidelines for Exercise Testing and Prescription*, ed 2 (Lea & Febiger, Philadelphia, 1993), for additional information.

A. Fitness Testing of Healthy Subjects

1. Field tests for the determination of cardiovascular fitness include time to run 1.5 miles or distance run in 12 minutes. These correlate well with $\dot{V}O_2$ max, but their use is limited to young persons or middle-aged individuals who have been carefully screened and have been jogging or running for some time.[2]
2. Multistage testing can provide a direct measurement of $\dot{V}O_2$ max.[1,2] Testing is usually completed in four to six treadmill stages, which progressively increase in speed and/or grade. Each stage is 3 to 6 minutes long. Electrocardiographic (ECG) monitoring is performed during the testing. Maximal oxygen uptake can be determined when the oxygen utilization plateaus despite an increase in workload.

B. Stress Testing for Convalescing Individuals and Individuals at Risk

Individuals undergoing stress testing should have a physical examination, be monitored by the ECG, and be closely observed at rest, during exercise, and during recovery (Fig. 4–5).

1. The *principles of stress testing* include[1,2,12,21,24]:
   a. Changing the workload by increasing the speed and/or grade of the treadmill or the resistance on the bicycle ergometer
   b. An initial workload that is low in terms of the individual's anticipated aerobic threshold
   c. Maintenance of each workload for 2 to 6 minutes
   d. Termination of the test at the onset of symptoms or a definable abnormality of the ECG
   e. When available, measurement of the individual's maximal oxygen consumption

2. In addition to serving as a basis for determining exercise levels or the exercise prescription, the stress test[2]:
   a. Helps establish a diagnosis of overt or latent heart disease.
   b. Evaluates cardiovascular functional capacity as a means of clearing individuals for strenuous work or exercise programs.

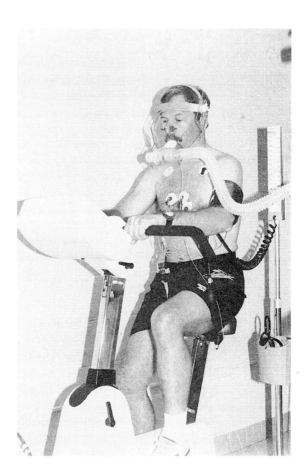

Figure 4–5. Placement of electrodes for the 12-lead exercise electrocardiogram used to determine heart rate and rhythm during the stress test.

  c. Determines the physical work capacity in kilogram-meters per minute (kg-m/min) or the functional capacity in METs.
  d. Evaluates responses to exercise training and/or preventive programs.
  e. Assists in the selection and evaluation of appropriate modes of treatment for heart disease.
  f. Increases individual motivation for entering and adhering to exercise programs.
  g. Is used clinically to evaluate patients with chest sensations or a history of chest pain to establish the probability that such patients have coronary disease. It can also evaluate the functional capacity of patients with chronic disease.

3. All individuals who are taking a stress test should:
  a. Have had a physical examination
  b. Be monitored by the ECG and closely observed at rest, during exercise, and during recovery
  c. Sign a consent form

4. *Precautions* to be taken are applicable for both stress testing and the exercise program.[2]
  a. Monitor the pulse to assess abnormal increases in heart rate.
  b. Blood pressure increases with exercise approximately 7 to 10 millimeters (mm) of mercury (Hg) per MET of physical activity.
    (1) Systolic pressure should not exceed 220 to 240 mm Hg.
    (2) Diastolic pressure should not exceed 120 mm Hg.
  c. Rate and depth of respiration increase with exercise.
    (1) Respiration should not be labored.
    (2) The individual should have no perception of shortness of breath.
  d. The increase in blood flow while exercising, which regulates core temperature and meets the demands of the working muscles, results in changes in the skin of the cheeks, nose, and earlobes. They become pink, moist, and warm to the touch.

5. End points requiring termination of the test period are[2]:
  a. Progressive angina.
  b. A significant drop in systolic pressure in response to an increasing workload.
  c. Lightheadedness, confusion, pallor, cyanosis, nausea, or peripheral circulatory insufficiency.
  d. Abnormal ECG responses including ST segment depression greater than 4 mm.
  e. Excessive rise in blood pressure.
  f. Subject wishes to stop.

C. Multistage Testing

Each of four to six stages is approximately 3 to 6 minutes. Differences in protocols involve the number of stages, magnitude of exercise (intensity), equipment used (bicycle, treadmill), duration of stages, end-points, position of body, muscle groups exercised, and types of effort (Fig. 4–6).

Protocols have been developed for multistage testing. The most popular treadmill protocol is the Bruce protocol.[9] Treadmill speed and grade are changed every 3 minutes. Speed increases from 1.7 mph up to 5.0 mph, whereas the initial grade of 10 percent increases up to 18 percent during the five stages.

Mr. Smith is a 55-yr-old sedentary male with a history of chest pain with exertion. He has undergone a stress test to assist in evaluating his angina. He is not taking any medications at the present time. He has been a smoker for 20 yr.

Resting Electrocardiogram (ECG): normal
Resting Heart Rate: 75 beats/min
Age-Predicted Maximal Heart Rate: 165 beats/min
Resting Blood Pressure: 128/86
Resting Respiration Rate: 20 breaths/min
Treadmill: Bruce protocol

Stage	Heart Rate	Blood Pressure	Comments
1	80		
	84		
	85	138/88	No complaints
2	88		
	90		
	88	142/90	No complaints
3	98		
	100		
	102	156/91	Complaining of leg fatigue
4	114		
	116		
	122	161/90	Complaining of minimal chest pain
5	133		
	135		
	137	174/89	Complaining of severe chest pain; test terminated

Conclusion: The stress test was terminated because of complaints of severe chest pain accompanied by a drop in the ST segment of the ECG to 4 mm. The symptom-limited maximal heart rate was determined to be 137 beats/min. Maximal oxygen consumption was determined to be 32 mL/kg/min.

Figure 4–6. Case example of an exercise stress test.

V. Determinants of an Exercise Program

Just as testing for fitness should be distinct from stress testing for patients or individuals at high risk, training programs for healthy individuals are distinct from the exercise prescription for individuals with cardiopulmonary disease.

Effective endurance training for any population must produce a conditioning or cardiovascular response. Elicitation of the cardiovascular response is dependent on three critical elements of exercise: *intensity, duration,* and *frequency.*[21,22,24,28]

A. Intensity[2,21,24]

Determination of the appropriate intensity of exercise to use is based on the overload principle and the specificity principle.

1. The *overload principle*

   Overload is a stress on an organism that is greater than the one regularly encountered during everyday life. To improve cardiovascular and muscular endurance, an overload must be applied to these systems. The exercise load (overload) must be above the training stimulus threshold (that stimulus that elicits a training or conditioning response) for adaptation to occur.

2. Once adaptation to a given load has taken place, for the individual to achieve further improvement, the training intensity (exercise load) must be increased.

3. Training stimulus thresholds are variable, depending on the individual's level of health, level of activity, age, and gender.

4. The higher the initial level of fitness, the greater the intensity of exercise needed to elicit a change.

5. A conditioning response occurs generally at 70 to 85 percent maximum heart rate (60 to 80 percent $\dot{V}o_2$ max).[2,8,12]

   a. Seventy percent maximum heart rate is a minimal level stimulus for eliciting a conditioning response in healthy young individuals.

   b. Eighty-five to 95 percent maximum heart rate is usually necessary to achieve a conditioning response for an athlete.

   c. The exercise does not have to be exhaustive to achieve a training response.

6. Determining maximum heart rate and exercise heart rate for training programs provides the basis for the initial intensity of the exercise.[1,2,21,28]

   a. When the individual is young and healthy, the *maximum heart rate* can be determined directly from a maximum performance multistage test, extrapolated from a heart rate achieved on a predetermined submaximal test, or less accurately calculated as 220 minus age.

   b. The *exercise heart race* is determined:

      (1) As a percentage of the maximum heart rate. The percentage used is dependent on the level of fitness of the individual.

      (2) Using the heart rate reserve (Karvonen's formula).[2]

         (a) It is based on the heart rate reserve (HRR), which is the difference between the resting heart rate (HR rest) and the maximal heart rate (HR max).

         (b) The exercise heart rate is determined as a percentage (usually 60 to 70 percent) of the heart rate reserve plus the resting heart rate:

   $$\textit{Exercise heart rate} = HR_{rest} + 60\%\text{--}70\% \, (HR_{max} - HR_{rest})$$

         (c) Utilizing Karnoven's formula, the exercise heart rate is higher than when using maximum heart rate alone.

7. Maximum heart rate and exercise heart rate used for the exercise prescription for individuals at risk for coronary artery disease, individuals with coronary artery disease or other chronic disease, and individuals who are elderly are ideally determined from performance on the stress test.[2,5,27]

   a. Maximum heart rate cannot be determined in the same manner as with the young and healthy.

      (1) Assuming that an individual has an average maximum heart rate, using the formula 220 minus age will produce substantial errors in prescribing exercise intensity for these individuals.[20]

(2) Maximum heart rate, which may be symptom limited, is considered maximum. At no time should the exercise heart rate exceed the symptom-limited heart rate achieved on the exercise test.

(3) Individuals with cardiopulmonary disease may start exercise programs, depending on their diagnosis, as low as 40 to 60 percent of their maximal heart rate.[8,17]

8. Exercising at a high intensity for a shorter period of time appears to elicit a greater improvement in $\dot{V}o_2$ max than exercising at a moderate intensity for a longer period of time. However, as exercise approaches the maximum limit, there is an increase in the relative risk of cardiovascular complications and the risk of musculoskeletal injury.

9. The higher the intensity and the longer the exercise intervals, the faster the training effect.[12]

10. Maximum oxygen consumption ($\dot{V}o_2$ max) is the best measure of intensity. Aerobic capacity and heart rate are linearly related and, therefore, maximum heart rate is a function of intensity.

11. The *specificity principle* as related to the specificity of training refers to adaptations in metabolic and physiologic systems depending on the demand imposed. There is no overlap when training for strength-power activities and training for endurance activities.[5,24,28] Workload and work-rest periods are selected so that training results in:
   a. Muscle strength without a significant increase in total oxygen consumption
   b. Aerobic or endurance training without training the anaerobic systems
   c. Anaerobic training without training the aerobic systems

12. Even when evaluating aerobic or endurance activities, there appears to be little overlap. When training for swimming events, the individual may not demonstrate an improvement in $\dot{V}o_2$ max when running.[21]

B. Duration[1,2,21,27]

1. The optimal duration of exercise for cardiovascular conditioning is dependent on the total work done, exercise intensity and frequency, and fitness level.

2. Generally speaking, the greater the intensity of the exercise, the shorter the duration needed for adaptation. The lower the intensity of exercise, the longer the duration needed.

3. A 20- to 30-minute session is generally optimal at 70 percent maximum heart rate. When the intensity is below the heart rate threshold, a 45-minute continuous exercise period may provide the appropriate overload. With high-intensity exercise, 10- to 15-minute exercise periods are adequate. Three 5-minute daily periods may be effective in some deconditioned patients.

4. Exercise of longer than 45 minutes duration increases the risk of musculoskeletal complications.

C. Frequency[21,22,27]

1. Like duration, there is no clear-cut information provided on the most effective frequency of exercise for adaptation to occur. Frequency may be a less important factor in exercise training than is intensity or duration.

2. Frequency varies, dependent on the health and age of the individual. Optimal frequency of training is generally three to four times a week. If training is at a low intensity, greater frequency may be beneficial. A frequency of two times a

week does not generally evoke cardiovascular changes, although older individuals and convalescing patients may benefit from a program of that frequency.[27]

3. As frequency increases beyond the optimal range, the risk of musculoskeletal complications increases.

4. For individuals who are in good general health, exercising 30 to 45 minutes at least three times a week (2000 kcal/week) appears to protect against coronary heart disease.

D. Mode[2,21-23]

1. Many types of activities provide the stimulus for improving cardiorespiratory fitness. The important factor is that exercise involve large muscle groups that are activated in a rhythmic, aerobic nature. However, the magnitude of the changes may be determined by the mode used.

2. For specific aerobic activities such as cycling and running, the overload must use the muscles required by the activity as well as stress the cardiorespiratory system (specificity principle). If endurance of the upper extremities is needed to perform activities on the job, then the upper extremity muscles must be targeted in the exercise program. The muscles trained develop a greater oxidative capacity with an increase in blood flow to the area. The increase in blood flow is due to increased microcirculation and more effective distribution of the cardiac output.

3. Training benefits are optimized when programs are planned to meet the individual needs and capacities of the participants. The skill of the individual, variations among individuals in competitiveness and aggressiveness, and variation in environmental conditions all must be considered.

E. The Reversibility Principle[21,24]

The beneficial effects of exercise training are transient and reversible.

1. Detraining occurs rapidly when a person stops exercising. After only 2 weeks of detraining, significant reductions in work capacity can be measured, and improvements can be lost within several months. In addition, a similar phenomenon occurs with individuals who are confined to bed with illness or disability. The individual becomes severely deconditioned, with loss of the ability to carry out normal daily activities as a result of inactivity.

2. The frequency or duration of physical activity required to maintain a certain level of aerobic fitness is less than that required to improve it.

VI. The Exercise Program

A carefully planned exercise program can result in higher levels of fitness for the healthy individual, slow the decrease in functional capacity of the elderly, and recondition those who have been ill or have chronic disease. There are three components of the exercise program: (1) a warm-up period, (2) the aerobic exercise period, and (3) a cool-down period.

A. The Warm-Up Period

Physiologically, a time lag exists between the onset of activity and the bodily adjustments needed to meet the physical requirements of the body.[1,2,13,21,27]

1. The purpose of the warm-up period is to enhance the numerous adjustments that must take place before physical activity. During this period there are:

a. An increase in muscle temperature; the higher temperature increases the efficiency of muscular contraction by reducing muscle viscosity and increasing the rate of nerve conduction.

b. An increased need for oxygen to meet the energy demands for the muscle. Extraction from hemoglobin is greater at higher muscle temperatures, facilitating the oxidative processes at work.

c. Dilatation of the previously constricted capillaries with increases in the circulation, augmenting oxygen delivery to the active muscles and minimizing the oxygen deficit and the formation of lactic acid.

d. Adaptation in sensitivity of the neural respiratory center to various exercise stimulants.

e. An increase in venous return; this occurs as blood flow is shifted centrally from the periphery.

2. The warm-up also prevents or decreases:

a. The susceptibility of the musculoskeletal system to injury by increasing flexibility

b. The occurrence of ischemic ECG changes and arrhythmias

3. The warm-up should be gradual and sufficient to increase muscle and core temperature without causing fatigue or reducing energy stores. Characteristics of the period include:

a. A 10-minute period of total body movement exercises such as calisthenics, static stretching, and running slowly.

b. The attainment of a heart rate within 20 beats per minute of the target heart tissue.

B. The Aerobic Exercise Period

The aerobic exercise period is the conditioning part of the exercise program. Attention to the determinants of intensity, frequency, duration, and mode of the program, as previously discussed, will have an impact on the effectiveness of the program. The main consideration when choosing a specific method of training is that the *intensity* be great enough to stimulate an increase in stroke volume and cardiac output and to enhance local circulation and aerobic metabolism within the appropriate muscle groups. The exercise period must be within the person's tolerance, above the threshold level for adaptation to occur, and below the level of exercise that evokes clinical symptoms.[2,3,5,18,21,27]

In aerobic exercise, submaximal, rhythmic, repetitive, dynamic exercise of large muscle groups is emphasized.

There are four methods of training that will challenge the aerobic system: continuous, interval (work relief), circuit, and circuit interval.

1. Continuous training[5,13,21]

a. A submaximal energy requirement, sustained throughout the training period, is imposed.

b. Once the steady state is achieved, the muscle obtains energy by means of aerobic metabolism. Stress is placed primarily on the slow-twitch fibers.

c. The activity can be prolonged for 20 to 60 minutes without exhausting the oxygen transport system.

d. Work rate is increased progressively as training improvements are achieved; overload can be accomplished by increasing the exercise duration.

e. In the healthy individual, continuous training is the most effective way to improve endurance.

2. Interval training[5,21,27]

In this type of training, the work or exercise is followed by a properly prescribed relief or rest interval. Interval training is perceived to be less demanding than continuous training. In the healthy individual, interval training tends to improve strength and power more than endurance.

a. The relief interval is either a rest relief (passive recovery) or a work relief (active recovery), and its duration ranges from a few seconds to several minutes. Work recovery involves continuing the exercise but at a reduced level from the work period. During the relief period, a portion of the muscular stores of ATP and the oxygen associated with myoglobin that were depleted during the work period are replenished by the aerobic system. An increase in $\dot{V}o_2$ max occurs.

b. The longer the work interval, the more the aerobic system is stressed. With a short work interval, the duration of the rest interval is critical if the aerobic system is to be stressed (a work-recovery ratio of 1:1 to 1:5 is appropriate). A rest interval equal to one and a half times the work interval allows the succeeding exercise interval to begin before recovery is complete and stresses the aerobic system. With a longer work interval, the duration of the rest is not as important.[21]

c. A significant amount of high-intensity work can be achieved with interval or intermittent work if there is appropriate spacing of the work-relief intervals. The total amount of work that can be completed with intermittent work is greater than the amount of work that can be completed with continuous training.

3. Circuit training[10,21]

Circuit training employs a series of exercise activities. At the end of the last activity, the individual starts from the beginning and again moves through the series. The series of activities is repeated several times.

a. Several exercise modes can be used involving large and small muscle groups and a mix of static or dynamic effort.

b. Use of circuit training can improve strength and endurance by stressing both the aerobic and anaerobic systems.

4. Circuit-interval training[21,22]

a. Combining circuit and interval training is effective because of the interaction of aerobic and anaerobic production of ATP.

b. In addition to the aerobic and anaerobic systems being stressed by the various activities, with the relief interval there is a delay in the need for glycolysis and the production of lactic acid prior to the availability of oxygen supplying the ATP.

C. The Cool-Down Period[3,27]

A cool-down period is necessary following the exercise period.
1. The purpose of the cool-down period is:
   a. To prevent pooling of the blood in the extremities by continuing to use the muscles to maintain venous return

b. To prevent fainting by increasing the return of blood to the heart and brain as cardiac output and venous return decreases

c. To enhance the recovery period with the oxidation of metabolic waste and replacement of the energy stores

d. To prevent myocardial ischemia, arrhythmias, or other cardiovascular complications

2. Characteristics of the cool-down period are similar to those of the warm-up period.

a. Total-body exercises such as calisthenics are appropriate.

b. The period should last 5 to 8 minutes.

VII. Physiologic Changes That Occur With Training

Changes in the cardiovascular and respiratory systems as well as changes in muscle metabolism occur following endurance training. These changes are reflected both at rest and with exercise. It is important to note that all of the following training effects cannot result from one training program.[21]

A. Cardiovascular Changes

1. **Changes at rest**[5,21-23]

a. A reduction in the resting pulse rate in some individuals because of:

(1) A decrease in sympathetic drive, with decreasing levels of norepinephrine and epinephrine

(2) A decrease in atrial rate secondary to biochemical changes in the muscles and levels of acetylcholine, norepinephrine, and epinephrine in the atria

(3) An increase in parasympathetic (vagal) tone secondary to decreased sympathetic tone

b. A decrease in blood pressure in some individuals

(1) This occurs with a decrease in peripheral vascular resistance.

(2) The largest decrease is in systolic blood pressure.

(3) This is most apparent in hypertensive individuals.

c. An increase in blood volume and hemoglobin, which facilitates the oxygen delivery capacity of the system

2. **Changes with exercise**

a. A reduction in the pulse rate because of the mechanisms listed in Section A.1.a

b. An increased stroke volume because of:

(1) An increase in myocardial contractility

(2) An increase in ventricular volume

c. An increased cardiac output

(1) The increased cardiac output is a result of the increased stroke volume.

(2) The increased cardiac output occurs with maximal exercise but not with submaximal exercise.

(3) The magnitude of the change is directly related to the increase in stroke volume and the magnitude of the reduced heart rate.

d. An increased extraction of oxygen by the working muscle because of enzymatic and biochemical changes in the muscle

e. An increased maximum oxygen uptake ($\dot{V}o_2$ max)

(1) Greater $\dot{V}O_2$ max results in a greater work capacity.

(2) The increased cardiac output increases the delivery of oxygen to the working muscles.

(3) The increased ability of the muscle to extract oxygen from the blood increases the utilization of the available oxygen.

f. A decreased blood flow per kilogram of the working muscle

(1) This occurs even though increasing amounts of blood are shunted to the exercising muscle.

(2) The increase in extraction of oxygen from the blood compensates for this change.

g. A decreased myocardial oxygen consumption (pulse rate times systolic blood pressure) for any given intensity of exercise

(1) This results from a decreased pulse rate, with or without a modest decrease in blood pressure.

(2) The product can be decreased significantly in the healthy subject without any loss of efficiency at a specific workload.

B. Respiratory Changes

These changes are observed at rest and with exercise after endurance training.[21-23]

1. Changes at rest

a. Larger lung volumes because of improved pulmonary function, with no change in tidal volume

b. Larger diffusion capacities because of:

(1) Larger lung volumes

(2) Greater alveolar-capillary surface area

2. Changes with exercise

a. Larger diffusion capacities for the same reasons as those listed in Section 1.b. Maximal capacity of ventilation is unchanged.

b. A lower amount of air ventilated at the same oxygen consumption. Maximum diffusion capacity is unchanged.

c. An increased maximal minute ventilation.

d. An increased ventilatory efficiency.

C. Metabolic Changes

These changes are observed at rest and with exercise following endurance training.

1. Changes at rest

a. Muscle hypertrophy and increased capillary density

b. An increased number and size of mitochondria increasing the capacity to generate ATP aerobically

c. Increases in muscle myoglobin concentration

(1) Myoglobin increases the rate of oxygen transport.

(2) Myoglobin possibly increases the rate of oxygen diffusion to the mitochondria.

2. Changes with exercise

a. A decreased rate of depletion of muscle glycogen at submaximal work levels

(1) This is due to:

(a) An increased capacity to mobilize and oxidize fat

(b) Increased fat mobilizing and metabolizing enzymes

(2) Another term for this phenomenon is glycogen sparing.

b. Lower blood lactate levels at submaximal work

(1) The mechanism is unclear.

(2) It does not appear to be related to a decrease in hypoxia of the muscles.

c. Less reliance on phosphocreatine (PC) and ATP in skeletal muscle

d. An increased capability to oxidize carbohydrate because of:

(1) An increased oxidative potential of the mitochondria

(2) An increased glycogen storage in the muscle

NOTE: Ill health may influence metabolic adaptations to exercise.

D. Other System Changes

Changes in other systems that occur with training include:

1. A decrease in body fat
2. A decrease in blood cholesterol and triglyceride levels
3. An increase in heat acclimatization
4. An increase in the breaking strength of bones, ligaments, and tendons

VIII. Application of Principles of an Aerobic Conditioning Program for the Patient With Coronary Disease

The use of the principles of aerobic conditioning in physical therapy has been most dominant in program planning for the individual following a myocardial infarction (MI) or following coronary artery bypass surgery.[1,2,8,17]

In the past 10 to 15 years, there have been major changes in the medical management of these patients. These changes have included shortened hospital stays, a more aggressive progression of activity for the patient following MI or cardiac surgery, and earlier initiation of an exercise program based on a low-level stress test prior to discharge from the hospital. An aerobic conditioning program, in addition to risk factor modification, is a dominant part of cardiac rehabilitation.

A. In-Patient Phase (Phase I)[1,2,8,17]

This phase of the program occurs in the hospital following stabilization of the patient's cardiovascular status after MI or coronary bypass surgery. Because the length of hospital care has decreased over the past few years, this time may be limited to 3 to 5 days. When hospital stays were longer, this phase often lasted 7 to 14 days and was referred to as phase 1 of the cardiac rehabilitation program.

1. The purpose of the early portion of cardiac rehabilitation is to:

a. Initiate risk factor education and address future modification of certain behaviors, such as eating habits and smoking.

b. Initiate self-care activities and progress from sitting to standing to minimize deconditioning (1 to 3 days postevent).

c. Provide an orthostatic challenge to the cardiovascular system (3 to 5 days postevent). This is usually accomplished by supervised ambulation. Ambulation is usually monitored electrocardiographically, as well as manually monitoring the heart rate, ventilation rate, and blood pressure.

d. Prepare patients and family for continued rehabilitation and for life at home after a cardiac event.

B. Out-Patient Phase (Phase II)[1,2,8,17]

This program is initiated either upon discharge from the hospital or, depending on the severity of the diagnosis, 6 to 8 weeks later. This delay will allow time for the myocardium to heal as well as time to monitor the patient's response to a new medical regimen. Participants are monitored via telemetry to determine heart rate and rhythm responses, blood pressure is recorded at rest and during exercise, and ventilation responses are noted. These programs usually last 8 to 12 weeks (Fig. 4–7).

1. The purpose of the program is to:
   a. Increase the person's exercise capacity in a safe and progressive manner so that adaptive cardiovascular and muscular changes occur. The early part of the program is referred to by some as "low-level" exercise training.
   b. Enhance cardiac functions and reduce the cardiac cost of work. This may help eliminate or delay symptoms such as angina and ST-segment changes in the patient with coronary heart disease.
   c. Produce favorable metabolic changes.
   d. Determine the effect of medications on increasing levels of activity.
   e. Relieve anxiety and depression.
   f. Progress the patient to an independent exercise program.
2. A symptom-limited test is performed 6 to 12 weeks after hospital discharge or as early as 2 to 4 weeks following discharge.
3. The exercise program is predominantly aerobic. Generally, for patients with functional capacities greater than 5 METs, the exercise prescription is based on the results of the symptom-limited exercise stress test.
   a. The initial level of activity or training intensity may be as low as 40 to 60 percent of the maximal heart rate or 40 to 70 percent of the functional capacity defined in METs. The starting intensity is dictated by the severity of the diagnosis in concert with the individual's age and prior fitness level. The intensity is progressed as the individual responds to the training program.

Mr. Smith is referred and undergoes further evaluation to determine the cause of his chest pain. He is diagnosed with single vessel coronary artery disease. He is referred to cardiac rehabilitation.

Medications: Nitroglycerin as needed to relieve angina.

Mr. Smith will attend cardiac rehabilitation 3 times/weekly for 8 to 12 weeks to improve his fitness level and attend smoking cessation classes. He will meet with a medical dietitian to discuss meal planning to lower his intake of fat and cholesterol.

Exercise Prescription: Mr. Smith will exercise at an intensity lower than his anginal threshold. This intensity will be initially established at 60 to 65 percent of his maximal heart rate or 50 percent of his $\dot{V}o_2$ max. He will exercise 3 times weekly for 20 to 40 minutes, depending on his tolerance.

Figure 4–7. Case example of a cardiac rehabilitation referral.

b. The duration of the exercise session may be limited to 10 to 15 minutes to start, progressing to 30 to 60 minutes as the patient's status improves. Each session usually includes 8- to 10-minute warm-up and cool-down periods.

c. Participants often attend sessions offered three times weekly.

d. The mode of exercise is usually continuous, using large muscle groups, such as stationary biking or walking. These activities allow for electrocardiographic monitoring via telemetry.

e. Circuit-interval exercise is a common method used with the patient in phase II. The patient can exercise on each modality at a defined workload, compared with exercising continuously on a bicycle or treadmill. As a result, the patient can:

(1) Perform more physical work.

(2) Exercise at a higher intensity. Fitness may improve in a shorter period of time.

(3) Maintain lactic acid and the oxygen deficit at minimum levels.

(4) Exercise at a lower rate of perceived exertion.

f. Low-level weight training may be initiated during the outpatient program, provided the individual has undergone a symptom-limited stress test. Resistive exercises should not produce ischemic symptoms associated with an increase in heart rate and systolic blood pressure. Therefore, heart rate and blood pressure should be monitored periodically throughout the exercise session. Starting weight may be calculated using 40 percent of a 1-RM effort.

g. Progression of the workload occurs when there have been three consecutive sessions (every-other-day sessions) during which the peak heart rate is below the target heart rate.

C. Out-Patient Program (Phase III)[1,2,8,17]

This phase of cardiac rehabilitation includes a supervised exercise conditioning program, which is often continued in a hospital or community setting. Heart rate and rhythm are no longer monitored via telemetry. Participants are reminded to monitor their own pulse rate, whereas a supervisory person is available to monitor blood pressure.

1. The purpose of the program is to continue to improve or maintain fitness levels achieved during the phase II program.

2. *Recreational activities* to maintain levels gained in phase II can include:

a. Swimming, which incorporates both arms and legs. However, there is a decreased awareness of ischemic symptoms while swimming, especially when skill level is poor.

b. Outdoor hiking, which is excellent if on level terrain.

3. Activities at 8 METs include:

a. Jogging approximately 5 miles per hour

b. Cycling approximately 12 miles per hour

c. Vigorous down-hill skiing

D. Special Considerations

There are special considerations related to types of exercise and patient needs that must be recognized when developing conditioning programs for patients with coronary disease.[1,2,5,27]

1. Arm exercises elicit different responses than leg exercises.
   a. Mechanical efficiency based on the ratio between output of external work and caloric expenditure is lower than with leg exercises.
   b. Oxygen uptake at a given external workload is significantly higher for arm exercises than for leg exercises.
   c. Myocardial efficiency is lower with leg exercises than with arm exercises.
   d. Myocardial oxygen consumption (heart rate times systolic blood pressure) is higher with arm exercises than with leg exercises.
2. Coronary patients complete 35 percent less work with arm exercises than with leg exercises before symptoms occur.

E. Adaptive Changes

Adaptive changes following training of individuals with cardiac disease include[17,24,27]:

1. An increased myocardial aerobic work capacity.
2. An increased maximum aerobic or functional capacity by predominantly widening the arteriovenous oxygen $(a-\bar{v}O_2)$ difference.
3. An increased stroke volume following high-intensity training 6 to 12 months into the training program.
4. A decreased myocardial demand for oxygen.
5. An increased myocardial supply by the decreased heart rate and prolongation of diastole.
6. An increased tolerance to a given physical workload before angina occurs.
7. A heart rate significantly lower at each submaximal workload and therefore a greater heart rate reserve. When muscles are used that are not directly involved in the activity, the reduction in heart rate will not be as great.
8. An improved psychologic orientation and, over time, an impact on depression scores, scores for hysteria, hypochondriasis, and psychoasthenia on the Minnesota Multiphasic Personality Inventory.

NOTE: Cardiovascular complications will be prevented and/or reduced if the program includes appropriate selection of patients, continuous evaluation of each patient, medical supervision of the exercise throughout the training period, regular communication with the physician, specific instructions to patients about adverse symptoms, class size limitations to 30 patients or fewer, and the maintenance of accurate records related to compliance to the program.[27]

IX. General Clinical Applications of Aerobic Training

A. Chronic Illness and Deconditioning

Deconditioned individuals, including those with chronic illness and the elderly, may have major limitations in pulmonary and cardiovascular reserve that severely curtail their daily activities.[24]

1. Implications of the changes due to deconditioning brought on by inactivity, resulting from any illness or chronic disease, are important to remember.[1,27]
   a. There is a decreased work capacity, which is a result of:
      (1) A decreased maximum oxygen uptake and decreased ability to use oxygen and perform work.
      (2) A decreased cardiac output. Cardiac output is the major limiting factor.

b. There is a decreased circulating blood volume that can be as much as 700 to 800 mL. For some individuals, this results in tachycardia along with orthostatic hypotension, dizziness, and episodes of syncope when initially attempting to stand.

c. There is a decrease in plasma and red blood cells, which increases the likelihood of life-threatening embothrombolic episodes and the prolongation of the convalescent period.

d. There is a decrease in lean body mass, which results in:
   (1) Decreased muscle size.
   (2) Decreased muscle strength and ability to perform activities requiring large muscle groups. For example, the individual may have difficulty walking with crutches or climbing stairs.

e. There is an increased excretion of urinary calcium, which results
   (1) From a decrease in the weight-bearing stimulus critical in maintaining bone integrity
   (2) In bone loss or osteoporosis
   (3) In an increased likelihood of fractures upon falling due to the osteoporosis

2. Through an exercise program, the negative cardiovascular, neuromuscular, and metabolic functions can be reversed. This results in[1,27]:

a. A decrease in resting heart rate, heart rate with any given exercise load, and urinary excretion of calcium

b. An increase in stroke volume at rest, stroke volume with exercise, cardiac output with exercise, total heart volume, lung volume (ventilatory volume), vital capacity, maximal oxygen uptake, circulating blood volume, plasma volume and red blood cells, and lean body mass

c. A reversal of the negative nitrogen and protein balance

d. An increase in levels of mitochondrial enzymes and energy stores

e. Less use of the anaerobic systems during activity

B. Disability, Functional Limitations, and Deconditioning

Individuals who have a physical disability or functional limitation should not be excluded from a conditioning program that will increase their fitness level. This includes individuals in wheelchairs or persons who have problems ambulating, such as those with paraplegia, hemiplegia, or amputation, and those with an orthopedic problem, such as arthrodesis.[7]

1. Adaptations must be made in testing the physically disabled using a wheelchair treadmill or more frequently using the upper extremity ergometer.

2. Exercise protocols may emphasize upper extremities and manipulation of the wheelchair.

3. It is important to remember that energy expenditure is increased when the gait is altered, and wheelchair use is less efficient than walking without impairment.

C. Problems, Goals, and Plan of Care

The goals of an aerobic exercise program are dependent on the initial level of fitness of the individual and on his or her specific clinical needs. The general goals are to decrease the deconditioning effects of disease and chronic illness and to improve the individual's cardiovascular and muscular fitness.

1. **Selected clinical problems**

   a. Increased susceptibility to thromboembolic episodes, pneumonia, atelectasis, and the likelihood of fractures

   b. Tachycardia, dizziness, and orthostatic hypotension when moving from sitting to standing

   c. A decrease in general muscle strength, with difficulty and shortness of breath in climbing stairs

   d. A decrease in work capacity that limits distances walked and activities tolerated

   e. Increased heart rate and blood pressure responses (rate-pressure product) to various activities

   f. A decrease in the maximum rate-pressure product tolerated with angina or other ischemic symptoms appearing at low levels of exercise

2. **Measurable short-term goals**

   a. Prevention of thromboembolic episodes, pneumonia, atelectasis, and fractures

   b. A decrease in the magnitude of the orthostatic hypotensive response

   c. Ability to climb stairs safely and without shortness of breath

   d. Tolerance for walking longer measured distances and completing activities without fatigue or symptoms

   e. A decrease in the heart rate and blood pressure (rate-pressure product) at a given level of activity

   f. An increase in the maximum rate-pressure product tolerated without ischemic symptoms

3. **Measurable long-term goals**

   a. An improved pulmonary, cardiovascular, and metabolic response to various levels of exercise

   b. An improved ability to complete selected activities with appropriate heart rate and blood responses to exercise

4. **Plan of care (convalescent)**

   a. Determine the exercise heart rate response that can be safely reached, based on the number of beats over the resting heart rate.

   b. Initiate a program of activities for the patient that will not elicit a cardiovascular response over the exercise heart rate (e.g., calisthenics, walking).

   c. Provide patients with clearly written instructions about any activity they perform on their own.

   d. Initiate an educational program that provides the patient with information about effort symptoms and exercise precautions, monitoring of heart rate, and modification, when indicated, of risk factors.

5. **Plan of care (with emphasis on adaptation)**

   a. Determine the maximum heart rate or symptom-limited heart rate by multistage testing with ECG monitoring.

   b. Decide on the threshold stimulus (percentage of maximum or symptom-limited heart rate) that will elicit a conditioning response for the individual tested and that will be used as the exercise heart rate.

   c. Determine the intensity, duration, and frequency of exercise that will result in attainment of the exercise heart rate and a conditioning response.

d. Determine the mode of exercise to be used based on the individual's physical capabilities and interest.

e. Initiate an exercise program with the patient and provide clearly written instructions regarding the details of the program.

f. Educate the patient about:

(1) Effort symptoms and the need to cease or modify exercise when these symptoms appear and to communicate with the physical therapist and/or physician about these problems

(2) Monitoring heart rate at rest as well as during and following exercise

(3) The importance of exercising within the guidelines provided by the physical therapist

(4) The importance of consistent long-term follow-up about the exercise program so that it can be progressed within safe limits

(5) The importance of modifying risk factors related to cardiac problems

X. Age Differences

Differences in endurance and physical work capacity among children, young adults, and middle-aged or elderly individuals are evident. Some comparisons are made between maximal oxygen uptake and the factors influencing it and among blood pressure, respiratory rate, vital capacity, and maximum voluntary ventilation in the different age categories.

A. Children[5,12,14,28]

Between the ages of 5 and 15 there is a threefold increase in body weight, lung volume, heart volume, and maximum oxygen uptake.

1. Heart rate

a. Resting heart rate is on the average above 125 (126 in girls, 135 in boys) at infancy.

b. Resting heart rate drops to adult levels at puberty.

c. Maximum heart rate is age related (220 minus age).

2. Stroke volume

a. Stroke volume is closely related to size.

b. Children 5 to 16 years of age have a stroke volume of 30 to 40 mL.

3. Cardiac output

a. Cardiac output is related to size.

b. Cardiac output increases with increasing stroke volume.

c. The increase in cardiac output for a given increase in oxygen consumption is a constant throughout life. It is the same in the child as in the adult.

4. Arteriovenous oxygen difference

a. Children tolerate a larger $a-\bar{v}O_2$ difference than adults.

b. The larger $a-\bar{v}O_2$ difference makes up for the smaller stroke volume.

5. Maximal oxygen uptake ($\dot{V}O_2$ max).

a. The $\dot{V}O_2$ max increases with age up to 20 years (expressed as liters per minute).

b. Before puberty, girls and boys show no significant difference in maximal aerobic capacity.

c. Cardiac output in children is the same as in the adult for any given oxygen consumption.

d. Endurance times increase with age until 17 to 18 years.

6. Blood pressure

a. Systolic blood pressure increases from 40 mm Hg at birth to 80 mm Hg at age 1 month to 100 mm Hg several years before puberty. Adult levels are observed at puberty.

b. Diastolic pressure increases from 55 to 70 mm Hg from 4 to 14 years of age, with little change during adolescence.

7. Respiration

a. Respiratory rate decreases from 30 breaths per minute at infancy to 16 breaths per minute at 17 to 18 years of age.

b. Vital capacity and maximum voluntary ventilation correlate with height, although the greater increase in boys than girls at puberty may be due to an increase in lung tissue.

8. Muscle mass and strength

a. Muscle mass increases through adolescence, primarily from muscle fiber hypertrophy and the development of sarcomeres. Sarcomeres are added at the musculotendinous junction to compensate for the required increase in length.

b. Girls develop peak muscle mass between 16 and 20 years, whereas boys develop peak muscle mass between 18 and 25 years.

c. Strength gains are associated with increased muscle mass in conjunction with neural maturation.

9. Anaerobic ability

a. Children generally demonstrate a limited anaerobic capacity. This may be due to a limited amount of phosphofructokinase, a controlling enzyme in the glycolytic pathway.

b. Children produce less lactic acid when performing anaerobically. This may be due to a limited glycolytic capacity.

B. Young Adult[21,22,28]

There are more data on the physiologic parameters of fitness for the young and the middle-aged adult than for the child or the elderly.

1. Heart rate

a. Resting heart rate reaches 60 to 65 beats per minute at 17 to 18 years of age (75 beats per minute in a sitting, sedentary young man).

b. Maximum heart rate is age related (190 beats per minute in the same sedentary young man).

2. Stroke volume

a. The adult values for stroke volume are 60 to 80 mL (75 mL in a sitting, sedentary young man).

b. With maximal exercise, stroke volume is 100 mL in that same sedentary young man.

3. **Cardiac output for the sedentary young man at rest**

   a. Cardiac output at rest is 75 beats per minute times 75 mL, or 5.6 liters per minute.

   b. With maximal exercise, cardiac output is 190 beats per minute times 100 mL, or 19 liters per minute.

4. **Arteriovenous oxygen difference (a−$\bar{v}O_2$ difference)**

   a. Twenty-five to 30 percent of the oxygen is extracted from blood as it runs through the muscles or other tissues at rest.

   b. In a normal, sedentary young man, it increases threefold (5.2 to 15.8 mL/100 mL blood) with exercise.

5. **Maximum oxygen uptake**

   a. The difference in $\dot{V}O_2$ max between male and female is greatest in the adult.

   b. Differences in $\dot{V}O_2$ max between the sexes is minimal when $\dot{V}O_2$ max is expressed relative to lean body weight.

   c. In the sedentary young man, maximum oxygen uptake equals 3000 mL/min (oxygen uptake at rest equals 300 mL/min).

6. **Blood pressure**

   a. Systolic blood pressure is 120 mm Hg (average). At peak effort of exercise, values may range from as low as 190 mm Hg to as high as 240 mm Hg.

   b. Diastolic blood pressure is 80 mm Hg (average). Diastolic pressure does not change markedly with exercise.

7. **Respiration**

   a. Respiratory rate is 12 to 15 breaths per minute.

   b. Vital capacity is 4800 mL in a man 20 to 30 years of age.

   c. Maximum voluntary ventilation varies considerably from laboratory to laboratory and is dependent on age and surface area of the body.

8. **Muscle mass and strength**

   a. Muscle mass increases with training as a result of hypertrophy. This hypertrophy can be the result of an increased number of myofibrils, increased actin and myosin, sarcoplasm, and/or connective tissue.

   b. There is limited evidence that suggests that the number of muscle fibers may increase, referred to as hyperplasia.

   c. As the nervous system matures, increased recruitment of motor units or decreased autogenic inhibition by Golgi tendon organs appears to also dictate strength gains.

9. **Anaerobic ability**

   a. Anaerobic training increases the activity of several controlling enzymes in the glycolytic pathway and enhances stored quantities of ATP and phosphocreatine.

   b. Anaerobic training increases the muscle's ability to buffer the hydrogen ions released when lactic acid is produced. Increased buffering allows the muscle to work anaerobically for longer periods of time.

C. Older Adult[21,22,28]

With increasing interest in the aged, data are appearing in the literature about this age group and their response to exercise.

1. **Heart rate**
   a. Resting heart rate is not influenced by age.
   b. Maximum heart rate is age related and decreases with age (in very general terms, 220 minus age). The average maximum heart rate for men 20 to 29 years of age is 190 beats per minute; for men 60 to 69 years of age, it is 164 beats per minute.
   c. The amount that the heart rate increases in response to static and maximum dynamic exercise (hand grip) decreases in the elderly.

2. **Stroke volume**

   Stroke volume decreases in the aged and results in decreased cardiac output.

3. **Cardiac output**

   Cardiac output decreases on an average of 7 to 3.4 liters per minute from age 19 to 86 years.

4. **a$-\bar{v}O_2$ difference**

   Arteriovenous oxygen difference decreases as a result of decreased lean body mass and low oxygen-carrying capacity.

5. **Maximum oxygen uptake**
   a. According to cardiorespiratory fitness classification,[3] if men 60 to 69 years of age of average fitness level are compared with men 20 to 29 years of age of the same fitness level, the maximal oxygen uptake for the older man is lower:
   20 to 29 years   31 to 37 mL/kg per minute
   60 to 69 years   18 to 23 mL/kg per minute
   b. Aerobic capacity decreases about 10 percent per decade when evaluating sedentary men. Maximum oxygen consumption decreases on an average from 47.7 mL/kg per minute at age 25 years to 25.5 mL/kg per minute at age 75 years. This decrease is not directly the result of age; athletes who continue exercising have a significantly lesser decrease in $\dot{V}o_2$ max when evaluated over a 10-year period.

6. **Blood pressure**

   Blood pressure increases because of increased peripheral vascular resistance.
   a. Systolic blood pressure of the aged is 150 mm Hg (average).
   b. Diastolic blood pressure is 90 mm Hg (average).
   c. If the definition of high blood pressure is 160/95, then 22 percent of men and 34 percent of women 65 to 74 years of age are hypertensive.
   d. Using 150/95 mm Hg as a cutoff, 25 percent of individuals are hypertensive at age 50 years and 70 percent between the ages of 85 and 95 years.

7. **Respiration**
   a. Respiratory rate increases with age.
   b. Vital capacity decreases with age. There is a 25 percent decrease in the vital capacity of the 50- to 60-year-old male compared with the 20- to 30-year-old male with the same surface area.
   c. Maximum voluntary ventilation decreases with age.

8. **Muscle mass and strength**
   a. Generally, strength decline with age is associated with a decrease in muscle mass and physical activity.

b. The decrease in muscle mass is primarily due to a decrease in protein synthesis, in concert with a decline in the number of fast-twitch muscle fibers.

c. Aging may also affect strength by slowing the nervous system's response time. This may alter the ability to effectively recruit motor units.

d. Continued training as one ages appears to reduce the effects of aging on the muscular system.

XI. Summary

This chapter has presented the topics of fitness and endurance and ways to achieve increased performance of physical activity in the healthy individual as well as the individual with coronary heart disease, a physical disability, or debilitating illness. Fitness, endurance, conditioning, deconditioning, and adaptation to exercise have been discussed. Energy expended for different levels of physical activity has been given, and the efficiency of the human being during activity has been included. A differentiation of fitness and stress testing has been emphasized, along with the development of training programs and the exercise prescription. Changes that occur with training and the mechanisms for their occurrence have been enumerated. Some basic information about comparing cardiovascular and respiratory parameters in the various age groups has been given.

References

1. American College of Sports Medicine: Resource Manual for Guidelines for Exercise Testing and Prescription, ed 2. Lea & Febiger, Philadelphia, 1993.
2. American College of Sports Medicine: Guidelines for Exercise Testing and Prescription, ed 4. Lea & Febiger, Philadelphia, 1991.
3. American Heart Association, The Committee on Exercise: Exercise Testing and Training of Apparently Healthy Individuals: A Handbook for Physicians. American Heart Association, 1972.
4. Astrand, P-O, and Rhyming, I: A nomogram for calculation of aerobic capacity (physical fitness) from pulse rate during submaximal work. J Appl Physiol 7:218, 1954.
5. Astrand, P, and Rodahl, K: Textbook of Work Physiology. Physiological Basis of Exercise, ed 3. McGraw-Hill, New York, 1986.
6. Balke, B: A simple field test for the assessment of physical fitness. Report 63-6. Civic Aeronautic Research Institute, Federal Aviation Agency, Oklahoma City, 1963.
7. Blocker, W, and Kitowski, V: Cardiac rehabilitation of the physically handicapped (amputee, hemiplegic, spinal cord injury patient and obese patient). In Blocker, W, and Cardus, D (eds): Rehabilitation in Ischemic Heart Disease. SP Medical and Scientific, New York, 1983.
8. Brannon, FJ, Foley, MW, Starr, JA, and Black, MG: Cardiopulmonary Rehabilitation: Basic Theory and Application, ed 2. FA Davis, Philadelphia, 1993.
9. Bruce, RA: Exercise testing for ventricular function. N Engl J Med 296:671–675, 1977.
10. Butler, RM, et al: The cardiovascular response to circuit weight training in patients with cardiac disease. J Cardiopulm Rehabil 7:402, 1987.
11. Cooper, KH, and Robertson, JW: Aerobics in Action.

In Long, C (ed): Prevention and Rehabilitation in Ischemic Heart Disease. Rehabilitation Medicine Library. Williams & Wilkins, Baltimore, 1980.
12. Ellestad, MH: Stress Testing: Principles and Practice, ed 2. FA Davis, Philadelphia, 1986.
13. Fox, EL, and Mathews, DK: Physiological Basis of Physical Education and Athletics, ed 3. Saunders College Publishing, Philadelphia, 1981.
14. Godfrey, S: Exercise Testing in Children. WB Saunders, Philadelphia, 1974.
15. Golding, LA, Myers, CR, and Sinning, WE (eds): Y's Way to Physical Fitness, ed 3. Human Kinetics, Champaign, IL, 1989.
16. Howley, ET, and Franks, BD: Health/Fitness Instructors Handbook. Human Kinetics, Champaign, IL, 1986.
17. Irwin, S, and Tecklin, JS: Cardiopulmonary Physical Therapy, ed 3. CV Mosby, St Louis, 1995.
18. Kenney, RA: Physiology of Aging: A Synopsis. Year Book Medical Publishers, Chicago, 1982.
19. Kline, GM, et al: Estimation of VO_2 max from a one-mile track walk, gender age, and body weight. Med Sci Sports Exerc 19:253–259, 1987.
20. Londeree, BR, and Moeschberger, ML: Influence of age and other factors on maximal heart rate. J Cardiac Rehabil 4:44, 1984.
21. McArdle, WD, Katch, FI, and Katch, VL: Exercise Physiology: Energy, Nutrition, and Human Performance, ed 3. Lea & Febiger, Philadelphia, 1991.
22. McArdle, WD, Katch, FI, and Katch, VL: Essentials of Exercise Physiology, Lea & Febiger, Philadelphia, 1994.
23. Powers, SK, and Howley, ET: Exercise Physiology: Theory and Application to Fitness and Performance, WC Brown, Dubuque, IA, 1990.
24. Skinner, JS: Exercise Testing and Exercise Prescrip-

tion for Special Cases. Theoretical Basis and Clinical Application. Lea & Febiger, Philadelphia, 1987.

25. Smith, JJ, and Kampine, JP: Circulatory Physiology: The Essentials. Williams & Wilkins, Baltimore, 1984.

26. US Department of Health and Human Services, Public Health Service: Healthy People 2000: National Health Promotion and Disease Prevention Objectives. US Government Printing Office, Washington, DC, 1990.

27. Wenger, NK, and Hellerstein, HK: Rehabilitation of the Coronary Patient. Wiley, New York, 1984.

28. Wilmore, JH, and Costill, DL: Physiology of Sport and Exercise. Human Kinetics, Champaign, IL, 1994.

Chapter

5

Stretching

Mobility and flexibility of the soft tissues that surround a joint, that is, muscles, connective tissue, and skin, in conjunction with adequate joint mobility are necessary for normal range of motion. Unrestricted, pain-free range of motion (ROM) is often required to perform many functional daily living tasks as well as occupational or recreational activities. Adequate mobility of soft tissues and joints is also thought to be an important factor in prevention of injury or reinjury to soft tissues. Conditions that may produce adaptive shortening of soft tissues around a joint and subsequent loss of range of motion include (1) prolonged immobilization, (2) restricted mobility, (3) connective tissue or neuromuscular diseases, (4) tissue pathology due to trauma, and (5) congenital and acquired bony deformities.

Prolonged immobilization can occur when a patient must wear a cast or a splint for an extended period of time after a fracture or surgery. An individual's mobility may be restricted because of prolonged bed rest or confinement to a wheelchair. This can lead to long-term static and often faulty positioning of joints and soft tissue. Neuromuscular diseases or trauma can lead to paralysis, spasticity, weakness, muscle imbalance, and pain, all of which make it difficult or impossible for a patient to move joints through a full range of motion. Connective tissue diseases (collagen diseases) such as scleroderma, dermatomyositis, and polymyositis as well as joint diseases such as rheumatoid arthritis and osteoarthritis can cause pain, muscle spasm, inflammation, and weakness and can alter the structure of soft tissues. Tissue pathology from trauma, inflammation, edema, ischemia, hemorrhage, surgical incision, laceration, and burns can lead to the production of dense fibrous tissue, which replaces normal soft tissue. These soft tissues then lose their normal elasticity and plasticity, resulting in loss of range of motion.

Muscle strength can also be altered when soft tissue adaptively shortens over time. As muscle loses its normal flexibility, a change in the length-tension relationship of the muscle also occurs. As the muscle shortens, it no longer is capable of producing peak tension,[24,36,58] and **tight weakness** develops. Loss of flexibility, for whatever reason, can also cause pain arising from muscle, connective tissue, or periosteum. This, in turn, also decreases muscle strength.

Limitation of joint range of motion because of **contracture** (adaptive shortening) of soft tissue may be treated with passive stretching combined with relaxation procedures and active inhibition techniques. The stretching procedures described in this chapter are techniques designed to elongate the contractile and noncontractile tissues of the

143

musculotendinous unit. Limitations of motion because of joint immobility and capsular restrictions are treated with joint mobilization and manipulation and are dealt with in Chapter 6.

OBJECTIVES

After studying this chapter, the reader will be able to:

1 Define specific terms related to stretching such as contracture, tightness, irreversible contracture, overstretching, and selective stretching.
2 Identify the pathologic processes and clinical situations in which limitations of motion of soft tissues and joints can occur.
3 Describe the properties of contractile and noncontractile soft tissue that affect the application and success of stretching procedures.
4 Define and explain the different therapeutic techniques used to elongate muscle, including active inhibition and passive stretching.
5 Describe the indications, goals, precautions, and contraindications to stretching.
6 Discuss the correct procedures a therapist should follow when setting up and carrying out stretching exercises.
7 Identify the general principles of relaxation exercises and apply them in preparation for stretching.
8 Describe proper patient positioning, hand placement, and stabilization used when applying stretching techniques to the upper and lower extremities.
9 Describe the appropriate application of active inhibition techniques.

I. Definition of Terms Related to Stretching

A. Flexibility[46,53,67,75,76]

Flexibility is the ability to move a single joint or series of joints through an unrestricted, pain-free range of motion. It is dependent upon the *extensibility* of muscles, which allows muscles that cross a joint to relax, lengthen, and yield to a stretch force. The arthrokinematics of the moving joint as well as the ability of periarticular connective tissues to deform also affect joint ROM and an individual's overall flexibility. Often the term "flexibility" is used to refer more specifically to the ability of the musculotendinous unit to elongate as a body segment or joint moves through the ROM.

Dynamic flexibility refers to the active range of motion of a joint. This aspect of flexibility is dependent upon the degree to which a joint can be moved by a muscle contraction and the amount of tissue resistance met during the active movement. *Passive flexibility* is the degree to which a joint can be passively moved through the available ROM and is dependent upon the extensibility of muscles and connective tissues that cross and surround a joint. Passive flexibility is a prerequisite for but does not ensure dynamic flexibility.

B. Stretching

Stretching is a general term used to describe any therapeutic maneuver designed to lengthen (elongate) pathologically shortened soft tissue structures and thereby to increase range of motion.

1. **Passive stretching**

   While the patient is relaxed, an external force, applied either manually or mechanically, lengthens the shortened tissues.

2. **Active inhibition**

   The patient participates in the stretching maneuver to inhibit tonus in a tight muscle.

3. **Flexibility exercises**

   The terms stretching and flexibility exercises are often used interchangeably.

C. Selective Stretching

Selective stretching is a process whereby the overall function of a patient may be improved by applying stretching techniques selectively to some muscles and joints but allowing limitation of motion to develop in other muscles or joints.

1. For example, in the patient with spinal cord injury, stability of the trunk is necessary for independence in sitting. With thoracic and cervical lesions, the patient will not have active control of the back extensors. If moderate tightness is allowed to develop in the extensors of the low back, the patient will be able to lean into the slightly tight structures and will have some trunk stability in sitting.

   NOTE: The patient must also have adequate range for independence in dressing and transfers. Too much tightness in the low back can decrease function.

2. Allowing slight contractures to develop in the long flexors of the fingers will enable the patient with spinal cord injury who lacks innervation of the intrinsic finger muscles to develop grasp through a tenodesis action.

D. Overstretch[39,53]

Overstretch is a stretch well beyond the normal range of motion of a joint and the surrounding soft tissues, resulting in hypermobility.

1. Overstretching may be necessary for certain healthy individuals with normal strength and stability participating in sports that require extensive flexibility.

2. Overstretching becomes detrimental when the supporting structures of a joint and the strength of the muscles around a joint are insufficient and cannot hold a joint in a stable, functional position during activities. This is often referred to as **stretch weakness.**

E. Contracture

Contracture is defined as the adaptive shortening of muscle or other soft tissues that cross a joint, which results in a limitation of range of motion.[14,35,36]

1. Contractures are described by identifying the tight muscle action. If a patient has tight elbow flexors and cannot fully extend the elbow, he or she is said to have an elbow flexion contracture. When a patient cannot fully abduct the leg because of tight adductors of the hip, he or she is said to have an adduction contracture of the hip.

2. The terms *contracture* and *contraction* (the process of tension developing in a muscle during shortening or lengthening)[32] are *not* synonymous and should not be used interchangeably.

F. Types of Contractures

Contractures can be more specifically defined and classified by the soft tissue structures involved.

1. Myostatic contracture[13]

a. There is no specific tissue pathology present. The musculotendinous unit has adaptively shortened and there is a significant loss of range of motion.

b. *Tightness* is a nonspecific term referring to mild shortening of an otherwise healthy musculotendinous unit. The term "tightness" is sometimes used to describe a mild transient contracture. A muscle that is "tight" can be lengthened to all but the outer limits of its range. Normal individuals who do not regularly participate in a flexibility program can develop mild myostatic contractures or tightness, particularly in two-joint muscles such as the hamstrings, rectus femoris, or gastrocnemius.

c. Myostatic contractures can be resolved in a relatively short time with gentle stretching exercises.

2. Adhesions

Motion is necessary to maintain tissue health and flexibility. Lack of motion results in increased cross bonding or adherence between collagen fibers. If tissue is immobilized in the shortened position for extended periods of time, loss of normal mobility occurs; that is, contractures develop from the architectural changes in the connective tissue.[14]

3. Scar tissue adhesions

a. Scar tissue develops in response to injury and the inflammatory response. The new fibers initially develop in randomized fashion; if they adhere to each other and to surrounding normal tissue in a disorganized pattern, the scar will restrict motion unless remodeled along the lines of stress.[28,64]

b. Chronic inflammation from continued mechanical or chemical irritation perpetuates fiber deposition, leading to significant scar development and restricted motion.[64]

4. Irreversible contracture

A permanent loss of extensibility of soft tissues that cannot be released by nonsurgical treatment occurs when normal soft tissue and organized connective tissue are replaced by an excessive amount of nonextensible tissue such as bone or fibrotic tissue.

5. Pseudomyostatic contracture[13]

Limitation of motion may also develop as the result of hypertonicity caused by a central nervous system lesion. The muscle appears to be in an inappropriate and constant state of contraction, resulting in an apparent limitation of motion.

II. Properties of Soft Tissue That Affect Elongation

As mentioned earlier, the soft tissues that can restrict joint motion are muscles, connective tissue, and skin. Each has unique qualities that affect its extensibility, that is, its ability to elongate. When stretching procedures are applied to these soft tissues, the velocity, intensity, and duration of the stretch force as well as temperature of the soft tissues all affect the response of the different types of soft tissues. Mechanical characteristics of contractile and noncontractile tissue as well as the neurophysiologic properties of contractile tissue all affect soft tissue lengthening.

When soft tissue is stretched, either elastic or plastic changes occur. **Elasticity** is the ability of soft tissue to return to its resting length after passive stretch. **Plasticity** is the tendency of soft tissue to assume a new and greater length after the stretch force has been removed.[55] Both contractile and noncontractile tissues have elastic and plastic qualities.[39,55]

A. Mechanical Properties of Contractile Tissue

Muscle is primarily composed of contractile tissue but is attached to and interwoven with noncontractile tissue such as tendon and fascia. The connective tissue framework in muscle, not active contractile components, is the primary source of resistance to passive elongation of muscle.

1. Contractile elements of muscle (Fig. 5-1)

Individual muscles are composed of many *muscle fibers*. A single muscle fiber is made up of many *myofibrils*. A myofibril is composed of *sarcomeres*, which lie in series. The sarcomere is the contractile unit of the myofibril and is composed of overlapping cross-bridges of actin and myosin. The sarcomere gives a muscle its ability to contract and relax. When a muscle contracts, the actin-myosin filaments slide together and the muscle shortens. When a muscle relaxes, the cross-bridges slide apart slightly, and the muscle returns to its resting length (Fig. 5-2).

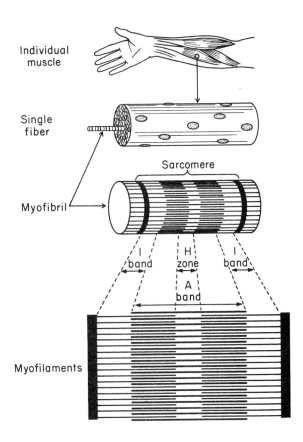

Figure 5-1. Structure of skeletal muscle.

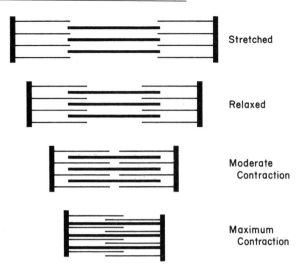

Stretched

Relaxed

Moderate
Contraction

Maximum
Contraction

Figure 5–2. Elongation and shortening of the sarcomere, the contractile unit of muscle.

2. Mechanical response of the contractile unit to stretch

a. When a muscle is passively stretched, initial lengthening occurs in the series elastic component and tension rises sharply. After a point there is a mechanical disruption of the cross-bridges as the filaments slide apart and an abrupt lengthening of the sarcomeres occurs (*sarcomere give*).[19] When the stretch force is released, the individual sarcomeres return to their resting length (Fig. 5–2). The tendency of muscle to return to its resting length after short-term stretch is called elasticity.[55,60,63]

b. After a muscle is immobilized for a period of time, a decrease in muscle protein and mitochondria occurs, resulting in atrophy and weakness.[2,13,58]

c. If a muscle is immobilized in a lengthened position over a prolonged period of time, the number of sarcomeres in series will increase, giving rise to a more permanent (plastic) form of muscle lengthening. A muscle will adjust its length over time to maintain the greatest functional overlap of actin-myosin.[60,62,73]

d. A muscle that has been immobilized in a shortened position produces increased amounts of connective tissue that serves to protect the muscle when it stretches. There is a reduction in the number of sarcomeres as the result of sarcomere absorption.[60,62,73]

e. The sarcomere adaptation to prolonged positions (either lengthened or shortened) is transient if the muscle is allowed to resume its normal length after immobilization.

B. Neurophysiologic Properties of Contractile Tissue

1. The muscle spindle (Fig. 5–3)

The muscle spindle is the major sensory organ of muscle and is composed of microscopic intrafusal fibers that lie in parallel to the extrafusal fiber. The muscle spindle monitors the velocity and duration of stretch and senses length changes in muscle.[6,53,67,75,76] Fibers of the muscle spindle sense how quickly a muscle is stretched. Primary (type Ia) and secondary (type II) afferent fibers arise from

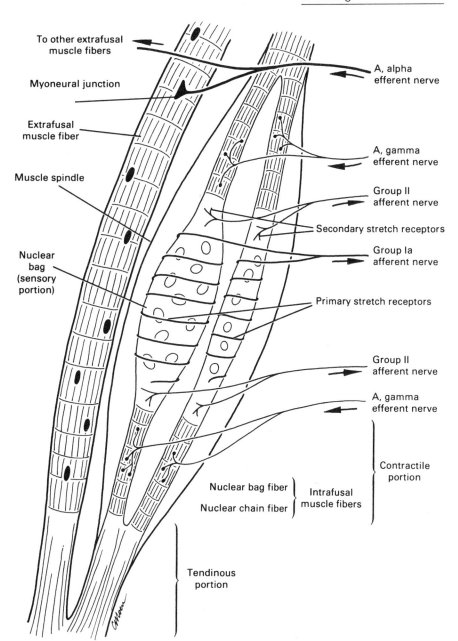

To other extrafusal
muscle fibers

Myoneural junction

Extrafusal
muscle fiber

Muscle spindle

Nuclear
bag
(sensory
portion)

A, alpha
efferent nerve

A, gamma
efferent nerve

Group II
afferent nerve

Secondary stretch receptors

Group Ia
afferent nerve

Primary stretch receptors

Group II
afferent nerve

A, gamma
efferent nerve

Contractile
portion

Nuclear bag fiber
Nuclear chain fiber
Intrafusal
muscle fibers

Tendinous
portion

Figure 5–3. Muscle spindle. Diagram shows intrafusal and extrafusal muscle fibers. The muscle spindle acts as a stretch receptor. (From Lemkuhl, LD, and Smith, LK: Brunnstrom's Clinical Kinesiology, ed 4. FA Davis, Philadelphia, 1983, p 97, with permission.)

muscle spindles, synapse on either the alpha or gamma motoneurons, respectively, and facilitate contraction of the extrafusal and intrafusal fibers.[67,75,76]

2. The Golgi tendon organ (GTO)

The GTO is located near the musculotendinous junction, wraps around the ends of the extrafusal fibers of a muscle, and is sensitive to the tension in a muscle caused by either passive stretch or active muscle contraction.

a. The GTO is a protective mechanism that inhibits contraction of the muscle in which it lies. It has a very low threshold for firing (fires easily) after an active muscle contraction and has a high threshold for firing with passive stretch.[20,75,76]

b. When excessive tension develops in a muscle, the GTO fires, inhibits alpha motoneuron activity, and decreases tension in the muscle. During stretching procedures the tension within the tendon determines if the individual sarcomeres in muscle are lengthened.[53,75,76]

3. The neurophysiologic response of muscle to stretch[6,46,53,67,75,76]

a. When a muscle is stretched very quickly, the primary afferent fibers stimulate alpha motoneurons in the spinal cord and facilitate contraction of extrafusal fibers, increasing tension in a muscle.[67,75,76] This is called the *monosynaptic stretch reflex.* Stretching procedures that are performed at too high a velocity may actually increase the tension in a muscle that is to be lengthened.

b. If a slow stretch force is applied to muscle, the GTO fires and inhibits the tension in the muscle, allowing the parallel elastic component (the sarcomere) of the muscle to lengthen.

C. Mechanical Characteristics of Noncontractile Soft Tissue

Noncontractile soft tissue permeates the entire body and is organized into various types of connective tissue to support the structures of the body. Ligaments, tendons, joint capsules, fasciae, noncontractile tissue within muscles, and skin all have characteristics that will lead to the development of adhesions and contractures and thus affect the flexibility of the tissues crossing the joint. When these tissues restrict range of motion and require stretching, it is important to understand how they respond to various intensities and duration of stretch forces and to recognize that the only way to increase flexibility in connective tissue is by remodeling its basic architecture.[14]

1. Material strength

The material strength of each tissue is related to its ability to resist a load or stress.[12,43]

a. **Stress** is force per unit area. Mechanical stress is the internal reaction or resistance to an external load. There are three kinds of stress.

(1) *Tension:* a tensile force that is applied perpendicular to the cross-sectional area of the tissue in a direction away from the tissue. Tension stress is a stretching force.

(2) *Compression:* a compressive force that is applied perpendicular to the cross-sectional area of the tissue in a direction toward the tissue. Compression stress occurs within joints, with muscle contraction and on weight bearing when a joint is loaded.

(3) *Shear:* a force that is parallel to the cross-sectional area of the tissue.

b. **Strain** is the amount of deformation that occurs when a load (stress) is applied.

c. A *stress-strain curve* depicts the mechanical strength of structures (Fig. 5–4).

(1) *Elastic range:* initially the strain is directly proportional to the ability of the material to resist the force. The tissue returns to its original size and shape when the load is released.

(2) *Elastic limit:* the point beyond which the tissue will not return to its original shape and size.

Figure 5–4. Stress-strain curve. When stressed, initially the wavy collagen fibers straighten (toe region). With additional stress, recoverable deformation occurs in the elastic range. Once the elastic limit is reached, sequential failure of the collagen fibers and tissue occurs in the plastic range, resulting in release of heat (hysteresis) and new length when the stress is released. The length from the stress point (X) results in a new length when released (X′); the heat released is represented by the area under the curve between these two points (hysteresis loop). (Y to Y′ represents additional length from additional stress with more heat released.) Necking is the region in which there is considerable weakening of the tissue and less force is needed for deformation. Total failure quickly follows even under smaller loads.

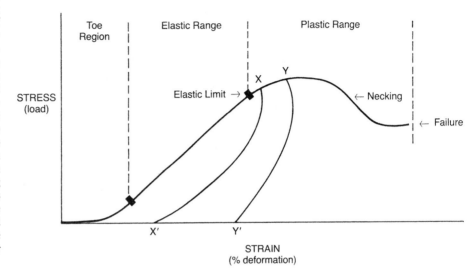

(3) *Plastic range:* the range beyond the elastic limit extending to the point of rupture. Tissue strained within this range will have permanent deformation.

(4) *Yield strength:* the load beyond the elastic limit that produces permanent deformation within the tissue. Once the yield point is reached, there is sequential failure of the tissue with permanent deformation (remodeling), and the tissue passes into the plastic range of the stress-strain curve. The deformation may be from a single load or the summation of several subcritical loads.[12]

(5) *Ultimate strength:* the greatest load the tissue can sustain. Once the maximum load is reached, there is increased strain (deformation) without an increase in stress.

(6) *Necking:* the region in which there is considerable weakening of the tissue; less force is needed for deformation, and failure rapidly approaches.

(7) *Breaking strength:* the load at the time the tissue fails.

(8) *Failure:* rupture of the integrity of the tissue.

d. Influences on the stress-strain curve.

(1) *Resilience:* the ability to absorb energy within the elastic range as work is accomplished. Energy is released when the load is removed and the tissue returns to its original shape.

(2) *Toughness:* the ability to absorb energy within the plastic range without breaking (failing). If too much energy is absorbed with the stress, there will be rupture.

(3) *Creep:* when a load is applied for an extended period of time, the tissue elongates, resulting in permanent deformation or failure. It is related to the viscosity of the tissue and is therefore time dependent. Deformation depends on the amount of force and the rate at which the force is applied. Creep occurs with low-magnitude load, usually in the elastic range, over a long time. The greater the load, the more rapid the rate of creep, but not in proportion to strain; therefore, a lesser load applied for a longer time will result in greater deformation. Increased temperature increases creep and therefore distensibility of the tissue.[40,70,71]

(4) *Structural stiffness:* tissue with greater stiffness will have a higher slope in the elastic region of the curve, indicating there is less elastic deformation with greater stress. Contractures and scar tissue have greater stiffness, probably because of a greater degree of bonding between collagen fibers and their surrounding matrix.

(5) *Heat production:* energy is released as heat when stress is applied. It is depicted by the area under the curve (hysteresis loop) in the plastic range. As the tissue is heated, it more easily distends.

(6) *Fatigue:* cyclic loading of the tissue increases heat production and may cause failure below the yield point. The greater the applied load, the fewer number of cycles are needed for failure. A minimum load is required for this failure; below the minimum load an apparent infinite number of cycles will not cause failure. This is the *endurance limit.* Examples of fatigue are stress fractures and overuse syndromes. Biologic tissue has the ability to repair itself after cyclic loading if the load is not too great and time is allowed before the cyclic loading is again applied.

2. Composition of connective tissue

Connective tissue is composed of three types of fibers and nonfibrous ground substance.[12,28,64]

a. *Collagen fibers* resist tensile deformation and are responsible for the strength and stiffness of tissue. Collagen fibers are composed of tropocollagen crystals, which form the building blocks of collagen microfibrils. Each additional level of composition of the fibers is arranged in an organized relationship and dimension (Fig. 5–5). There are five classes of collagen; the fibers of tendons and ligaments mostly contain type I collagen, which is highly resistant to tension.[64] As collagen fibers develop and mature, they bind together, initially with unstable hydrogen bonding, which then converts to stable covalent bonding. The stronger the bonds, the greater the mechanical stability of the tissue.

b. *Elastin fibers* provide extensibility. They show a great deal of elongation with small loads and fail abruptly without deformation at higher loads. Tissues with greater amounts of elastin have greater flexibility.

c. *Reticulin fibers* provide tissue with bulk.

d. *Ground substance*, mostly an organic gel containing water, reduces friction between fibers, transports nutrients and metabolites, and may help prevent excessive cross-linking between fibers by maintaining space between fibers.[15,64]

3. Mechanical behavior of noncontractile tissue

The mechanical behavior of the various noncontractile tissues is determined by the proportion of collagen and elastin fibers and by the structural orientation of

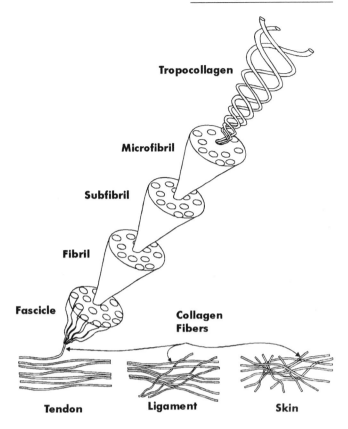

Figure 5–5. Composition of collagen fibers showing the aggregation of tropocollagen crystals as the building blocks of collagen. Organization of the fibers within connective tissue is related to the function of the tissue. Tissues with parallel fiber orientation, such as tendons, are able to withstand greater tensile loads than tissue such as skin where the fiber orientation appears more random.

the fibers. Collagen is the structural element that absorbs most of the tensile stress. Collagen elongates quickly under light loads (wavy fibers straighten within the toe region); with increasing tension, the fibers continue to stiffen. They strongly resist the deforming force that begins to break the bonds between collagen fibrils and molecules. When a substantial number of bonds are broken, the fibers fail. Tissue with greater proportion of collagen provides greater stability. Collagen is five times as strong as elastin.

a. In tendons, collagen fibers are parallel and can resist the greatest tensile load.

b. In skin, collagen fibers are random and weakest in resisting tension.

c. In ligaments, joint capsules, and fasciae, the collagen fibers vary between the two extremes. Ligaments that resist the major joint stresses have more parallel orientation of collagen fibers and a larger cross-sectional area.[51]

4. **Interpreting the stress-strain curve**[63,64,77]

a. Collagen fibers at rest are wavy, so initially they straighten as stress is applied. Little force is required for elongation in this range (toe region), where most functional activity normally occurs. Additionally, in the toe region, stress removes any macroscopic slack in the three-dimensional matrix of collagenous tissues.

b. As the tissue is taken to the end of the full normal range of motion and a gentle stretch is applied, the tissue functions in the elastic portion (linear phase) of the curve. With this stress the collagen fibers line up with the applied force; the bonds between fibers and between the surrounding matrix are strained, some microfailure between the collagen bonds begins, and some water may be displaced from the ground substance. There is complete recovery from this normal deformation if the stress is not maintained.

c. If stress continues, the tissue reaches the yield point and sequential failure of the bonds between collagen fibrils and eventually of collagen fibers occurs. Heat is released and absorbed in the tissue and there is permanent deformation. Because collagen is crystalline, individual fibers do not stretch but they rupture. In the plastic range it is the rupturing of fibers that results in increased length.

d. If maximum load and point of ultimate strength are reached, there is increased strain without an increase in stress. If necking is reached, the tissue rapidly fails. The therapist must be cognizant of the tissue feel when stretching because as the tissue begins necking and the stress is maintained, there will be complete failure (rupture). Experimentally, maximum tensile deformation of isolated collagen fibers prior to failure is 7 to 8 percent; whole ligaments may withstand strain of 20 to 40 percent.[51]

e. Using the principle of creep, low-magnitude loads over long periods increase the deformation of noncontractile tissue, allowing a gradual rearrangement of collagen fiber bonds (remodeling) and redistribution of water to surrounding tissues.[59,63] Increasing the temperature of the part will increase the creep.[40,71,72] Complete recovery from creep may occur over time, but not as rapidly as a single strain. A low load applied for a prolonged period is better tolerated by people and allows for remodeling of the collagen fibers. Patient reaction dictates the time a specific load is tolerated. Fifteen to 20 minutes of low-intensity sustained stretch, repeated on 5 consecutive days, has been documented to cause a change in the length of the hamstring muscles.[47]

f. *Cyclic loading*, or repetitive submaximal stress, increases heat production and the effects of the tissue adapting (remodeling) to a new length. Starring and coworkers[59] documented increased hamstring length using a 10-second hold followed by an 8-second rest, repeated for 15 minutes on 5 consecutive days.

g. Tissue failure can occur as a single maximal event (acute tear from injury or manipulation that exceeds the failure point) or from repetitive submaximal stress (fatigue or stress failure from cyclic loading).

h. Healing and adaptive (remodeling) capabilities of biologic tissue allow tissue to respond to repetitive loads if time is allowed between bouts. This is important for increasing both flexibility and tensile strength of the tissue.

   (1) If healing and remodeling time is not allowed, a breakdown of tissue (failure) will occur, as in overuse syndromes and stress fractures.

   (2) Intensive stretching is usually not done every day in order to allow time for healing. If the inflammation from the microruptures is excessive, additional scar tissue is laid down, which could become more restrictive.[14]

   (3) Greater precaution is required with aging because collagen loses its elasticity, and there is decreased capillary blood supply that reduces the healing capability.

5. Changes in collagen affecting stress-strain response

a. *Effects of immobilization*

   There is weakening of the tissue because of collagen turnover and weak bonding between the new, nonstressed fibers. There is also adhesion formation because of greater cross-linking between disorganized collagen fibers and because of decreased effectiveness of the ground substance maintaining space and lubrication between the fibers.[15,63] Rate of return to normal tensile strength is slow. Following 8 weeks of immobilization the anterior cruciate ligament in monkeys failed at 61 percent of maximum load; after 5 months of reconditioning, failed at 79 percent; after 12 months of reconditioning, failed at 91 percent.[49,50] There was also a reduction in energy absorbed and an increase in compliance (decreased stiffness) prior to failure following immobilization. Partial and near-complete recovery followed the same 5-month and 12-month pattern.[50]

b. *Effects of inactivity (decrease of normal activity)*
There is a decrease in size and amount of collagen fibers, resulting in weakening of the tissue; there is a proportional increase in the predominance of elastin fibers, resulting in an increased compliance. Recovery takes about 5 months of regular cyclic loading.

c. *Effects of age*
There is a decrease in the maximum tensile strength and in the elastic modulus, and the rate of adaptation to stress is slower.[51] There is an increased tendency for overuse syndromes, fatigue failures, and tears with stretching.[77]

d. *Effects of corticosteroids*
There is a long-lasting deleterious effect on mechanical properties of collagen with a decrease in tensile strength.[77] There is fibrocyte death next to the injection site with delay in reappearance up to 15 weeks.[51]

An understanding of the qualities of contractile and noncontractile tissues and their responses to immobilization and stretch will assist the therapist in selecting the safest and most effective stretching procedures for patients.

III. Therapeutic Methods to Elongate Soft Tissues

There are three basic methods to elongate the contractile or noncontractile components of the musculotendinous unit: manually or mechanically applied passive stretching, active inhibition, and self-stretching.[5,10,32,39,65] Self-stretching may involve passive stretch, active inhibition, or both. All stretching procedures should be preceded by some low-intensity active exercise or therapeutic heat to warm up the tissues that are to be stretched. Soft tissue yields more easily to stretch if the muscle is warm when the stretch force is applied.

A. Passive Stretching

Passive stretching procedures are classified by the type of stretch force applied, the intensity of the stretch, and the duration of the stretch. Both contractile and noncontractile tissues can be elongated by passive stretching.

1. Manual passive stretching

a. The therapist applies the external force and controls the direction, speed, intensity, and duration of the stretch to the soft tissues that have caused the contracture and restriction of joint motion. The tissues are elongated beyond their resting length.

b. This technique should not be confused with passive range of motion exercises. Passive stretching takes the structures beyond the free range of motion.

Passive range of motion, as defined in Chapter 2, is applied only within the unrestricted available range.

c. The patient must be as relaxed as possible during passive stretching.

d. The stretch force is usually applied for no less than 6 seconds but preferably for at least 15 to 30 seconds and repeated several times in an exercise session. Manual passive stretching is generally considered to be a short-duration stretch.[32,67]

(1) No specific number of seconds has been determined to be the most effective duration for passive stretching.

(2) In one study,[45] passive stretching was applied to the hip abductors of healthy subjects for 15 seconds, 45 seconds, and 2 minutes at the same intensity. The 15-second stretch was just as effective as the 2-minute stretch. In another study,[3] in which daily stretching of the hamstring muscles was carried out for 15, 30, or 60 seconds, it was determined that 30- and 60-second stretches increased ROM more than a 15-second stretch but there was no significant difference in the effectiveness of 30- and 60-second stretches.

e. The intensity and duration of the stretch are dependent on the patient's tolerance and the therapist's strength and endurance. A low-intensity manual stretch applied for as long as possible will be more comfortable and more readily tolerated by the patient and will result in optimal rates of improvement without exposing weakened tissue to excessive force and jeopardizing its structure.[14]

f. Maintained versus ballistic stretching.[46,54]

(1) When manual passive stretching is appropriately applied, the stretch is very slow and gentle. The stretch force is *maintained*, as previously mentioned, for 15 seconds, 30 seconds, or longer. A low-intensity maintained stretch that is applied gradually is less likely to facilitate the stretch reflex and increase tension in the muscle being lengthened. This is often called a *static stretch*.[21,23]

(2) *Ballistic stretching* is a high-intensity very short-duration "bouncing" stretch. It is usually achieved when a patient actively bounces by contracting the muscle group opposite the tight muscle group and using body weight and momentum as the force to elongate the tight muscle. Although ballistic stretching has been shown to increase ROM, it is considered unsafe because of poor control and the potential of inappropriately rupturing weakened tissues. The elderly, sedentary individuals, and persons with early healing of injuries (including surgery) or after immobilization are particularly at risk of undesirable tissue trauma with ballistic stretching because of the weakened state of the connective tissue. In addition, a ballistic stretch quickly lengthens the muscle spindle and facilitates the stretch reflex, causing an increase in tension in the muscle that is being stretched. Muscles and connective tissues are more susceptible to microtrauma with ballistic stretching than with a low-intensity maintained stretch.

(3) It has been shown that the tension created in a muscle during ballistic stretching is almost twice that created with a low-intensity maintained stretch.[69]

g. In comparison to the long-duration mechanical stretching procedure, applied for 20 minutes or more, manual passive stretching is a rather short-duration stretch. It is common for a therapist to manually apply an end-range static stretch for 15 to 30 seconds. If this procedure is repeated eight times, for ex-ample, the total duration of the stretching treatment would be only 2 to 4 minutes. Some investigators have suggested that the temporary gains in ROM achieved as the result of short-duration manual passive stretching techniques are transient and are attributed to temporary sarcomere give (elastic changes in actin-myosin overlap)[25] or to connective tissue recovery from the creep re-sponse (return of water and realigning of collagen bonds).[64]

2. Prolonged mechanical passive stretching[40,55,59,70,71]

a. A low-intensity external force (5 to 15 lb or 5 to 10 percent of body weight) is applied to shortened tissues over a prolonged period with mechanical equipment.

b. The stretch force is applied through positioning of the patient, with weighted traction and pulley systems or with dynamic splints or serial casts.

c. The prolonged stretch may be maintained for 20 to 30 minutes or as long as several hours.

   (1) Several authors have suggested that a period of 20 minutes or longer is necessary for a stretch to be effective and increase range of motion when low-intensity prolonged mechanical stretch is used.[8,39,55] Bohannon[8] eval-uated the effectiveness of an 8-minute stretch of the hamstrings in com-parison to a 20-minute or longer stretch using an overhead cable-pulley system. The 8-minute stretch resulted in only a small increase in ham-string flexibility, which was lost within 24 hours. It was suggested that a 20-minute or longer stretch is necessary to effectively increase range of motion on a more permanent basis. Significant increases in range of mo-tion in subjects who were healthy but had tight lower extremity muscula-ture have also been reported using only 10 minutes of low-intensity pro-longed mechanical stretch.[23]

   (2) Bohannon and Larkin[9] also used a regimen of tilt table–wedge board standing for 30 minutes daily to increase the range of ankle dorsiflexion in patients with neurologic disorders.

   (3) Prolonged, low-intensity stretch and an increase in range can also be ac-complished with a dynamic splint[30] such as the Dynasplint (Fig. 5–6). The splint is applied for 8 to 10 hours. Units are available for the elbow, wrist, knee, and ankle.

d. Low-intensity prolonged stretch (5- to 12-lb stretch force applied 1 hour per day) has been shown to be significantly more effective than manual passive stretching over a 4-week period in patients with long-standing bi-lateral knee flexion contractures.[44] The patients also reported that the pro-longed mechanical stretch was more comfortable than the manual stretch-ing procedure.

e. Plastic changes in noncontractile and contractile tissues may be the basis of "permanent" or long-term improvements in flexibility.[8,14]

   (1) When muscles are held in a lengthened position for several weeks, sar-comeres are added in series.[60,62,73]

   (2) When noncontractile connective tissues are stretched with a low-intensity prolonged stretch force, plastic deformation occurs and the length of the tissue increases.[40,70,71]

   NOTE: The term *permanent lengthening* means that length is maintained after the stretch force is removed. The increase in length will be "perma-nent" only if the new length is used regularly.

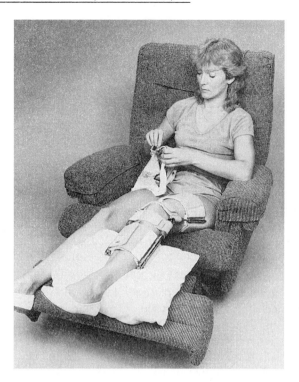

Figure 5–6. The Dynasplint Systems® Unit places a prolonged stretch on soft tissue to reduce a knee flexion contracture. (Reprinted by permission of Dynasplint Systems, Inc., Baltimore, MD.)

3. Cyclic mechanical stretching

Passive stretching using a mechanical device such as the Autorange (Valley City, ND) can also be done in a cyclic mode. The intensity of the stretch, the length of each stretch cycle, and the number of stretch cycles per minute can all be adjusted on this mechanical stretching unit.

Starring et al[59] used the term **cyclic stretching** to describe a repeated stretch applied by means of a mechanical device. She compared cyclic stretching, using a repeated, 10-second end-range mechanical stretch force followed by a brief rest, with a sustained (maintained) mechanical stretch. The intensity of the stretch force was applied to the level of the patient's tolerance and ability to remain relaxed. The stretching procedures were applied to the hamstrings of healthy subjects for 15 minutes per day for 5 consecutive days. Significant increases in hamstring extensibility were achieved using both stretching techniques. One week after stretching was discontinued, both groups maintained most of the gained ROM. Although both stretching techniques were effective, subjects reported that cyclic stretching was more comfortable and more tolerable than sustained stretching. Therefore the authors advocated cyclic over sustained stretching.

This study of cyclic and sustained stretching supports the importance of imposing a prolonged stretch on tight muscles and connective tissue to achieve plastic deformation and lengthening of soft tissues. A prolonged stretch is more likely to effect long-term gains in ROM. Prolonged mechanical stretching, either cyclic or sustained, seems to be consistently more effective than manual passive stretching because the stretch force is applied for a far longer duration than is practical with manual stretching.

B. Active Inhibition[3,18,39,54,61,65,68]

Active inhibition refers to techniques in which the patient reflexively relaxes the muscle to be elongated prior to or during the stretching maneuver. When a muscle is inhibited (relaxed), there is minimal resistance to elongation of the muscle. Active inhibition techniques relax only the contractile structures within muscle, not connective tissues. This type of stretching is possible only if the muscle to be elongated is normally innervated and under voluntary control. It cannot be used in patients with severe muscle weakness, spasticity, or paralysis from neuromuscular dysfunction.

Therapists have used active inhibition techniques, most of which have been adapted from proprioceptive neuromuscular facilitation (PNF) techniques,[68] for many years as an adjunct or alternative to manual passive stretching. Inhibition techniques increase muscle length by relaxing and elongating the contractile components of muscle. The assumption is that sarcomere give will occur more easily when the muscle is relaxed, with less active resistance (tension) in the muscle as it is elongated. An advantage of inhibition techniques is that muscle elongation is a more comfortable form of stretching than traditional high-intensity short-duration passive stretching. A disadvantage of active inhibition is that because it is a high-intensity stretch, it affects primarily the elastic structures of muscle and produces less permanent increase in soft tissue extensibility than more prolonged stretching methods.

Several variations of active inhibition techniques can be used to first relax (inhibit) and then elongate tight muscles. They include (1) hold-relax (HR), (2) hold-relax with agonist contraction (HR-AC), and (3) agonist contraction (AC). In classic PNF, these inhibition techniques are performed using diagonal patterns.[27,68] In this chapter inhibition techniques are described using anatomic planes of motion.

1. Hold-relax (HR)[11,18,52,54,61,67,68]

a. In the hold-relax procedure, the patient performs an *end-range isometric contraction* of the tight muscle before it is passively lengthened. The rationale behind this technique is that, after a prestretch contraction of the tight muscle, that same muscle will relax as the result of *autogenic inhibition* and therefore be more easily lengthened. The Golgi tendon organ (GTO) may fire and inhibit tension in the muscle so that it can be more easily lengthened.

b. A variation of the hold-relax technique is the *contract-relax* (CR) technique.[68] After the tight muscle has been passively lengthened, the patient performs a *concentric isotonic* contraction of the tight muscle against resistance before the muscle is elongated.

c. In the clinical and athletic training settings, practitioners have reported that both techniques appear to make passive elongation of muscle more comfortable for the patient than do manual passive stretching procedures.

d. Practitioners have assumed that the prestretch contraction causes a reflexive relaxation accompanied by a decrease in electromyographic (EMG) activity in the tight muscle. Some investigators[11,16,48] have refuted this assumption, whereas others have supported it. In two studies,[16,48] a postcontraction sensory discharge (increased EMG activity) was identified in the muscle to be lengthened. This indicated that the muscle to be stretched was not effectively relaxed. In another study, no postcontraction elevation in EMG activity was found with the use of the contract-relax technique.[11]

e. Obviously clinicians must evaluate the effectiveness of the hold-relax and contract-relax techniques and determine their usefulness with individual patients.

2. Hold-relax with agonist contraction (HR-AC)[11,17,18,48,68]

a. A variation of the hold-relax technique is a prestretch isometric contraction of the tight muscle and relaxation of the tight muscle followed by a concentric contraction of the muscle opposite the tight muscle. As the agonist muscle opposite the tight muscle shortens, the tight muscle lengthens. This technique combines *autogenic inhibition* and *reciprocal inhibition* to lengthen a tight muscle.

b. In one study,[17] the HR-AC technique produced a greater increase in ankle dorsiflexion range than did the HR technique. Both inhibition techniques produced a greater increase in range of ankle dorsiflexion than did manual passive stretching. In another study, there was no significant difference between HR and HR-AC techniques.[48]

3. Agonist contraction (AC)[3,10,11,18]

a. Another inhibition technique is agonist contraction. This term has been used in several studies, but it can be misunderstood. As with HR-AC, the "agonist" refers to the muscle opposite the tight muscle; "antagonist," therefore, refers to the tight muscle. During this procedure, the patient dynamically contracts (shortens) the muscle *opposite the tight muscle* against resistance. This causes a *reciprocal inhibition* of the tight muscle, and the tight muscle lengthens more easily as the extremity moves.

b. Therapists have found that this is an effective and very gentle way to lengthen a tight muscle, particularly if the tight muscle is painful or in the early stages of healing. This method is least effective when a patient has close to normal range.

C. Self-stretching

Self-stretching is a type of flexibility exercise that patients carry out themselves. Patients may passively stretch out their own contractures by using their body weight as the stretch force. They may also actively inhibit a muscle to increase its length. Self-stretching enables patients to independently maintain or increase ROM gained in treatment sessions. The guidelines for the intensity and duration of the stretch that apply to self-stretching are the same as those for passive stretching carried out by a therapist or mechanical stretching procedures.

Self-stretching techniques are an important aspect of a home exercise program and the long-term management of many musculoskeletal or neuromuscular problems. Educating the patient to safely carry out self-stretching procedures at home is important for the prevention of reinjury or future dysfunction. Specific self-stretching procedures will not be discussed or illustrated in this chapter. Illustrations and explanation for many self-stretching exercises can be found in Chapters 8 through 13 and 15, which all deal with exercises for the upper and lower extremities and trunk.

IV. Indications and Goals of Stretching[1,3,5,18,39,65]

A. Indications

1. When range of motion is limited as a result of contractures, adhesions, and scar tissue formation, leading to shortening of muscles, connective tissue, and skin.
2. When limitations may lead to structural (skeletal) deformities otherwise preventable.
3. When contractures interfere with everyday functional activities or nursing care.
4. When there is muscle weakness and opposing tissue tightness. Tight muscles must be elongated before weak muscles can be effectively strengthened.

B. Goals

1. The overall goal of stretching is to regain or re-establish normal range of motion of joints and mobility of soft tissues that surround a joint.
2. Specific goals are to:
   a. Prevent irreversible contractures.
   b. Increase the general flexibility of a part of the body in conjunction with strengthening exercises.
   c. Prevent or minimize the risk of musculotendinous injuries related to specific physical activities and sports.

V. Procedures for Applying Passive Stretching[1,5,18,32,46,53,61,67]

A. Evaluation of the Patient Prior to Stretching

1. Identify functional limitations that are the result of limited ROM.
2. Determine if soft tissue or joint limitation is the cause of decreased motion and choose appropriate stretching or joint mobilization techniques or a combination of both to correct the limitation. Always evaluate the joint for adequate joint play. Before beginning soft tissue stretching techniques at any treatment session, use joint mobilization techniques to re-establish some joint play.
3. Assess the underlying strength of muscles in which there is limitation of motion and realistically consider the value of stretching the limiting structures. The individual must have the capability of developing adequate strength to control the new range of motion.

B. Prior to the Initiation of Stretching

1. Consider the best type of stretching or alternative to stretching to increase range.
2. Explain the goals of stretching to the patient.
3. Position the patient in a comfortable and stable position that will allow the best plane of motion in which the stretching procedure can be done. The direction of stretch will be exactly opposite the direction of tightness.
4. Explain the procedure to the patient and be certain he or she understands.
5. Free the area to be stretched of any restrictive clothing, bandages, or splints.
6. Explain to the patient that it is important to be as relaxed as possible throughout the stretching period and that the stretching procedures will be geared to his or her tolerance level.
7. Employ relaxation techniques prior to stretching, if necessary. (See Section VI of this chapter for more specific information.)

8. Apply heat or any warm-up exercises to the soft tissues to be stretched. Warming tight structures increases their extensibility and decreases the possibility of injury.

C. When Applying the Stretch

1. Move the extremity slowly through the free range to the point of restriction.
2. Then grasp proximally and distally to the joint in which motion is to occur. The grasp should be firm but not uncomfortable to the patient. Use padding, if necessary, in areas with minimal subcutaneous tissue, over a bony surface, or with reduced sensitivity. Use the broad surfaces of the hands to apply all forces.
3. Firmly stabilize the proximal segment (manually or with equipment) and move the distal segment.
    a. To stretch a multijoint muscle, stabilize either the proximal or distal segment to which the tight muscle attaches.
    b. Stretch the muscle over one joint at a time, then over all joints simultaneously until optimum length of soft tissues is achieved.
    c. To minimize compressive forces in small joints, stretch the distal joints first and proceed proximally.
4. To avoid joint compression during the stretching procedure, apply very gentle (grade I) traction to the moving joint.
5. Apply the stretch force in a gentle, slow, and sustained manner. Take the restricted soft tissues to the point of tightness and then move just beyond.
    a. The force must be enough to place tension on the soft tissue structures, but not so great as to cause pain or injure the structures.
    b. Avoid ballistic stretching. Do not bounce the extremity at the end of the range. This will facilitate the stretch reflex and cause a reflex facilitation of the muscle being stretched. Ballistic stretching tends to cause the greatest amount of trauma and injury to tissues.
    c. In the stretched position, the patient should experience a sense of pulling or tightness of the structures being stretched, but not pain.
6. Hold the patient in the stretched position at least 15 to 30 seconds or longer.
    a. During this time the tension in the tissues should slowly decrease.
    b. When tension decreases, move the extremity or joint a little farther.
7. Gradually release the stretch force.
8. Allow the patient and therapist to rest momentarily and then repeat the maneuver.

NOTE: Do not attempt to gain full range in one or two treatment sessions. Increasing flexibility is a slow and gradual process. It may take several weeks of treatment to see significant results.

D. After Stretching

1. Apply cold to the soft tissues that have been stretched and allow these structures to cool in a lengthened position. This will minimize poststretch muscle soreness that can occur as the result of microtrauma during stretching. When soft tissues are cooled in a lengthened position, increases in range of motion are more readily maintained.[42,55]
2. Have the patient perform active exercises and functional activities that use the gained range of motion.
3. Develop a balance in strength in the antagonistic muscles in the new range so that there is control and stability as flexibility increases.

VI. Inhibition and Relaxation

Inhibition and relaxation procedures have been used for years by a variety of professionals to relieve pain, muscle tension, and associated physical and mental dysfunctions, including tension headaches, high blood pressure, and respiratory distress.[32,34,37,56,74]

Active inhibition techniques are reflex relaxation procedures that therapists use to inhibit muscle tension or guarding prior to lengthening. The background for these techniques has been discussed in Section III.B of this chapter. The procedures for application of active inhibition techniques are outlined in this section.

A brief overview of other therapeutic modalities used to promote relaxation and extensibility of soft tissue is also covered in this section.

A. Active Inhibition Techniques: Procedures for Application

1. Hold-relax (HR)

  a. Procedure
    (1) Start with the tight muscle in a comfortably lengthened position.
    (2) Ask the patient to isometrically contract the tight muscle against substantial resistance for 5 to 10 seconds until the muscle begins to fatigue.
    (3) Then have the patient voluntarily relax.
    (4) The therapist then lengthens the muscle by passively moving the extremity through the gained range.
    (5) Repeat the entire procedure after several seconds of rest. Have the patient rest with the muscle in a comfortably lengthened position.

  b. ***Precautions***
    (1) The isometric contraction of the tight muscle should not be painful.
    (2) It is not necessary for the patient to perform a maximal isometric contraction of the tight muscle prior to stretch. A *submaximal* isometric contraction held for a longer period will adequately inhibit the tight muscle. Postcontraction sensory discharge (lingering tension in muscle after the prestretch contraction) may be a greater problem if a maximum contraction is performed. A submaximal long-duration contraction will also be easier for the therapist to control if the patient is strong.

  c. Example: tight ankle plantarflexors
    (1) Dorsiflex the ankle to a comfortable position to lengthen the tight muscles.
    (2) Place your hand on the plantar surface of the patient's foot.
    (3) Have the patient isometrically contract the plantarflexors against your resistance for 5 to 10 seconds.
    (4) Tell the patient to relax; then passively dorsiflex the patient's ankle to lengthen the plantarflexors.

2. Hold-relax with agonist contraction (HR-AC)

  a. Procedure
    (1) Follow the same procedure as done for hold-relax.
    (2) After the patient contracts the tight muscle, have the patient perform a concentric contraction of the agonist, the muscle opposite the tight muscle. The patient actively moves the extremity through the increased range.

b. **_Precautions_**: same as for hold-relax
c. Example: tight ankle plantarflexors
   (1) Follow the procedures described in hold-reflex.
   (2) After the patient isometrically contracts the plantarflexors, have the patient actively dorsiflex the foot to elongate the plantarflexors.

3. Agonist contraction (AC)

a. Procedure
   (1) Passively lengthen the tight muscle to a comfortable position.
   (2) Have the patient perform a concentric (shortening) contraction of the agonist, the muscle opposite the tight muscle.
   (3) Apply mild resistance to the contracting muscle, but allow joint movement to occur.
   (4) The tight muscle will relax and lengthen as the result of reciprocal inhibition as joint movement occurs.
b. **_Precautions_**
   (1) Do not apply excessive resistance to the contracting muscle. This may cause irradiation of tension to the tight muscle rather than relaxation and may restrict movement of the joint or cause pain.
   (2) Remember: This procedure is often used when muscle spasm restricts joint movement. This type of active inhibition is very useful if a patient cannot generate a strong pain-free contraction of the tight muscle, which must be done in the hold-relax procedure.
c. Example: painful and tight ankle plantarflexors
   (1) Place the patient's ankle in a comfortable position.
   (2) Apply mild resistance to the dorsum of the foot as the patient dynamically contracts the dorsiflexors. Allow joint movement (increased dorsiflexion) with relaxation and elongation of the plantarflexors to occur.

B. Local Relaxation

1. Heat*

Warming up soft tissue prior to stretching will increase the extensibility of the shortened tissue. Warm muscles relax and lengthen more easily, making stretching more comfortable for the patient. As the temperature of muscle increases, the amount of force required to elongate noncontractile and contractile tissues and the time the stretch force must be applied decrease. As intramuscular temperature increases, connective tissue yields more easily to passive stretch, and the sensitivity of the GTO increases (which makes it more likely to fire and inhibit muscle tension).[20] Heating also minimizes the chance of microtrauma to soft tissue during stretching and therefore may decrease postexercise delayed-onset muscle soreness.[29,42,75,76] Heating can be achieved with superficial or deep heat applied to soft tissue before or during stretching. Low-intensity active exercise performed prior to stretching will increase circulation to soft tissue and warm the tissues to be stretched. Although results of studies differ, a brief walk, nonfatiguing cycling on a stationary bicycle, or a few minutes of active arm ex-

---

*Refs. 20, 22, 29, 33, 41, 43, 52, 55, 57, 70, 71.

ercise can all be used to increase intramuscular temperature before stretching activities are initiated.[22,33,57]

Although stretching is often thought of as a warm-up activity and performed prior to vigorous exercise, the clinician and patient must always remember that an appropriate warm-up must also occur in the preparation for stretching. It is debatable whether heating should occur prior to or during the stretching procedure.

The use of heat alone without stretching has been shown to have either little effect or no effect on long-term improvement in muscle flexibility.[29,59] The combination of heat and stretching produces greater long-term gains in tissue length than stretching without the application of prestretch heating.[29]

NOTE: The application of cold prior to stretching (cryostretching) has been advocated to decrease muscle tone and make the muscle less sensitive to stretch in healthy subjects[26] and in patients with spasticity or rigidity secondary to upper motor neuron lesions.[68] The use of cold immediately after soft tissue injury effectively decreases pain and muscle spasm.[38,52] Once soft tissue healing and scarring begin, cold makes healing tissues less extensible and more susceptible to microtrauma during stretching.[14,38] Cooling soft tissues in a lengthened position after stretching has also been shown to promote more permanent increases in soft tissue length and minimize poststretch muscle soreness.[42,55]

It is the authors' recommendation that cold be applied to injured soft tissues in the first 24 to 48 hours after injury to minimize swelling, muscle spasm, and pain. When stretching is indicated, soft tissues should be heated prior to or during the stretching maneuver. After stretching, cold should be applied to muscles held in a lengthened position to minimize poststretch muscle soreness and to promote longer lasting gains in ROM.

2. Massage[4,37]

It is well documented that massage, particularly deep massage, can be used to increase local circulation and to decrease muscle spasm and stiffness. Massage is often preceded by the application of heat to further improve the extensibility of soft tissues prior to stretching.

3. Biofeedback[37]

A patient, if properly trained, can monitor and reduce the amount of tension in a muscle through biofeedback. Through visual or auditory feedback, a patient can begin to sense or feel what muscle relaxation is. Biofeedback is just one tool that can be useful in helping the patient learn and practice the process of relaxation. By reducing muscle tension, pain can be decreased and flexibility increased.

4. Joint traction or oscillation[18,32]

a. Slight manual distraction of joint surfaces prior to or in conjunction with joint mobilization or stretching techniques can be used to inhibit joint pain and spasm of muscles around a joint (see Chapter 6).[18]

b. Pendular motions[32] of a joint, advocated by Codman, use the weight of the limb to distract the joint surfaces and thereby to oscillate and relax the limb (see Fig. 8–1). The joint may be further distracted by adding a 1- or 2-lb weight to the extremity, which will cause a stretch force on joint tissues.

C. General Relaxation[34,37,56]

1. General progressive relaxation techniques may also be a useful adjunct to a stretching program. A patient may learn to relax the total body or an extremity. Tension in muscles can be relieved by conscious effort and thought. Some techniques, such as autogenic relaxation advocated by Schultz,[56] suggest progressive conscious control and relaxation of muscle and body tension. Other techniques, such as Jacobson's progressive relaxation,[34] suggest a systematic distal-to-proximal progression of conscious contraction and relaxation of musculature.

2. Procedures for progressive relaxation training.[7,34,37,56]
   a. Place the patient in a quiet area and in a comfortable position, and be sure that he or she is free of restrictive clothing.
   b. Have the patient breathe in a deep, relaxed manner.
   c. Ask the patient to voluntarily contract the distal musculature in the hands or feet for a few seconds. Then have the patient consciously relax those muscles.
   d. Suggest that the patient try to feel a sense of heaviness in the hands or feet.
   e. Suggest to the patient that he or she feels a sense of warmth in the muscles just relaxed.
   f. Progress to a more proximal area of the body. Have the patient actively contract and then actively relax more proximal musculature. Eventually have the patient isometrically contract and then consciously relax the entire extremity.
   g. Suggest to the patient that he or she should feel a sense of heaviness and warmth throughout the entire limb and eventually throughout the whole body.

NOTE: Any combination of local and general relaxation may be used by the therapist to promote maximum muscle relaxation and therefore the potential for maximum muscle flexibility in a stretching program.

VII. Precautions and Contraindications

A. Precautions for Stretching[1,5,18,31,39,66]

1. Do not passively force a joint beyond its normal range of motion. Remember, normal range of motion varies among individuals.
2. Newly united fractures should be protected by stabilization between the fracture site and the joint in which the motion takes place.
3. Use extra caution in patients with known or suspected osteoporosis due to disease, prolonged bed rest, age, and prolonged use of steroids.
4. Avoid vigorous stretching of muscles and connective tissues that have been immobilized over a long time. Connective tissues (tendons and ligaments) lose their tensile strength after prolonged immobilization.
   a. High-intensity short-duration stretching procedures tend to cause more trauma and resulting weakness of soft tissues than low-intensity long-duration stretch.
   b. Strengthening exercises should be concurrently built into a stretching program as range of motion increases so that a patient can develop an appropriate balance between flexibility and strength.
5. If a patient experiences joint pain or muscle soreness lasting more than 24 hours after stretching, too much force has been used during stretching and an inflammatory response is occurring that will cause increased scar tissue formation. Pa-

tients should experience no more residual discomfort than a transitory feeling of tenderness.

6. Avoid stretching edematous tissue, as it is more susceptible to injury than normal tissue. Continued irritation of edematous tissues usually causes increased pain and edema.

7. Avoid overstretching weak muscles, particularly those that support body structures in relation to gravity.

B. Contraindications to Stretching

1. When a bony block limits joint motion
2. After a recent fracture
3. Whenever there is evidence of an acute inflammatory or infectious process (heat and swelling) in the tight tissues and surrounding region
4. Whenever there is sharp, acute pain with joint movement or muscle elongation
5. When a hematoma or other indication of tissue trauma is observed
6. When contractures or shortened soft tissues are providing increased joint stability in lieu of normal structural stability or muscle strength
7. When contractures or shortened soft tissues are the basis for increased functional abilities, particularly in patients with paralysis or severe muscle weakness

VIII. Techniques of Stretching Using Anatomic Planes of Motion

As with range of motion (ROM) exercises described in Chapter 2, the following techniques are described with the patient in a supine position. Alternate patient positions such as prone or seated are indicated for some motions and are noted when necessary.

Effective manual stretching techniques require adequate stabilization of the patient and sufficient strength and good body mechanics of the therapist. Depending on the size (height and weight) of the therapist and the patient, variations in the position of the patient and suggested hand placements may have to be made by the therapist.

Each description of a stretching technique is identified by the plane of motion that is to be increased and followed by a notation of the muscle group being stretched. Each section contains a discussion of special considerations for each joint being stretched.

Prolonged passive stretching techniques using mechanical equipment are applied in the same positions and using the same points of stabilization as manual passive stretching. The stretch force is applied at a lower intensity and is applied over a much longer period than with manual passive stretching. The stretch force is provided by a weighted pulley system rather than the strength of a therapist. The patient is stabilized with belts, straps, or counterweights.

Self-stretching techniques of the extremities and trunk, which the patient can do without assistance from the therapist, are not covered in this chapter. These techniques are found for each joint of the extremities in Chapters 8 through 13. Stretching procedures for the musculature of the cervical, thoracic, and lumbar spine are found in Chapter 15.

A. The Upper Extremity

1. The shoulder: special considerations

Many muscles involved with shoulder motion attach to the scapula rather than the thorax. Therefore, when most muscles of the shoulder girdle are stretched, it is mandatory to stabilize the scapula. Without scapular stabilization the stretch force will be transmitted to those muscles that normally stabilize the scapula during movement of the arm. This subjects these muscles to possible over-stretching and disguises the true range of motion of the glenohumeral joint.

Remember:

—When the scapula is stabilized and not allowed to abduct or up-wardly rotate, only 120 degrees of shoulder flexion and abduction can occur at the glenohumeral joint.

—When scapular movement is stabilized, the humerus must be exter-nally rotated to gain full range of motion.

—Muscles most apt to exhibit tightness are those that *prevent* full shoulder flexion, abduction, and rotation. It is rare to find tightness in structures that prevent shoulder adduction and extension to neu-tral.

a. **To increase flexion of the shoulder** (to stretch the shoulder extensors) (Fig. 5–7)

(1) Hand placement

Grasp the posterior aspect of the distal humerus, just above the elbow.

(2) Stabilize the axillary border of the scapula to stretch the teres major, or stabilize the lateral aspect of the thorax and superior aspect of the pelvis to stretch the latissimus dorsi.

(3) Move the patient into full shoulder flexion to elongate the shoulder ex-tensors.

b. **To increase hyperextension of the shoulder** (to stretch the shoulder flex-ors) (Fig. 5–7)

(1) Alternate position

Place the patient in a prone position.

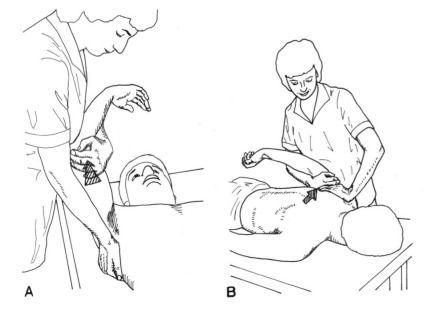

Figure 5–7. (*A*) Hand placement and stabilization of the scapula for stretch-ing procedure to elongate the teres major. (*B*) Hand placement and stabi-lization of the scapula to increase hy-perextension of the shoulder.

A   B

    (2) Hand placement

        Support the forearm and grasp the distal humerus.

    (3) Stabilize the posterior aspect of the scapula to prevent substitute movements.

    (4) Move the patient's arm into full hyperextension of the shoulder to elongate the shoulder flexors.

c. **To increase abduction of the shoulder** (to stretch the adductors) (Fig. 5–8)

    (1) Hand placement

        With the elbow flexed to 90 degrees, grasp the distal humerus.

    (2) Stabilize the axillary border of the scapula.

    (3) Move the patient into full shoulder abduction to lengthen the adductors of the shoulder.

d. **To increase adduction of the shoulder** (to stretch the abductors)

    (1) It is rare that a patient will not be able to fully adduct the shoulder to 0 degrees (so the upper arm is at the patient's side).

    (2) Even if a patient has worn an abduction splint after a soft tissue or joint injury of the shoulder, when the patient is upright the constant pull of gravity will elongate the shoulder abductors so the patient can adduct to a neutral position.

e. **To increase external rotation of the shoulder** (to stretch the internal rotators) (Fig. 5–9)

    (1) Hand placement

        Abduct the shoulder to 45 to 90 degrees or place the arm at the side and flex the elbow to 90 degrees. Grasp the distal forearm with one hand and stabilize the elbow with the other hand.

    (2) Stabilization of the scapula will be provided by the table upon which the patient is lying.

    (3) Externally rotate the patient's shoulder by moving the patient's forearm closer to the table. This will fully lengthen the internal rotators.

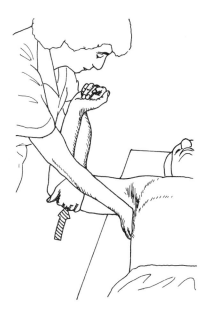

Figure 5–8. Hand placement and stabilization of the scapula for stretching procedure to increase shoulder abduction.

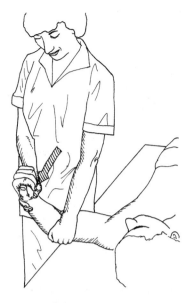

Figure 5–9. Hand placement and stabilization of the scapula for stretching procedure to increase external rotation of the shoulder.

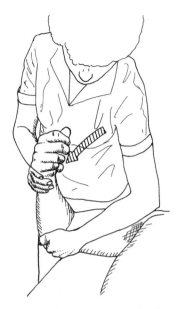

Figure 5–10. Hand placement and stabilization of the shoulder to increase internal rotation of the shoulder.

NOTE: It is necessary to apply the stretch forces across the intermediate elbow joint when elongating the internal and external rotators of the shoulder. Therefore, be sure the elbow joint is stable and pain free.

f. **To increase internal rotation of the shoulder** (to stretch the external rotators) (Fig. 5–10)
   (1) Hand placement
   Same as when increasing external rotation of the shoulder.
   (2) Stabilize the anterior aspect of the shoulder.
   (3) Move the patient into internal rotation to lengthen the external rotators of the shoulder.

g. **To increase horizontal abduction of the shoulder** (to stretch the pectoralis muscles)
   (1) Alternate position
   To reach full horizontal abduction in supine position, the patient's shoulder must be at the edge of the table. As with passive ROM (see Fig. 2–5A), begin with the shoulder in 90 degrees of abduction; the patient's elbow may also be flexed.
   (2) Hand placement
   Grasp the anterior aspect of the distal humerus.
   (3) Stabilize the anterior aspect of the shoulder.
   (4) Move the patient's arm into full horizontal abduction to stretch the horizontal adductors.

   NOTE: The horizontal adductors are usually tight bilaterally. Stretching techniques can be applied bilaterally by the therapist, or a bilateral self-stretch can be done by the patient by using a corner or wand (see Figs. 8–18 through 8–20).

h. **Scapular mobilization**
  (1) To have full shoulder motion, a patient must have normal scapular mobility.
  (2) See scapular mobilization techniques in Chapter 6.

2. **Elbow and forearm: special considerations**

   Several muscles that cross the elbow, such as the biceps brachii and brachioradialis, also influence supination and pronation of the forearm. Therefore, when stretching the elbow flexors and extensors, the forearm should be pronated and supinated.

   Precaution: Vigorous stretching of the elbow flexors may cause internal trauma to these muscles. This may precipitate myositis ossificans, especially in children. Passive stretching should be done gently, or the use of active inhibition techniques should be considered.

   a. **To increase elbow flexion** (to stretch the elbow extensors) (see Fig. 2–7).
      (1) Hand placement
          Grasp the distal forearm just proximal to the wrist.
      (2) Stabilize the humerus.
      (3) Flex the patient's elbow just past the point of tightness to lengthen the elbow extensors.

   b. **To increase elbow extension** (to stretch the elbow flexors) (Fig. 5–11).
      (1) Hand placement
          Grasp the distal forearm.
      (2) Stabilize the scapula and anterior aspect of the proximal humerus.
      (3) Extend the elbow as far as possible to lengthen the elbow flexors.

          NOTE: Be sure to do this with the forearm in supination, pronation, and a neutral position to stretch each of the elbow flexors.

   c. **To increase supination or pronation of the forearm** (see Fig. 2–10)
      (1) Hand placement
          With the patient's humerus supported on the table and the elbow flexed to 90 degrees, grasp the distal forearm.

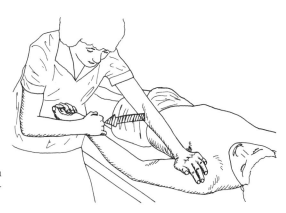

Figure 5–11. Hand placement and stabilization of the scapula and proximal humerus for stretching procedures to increase elbow extension.

(2) Stabilize the humerus.

(3) Supinate or pronate the forearm just beyond the point of tightness as indicated. Be sure the force is applied to the radius rotating around the ulna. Do not twist the hand.

(4) Repeat the procedure with the elbow extended. Be sure to stabilize the humerus to prevent internal or external rotation of the shoulder.

3. The wrist: special considerations

The extrinsic muscles of the fingers cross the wrist joint and therefore may influence the range of motion of the wrist. Wrist motion may also be influenced by the position of the elbow and forearm because the wrist flexors and extensors attach proximally to the epicondyles of the humerus.

When stretching the musculature of the wrist, the stretch force should be applied proximal to the metacarpophalangeal (MCP) joints, and the fingers should be relaxed.

Alternate position: It may be easier to have the patient sitting in a chair adjacent to the therapist, with the forearm supported on the table, rather than lying supine.

a. **To increase wrist flexion** (see Fig. 2–11)

(1) Hand placement

Supinate the forearm and grasp the patient at the dorsal aspect of the hand.

(2) Stabilize the forearm.

(3) To elongate the wrist extensors, flex the patient's wrist and allow the fingers to extend passively. To further elongate the wrist extensors, extend the patient's elbow.

(4) Alternate position

The patient's forearm may also be in mid-position and supported along the ulna.

b. **To increase wrist extension** (Fig. 5–12)

(1) Hand placement

Pronate the forearm and grasp the patient at the palmar aspect of the hand.

(2) Stabilize the forearm.

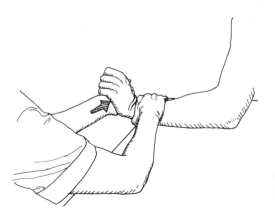

Figure 5–12. Hand placement and stabilization of the forearm for stretching procedure to increase extension of the wrist.

(3) To lengthen the wrist flexors, extend the patient's wrist, allowing the fingers to passively flex.

(4) Alternate position

Support the patient's forearm on the table but allow the hand to drop over the edge of the table. Then passively extend the wrist. This may be more comfortable for the therapist or necessary if the patient has a severe wrist flexion contracture.

(5) Alternate position

The patient's forearm may also be in mid-position and supported along the ulna.

c. **To increase radial deviation**

(1) Hand placement

Grasp the ulnar aspect of the hand along the fifth metacarpal. Hold the wrist in mid-position.

(2) Stabilize the forearm.

(3) Radially deviate the wrist to lengthen the ulnar deviators of the wrist.

d. **To increase ulnar deviation**

(1) Hand placement

Grasp the radial aspect of the hand along the second metacarpal, not the thumb.

(2) Stabilize the forearm.

(3) Ulnarly deviate the wrist to lengthen the radial deviators.

4. **The fingers: special considerations**

The complexity of joints and multijoint muscles of the fingers requires careful evaluation of the factors limiting motion and specifically the location of the limited motion. Fingers should always be stretched individually, not grossly stretched.

If an extrinsic muscle limits motion, lengthen it over one joint while stabilizing the other joints. Then lengthen it over two joints simultaneously, and so forth, until normal length is obtained. As noted in Chapter 2, begin the motion with the most distal joint to minimize joint compression of the small joints of the fingers.

Do not produce hypermobility in one joint while stretching a tendon across two more joints simultaneously. This is particularly important at the MCP joints when stretching the flexor digitorum profundus.

The web space between the first and second metacarpals is crucial for a functional hand. Stretch this area by applying force to the heads of the first and second metacarpals, not the phalanges.

a. **To increase flexion and extension and abduction and adduction of the MCP joints** (see Fig. 2–13A)

(1) Hand placement

Grasp the proximal phalanx with your thumb and index finger.

(2) Stabilize the metacarpal with your other thumb and index finger. Keep the wrist in mid-position.

(3) Move the MCP joint in the desired direction for stretch. Allow the PIP and DIP joints to passively flex or extend.

b. **To increase flexion and extension of the PIP and DIP joints** (see Fig. 2–13B)

(1) Hand placement

Grasp the middle or distal phalanx with your thumb and finger.

(2) Stabilize the proximal or middle phalanx with your other thumb and finger.

(3) Move the PIP or DIP joint in the desired direction for stretch.

c. **Stretching specific extrinsic and intrinsic muscles of the fingers**

In Chapter 2 (Section VI.A.13) elongation of extrinsic and intrinsic muscles of the hand is described. To stretch these muscles beyond their available range, the same hand placement and stabilization are used as with passive ROM. The only difference in technique is that the therapist moves the patient beyond the point of tightness.

B. The Lower Extremity

1. The hip: special considerations

Because muscles of the hip attach to the pelvis or lumbar spine, the pelvis must always be stabilized when lengthening muscles about the hip. If the pelvis is not stabilized, the stretch force will be transferred to the lumbar spine, in which unwanted compensatory motion will occur.

a. **To increase flexion of the hip with the knee flexed** (to stretch the gluteus maximus) (see Fig. 2–15B)

(1) Hand placement

Flex the hip and knee simultaneously.

(2) Stabilize the opposite femur in extension to prevent a posterior tilt of the pelvis.

(3) Move the patient's hip and knee into full flexion to lengthen the one-joint hip extensor.

b. **To increase flexion of the hip with the knee extended** (to stretch the hamstrings [Fig. 5–13A])

(1) Hand placement

With the patient's knee fully extended, support the patient's lower leg with your arm or shoulder.

(2) Stabilize the opposite extremity along the anterior aspect of the thigh with your other hand or a belt or with the assistance of another person.

(3) With the knee in maximum extension, flex the hip as far as possible.

(4) Alternate position (Fig. 5–13B).

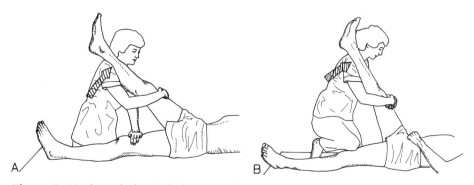

Figure 5–13. (*A* and *B*) Hand placement and stabilization of the pelvis and low back for stretching procedures to increase hip flexion with knee extension (stretch the hamstrings).

    (a) Kneel on the mat and place the patient's heel against your shoulder. Place both of your hands along the anterior aspect of the distal femur to keep the knee extended.

    (b) The opposite extremity is stabilized in extension by a belt or towel and held in place by the therapist's knee.

  c. **To increase hip extension** (to stretch the iliopsoas) (Fig. 5–14)

    (1) Stabilize the pelvis by flexing the opposite hip and knee to the patient's chest. Maintain that position to prevent an anterior tilt of the pelvis during stretching.

    (2) Hand placement and position of patient

       (a) Have the patient close to the edge of the bed so that the hip being stretched can be hyperextended.

       (b) While stabilizing the opposite hip and pelvis with one hand, move the hip to be stretched into extension or hyperextension by placing a downward pressure on the anterior aspect of the distal femur with your other hand.

    (3) Alternate position

    Patient lying prone (Fig. 5–15)

       (a) Hand placement

       Support and grasp the anterior aspect of the patient's distal femur.

       (b) Stabilize the patient's buttocks to prevent movement of the pelvis.

       (c) Hyperextend the patient's hip by lifting the femur off the table.

  d. **To increase hip extension and knee flexion simultaneously** (to stretch the rectus femoris)

    (1) Position of patient (see Fig. 5–14)

    Flex the opposite hip and knee to the patient's chest to stabilize the pelvis.

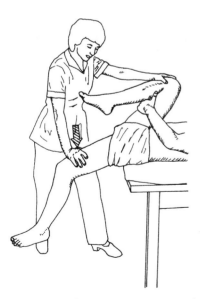

Figure 5–14. Hand placement and stabilization of the pelvis to increase hyperextension of the hip (stretch the iliopsoas) with the patient lying supine.

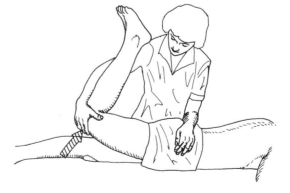

Figure 5–15. Hand placement and stabilization to increase hyperextension of the hip with the patient lying prone.

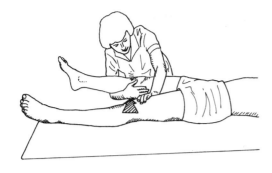

Figure 5–16. Hand placement and stabilization of the opposite extremity and pelvis for stretching procedure to increase abduction of the hip.

    (2) Hand placement

        With the hip to be stretched in full extension, place your hand on the distal tibia and gently flex the knee of that extremity as far as possible.

  e. **To increase abduction of the hip** (to stretch the adductors [Fig. 5–16])

    (1) Hand placement

        Support the distal thigh with your arm and forearm.

    (2) Stabilize the pelvis by placing pressure on the opposite anterior iliac crest or by maintaining the opposite lower extremity in slight abduction.

    (3) Abduct the hip as far as possible to stretch the adductors.

        NOTE: You may apply your stretch force cautiously at the medial malleolus only if the knee is stable and pain free. This creates a great deal of stress to the medial supporting structures of the knee and is generally not recommended by the authors.

  f. **To increase adduction of the hip** (to stretch the tensor fasciae latae)

    (1) Alternate position (Fig. 5–17)

        Place the patient in a side-lying position with the hip to be stretched uppermost. Flex the bottom hip and knee to stabilize the patient.

    (2) Hand placement

        Extend the patient's hip to neutral or into slight hyperextension, if possible. Place your hand on the lateral aspect of the distal femur.

    (3) Stabilize the pelvis at the iliac crest with your other hand.

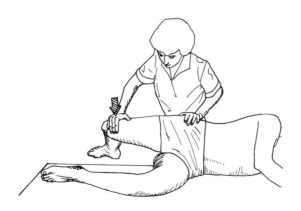

Figure 5–17. Patient positioned side-lying. Hand placement and procedure to stretch the tensor fasciae latae.

(4) Let the patient's hip adduct with gravity and apply the stretch force to the lateral aspect of the distal femur to further adduct the hip.

NOTE: If the patient's hip cannot be extended to neutral, the hip flexors must be stretched before the tensor fasciae latae can be stretched.

g. **To increase external rotation of the hip** (to stretch the internal rotators)
   (1) Alternate position (Fig. 5–18)
       Place the patient in a prone position, hips extended and knee flexed to 90 degrees.
   (2) Hand placement
       Grasp the distal tibia of the extremity to be stretched.
   (3) Stabilize the pelvis by applying pressure with your other hand across the buttocks.
   (4) Apply pressure to the lateral malleolus and externally rotate the hip as far as possible.

   NOTE: You must apply your stretch force at the ankle, thus crossing the knee joint. If you stretch the hip rotators in this manner, the knee must be stable and pain free.

h. **To increase internal rotation of the hip** (to stretch the external rotators)
   (1) Alternate position and stabilization (Fig. 5–18)
       Same as when increasing external rotation described previously.
   (2) Hand placement
       Apply pressure to the medial malleolus and internally rotate the hip as far as possible.

2. **The knee: special considerations**

The position of the hip during stretching will influence the flexibility of the flexors and extensors of the knee. The flexibility of the hamstrings and the rectus femoris must be evaluated separately from the one-joint muscles that affect knee motion.

a. **To increase knee flexion** (to stretch the knee extensors)

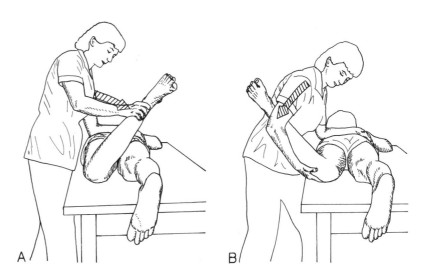

Figure 5–18. (*A* and *B*) Hand placement and stabilization to increase external and internal rotation of the hip with patient prone.

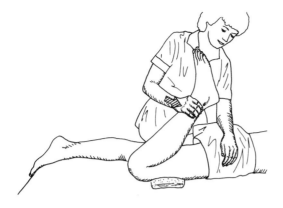

Figure 5–19. Hand placement and stabilization to increase knee flexion (stretch the rectus femoris and quadriceps) with the patient lying prone.

    (1) Alternate position
      Patient lying prone (Fig. 5–19).
      (a) Stabilize the pelvis by applying a downward pressure across the buttocks.
      (b) Hand placement
          Grasp the anterior aspect of the distal tibia and flex the patient's knee.

          NOTE: Place a rolled towel under the thigh just above the knee to prevent compression of the patella against the table during the stretch.

          Precaution: Stretching the knee extensors too vigorously in the prone position can traumatize the knee joint and cause edema.
    (2) Alternate position
      (a) Have the patient sit over the edge of a table (hips flexed to 90 degrees and knee flexed as far as possible).
      (b) Stabilize the anterior aspect of the proximal femur with one hand.
      (c) Apply the stretch force to the anterior aspect of the distal tibia and flex the patient's knee as far as possible.
          NOTE:
          i. This position is useful when working in the 0- to 100-degree range of knee flexion.
          ii. The prone position is best for increasing knee flexion from 90 to 135 degrees.

  b. **To increase knee extension in the mid-range** (to stretch the knee flexors)
    (1) Alternate position (Fig. 5–20)
      Place the patient in a prone position and put a small, rolled towel under the patient's distal femur, just above the patella.
    (2) Hand placement and stabilization
      Grasp the distal tibia with one hand and stabilize the buttocks to prevent hip flexion with the other hand. Slowly extend the knee to stretch the knee flexors.

  c. **To increase knee extension at the end of the range** (Fig. 5–21)
    (1) Hand placement
      Grasp the distal tibia of the knee to be stretched.

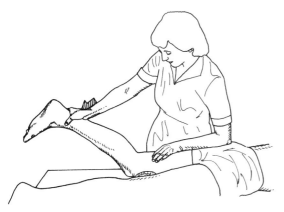

Figure 5-20. Hand placement and stabilization to increase mid-range knee extension with the patient lying prone.

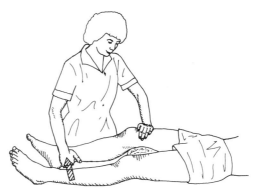

Figure 5-21. Hand placement and stabilization to increase knee extension at the end of the range.

(2) Stabilize the hip by placing your hand or forearm across the anterior thigh. This will prevent hip flexion during stretching.

(3) Apply the stretch force to the posterior aspect of the distal tibia and extend the patient's knee.

3. The ankle: special considerations

The ankle is composed of multiple joints. Consider the mobility of these joints (see Chapter 6) as well as the soft tissues around these joints when increasing range of motion of the ankle.

a. **To increase dorsiflexion of the ankle with the knee extended** (to stretch the gastrocnemius muscle) (see Fig. 2-20)

   (1) Hand placement

       Grasp the patient's heel (calcaneus) with one hand.

   (2) Stabilize the anterior aspect of the tibia with your other hand.

   (3) Pull the calcaneus downward with your thumb and fingers and gently push upward on the heads of the metatarsals.

b. **To increase dorsiflexion of the ankle with the knee flexed** (to stretch the soleus muscle)

   (1) To eliminate the effect of the two-joint gastrocnemius muscle, the knee must be flexed.

   (2) Hand placement, stabilization, and stretch force are the same as when stretching the gastrocnemius.

       Precaution: Avoid placing too much pressure against the heads of the metatarsals and stretching the long arch of the foot. Overstretching the long arch of the foot can cause a rocker-bottom foot.

c. **To increase plantarflexion of the ankle**

   (1) Hand placement

       (a) Support the posterior aspect of the distal tibia with one hand.

       (b) Grasp the foot along the tarsal and metatarsal areas.

   (2) Apply the stretch force to the anterior aspect of the foot and plantarflex the foot as far as possible.

d. **To increase inversion and eversion of the ankle**

Inversion and eversion of the ankle occur at the subtalar joint. Mobility of the subtalar joint (with appropriate strength) is important for walking on uneven surfaces.

(1) To increase motion in this joint, grasp the calcaneus and move it medially and laterally while stabilizing the talus (see Figs. 2–21A and B).

(2) To stretch the tibialis anterior (which inverts and dorsiflexes the ankle).

(a) Grasp the anterior aspect of the foot.

(b) Plantarflex and evert the ankle.

(3) To stretch the tibialis posterior (which plantarflexes and inverts the foot).

(a) Grasp the plantar surface of the foot.

(b) Dorsiflex and evert the foot.

(4) To stretch the peroneals (which evert the foot).

(a) Grasp the tarsal region of the foot.

(b) Invert the foot.

e. **To increase flexion and extension of the toes** (see Fig. 2–23)

NOTE: It is best to individually stretch any tight musculature that affects motion in the toes. With one hand, stabilize the bone proximal to the tight joint, and with the other hand move the joint in the desired direction.

C. The Trunk

Stretching techniques to increase motion in the cervical, thoracic, and lumbar spine can be found in Chapter 15.

IX. Summary

This chapter has provided an overview of background, principles, and procedures for the application of stretching techniques. Causes of soft tissue contractures related to immobilization, trauma, and disease and the changes that occur in muscle and connective tissue when immobilized have been reviewed.

The mechanical and neurophysiologic properties of contractile and noncontractile tissues have been described. The response of these tissues to stretching procedures have also been discussed. Indications and goals for stretching as well as precautions and contraindications have been reviewed.

Various methods of active inhibition and passive stretching have been explained. Procedures and techniques of relaxation, active inhibition, and passive stretching have been covered in detail. Emphasis has been placed on positioning of patient, stabilization of joints, and placement of the therapist's hand.

References

1. Agre, JC: Static stretching for athletes. Arc d Rehabil 59:561, 1978.
2. Astrand, PO, and Rodahl, K: Textbook of Work Physiology, ed 2. McGraw-Hill, New York, 1977.
3. Bandy, WB, and Irion, JM: The effects of time on static stretch on the flexibility of the hamstring muscles. Phys Ther 74:845–850, 1994.
4. Beard, G, and Wood, E: Massage: Principles and Techniques, ed 3. WB Saunders, Philadelphia, 1981.
5. Beaulieu, JA: Developing a stretching program. The Physician and Sportsmedicine 9:59, 1981.
6. Becker, RO: The electrical response of human skeletal muscle to passive stretch. Surg Forum 10:828, 1960.

7. Benson, H, Beary, JF, and Carol, MP: The relaxation response. Psychiatry 37:37, 1974.

8. Bohannon, RW: Effect of repeated eight minute muscle loading on the angle of straight leg raising. Phys Ther 64:491, 1984.

9. Bohannon, RW, and Larkin, PA: Passive ankle dorsiflexion increases in patients after a regimen of tilt table: Wedge board standing. Phys Ther 65:1676, 1985.

10. Cherry, D: Review of physical therapy alternatives for reducing muscle contracture. Phys Ther 60:877, 1980.

11. Condon, SN, and Hutton, RS: Soleus muscle electromyographic activity and ankle dorsiflexion range of motion during four stretching procedures. Phys Ther 67:24, 1987.

12. Cornwall, M: Biomechanics of noncontractile tissue: A review. Phys Ther 64:1869, 1984.

13. Cummings, GS, Crutchfeld, CA, and Barnes, MR: Soft Tissue Changes in Contractures, Vol 1. Stokesville, Atlanta, 1983.

14. Cummings, GS, and Tillman, LJ: Remodeling of dense connective tissue in normal adult tissues. In Currier, DP, and Nelson, RM (eds): Dynamics of Human Biologic Tissues. FA Davis, Philadelphia, 1992.

15. Donatelli, R, and Owens-Burkhart, H: Effects of immobilization on the extensibility of periarticular connective tissue. Journal of Orthopaedic and Sports Physical Therapy 3:67, 1981.

16. Eldred, E, Hulton, RS, and Smith, JL: Nature of persisting changes in afferent discharge from muscle following its contraction. Prog Brain Res 44:157, 1976.

17. Etnyre, BR, and Abraham, LD: Gains in range of ankle dorsiflexion using three popular stretching techniques. Am J Phys Med 65:189, 1986.

18. Evjenth, O, and Hamberg, J: Muscle Stretching in Manual Therapy: A Clinical Manual, Vol 1. Alfta, Rehab, Alfta, Sweden, 1984.

19. Flitney, FW, and Hirst, DG: Cross bridge detachment and sarcomere "give" during stretch of active frog's muscle. J Physiol 276:449, 1978.

20. Fukami, Y, and Wilkinson, RS: Responses of isolated golgi tendon organs of the cat. J Physiol 265:673–689, 1977.

21. Gajdosik, RL: Effects of static stretching on the maximal length and resistance to passive stretch of short hamstring muscles Journal of Orthopaedic and Sports Physical Therapy 14(6):250–255, 1991.

22. Gillette, TM, et al: Relationship of body core temperature and warm-up to knee range of motion. Journal of Orthopaedic and Sports Physical Therapy 13(3):126–131, 1991.

23. Godges, JJ, et al: The effects of two stretching procedures on hip range of motion and gait economy. Journal of Orthopaedic and Sports Physical Therapy 10(9):350–356, 1989.

24. Gossman, M, Sahrmann, S, and Rose, S: Review of length-associated changes in muscle. Phys Ther 62:1799, 1982.

25. Griffiths, PJ, et al: Cross bridge slippage in skinned frog muscle fibers. Biophys Struct Mech 7:107, 1980.

26. Halkovich, LR, et al; Effect of Fluori-Methane® spray on passive hip flexion. Phys Ther 61:185–189, 1981.

27. Hanten, WP, and Chandler, SD: The effect of myofascial release leg pull and saggital plane isometric contract-relax technique on passive straight-leg raise an-

gle. Journal of Orthopaedic and Sports Physical Therapy 20:138–144, 1994.

28. Hardy, MA: The biology of scar formation. Phys Ther 69:1015, 1989.

29. Henricson, AS, et al: The effect of heat and stretching on range of hip motion. Journal of Orthopaedic and Sports Physical Therapy 6(2):110–115, 1985.

30. Hepburn, G, and Crivelli, K: Use of elbow Dynasplint for reduction of elbow flexion contracture: A case study. J Orthop Sports Phys Ther 5:269, 1984.

31. Hlasney, J: Effect of flexibility exercises on muscle strength. Phys Ther Forum 7:3, 15, 1988.

32. Hollis, M: Practical Exercise Therapy, ed 2. Blackwell Scientific, Oxford, 1982.

33. Hubley, CL, Korzey, JW, and Stansih, WD: The effects of static stretching exercise and stationary cycling on range of motion at the hip joint. Journal of Orthopaedic and Sports Physical Therapy 6(2):104–109, 1984.

34. Jacobson, E: Progressive Relaxation. University of Chicago Press, Chicago, 1929.

35. Kendall, F, and McCreary, E: Muscles: Testing and Function, ed 3. Williams & Wilkins, Baltimore, 1983.

36. Kendall, H, and Kendall, F: Posture and Pain. Williams & Wilkins, Baltimore, 1952.

37. Kessler, R, and Hertling, D: Management of Common Musculoskeletal Disorders. Harper & Row, Philadelphia, 1983.

38. Knight, KL: Cryotherapy: Theory, Technique and Physiology. Chattanooga Corp, Chattanooga, TN, 1989.

39. Kottke, F: Therapeutic exercise. In Krusen, F, Kottke, F, and Ellwood, M (eds): Handbook of Physical Medicine and Rehabilitation, ed 2. WB Saunders, Philadelphia, 1971.

40. Kottke, FJ, Pauley, DL, and Park, KA: The rationale for prolonged stretching for correction of shortening of connective tissue. Arch Phys Med Rehabil 47:345, 1966.

41. Lehmann, JF, et al: The effect of therapeutic temperatures on tendon extensibility. Arch Phys Med Rehabil 51:481, 1970.

42. Lentell, G, et al: The use of thermal agents to influence the effectiveness of a low-load prolonged stretch. Journal of Orthopaedic and Sports Physical Therapy 16(5):200–207, 1992.

43. Leveau, B: Basic biomechanics in sports and orthopedic therapy. In Gould, J, and Davies, G (eds): Orthopedic and Sports Physical Therapy. CV Mosby, St Louis, 1985.

44. Light, KE, et al: Low-load prolonged stretch vs. high-load brief stretch in treating knee contractures. Phys Ther 64:330, 1984.

45. Madding, SW, et al: Effect of duration of passive stretch on hip abduction range of motion. Journal of Orthopaedic and Sports Physical Therapy 8:409, 1987.

46. McClure, M: Exercise and training for spinal patients. Part B: Flexibility training. In Basmajian, JV, and Nyberg, R (eds): Rational Manual Therapies. Williams & Wilkins, Baltimore, 1993.

47. Medeiros, J, et al: The influence of isometric exercise and passive stretch on hip joint motion. Phys Ther 57:518, 1977.

48. Moore, MA, and Hutton, R: Electromyographic inves-

tigation of muscle stretching techniques. Med Sci Sports Exer 12:322, 1980.

49. Noyes, FR, et al: Biomechanics of ligament failure. J Bone Joint Surg Am 56:1406, 1974.

50. Noyes, FR: Functional properties of knee ligaments and alterations induced by immobilization. Clin Orthop Rel Res 123:210, 1977.

51. Noyes, FR, Keller, CS, Grood, ES, and Butler, DL: Advances in understanding of knee ligament injury, repair and rehabilitation. Med Sci Sports Exerc 16:427, 1984.

52. Prentice, WE: A electromyographic analysis of the effectiveness of heat or cold and stretching for inducing relaxation in an injured muscle. Journal of Orthopaedic and Sports Physical Therapy 3:133–140, 1982.

53. Prentice, WE: Rehabilitation Techniques in Sports Medicine. Times Mirror/Mosby, St Louis, 1990.

54. Sady, SP, Wortman, M, and Blanke, D: Flexibility training: Ballistic, static or proprioceptive neuromuscular facilitation. Arch Phys Med Rehabil 63:261, 1982.

55. Sapega, A, et al: Biophysical factors in range of motion exercises. The Physician and Sportsmedicine 9:57, 1981.

56. Schultz, JH, and Luthe, W: Autogenic Training: A Psychophysiologic Approach in Psychotherapy. Grune & Stratton, New York, 1959.

57. Smith, CA: The warm-up procedure: To stretch or not to stretch. A brief review. Journal of Orthopaedic and Sports Physical Therapy 19(1):12–17, 1994.

58. Sotoberg, GL: Skeletal muscle function. In Currier, DP, and Nelson, RM (eds): Dynamics of Human Biologic Tissues, FA Davis, Philadelphia, 1992.

59. Starring, DT, et al: Comparison of cyclic and sustained passive stretching using a mechanical device to increase resting length of hamstring muscles. Phys Ther 68:314, 1988.

60. Tabary, JC, et al: Physiological and structural changes in the cat soleus muscle due to immobilization at different lengths by plaster casts. J Physiol (Lond) 224:231, 1972.

61. Tannigawa, M: Comparison of the hold-relax procedure and passive mobilization on increasing muscle length. Phys Ther 52:725, 1972.

62. Tardieu, C, et al: Adaptation of connective tissue length to immobilization in the lengthened and shortened position in cat soleus muscle. J Physiol (Paris) 78:214, 1982.

63. Threlkeld, AJ: The effects of manual therapy on connective tissue. Phys Ther 72:893, 1992.

64. Tillman, LJ, and Cxummings, GS: Biologic mechanisms of connective tissue mutability. In Currier, DP, and Nelson, RM (eds): Dynamics of Human Biologic Tissues. FA Davis, Philadelphia, 1992.

65. Trombly, CA: Occupational Therapy for Physical Dysfunction, ed 2. Williams & Wilkins, Baltimore, 1983.

66. Van Beveren, PS: Effects of muscle stretching program on muscle strength. Empire State Phys Ther 20:5, 1979.

67. Vesco, JJ: Principles of stretching. In Torg, JS, Welsh, RP, and Shephard, RJ (eds): Current Therapy in Sports Medicine, Vol 2. BC Decker, Toronto, 1990.

68. Voss, DE, Ionla, MK, and Myers, BJ: Proprioceptive Neuromuscular Facilitation, ed 3. Harper & Row, Philadelphia, 1985.

69. Walker, SM: Delay of twitch relaxation induced by stress and stress relaxation. J Appl Physiol 16:801, 1961.

70. Warren, CG, Lehmann, JF, and Koblanski, JN: Heat and stretch procedures: An evaluation using rat tail tendon. Arch Phys Med Rehabil 57:122, 1976.

71. Warren, CG, Lehmann, JF, and Koblanski, JN: Elongation of rat tail tendon: Effect of load and temperature. Arch Phys Med Rehabil 51:481, 1970.

72. Wessling, KC, Derane, DA, and Hylton, CR: Effect of static stretch vs. static stretch and ultrasound combined on triceps surae muscle extensibility in healthy women. Phys Ther 67:674, 1987.

73. Wiliams, PR, and Goldspink, G: Changes in sarcomere length and physiological properties in immobilized muscle. J Anat 127:459, 1978.

74. Wolpe, J: Psychotherapy by Reciprocal Inhibition. Stanford University Press, Stanford, 1958.

75. Zachazewski, JE: Flexibility in sports. In Sanders, B (ed): Sports Physical Therapy. Appleton & Lange, Norwalk, CT, 1990.

76. Zachazewski, JE: Improving flexibility. In Scully, RM, and Barnes, MR (eds): Physical Therapy, JB Lippincott, Philadelphia, 1989.

77. Zarins, B: Soft tissue injury and repair: Biomechanical aspects. Int J Sports Med 3:9, 1982.

Peripheral Joint Mobilization

Historically, when a patient had limited range of motion (ROM), the therapeutic approach was to stretch the region with passive stretching techniques (see Chapter 5). Over the past 30 years, therapists have identified and learned techniques that deal more directly with stretching the *source* of the limitation, and thus they are managing dysfunctions better and with less trauma. Muscle elongation or active inhibition techniques are used to counteract loss of flexibility in the contractile elements of muscle (see Chapter 5); cross-fiber massage techniques are used to increase mobility in selected ligaments and tendons; and joint mobilization and manipulation techniques are used to safely stretch or snap structures to restore normal joint mechanics with less trauma than passive stretching.

Joint mobilization refers to techniques that are used to treat joint dysfunction such as stiffness, reversible joint hypomobility, or pain.[8] Currently several schools of thought and treatment techniques are popular in the United States, and leading practitioners and educators are attempting to blend common points to yield more uniform treatment from the various approaches.[2,9]

To effectively use joint mobilization for treatment, the practitioner must know and be able to evaluate the anatomy, arthrokinematics, and pathology of the neuromusculoskeletal system[8] and to recognize when the techniques are indicated or when other stretching techniques would be more effective for regaining lost motion. Indiscriminate use of joint mobilization techniques when not indicated could lead to potential harm to the patient's joints.

The importance of evaluation skills and of the ability to identify the various structures that can cause decreased range of motion and pain underlies the presentation of material in this chapter. We assume that, prior to learning the joint mobilization techniques presented here, the student or therapist will have had (or will be concurrently taking) a course in orthopedic evaluation and therefore is able to choose appropriate, safe techniques for treating the patient's functional limitation. (See evaluation outline in Chapter 1 and guidelines in Chapter 7.) The reader is referred to several resources for additional study of evaluation procedures.[2,3,7–9,11,19,20]

When indicated, joint mobilization is a safe and effective means of restoring or maintaining joint play within a joint and can also be used for treating pain.[8,10,13]

OBJECTIVES

After studying this chapter, the reader will be able to:

1　Define terminology of joint mobilization.
2　Summarize basic concepts of joint motion.
3　Identify indications and goals for joint mobilization.
4　Identify limitations of joint mobilization.
5　Identify contraindications for joint mobilization.
6　Describe procedures for applying joint mobilization.
7　Apply basic techniques of joint mobilization to the extremity joints.

I. Definitions of Joint Mobilization

A. Mobilization

A passive movement performed by the therapist at a speed slow enough that the patient can stop the movement. The technique may be applied with an oscillatory motion or a sustained stretch intended to decrease pain or increase mobility. The techniques may use physiologic movements or accessory movements.[8,11]

1. Physiologic movements

Movements that the patient can do voluntarily; for example, the classic or traditional movements such as flexion, abduction, and rotation. The term *osteokinematics* is used when these motions of the bones are described.

2. Accessory movements

Movements within the joint and surrounding tissues that are necessary for normal range of motion but that cannot be actively performed by the patient.[13] Terms that relate to accessory movements are component motions and joint play.

a. **Component motions** are those motions that accompany active motion but are not under voluntary control; the term is often used synonymously with accessory movement.[9] Motions such as upward rotation of the scapula and clavicle, which occurs with shoulder flexion, and rotation of the fibula, which occurs with ankle motions, are component motions.

b. **Joint play** describes the motions that occur between the joint surfaces as well as the distensibility or "give" in the joint capsule, which allows the bones to move. The movements are necessary for normal joint functioning through the range of motion and can be demonstrated passively, but they cannot be performed actively by the patient.[13] The movements include distractions, sliding, compression, rolling, and spinning of the joint surfaces (see Section II).[9] The term *arthrokinematics* is used when these motions of the bone surfaces within the joint are described.

NOTE: Procedures to distract or slide the joint surfaces to decrease pain or restore joint play are the fundamental joint mobilization techniques described in this text.

B. Manipulation

A passive movement using physiologic or accessory motions, which may be applied with a thrust or when the patient is under anesthesia.

1. **Thrust**

   A sudden movement performed with a high-velocity, short-amplitude motion such that the patient cannot prevent the motion.[11,13] The motion is performed at the end of the pathologic limit of the joint and is intended to alter positional relationships, to snap adhesions, or to stimulate joint receptors.[13] Pathologic limit means the end of the available range of motion when there is restriction. *Thrust techniques are beyond the scope of this text.*

2. **Manipulation under anesthesia**

   A medical procedure used to restore full range of movement by breaking adhesions around a joint while the patient is anesthetized. The technique may be a rapid thrust or a passive stretch using physiologic or accessory movements.

II. Basic Concepts of Joint Motion: Arthrokinematics

A. Joint Shapes

The type of motion occurring between bony partners within a joint is influenced by the shapes of the joint surfaces. The shapes may be described as *ovoid* or *sellar.*[14]

1. **Ovoid**

   One surface is convex; the other is concave (Fig. 6–1A).

2. **Sellar (Saddle)**

   One surface is concave in one direction and convex in the other, with the opposing surface convex and concave, respectively; similar to a horseback rider being in complementary opposition to the shape of a saddle (Fig. 6–1B).

B. Types of Motion

As a bony lever moves about an axis of motion, there is also movement of the bone surface on the opposing bone surface within the joint.

1. The movement of the bony lever is called *swing* and is classically described as flexion, extension, abduction, adduction, and rotation. The amount of movement can be measured in degrees with a goniometer and is called range of motion.

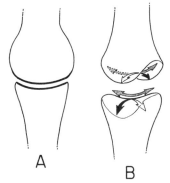

Figure 6–1. (*A*) With ovoid joints, one surface is convex and the other, concave. (*B*) With sellar joints, one surface is concave in one direction and convex in the other, with the opposing surface convex and concave, respectively.

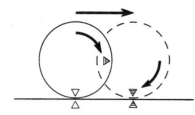

Figure 6–2. Diagrammatic representation of one surface rolling on another. New points on one surface meet new points on the opposing surface.

2. Motion of the bone surfaces within the joint is a variable combination of *rolling, sliding,* or *spinning.*[8,9,12,15] These accessory motions allow for greater angulation of the bone as it swings. For the rolling, sliding, or spinning to occur, there must be adequate capsule laxity or joint play.

   a. *Roll*

   Characteristics of one bone rolling on another (Fig. 6–2).

   (1) The surfaces are incongruent.

   (2) New points on one surface meet new points on the opposing surface.

   (3) Rolling results in angular motion of the bone (swing).

   (4) Rolling is always in the same direction as the angulating bone motion (Figs. 6–3A and B), whether the surface is convex or concave.

   (5) Rolling, if it occurs alone, causes compression of the surfaces on the side to which the bone is angulating and separation on the other side. Passive stretching using bone angulation alone may cause stressful compressive forces to portions of the joint surface, potentially leading to joint damage.

   (6) In normally functioning joints, pure rolling does not occur alone but in combination with joint sliding and spinning.

   b. *Slide*

   Characteristics of one bone sliding across another.

   (1) For a pure slide, the surfaces must be congruent, either flat (Fig. 6–4A) or curved (Fig. 6–4B).

   (2) The same point on one surface comes into contact with new points on the opposing surface.

   (3) Pure sliding does not occur in joints, because the surfaces are not completely congruent.

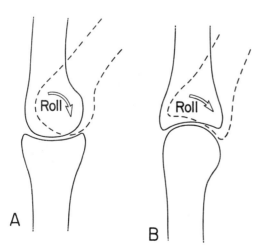

A   B

Figure 6–3. Rolling is always in the same direction as bone motion, whether the moving bone is (*A*) convex or (*B*) concave.

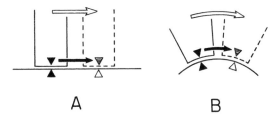

Figure 6–4. Diagrammatic representation of one surface sliding on another, whether (*A*) flat or (*B*) curved. The same point on one surface comes into contact with new points on the opposing surface.

    (4) The direction in which sliding occurs depends on whether the moving surface is concave or convex. Sliding is in the opposite direction of the angular movement of the bone if the moving joint surface is convex (Fig. 6–5A). Sliding is in the same direction as the angular movement of the bone if the moving surface is concave (Fig. 6–5B).

    NOTE: This mechanical relationship is known as the *convex-concave rule* and is the basis for determining the direction of the mobilizing force when joint mobilization gliding techniques are used.[8]

  c. *Combined roll-sliding in a joint*[8]
    (1) The more congruent the joint surfaces are, the more sliding there is of one bony partner on the other with movement.
    (2) The more incongruent the joint surfaces are, the more rolling there is of one bony partner on the other with movement.
    (3) When muscles actively contract to move a bone, some of the muscles may cause or control the sliding movement of the joint surfaces. For example, the caudal sliding motion of the humeral head during shoulder abduction is caused by the rotator cuff muscles, and the posterior sliding of the tibia during knee flexion is caused by the hamstring muscles. If this function is lost, the resulting abnormal joint mechanics may cause microtrauma and joint dysfunction.
    (4) The joint mobilization techniques described in this chapter use the sliding component of joint motion to restore joint play and reverse joint hypo-

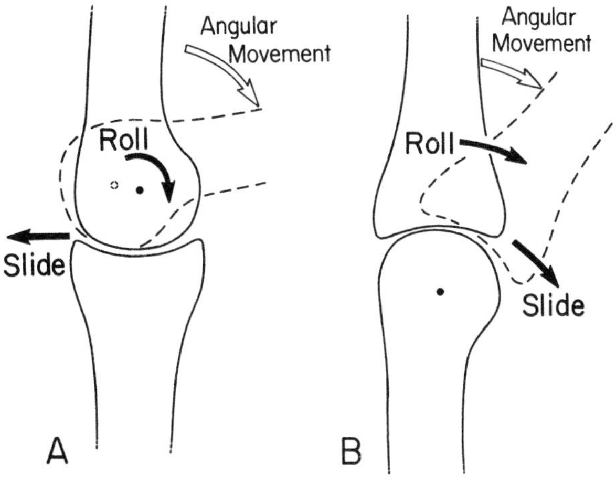

Figure 6–5. Diagrammatic representation of the concave-convex rule. (*A*) If the surface of the moving bone is convex, sliding is in the opposite direction of the angular movement of the bone. (*B*) If the surface of the moving bone is concave, sliding is in the same direction as the angular movement of the bone.

mobility. Rolling (passive angular stretching) is not used to stretch tight joint capsules because it causes joint compression.

NOTE: When the therapist passively moves the articulating surface in the direction in which the slide normally occurs, the technique is called translatoric glide or, simply, glide.[8] It is used to control pain when applied gently or to stretch the capsule when applied with a stretch force.

d. *Spin*

Characteristics of one bone spinning on another.

(1) There is rotation of a segment about a stationary mechanical axis (Fig. 6–6).

(2) The same point on the moving surface creates an arc of a circle as the bone spins.

(3) Spinning rarely occurs alone in joints but in combination with rolling and sliding.

(4) Three examples of spin occurring in joints of the body are the shoulder with flexion/extension, the hip with flexion/extension, and the radiohumeral joint with pronation/supination (Fig. 6–7).

C. Passive-Angular Stretching Versus Joint-Glide Stretching[10]

1. Passive-angular stretching procedures, as when the bony lever is used to stretch a tight joint capsule, may cause increased pain or joint trauma because:

a. The use of a lever significantly magnifies the force at the joint.

b. The force causes excessive joint compression in the direction of the rolling bone (see Fig. 6–3).

c. The roll without a slide does not replicate normal joint mechanics.

2. Joint glide (mobilization) stretching procedures, as when the translatoric slide component of the bones is used to stretch a tight capsule, are safer and more selective because:

a. The force is applied close to the joint surface and controlled at an intensity compatible with the pathology.

b. The direction of the force replicates the sliding component of the joint mechanics and does not compress the cartilage.

c. The amplitude of the motion is small yet specific to the restricted or adhered portion of the capsule or ligaments; thus, the forces are selectively applied to the desired tissue.

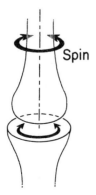

Figure 6–6. Diagrammatic representation of spinning. There is rotation of a segment about a stationary mechanical axis.

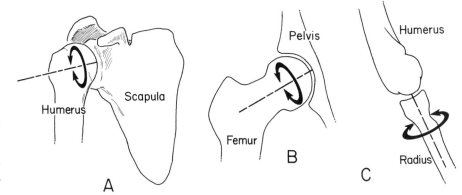

Figure 6–7. Examples of joint spin location in the body. (*A*) Humerus with flexion/extension. (*B*) Femur with flexion/extension. (*C*) Head of the radius with pronation/supination.

D. Other Accessory Motions That Affect the Joint Include Compression and Traction

1. **Compression** is the decrease in the joint space between bony partners.
   a. Compression normally occurs in the extremity and spinal joints when weight bearing.
   b. Some compression occurs as muscles contract; this provides stability to the joints.
   c. As one bone rolls on the other (see Fig. 6–13), some compression also occurs on the side to which the bone is angulating.
   d. Normal intermittent compressive loads help move synovial fluid and thus help maintain cartilage health.
   e. Abnormally high compression loads may lead to articular cartilage changes and deterioration.[6]
2. **Traction** is the distraction or separation of the joint surfaces.
   a. For distraction to occur within the joint, the surfaces must be pulled apart. The movement is not always the same as pulling on the long axis of one of the bony partners. For example, if traction is applied to the shaft of the humerus, it will result in a glide of the joint surface (Fig. 6–8A). Distraction of the glenohumeral joint requires a pull at right angles to the glenoid fossa (Fig. 6–8B).
   b. For clarity, whenever there is pulling on the long axis of a bone, the term *long-axis traction* will be used. Whenever the surfaces are to be pulled apart

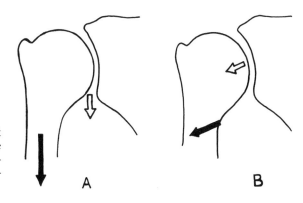

Figure 6–8. (*A*) Traction applied to the shaft of the humerus results in caudal gliding of the joint surface. (*B*) Distraction of the glenohumeral joint requires separation at right angles to the glenoid fossa.

at right angles, the terms *distraction, joint traction,* or *joint separation* will be used.

NOTE: For joint mobilization techniques, distraction is used to control or relieve pain when applied gently or to stretch the capsule when applied with a stretch force.

E. Effects of Joint Motion

1. Joint motion stimulates biologic activity by moving synovial fluid, which brings nutrients to the avascular articular cartilage of the joint surfaces and intra-articular fibrocartilage of the menisci.[9] Atrophy of the articular cartilage begins soon after immobilization is imposed on joints.[1,4–6]

2. Joint motion maintains extensibility and tensile strength of the articular and periarticular tissues. With immobilization there is fibrofatty proliferation, which causes intra-articular adhesions, as well as biochemical changes in tendon, ligament, and joint capsule tissue, which causes joint contractures and ligamentous weakening.[1]

3. Afferent nerve impulses from joint receptors transmit information to the central nervous system and therefore provide for awareness of position and motion. With injury or joint degeneration, there is a potential decrease in an important source of proprioceptive feedback that may affect an individual's balance response.[21] Joint motion provides sensory input relative to[16,17]:
   a. Static position and sense of speed of movement (type I receptors found in the superficial joint capsule)
   b. Change of speed of movement (type II receptors found in deep layers of the joint capsule and articular fat pads)
   c. Sense of direction of movement (type I and III receptors; type III found in joint ligaments)
   d. Regulation of muscle tone (type, I, II, and III receptors)
   e. Nociceptive stimuli (type IV receptors found in the fibrous capsule, ligaments, articular fat pads, periosteum, and walls of blood vessels)

III. Indications for Joint Mobilization

A. Pain, Muscle Guarding, and Spasm

Painful joints, reflex muscle guarding, and muscle spasm can be treated with *gentle joint-play* techniques to stimulate neurophysiologic and mechanical effects.[6,9,11]

1. Neurophysiologic effects

Small-amplitude oscillatory and distraction movements are used to stimulate the mechanoreceptors that may inhibit the transmission of nociceptive stimuli at the spinal cord or brain stem levels.[9,13,15]

2. Mechanical effects

Small-amplitude distraction or gliding movements of the joint are used to cause synovial fluid motion, which is the vehicle for bringing nutrients to the avascular portions of the articular cartilage (and intra-articular fibrocartilage when present).[6,9] Gentle joint-play techniques help maintain nutrient exchange and thus prevent the painful and degenerating effects of stasis when a joint is swollen or painful and cannot move through a range of motion.

NOTE: The small-amplitude joint techniques used to treat pain, muscle guarding, or muscle spasm should not place a stretch on the reactive tissues (see Contraindications and Precautions under Section V).

B. Reversible Joint Hypomobility

Reversible joint hypomobility can be treated with *progressively vigorous joint-play stretching* techniques to elongate hypomobile capsular and ligamentous connective tissue. Sustained or oscillatory stretch forces are used to mechanically distend the shortened tissue.[8,9,11]

C. Progressive Limitation

Diseases that progressively limit movement can be treated with joint-play techniques to maintain available motion or retard progressive mechanical restrictions. The dosage of distraction or glide is dictated by the patient's response to treatment and the state of the disease.

D. Functional Immobility

When a patient cannot functionally move a joint for a period of time, the joint can be treated with nonstretch gliding or distraction techniques to maintain available joint play and prevent the degenerating and restricting effects of immobility.

IV. Limitations of Joint Mobilization Techniques

A. Mobilization techniques cannot change the disease process of disorders such as rheumatoid arthritis or the inflammatory process of injury. In these cases treatment is directed toward minimizing pain, maintaining available joint play, and reducing the effects of any mechanical limitations (see Chapter 7).

B. The skill of the therapist will affect the outcome. The techniques described in this text are relatively safe if directions are followed and precautions are heeded, but if these techniques are used indiscriminately on patients not properly evaluated and screened for such maneuvers or if they are applied too vigorously for the condition, joint trauma or hypermobility may result.

V. Contraindications and Precautions

A. The Only True Contraindications to Stretching Techniques Are Hypermobility, Joint Effusion, and Inflammation[8]

1. Hypermobility

a. The joints of patients with potential necrosis of the ligaments or capsule should not be stretched.

b. Patients with painful hypermobile joints may benefit from gentle joint-play techniques (see Section III.A) if kept within the limits of motion. Stretching is not done.

2. Joint effusion

There may be joint swelling (effusion) from trauma or disease. Rapid swelling of a joint usually indicates bleeding within the joint and may occur with trauma or in diseases such as hemophilia. Medical intervention is required for aspiration of the blood to minimize its necrotizing effect on the articular cartilage. Slow swelling (greater than 4 hours) usually indicates serous effusion (a buildup of excess synovial fluid) or edema within the joint from mild trauma, irritation, or a disease such as arthritis.

a. Never stretch a swollen joint with mobilization or passive stretching techniques. The capsule is already on a stretch by being distended to accommodate the extra fluid. The limited motion is from the extra fluid and muscle response to pain, not from shortened fibers.

b. Gentle oscillating motions that do not stress or stretch the capsule may help block the transmission of a pain stimulus so that it is not perceived and may also help improve fluid flow while maintaining available joint play (see Section III.A).

c. If the patient's response to gentle techniques results in increased pain or joint irritability, the techniques were applied too vigorously or should not be done with the current state of pathology.

3. Inflammation

Whenever inflammation is present, stretching will increase pain and muscle guarding and will result in greater tissue damage. Gentle oscillating or distraction motions may temporarily inhibit the pain response. See Chapter 7 for an appropriate approach to treatment when inflammation is present.

B. Conditions Requiring Special Precautions for Stretching

In most cases, joint mobilization techniques are safer than passive angular stretching, in which the bony lever is used to stretch tight tissue and joint compression results. Mobilization may be used with extreme care in the following conditions if signs and the patient's response are favorable:

1. Malignancy
2. Bone disease detectable on x ray
3. Unhealed fracture (depends on the site of the fracture and stabilization provided)
4. Excessive pain (determine the cause of pain and modify treatment accordingly)
5. Hypermobility in associated joints (associated joints must be properly stabilized so the mobilization force is not transmitted to them)
6. Total joint replacements (the mechanism of the replacement is self-limiting, and therefore the mobilization gliding techniques may be inappropriate)
7. Newly formed or weakened connective tissue such as immediately following injury, surgery, or disuse or when the patient is taking certain medications such as corticosteroids (gentle progressive techniques within the tolerance of the tissue help align the developing fibrils, but forceful techniques are destructive)
8. Systemic connective tissue diseases such as rheumatoid arthritis, in which the disease weakens the connective tissue (gentle techniques may benefit restricted tissue, but forceful techniques may rupture tissue and result in instabilities)
9. Elderly individuals with weakened connective tissue and diminished circulation (gentle techniques within the tolerance of the tissue may be beneficial to increase mobility)

VI. Procedures for Applying Joint Mobilization Techniques

A. Evaluation and Assessment

If the patient has limited or painful motion, evaluate and decide which tissues are limiting function and the state of pathology (see Chapter 1). Determine whether treatment will be directed primarily toward relieving pain or stretching a joint or soft tissue limitation.[3,11]

1. The quality of pain when testing the range of motion helps determine the stage of recovery and the dosage of techniques used for treatment. (See Figs. 7–2 and 7–3.)

    a. If pain is experienced before tissue limitation—such as the pain that occurs with muscle guarding following an acute injury or during the active stage of a disease—gentle pain-inhibiting joint techniques may be used. The same techniques will also help maintain joint play. (See Section B, Grades or Dosages of Movement.) Stretching under these circumstances is contraindicated.

    b. If pain is experienced concurrently with tissue limitation—such as the pain and limitation that occur when damaged tissue begins to heal—the limitation is treated cautiously. Gentle stretching techniques specific to the tight structure are used to gradually improve movement yet not exacerbate the pain by reinjuring the tissue.

    c. If pain is experienced after tissue limitation is met because of stretching of tight capsular or periarticular tissue, the stiff joint can be aggressively stretched with joint-play techniques and the periarticular tissue with the stretching techniques described in Chapter 5.

2. The joint capsule is limiting motion and should respond to mobilization techniques if the following signs are present:

    a. The passive range of motion for that joint is limited in a capsular pattern. (These patterns are described for each peripheral joint under the respective sections on joint problems in Chapters 8 through 13.)

    b. There is a firm capsular end-feel when overpressure is applied to the tissues limiting the range.

    c. There is decreased joint-play movement when mobility tests (articulations) are performed.

3. An adhered or contracted ligament is limiting motion if there is decreased joint play and pain when the fibers of the ligament are stressed. Ligaments often respond to joint mobilization techniques if applied specific to their line of stress.

4. Subluxation or dislocation of one bony part on another and loose intra-articular structures that block normal motion may respond to joint manipulation or thrust techniques. Some of the simpler manipulations are described in appropriate sections in this text. Others require more advanced training and are beyond the scope of this book.

B. Grades or Dosages of Movement

Two systems of grading dosages for mobilization are used.

1. Graded oscillation techniques[11] (Fig. 6–9)

   a. *Dosages*

      (1) Grade I

      Small-amplitude rhythmic oscillations are performed at the beginning of the range.

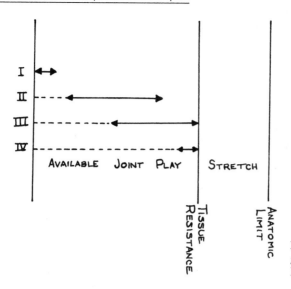

Figure 6-9. Diagrammatic representation of graded oscillation techniques. (Adapted from Maitland,[11] p 29.)

(2) Grade II

Large-amplitude rhythmic oscillations are performed within the range, not reaching the limit.

(3) Grade III

Large-amplitude rhythmic oscillations are performed up to the limit of the available motion and are stressed into the tissue resistance.

(4) Grade IV

Small-amplitude rhythmic oscillations are performed at the limit of the available motion and stressed into the tissue resistance.

(5) Grade V

A small-amplitude, high-velocity thrust technique is performed to snap adhesions at the limit of the available motion. Thrust techniques used for this purpose require advanced training and are beyond the scope of this book.

b. *Uses*

(1) Grades I and II are primarily used for treating joints limited by pain. The oscillations may have an inhibitory effect on perception of painful stimuli by repetitively stimulating mechanoreceptors that block nociceptive pathways at the spinal cord or brain stem levels.[13,18] These nonstretch motions help move synovial fluid to improve nutrition to the cartilage.

(2) Grades III and IV are primarily used as stretching maneuvers.

c. *Techniques*

The oscillations may be performed using physiologic (osteokinematic) motions or joint-play (arthrokinematic) techniques.

2. Sustained translatory joint-play techniques[8] (Fig. 6-10)

a. *Dosages*

(1) Grade I (loosen)

Small-amplitude distraction is applied where no stress is placed on the capsule. It equalizes cohesive forces, muscle tension, and atmospheric pressure acting on the joint.

(2) Grade II (tighten)

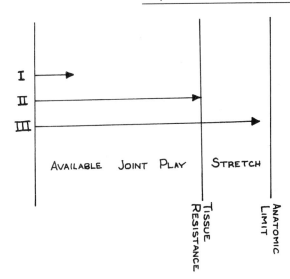

Figure 6–10. Diagrammatic representation of sustained translatory joint-play techniques. (Adapted from Kaltenborn,[8] p 22.)

Enough distraction or glide is applied to tighten the tissues around the joint. Kaltenborn[8] calls this "taking up the slack."

(3) Grade III (stretch)

A distraction or glide is applied with an amplitude large enough to place a stretch on the joint capsule and on surrounding periarticular structures.

b. *Uses*

(1) Grade I distraction is used with all gliding motions and may be used for relief of pain.

(2) Grade II distraction is used for the initial treatment to determine how sensitive the joint is. Once joint reaction is known, the dosage of treatment is either increased or decreased accordingly.

(3) Gentle grade II distraction applied intermittently may be used to inhibit pain; grade II glides may be used to maintain joint play when range of motion is not allowed.

(4) Grade III joint distraction or glides are used to stretch the joint structures and thus increase joint play.

c. *Techniques*

This grading system describes only joint-play techniques that separate (distract) or glide (slide) the joint surfaces.

3. Comparison

When using either grading system, dosages I and II are low intensity and so do not cause a stretch force on the joint capsule or surrounding tissue, although, by definition, sustained grade II techniques take up the slack of the tissues whereas grade II oscillation techniques stay within the slack. Grades III and IV oscillations and Grade III sustained stretch techniques are similar in intensity in that they all are applied with a stretch force at the limit of motion. The differences are related to the rhythm or speed of repetition of the stretch force.

a. For clarity and consistency, when referring to dosages in this text:

(1) The notation *graded oscillations* means: use the dosages as described in the section on graded oscillation techniques.

(2) The notation *sustained grade* means: use the dosages as described in the section on sustained translatory joint-play techniques.

b. The choice of using oscillating or sustained techniques depends on the patient's response.

(1) When dealing with managing pain, either grade I or II oscillation techniques or slow intermittent grade I or II sustained joint distraction techniques are recommended. The patient's response dictates the intensity and frequency of the joint-play technique.

(2) When dealing with loss of joint play and thus decreased functional range, sustained techniques applied in a cyclic manner are recommended. The longer the stretch force can be maintained, the greater the creep and plastic deformation of the connective tissue.

(3) When attempting to maintain available range by using joint-play techniques, either grade II oscillating or sustained grade II techniques can be used.

C. Patient Position

The patient and the extremity to be treated should be positioned so the patient can relax. Techniques of relaxation or inhibition (see Chapter 5) may be appropriately used prior to or between stretching.

D. Joint Position

Evaluation of joint play and the first treatment are performed in the **resting position** for that joint, that is, that position in which the capsule has greatest laxity. Maximum joint traction and joint play are available in that position (see Section H). In some cases, the position to use is the one in which the joint is least painful.

E. Stabilization

Firmly and comfortably stabilize one joint partner, usually the proximal bone. Stabilization may be provided by a belt, one of the therapist's hands, or an assistant holding the part. Appropriate stabilization prevents unwanted stress to surrounding tissues and joints and makes the stretch force more specific and effective.

F. Treatment Force

The treatment force (either gentle or strong) is applied as close to the opposing joint surface as possible. The larger the contact surface is, the more comfortable the procedure will be. For example, instead of forcing with your thumb, use the flat surface of your hand.

G. Direction of Movement

1. The direction of movement during treatment is either parallel to or perpendicular to the treatment plane. *Treatment plane* is described by Kaltenborn[8] as a plane perpendicular to a line running from the axis of rotation to the middle of the concave articular surface. The plane is in the concave partner so its position is determined by the position of the concave bone (Fig. 6–11).

2. Joint traction techniques are applied perpendicular to the treatment plane. The entire bone is moved so that the joint surfaces are separated.

3. Gliding techniques are applied parallel to the treatment plane.

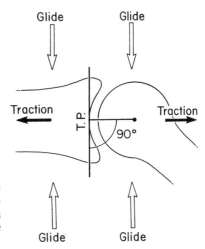

Figure 6–11. Treatment plane (T.P.) is at right angles to a line drawn from the axis of rotation to the center of the concave articulating surface and lies in the concave surface. Joint traction is applied perpendicular and glides are applied parallel to the treatment plane.

    a. Glide in the direction in which the slide would normally occur for the desired motion. Direction of sliding is easily determined by using the convex-concave rule (see Section II.B.2). If the surface of the moving bony partner is convex, the treatment glide should be opposite to the direction in which the bone swings. If the surface of the moving bony partner is concave, the treatment glide should be in the same direction (see Figs. 6–5A and B).

    b. The entire bone is moved so that there is gliding of one joint surface on the other. The bone should not be used as a lever; it should have no arcing motion (swing) that would cause rolling and thus compression of the joint surfaces.

H. Initiation and Progression of Treatment (Fig. 6–12)

    1. The initial treatment is the same whether treating to decrease pain or to increase joint play. The purpose is to determine joint reactivity before proceeding. Use a sustained grade II distraction of the joint surfaces with the joint held in resting position or the position of greatest relaxation.[8] Note the immediate joint response relative to irritability and range.

    2. The next day, evaluate joint response.

        a. If there is increased pain and sensitivity, reduce the amplitude of treatment to grade I oscillations.

        b. If the joint is the same or better, perform either of the following:

            (1) Repeat the same maneuver if the goal of treatment is to maintain joint play.

            (2) Progress the maneuver to sustained grade III traction or glides if the goal of treatment is to increase joint play.

    3. To progress the stretch technique, move the bone to the end of the available range of motion, then apply the sustained grade III distraction or glide techniques. Advanced progressions include pre-positioning the bone at the end of the available range and rotating it prior to applying grade III distraction or glide techniques (not illustrated in this chapter).

    4. Hints.[8]

        a. Warm the tissue around the joint prior to stretching. Modalities, massage, or gentle muscle contractions will increase the circulation and warm the tissues.

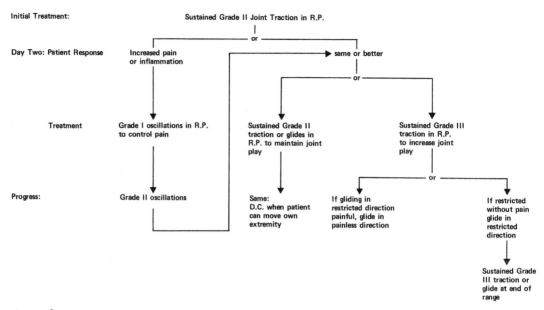

Figure 6–12. Initiation and progression of treatment.

b. Muscle relaxation techniques and oscillation techniques may inhibit muscle guarding and should be alternated with the stretching techniques, if necessary.

c. When using sustained gliding techniques, a grade I distraction should be used with it. A grade II or III distraction should not be used with a grade III glide to avoid excessive trauma to the joint.

d. If gliding in the restricted direction is too painful, begin gliding mobilizations in the painless direction. Progress to gliding in the restricted direction when mobility improves a little and it is not painful.

e. When applying stretching techniques, move the bony partner through the available range of joint play first; that is, "take up the slack." When tissue resistance is felt, apply the stretch force against the restriction.

5. To maintain joint play by using gliding techniques when range of motion techniques are contraindicated or not possible for a period of time, use sustained grade II or grade II oscillation techniques.

I. Speed, Rhythm, and Duration of Movements

1. Oscillations[11]

a. Grades I and IV are usually rapid oscillations, like manual vibrations.

b. Grades II and III are smooth, regular oscillations at two or three per second for 1 to 2 minutes.

c. Vary the speed of oscillations for different effects such as low amplitude and high speed to inhibit pain or slow speed to relax muscle guarding.

2. Sustained[8]

a. For painful joints, apply intermittent distraction for 7 to 10 seconds with a few seconds of rest in between for several cycles. Note response and either repeat or discontinue.

b. For restricted joints, apply a minimum of a 6-second stretch force, followed by partial release (to grade I or II), then repeat with slow, intermittent stretches at 3- to 4-second intervals.

J. Treatment Soreness

Stretching maneuvers usually cause soreness. Perform the maneuvers on alternate days to allow soreness to decrease and tissue healing to occur between stretching sessions. The patient should perform range of motion into any newly gained range during this time. If there is increased pain after 24 hours, the dosage (amplitude) or duration of treatment was too vigorous. Decrease the dosage or duration until the pain is under control.

K. Reassessment

The patient's joint and range of motion should be reassessed after treatment and again before the next treatment. Alterations in treatment are dictated by the joint response.

L. Total Program

Mobilization techniques are one part of a total treatment program when there is decreased function. If muscles or connective tissues are also limiting motion, inhibition and passive stretching techniques are alternated with joint mobilization in the same treatment session. Therapy should also include appropriate range of motion, strengthening, and functional techniques (see Chapters 8 through 13).

VII. Peripheral Joint Mobilization Techniques

The following are suggested joint distraction and gliding techniques for use by entry level therapists and those attempting to gain a foundation in joint mobilization. A variety of adaptations can be made from these techniques. The distraction and glide techniques should be applied with respect to the dosage, frequency, progression, precautions, and procedures as described in the previous sections.

NOTE: Terms such as proximal hand, distal hand, lateral hand, or other descriptive terms indicate that the therapist should use the hand that is more proximal, distal, or lateral to the patient or the patient's extremity.

A. Shoulder Girdle Complex (Fig. 6–13)

1. Glenohumeral joint

Concave glenoid fossa receives the convex humeral head.

RESTING POSITION
Shoulder abducted 55 degrees, horizontally adducted 30 degrees, and rotated so that the forearm is in the horizontal plane.

TREATMENT PLANE
In the glenoid fossa and moves with the scapula. (See definition in Section VI.G.)

STABILIZATION
Fixate the scapula with a belt or have an assistant help.

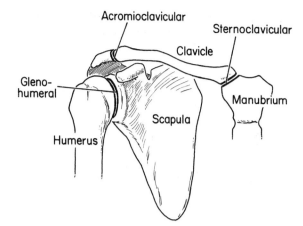

Figure 6–13. Bones and joint of the shoulder girdle complex.

a. **Joint traction** (distraction) (Fig. 6–14)

INDICATIONS

Testing; initial treatment (sustained grade II); pain control (grade I or II oscillations); general mobility (sustained grade III).

POSITION OF PATIENT

Supine, with arm in resting position; support the forearm between your trunk and elbow.

HAND PLACEMENT

Use the hand nearer the part being treated (for example, left hand if treating the patient's left shoulder) and place it in the patient's axilla with your thumb just distal to the joint margin anteriorly and fingers posteriorly. Your other hand supports the humerus from the lateral surface.

MOBILIZING FORCE

With the hand in the axilla, move the humerus laterally.

NOTE: The entire arm moves in a translatoric motion away from the plane of the glenoid fossa. Distractions may be performed with the humerus in any position (see Figs. 6–17, 6–19, and 8–7). The therapist must be aware of the

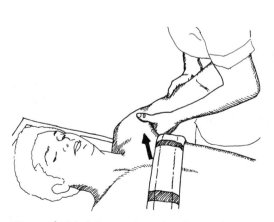

Figure 6–14. Joint traction; glenohumeral joint.

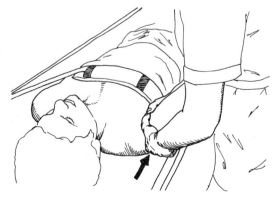

Figure 6–15. Caudal glide; glenohumeral joint.

amount of scapular rotation and adjust the distraction force against the humerus so it is perpendicular to the plane of the glenoid fossa.

b. **Caudal glide** (Fig. 6–15)

INDICATIONS

To increase abduction (sustained grade III); to reposition humeral head if superiorly positioned.

PATIENT POSITION

Same as with distraction.

HAND PLACEMENT

Place one hand in the patient's axilla (as in Section a) to provide the grade I distraction; the web space of your other hand is placed just distal to the acromion process.

MOBILIZING FORCE

With the superiorly placed hand, glide the humerus in an inferior direction.

c. **Caudal glide: alternate**

HAND PLACEMENT

Same as with distraction (see Fig. 6–14).

MOBILIZING FORCE

Comes from the hand around the arm, pulling caudally as you lean backward.

NOTE: This glide is also called long-axis traction.

d. **Caudal glide progression** (Fig. 6–16A)

INDICATION

To increase abduction when range approaches 90 degrees.

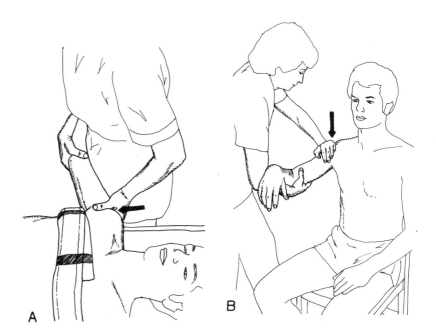

Figure 6–16. Caudal glide with the shoulder near 90 degrees, (*A*) supine and (*B*) sitting.

POSITION OF PATIENT

Supine, with the arm abducted to the end of its available range. External rotation of the humerus should be added to the end-range position as the arm approaches and goes beyond 90 degrees.

POSITION OF THERAPIST AND HAND PLACEMENT

Stand facing the patient's feet, and stabilize the patient's arm against your trunk with the hand farther from the patient. A slight lateral motion of your trunk will provide the grade I distraction. Place the web space of your other hand just distal to the acromion process on the proximal humerus.

MOBILIZING FORCE

With the hand on the proximal humerus, glide the humerus in an inferior direction.

ALTERNATE POSITION

Sitting (Fig. 6–16B).

e. **Elevation progression** (Fig. 6–17A)

INDICATION

To increase elevation beyond 90 degrees of abduction.

POSITION OF PATIENT

Supine, with the arm abducted and elevated to the end of its available range. The humerus is then externally rotated to its limit.

POSITION OF THERAPIST AND HAND PLACEMENT

Same as caudal glide progression; the therapist adjusts his or her body position so that the hand applying the mobilizing force is aligned with the treatment plane. The hand grasping the elbow applies a grade I distraction force.

MOBILIZING FORCE

With the hand on the proximal humerus, glide the humerus in a progressively anterior direction. The direction of force will depend on the amount of upward rotation and protraction of the scapula. The force directs the head of the humerus against the inferior folds of the capsule in the axilla.

ALTERNATE POSITION

Sitting (Fig. 6–17B).

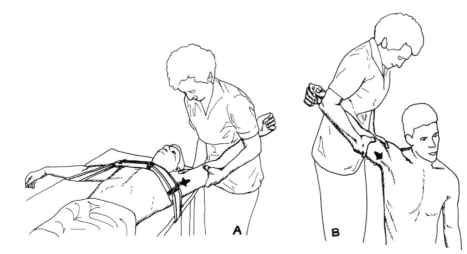

Figure 6–17. Elevation progression; glenohumeral joint (*A*) supine and (*B*) sitting. Used when the range is greater than 90 degrees. Note the externally rotated position of the humerus.

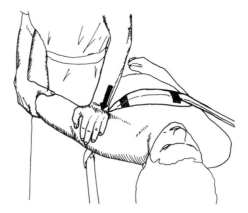

Figure 6–18. Posterior glide; glenohumeral joint.

f. **Posterior glide** (Fig. 6–18)

INDICATIONS

To increase flexion; to increase internal rotation.

POSITION OF PATIENT

Supine, with the arm in resting position.

POSITION OF THERAPIST AND HAND PLACEMENT

Stand with your back to the patient, between the patient's trunk and arm; support the arm against your trunk, grasping the distal humerus with your lateral hand. This position provides grade I distraction to the joint. Place the lateral border of your top hand just distal to the anterior margin of the joint, with your fingers pointing superiorly. This hand gives the mobilizing force.

MOBILIZING FORCE

Glide the humeral head posteriorly by moving the entire arm as you bend your knees.

g. **Posterior glide progression** (Fig. 6–19)

INDICATIONS

To increase posterior gliding when flexion approaches 90 degrees; to increase horizontal adduction.

POSITION OF PATIENT

Supine, with arm flexed to 90 degrees, internally rotated, with elbow flexed. The arm may also be placed in horizontal adduction.

HAND PLACEMENT

Place padding under the scapula for stabilization. Place one hand across the proximal surface of the humerus to apply a grade I distraction. Place your other hand over the patient's elbow. A belt placed around your pelvis and the patient's humerus may be used to apply the distraction force.

MOBILIZING FORCE

Glide the humerus posteriorly by pushing down at the elbow through the long axis of the humerus.

h. **Anterior glide** (Fig. 6–20)

INDICATIONS

To increase extension; to increase external rotation.

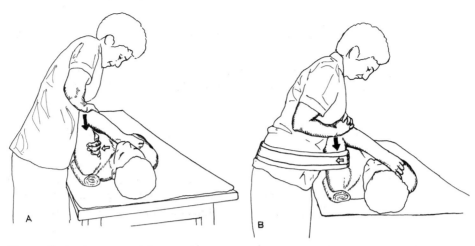

Figure 6–19. Posterior glide progression; glenohumeral joint. (*A*) Using one hand or (*B*) using a belt to give a grade I distraction force.

POSITION OF PATIENT

Prone, with arm in resting position over the edge of the treatment table, supported on your thigh. Stabilize the acromion with padding.

POSITION OF THERAPIST AND HAND PLACEMENT

Stand facing the top of the table with the leg closer to the table in a forward stride position. Support the patient's arm against your thigh with your outside hand. The arm positioned on your thigh provides a grade I distraction. Place the ulnar border of your other hand just distal to the posterior angle of the acromion process, with your fingers pointing superiorly. This hand gives the mobilizing force.

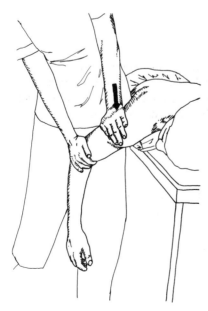

Figure 6–20. Anterior glide; glenohumeral joint.

MOBILIZING FORCE

Apply in an anterior and slightly medial direction. Bend both knees so the entire arm moves anteriorly.

Precaution. Do not lift the arm at the elbow and thereby cause an angulation of the humerus; such angulation could lead to an anterior subluxation of the humeral head.

i. **Anterior glide progression**

INDICATION

To increase external rotation.

Precaution: Do not place the shoulder in 90 degrees abduction and then progress to externally rotating the arm while applying an anterior glide. Such a technique may lead to anterior subluxation of the humeral head.

TECHNIQUES

Use a distraction progression of the humerus. Begin with the shoulder in resting position, externally rotate the humerus, then apply a grade III distraction perpendicular to the plane of the glenoid fossa (see Fig. 8–7).

Use elevation progression (see Fig. 6–17) because external rotation is incorporated into that technique.

NOTE: To gain full elevation of the humerus, the accessory and component motions of clavicular elevation and rotation, scapular rotation, and external rotation of the humerus as well as adequate joint play anteriorly and inferiorly are necessary. The clavicular and scapular mobilizations are described in the following sections.

2. **Acromioclavicular joint: anterior glide (Fig. 6–21)**

INDICATION

To increase mobility of the joint.

STABILIZATION

Fixate the scapula at the acromion process.

POSITION OF PATIENT

Sitting or prone.

HAND PLACEMENT

With the patient sitting, stand behind the patient and stabilize the acromion process with the fingers of your lateral hand. The thumb of your other hand is placed posteriorly on the clavicle, just medial to the joint space. With the patient prone, stabilize the acromion with a towel roll under the shoulder.

MOBILIZING FORCE

Your thumb pushes the clavicle anteriorly.

3. **Sternoclavicular joint**

The proximal articulating surface of the clavicle is convex superiorly/inferiorly and concave anteriorly/posteriorly.

POSITION OF PATIENT AND STABILIZATION

Supine. The thorax provides stability to the sternum.

a. **Posterior glide** (Fig. 6–22)

INDICATION

To increase retraction.

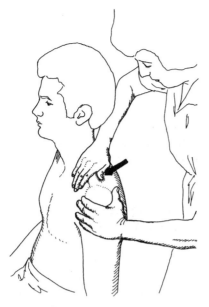

Figure 6–21. Anterior glide; acromio-clavicular joint.

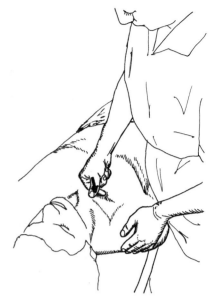

Figure 6–22. Posterior glide of the sternoclavicular joint; the same hand placement is used for superior glide.

HAND PLACEMENT

Place your thumb on the anterior surface of the proximal end of the clavicle; flex your index finger and place the middle phalanx along the caudal surface of the clavicle to support the thumb.

MOBILIZING FORCE

Push with your thumb in a posterior direction.

b. **Anterior glide** (Fig. 6–23)

INDICATION

To increase protraction.

HAND PLACEMENT

Your fingers are placed superiorly and thumb inferiorly around the clavicle.

MOBILIZING FORCE

The fingers and thumb lift the clavicle anteriorly.

c. **Inferior glide** (Fig. 6–23)

INDICATION

To increase elevation.

HAND PLACEMENT

Your fingers are placed superior to the clavicle as in Section b.

MOBILIZING FORCE

Your fingers pull the proximal clavicle caudally.

d. **Superior glide** (see Fig. 6–22)

INDICATION

To increase depression.

HAND PLACEMENT

Same as Section a previously.

MOBILIZING FORCE

Your index finger pushes in a superior direction.

4. Scapulothoracic articulation

This is not a true joint, but the soft tissue is stretched to obtain normal shoulder girdle mobility (Fig. 6–24).

INDICATIONS

To increase scapular motions of elevation, depression, protraction, retraction, rotation, and winging. (Winging is an accessory motion that occurs when a person attempts to place the hand behind the back, accompanying shoulder internal rotation and scapular downward rotation.)

POSITION OF PATIENT

If there is little mobility, begin prone (see Fig. 2–6), and progress to side-lying, with the patient facing you. The patient's arm is draped over your inferior arm and allowed to hang so that the muscles are relaxed.

HAND PLACEMENT

Your superior hand is placed across the acromion process to control the direction of motion. The fingers of your inferior hand scoop under the medial border and inferior angle of the scapula.

MOBILIZING FORCE

The scapula is moved in the desired direction by lifting from the inferior angle or by pushing on the acromion process.

B. The Elbow and Forearm Complex (Fig. 6–25)

1. The humeroulnar articulation

The convex trochlea articulates with the concave olecranon fossa.

RESTING POSITION

Elbow flexed 70 degrees, forearm supinated 10 degrees.

TREATMENT PLANE

In the olecranon fossa, angled approximately 45 degrees from the long axis of the ulna (Fig. 6–26).

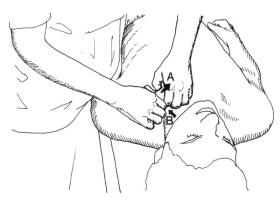

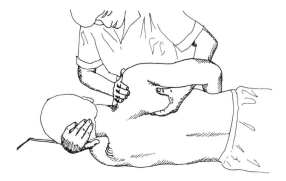

Figure 6–23. (*A*) Anterior glide of the sternoclavicular joint. (*B*) Same hand placement is used for inferior glide.

Figure 6–24. Scapulothoracic mobilization.

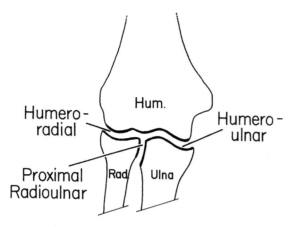

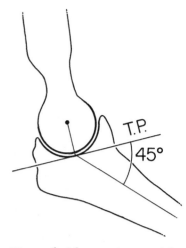

Figure 6–25. Bones and joints of the elbow complex.

Figure 6–26. Lateral view of the humeroulnar joint, depicting the treatment plane (T.P.).

STABILIZATION

Fixate the humerus against the treatment table with a belt or use an assistant to hold it.

a. **Joint traction** (Fig. 6–27A)

INDICATIONS

Testing; initial treatment (sustained grade II); pain control (grade I or II oscillation); to increase flexion or extension.

POSITION OF PATIENT

Supine, elbow over the edge of the treatment table or supported with padding just proximal to the olecranon process. The wrist rests against the therapist's shoulder, allowing the elbow to be in resting position.

HAND PLACEMENT

Using your medial hand, place your fingers over the proximal ulna on the volar surface; reinforce it with your other hand.

MOBILIZING FORCE

Force against the proximal ulna at a 45-degree angle to the shaft.

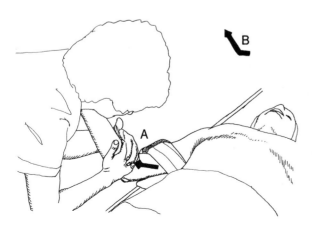

Figure 6–27. Joint traction. (*A*) Humeroulnar articulation. (*B*) Arrow indicating joint traction with distal glide.

b. **Traction progression**

INDICATIONS
To increase flexion or extension.

POSITION OF PATIENT
Same as in Section a, except that the elbow is positioned at the end of its available range of motion before applying the distracting force.

HAND PLACEMENT
Adjust your position to best apply the mobilization force and stabilize the forearm. When the elbow is near extension, stand and place the base of your hand against the proximal ulna.

MOBILIZING FORCE
Always force against the ulna at a 45-degree angle, no matter at what angle the elbow is.

c. **Distal glide** (Fig. 6–27B)

INDICATION
To increase flexion.

POSITION OF PATIENT AND HAND PLACEMENT
Same as in Section a.

MOBILIZING FORCE
Use a scooping motion in which distraction is applied to the joint first as in Section a; then pull along the long axis of the ulna (distal traction).

2. **The humeroradial articulation**

The convex capitulum articulates with the concave radial head.

RESTING POSITION
Elbow extended, forearm supinated.

TREATMENT PLANE
In the concave radial head perpendicular to the long axis of the radius.

STABILIZATION
Fixate the humerus with one of your hands.

a. **Joint traction** (Fig. 6–28)

INDICATIONS
To increase mobility of the radius; to correct a pushed elbow (proximal displacement of the radius).

POSITION OF PATIENT
Supine; or sitting, with the arm resting on the treatment table.

POSITION OF THERAPIST AND HAND PLACEMENT
Position yourself on the ulnar side of the patient's forearm. Stabilize the patient's humerus with your superior hand; grasp around the distal radius with the fingers and thenar eminence of your inferior hand; be sure you are not grasping around the distal ulna.

MOBILIZING FORCE
Pull the radius distally (long-axis traction will cause joint traction).

b. **Dorsal or volar glide of the radius** (Fig. 6–29)

INDICATIONS
Dorsal glide, to increase extension; volar glide, to increase flexion.

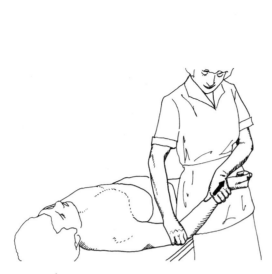

Figure 6–28. Joint traction; humeroradial articulation.

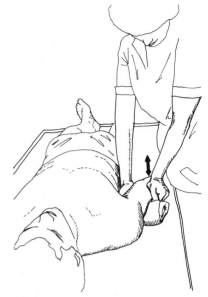

Figure 6–29. Dorsal and volar glide; humeroradial articulation.

POSITION OF PATIENT

Supine, or sitting with the elbow extended and supinated as far as possible.

HAND PLACEMENT

Stabilize the humerus from the medial side of the patient's arm. Place the palmar surface of your lateral hand on the volar aspect and your fingers on the dorsal aspect of the radial head.

MOBILIZING FORCE

Force the radial head dorsally with the palm of your hand or volarly with your fingers. If a stronger force is needed for the volar glide, realign your body, and push with the base of your hand against the dorsal surface in a volar direction.

c. **Joint compression** (Fig. 6–30)

INDICATION

To reduce a pulled elbow subluxation.

POSITION OF PATIENT

Sitting or supine.

HAND PLACEMENT

Using the same hand as that of the patient, place your thenar eminence against the patient's thenar eminence (locking thumbs). Fixate the humerus and proximal ulna against a firm object (treatment table or your other hand).

MOBILIZING FORCE

Push along the long axis of the radius by putting pressure against the thenar eminence; simultaneously supinate the forearm.

NOTE: To replace an acute subluxation, a quick motion (manipulation) is used.

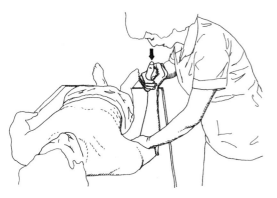

Figure 6–30. Joint compression; humeroradial articulation.

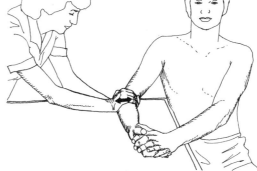

Figure 6–31. Dorsal-volar glide; proximal radioulnar joint.

3. **Radioulnar articulations**

   a. **Proximal radioulnar joint** (Fig. 6–31). (Convex rim of the radial head articulates with the concave radial notch on the ulna.)

     RESTING POSITION
     Elbow flexed 70 degrees, forearm supinated 35 degrees.

     TREATMENT PLANE
     In the radial notch of the ulna, parallel to the long axis of the ulna.

     STABILIZATION
     Proximal ulna.

     INDICATIONS
     Dorsal glide, to increase pronation; volar glide, to increase supination.

     POSITION OF PATIENT
     Sitting or supine, with the elbow and forearm in resting position.

     HAND PLACEMENT
     Fixate the ulna with your medial hand around the medial aspect of the forearm; place your other hand around the head of the radius with the fingers on the volar surface and the palm on the dorsal surface.

     MOBILIZING FORCE
     Force the radial head volarly by pushing with your palm or dorsally by pulling with your fingers. If a stronger force is needed for the dorsal glide, move around to the other side of the patient, switch hands, and push from the volar surface with the base of your hand against the radial head.

   b. **Distal radioulnar joint** (Fig. 6–32). (The concave ulnar notch of the radius articulates with the convex head of the ulna.)

     RESTING POSITION
     Supinated 10 degrees.

     TREATMENT PLANE
     Articulating surface of the radius, parallel to the long axis of the radius.

     STABILIZATION
     Distal ulna.

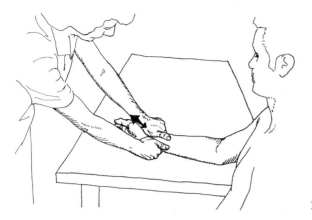

Figure 6–32. Dorsal-volar glide; distal radioulnar joint.

INDICATIONS

Dorsal glide, to increase supination; volar glide, to increase pronation.

POSITION OF PATIENT

Sitting, with arm on the treatment table; forearm in resting position.

HAND PLACEMENT

Stabilize the distal ulna by placing the fingers of one hand on the dorsal surface and the thenar eminence and thumb on the volar surface. Place your other hand in the same manner around the distal radius.

MOBILIZING FORCE

Glide the distal radius dorsally or volarly parallel to the ulna.

C. The Wrist Complex (Fig. 6–33)

1. Radiocarpal joint

Concave distal radius articulates with the convex proximal row of carpals, which is composed of the scaphoid, lunate, and triquetrum.

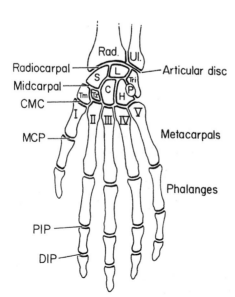

Figure 6–33. Bones and joints of the wrist and hand.

RESTING POSITION

Straight line through the radius and third metacarpal with slight ulnar deviation.

TREATMENT PLANE

In the articulating surface of the radius perpendicular to the long axis of the radius.

STABILIZATION

Distal radius and ulna.

a. **Joint traction (distraction)** (Fig. 6–34)

INDICATIONS

Testing; initial treatment; pain control; general mobility of the wrist.

POSITION OF PATIENT

Sitting, with forearm supported on the treatment table, wrist over the edge of the table.

HAND PLACEMENT

With the hand closest to the patient, grasp around the styloid processes and fixate the radius and ulna against the table. Your other hand grasps around the distal row of carpals.

MOBILIZING FORCE

Pull in a distal direction with respect to the arm.

b. **General glides**

INDICATIONS

Dorsal glide to increase flexion (Fig. 6–35); volar glide to increase extension (Fig. 6–36); radial glide to increase ulnar deviation; ulnar glide to increase radial deviation (Fig. 6–37).

POSITION OF PATIENT AND HAND PLACEMENT

Same as in Section a, except rotate the forearm when performing radial or ulnar glide for ease in accomplishing the technique.

MOBILIZING FORCE

Comes from the hand around the distal carpals.

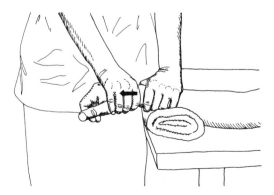

Figure 6–34. Joint traction; wrist joint.

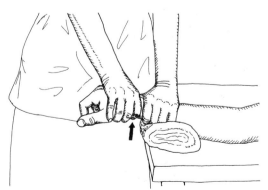

Figure 6–35. Dorsal glide; general mobilization of the wrist joint.

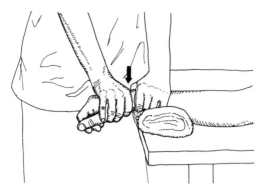

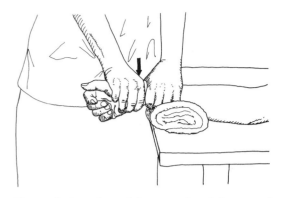

Figure 6–36. Volar glide; general mobilization of the wrist joint.

Figure 6–37. Ulnar glide; general mobilization of the wrist joint.

2. Specific glides of the carpals in the proximal row with the radius and ulna

POSITION OF PATIENT

Sitting, with the hand being held by the therapist so that the elbow hangs unsupported. The weight of the arm provides slight joint traction (grade I) so the therapist then needs only to apply the glides.

HAND PLACEMENT

Place your index fingers on the volar surface of the bone to be stabilized (see stabilization), the thumbs on the dorsal surface of the bone to be mobilized.

STABILIZATION

To increase flexion, the index fingers stabilize the distal bone (scaphoid or lunate) (Fig. 6–38). To increase extension, the index fingers stabilize the proximal bone (radius) (Fig. 6–39).

MOBILIZING FORCE

In each case, the force comes from the thumbs on the dorsal surface of the bone to be mobilized. By mobilizing from the dorsal surface, pressure against the nerves, blood vessels, and tendons in the carpal tunnel and Guyon's canal is minimized and a stronger mobilizing force can be used without pain.

a. **Scaphoid-radius** (scaphoid convex, radius concave) and **lunate-radius** (lunate convex, radius concave)

INDICATIONS

To increase flexion, glide radius volarly on fixed scaphoid or glide radius volarly on fixed lunate (see Fig. 6–38). To increase extension, glide scaphoid volarly on fixed radius or glide lunate volarly on fixed radius (Fig. 6–39).

b. **Ulnar-meniscal triquetral articulation**

INDICATIONS

To unlock the articular disk, which may block motions of the wrist or forearm, glide ulna volarly on fixed triquetrum.

3. Specific glides of the intercarpal joints

POSITION OF PATIENT AND HAND PLACEMENT

Same as described in Section 2.

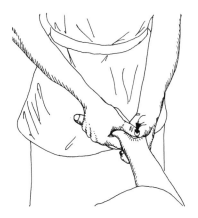

Figure 6–38. Stabilization of the distal bone; volar glide of the proximal bone; shown is stabilization of the scaphoid and lunate with volar glide to the radius.

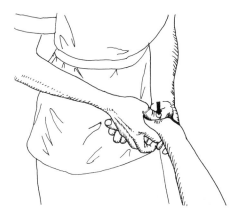

Figure 6–39. Stabilization of the proximal bone; volar glide of the distal bone; shown is stabilization of the radius with volar glide to the lunate.

STABILIZATION

In all cases the stabilization is applied with the index fingers overlapped on the volar surface.

MOBILIZATION FORCE

In all cases the force comes from the overlapped thumbs on the dorsal surface.

a. *Glides to increase extension*

Stabilize the bone that has the concave articulating surface, and apply the mobilizing force against the dorsal surface of the bone with the convex articulating surface. The force is in a volar direction.

EXAMPLES

(1) To increase extension and radial deviation at the trapezium-trapezoid/scaphoid articulation, glide the scaphoid volarly with your thumbs while stabilizing the trapezium-trapezoid unit with your index fingers.

(2) To increase extension at the capitate/lunate articulation, glide the capitate volarly with your thumbs while stabilizing the lunate with your index fingers.

b. *Glides to increase flexion*

Stabilize the bone that has the convex articulating surface and apply the mobilizing force against the dorsal surface of the bone with the concave articulating surface. The force is in a volar direction.

EXAMPLES

(1) To increase flexion at the trapezium-trapezoid/scaphoid articulation, glide the trapezium-trapezoid unit volarly with your thumbs while stabilizing the scaphoid with your index fingers.

(2) To increase flexion at the capitate/lunate articulation, glide the lunate volarly with your thumbs while stabilizing the capitate.

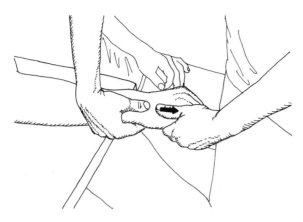

Figure 6–40. Joint traction; carpometacarpal joint.

D. The Hand and Finger Joints

1. The carpometacarpal and intermetacarpal joints of digits II through V

a. **Joint traction** (Fig. 6–40)

INDICATION
To increase mobility of the hand.

STABILIZATION AND HAND PLACEMENT
Stabilize the respective carpal with one hand; grasp with your thumb dorsal and index fingers volar. Your other hand grasps around the proximal portion of a metacarpal, thumb dorsal and fingers volar.

MOBILIZING FORCE
Apply long-axis traction to the metacarpal to separate the joint surfaces.

b. **Volar glide**

INDICATION
To increase mobility of the arch of the hand.

STABILIZATION AND HAND PLACEMENT
Same as in Section a.

MOBILIZING FORCE
The thumb on the dorsum of the metacarpal glides the proximal portion of the bone volarward.

c. See also the technique for cupping and flattening the arch of the hand described in Chapter 2.

2. The carpometacarpal joint of the thumb

A saddle joint: The trapezium is concave, proximal metacarpal convex for abduction/adduction; the trapezium is convex, proximal metacarpal concave for flexion/extension.

RESTING POSITION
Midway between flexion and extension and between abduction and adduction.

STABILIZATION
Fixate the trapezium with the hand that is closer to the patient.

TREATMENT PLANE

In the trapezium for abduction-adduction; in the proximal metacarpal for flexion-extension.

a. **Joint traction**

INDICATIONS

Testing; initial treatment; pain control; general mobility.

POSITION OF PATIENT

Forearm and hand resting on the treatment table.

HAND PLACEMENT

Fixate the trapezium with the hand that is closer to the patient; grasp the patient's metacarpal by wrapping your fingers around it (similar to Fig. 6–41A).

MOBILIZING FORCE

Apply long-axis traction to separate the joint surfaces.

b. **Glides** (Fig. 6–41)

INDICATIONS

To increase flexion, ulnar glide; to increase extension, radial glide; to increase abduction, dorsal glide; to increase adduction, volar glide.

POSITION OF PATIENT AND HAND PLACEMENT

The trapezium is stabilized by grasping it directly or by wrapping your fingers around the distal row of carpals. Place the thenar eminence of your other hand against the base of the patient's first metacarpal on the side opposite the desired glide. (In Fig. 6–41A, the surface of the hand is on the radial side of the metacarpal to cause an ulnar glide.)

MOBILIZING FORCE

Comes from your thenar eminence on the metacarpal. Adjust your body position to line up the force as illustrated in Figure 6–41A through D.

3. The metacarpophalangeal and interphalangeal joints of the fingers

In all cases, the distal end of the proximal articulating surface is convex, and the proximal end of the distal articulating surface is concave.

NOTE: Because all the articulating surfaces are the same for the digits, all techniques are applied in the same manner to each joint.

RESTING POSITION

Slight flexion in all joints.

TREATMENT PLANE

In the distal articulating surface.

STABILIZATION

Rest the forearm and hand on the treatment table; fixate the proximal articulating surface with the fingers of one hand.

a. **Joint traction** (Fig. 6–42)

INDICATIONS

Testing; initial treatment; pain control; general mobility.

HAND PLACEMENT

Use your proximal hand to stabilize the proximal bone; wrap the fingers and thumb of your other hand around the distal bone close to the joint.

MOBILIZING FORCE

Apply long-axis traction to separate the joint surface.

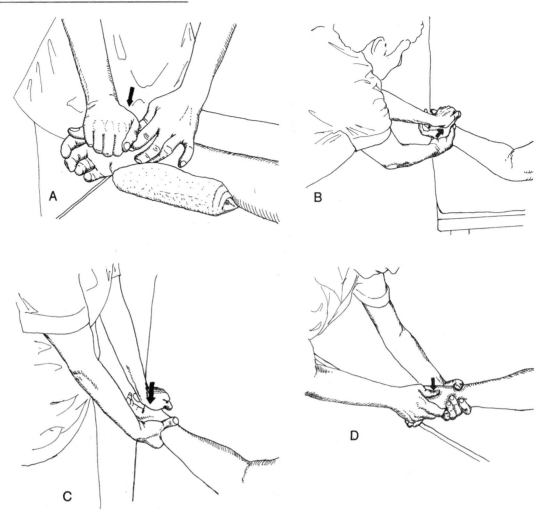

Figure 6–41. Carpometacarpal joint of the thumb. (*A*) Ulnar glide to increase flexion. (*B*) Radial glide to increase extension. (*C*) Dorsal glide to increase abduction. (*D*) Volar glide to increase adduction. Note that the thumb of the therapist is placed in the web space between the index and thumb of the patient's hand in order to apply a volar glide.

b. **Glides**

INDICATIONS

To increase flexion, volar glide (Fig. 6–43); to increase extension, dorsal glide; to increase abduction or adduction, radial or ulnar glide (depending on finger).

MOBILIZING FORCE

The glide force is applied by the thumb against the proximal end of the bone to be moved.

c. **Rotations** (Fig. 6–44)

INDICATIONS

To increase final degrees of motion.

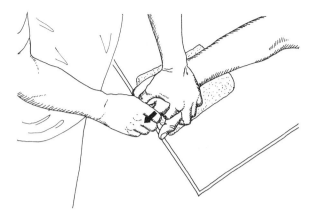

Figure 6–42. Joint traction of a metacarpophalangeal joint.

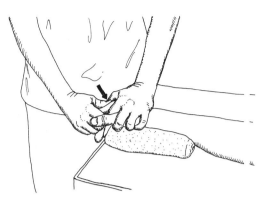

Figure 6–43. Volar glide of a metacarpophalangeal joint.

MOBILIZING FORCE
Initially, rotate the distal bone on the stabilized proximal bone, then apply a traction force.

E. The Hip Joint (Fig. 6–45)

The concave acetabulum receives the convex femoral head.

RESTING POSITION
Hip flexion 30 degrees, abduction 30 degrees, and slight external rotation.

STABILIZATION
Fixate the pelvis to the treatment table with belts.

1. Distraction of the weight-bearing surface: caudal glide (Fig. 6–46)

NOTE: Because of the deep configuration of this joint, traction applied perpendicular to the treatment plane causes a lateral glide of the superior, weight-bearing surface. To get separation of the weight-bearing surface, a caudal glide is used.

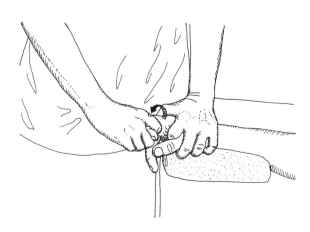

Figure 6–44. Rotation of a metacarpophalangeal joint.

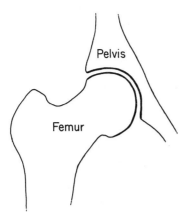

Figure 6–45. Bones of the hip joint.

INDICATIONS
Testing; initial treatment; pain control; general mobility.

POSITION OF PATIENT
Supine, with hip in resting position and the knee extended.

    Precaution: With knee dysfunction, this position should not be used; see alternate position under Section 2.

POSITION OF THERAPIST AND HAND PLACEMENT
Stand at the end of the treatment table; place a belt around your trunk, then cross the belt over the patient's foot and around the ankle. Place your hands proximal to the malleoli, under the belt. The belt allows you to use your body weight to apply the mobilizing force.

MOBILIZING FORCE
A long-axis traction is applied by pulling on the leg as you lean backward.

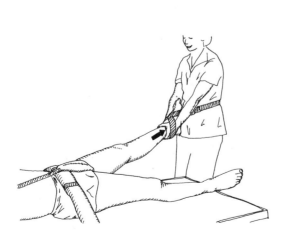

Figure 6–46. Distraction of the weight-bearing surface of the hip joint: caudal glide.

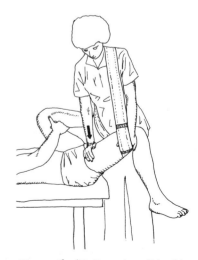

Figure 6–47. Posterior glide; hip joint.

2. Alternate position for caudal glide

INDICATION

Same as in Section 1, to apply distraction to the weight-bearing surface of the hip when there is knee dysfunction.

POSITION OF PATIENT

Supine, with the hip and knee flexed.

POSITION OF THERAPIST AND HAND PLACEMENT

Wrap your hands around the epicondyles of the femur and distal thigh. Do not compress the patella.

MOBILIZING FORCE

Comes from your hands and is applied in a caudal direction as you lean backward.

3. Posterior glide (Fig. 6–47)

INDICATIONS

To increase flexion; to increase internal rotation.

POSITION OF PATIENT

Supine, with hips at the end of the table. The patient helps stabilize the pelvis by flexing the opposite hip and holding the thigh with the hands. The hip to be mobilized is in resting position.

POSITION OF THERAPIST AND HAND PLACEMENT

Stand on the medial side of the patient's thigh. Place a belt around your shoulder and under the patient's thigh to help hold the weight of the lower extremity. Place your distal hand under the belt and distal thigh. Place your proximal hand on the anterior surface of the proximal thigh.

MOBILIZING FORCE

Keep your elbows extended and flex your knees; apply the force through your proximal hand in a posterior direction.

4. Anterior glide (Fig. 6–48)

INDICATIONS

To increase extension; to increase external rotation.

POSITION OF PATIENT

Prone, with trunk resting on the table and hips over the edge. The opposite foot is on the floor.

POSITION OF THERAPIST AND HAND PLACEMENT

Stand on the medial side of the patient's thigh; place a belt around your shoulder and the patient's thigh to help support the weight of the leg. With your distal hand, hold the patient's leg. Place your proximal hand posteriorly on the proximal thigh, just below the buttock.

MOBILIZING FORCE

Keep your elbow extended and flex your knees; apply the force through your proximal hand in an anterior direction.

ALTERNATE POSITION (Fig. 6–48B)

Position patient side-lying with the thigh comfortably flexed and supported by pillows. Stand posterior to the patient and stabilize the pelvis across the anterior

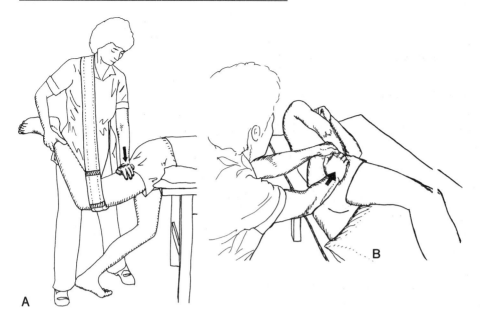

Figure 6–48. Anterior glide; hip joint (*A*) prone and (*B*) side-lying.

superior iliac spine with your cranial hand. Push against the posterior aspect of the greater trochanter in an anterior direction with your caudal hand.

F. The Knee and Leg (Fig. 6-49)

1. The tibiofemoral articulation

Concave tibial plateaus articulate on the convex femoral condyles.

RESTING POSITION
Flexion 25 degrees.

TREATMENT PLANE
Along the surface of the tibial plateaus. Therefore, it moves with the tibia as the knee angle changes.

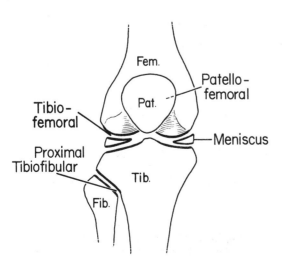

Figure 6–49. Bones and joints of the knee and leg.

STABILIZATION

In most cases, the femur is stabilized with a belt or by the table.

a. **Joint traction: long-axis traction** (Figs. 6–50A, B, and C)

INDICATIONS

Testing; initial treatment; pain control; general mobility.

POSITION OF PATIENT

Sitting, supine, or prone, beginning with the knee in resting position.

HAND PLACEMENT

Grasp around the distal leg, proximal to the malleoli with both hands.

MOBILIZING FORCE

Pull on the long axis of the tibia to separate the joint surfaces.

b. **Posterior glide: drawer test** (Fig. 6–51)

INDICATIONS

Testing; to increase flexion.

POSITION OF PATIENT

Supine, with the foot resting on the table. The position for the drawer test can be used to mobilize the tibia either anteriorly or posteriorly, although no grade I distraction can be applied with the glides.

POSITION OF THERAPIST AND HAND PLACEMENT

Sit on the table with your thigh fixating the patient's foot. With both hands, grasp around the tibia, fingers pointing posteriorly and thumbs anteriorly.

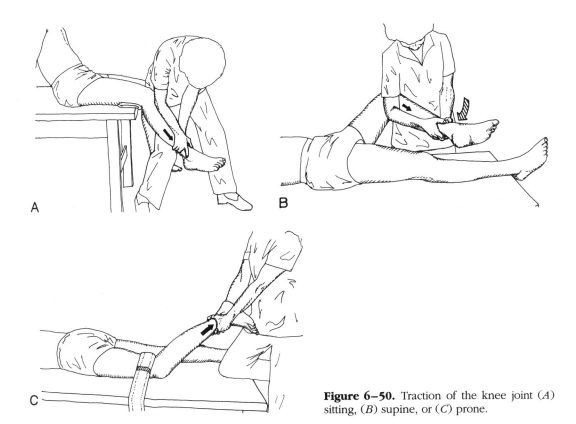

A   B   C

Figure 6–50. Traction of the knee joint (*A*) sitting, (*B*) supine, or (*C*) prone.

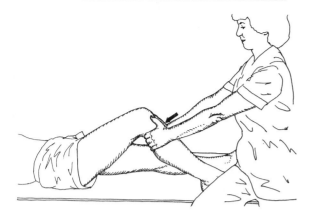

Figure 6–51. Posterior glide (drawer); knee joint.

MOBILIZING FORCE

Extend your elbows and lean your body weight forward; push the tibia posteriorly with your thumbs.

c. **Posterior glide, alternate position, and progression** (Fig. 6–52)

INDICATION

To increase flexion.

POSITION OF PATIENT

Sitting, with the knee flexed over the edge of the treatment table, beginning in resting position (Fig. 6–52A) and progressing to near 90 degrees (Fig. 6–52B).

POSITION OF THERAPIST AND HAND PLACEMENT

When in resting position, stand on the medial side of the patient's leg. Hold the distal leg with your distal hand and place the palm of your proximal hand along the anterior aspect of the tibia. When near 90 degrees, sit on a low stool; stabilize the leg between your knees and place one hand on the anterior aspect of the tibia. Progression beyond 90 degrees requires the patient to lie prone.

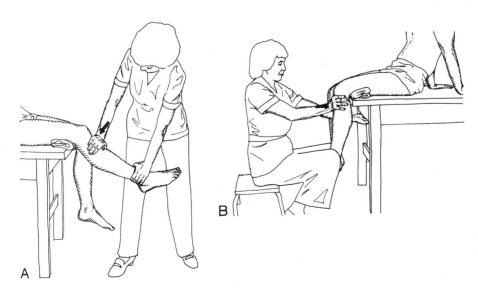

Figure 6–52. Posterior glide of the knee joint (*A*) in resting position and (*B*) near 90 degrees.

MOBILIZING FORCE

Extend your elbow and lean your body weight onto the tibia, gliding it posteriorly.

d. **Anterior glide** (Fig. 6–53)

INDICATION

To increase extension.

POSITION OF PATIENT

Prone, with the knee in resting position. Place a small pad under the distal femur to prevent patellar compression.

HAND PLACEMENT

Grasp the distal tibia with the hand that is closer to it, and place the palm of the proximal hand on the posterior aspect of the proximal tibia.

MOBILIZING FORCE

Force with the hand on the proximal tibia in an anterior direction.

NOTE: The drawer test position can also be used (see Section b). The mobilizing force comes from the fingers on the posterior tibia as you lean backward (see Fig. 6–51).

2. **Patellofemoral joint**

a. **Distal glide** (Fig. 6–54)

INDICATION

To increase patellar mobility for knee flexion.

POSITION OF PATIENT

Supine, with knee extended.

HAND PLACEMENT

Stand next to the patient's thigh, facing the patient's feet. Place the web space of the hand that is closer to the thigh around the superior border of the patella. Use the other hand for reinforcement.

MOBILIZING FORCE

Glide the patella in a caudal direction, parallel to the femur.

Precaution: Do not compress the patella into the femoral condyles while performing this technique.

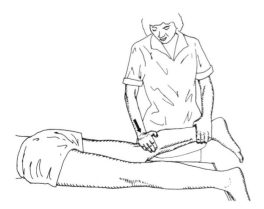

Figure 6–53. Anterior glide; knee joint.

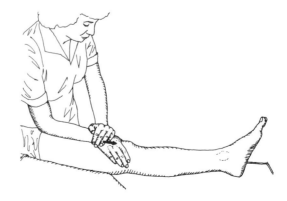

Figure 6–54. Distal glide; patellofemoral joint.

b. **Medial-lateral glide** (Fig. 6–55)

INDICATION

To increase patellar mobility.

POSITION OF PATIENT

Supine, with knee extended.

HAND PLACEMENT

Place your fingers medially and thumbs laterally around the medial and lateral borders of the patella, respectively.

MOBILIZING FORCE

Glide the patella in a medial or lateral direction, against the restriction.

3. **Proximal tibiofibular articulation: anterior (ventral) glide (Fig. 6–56)**

INDICATIONS

To increase movement of the fibular head; to reposition a posteriorly positioned head.

POSITION OF PATIENT

Side-lying, with the trunk and hips rotated partially toward prone; the top leg is flexed forward so that the knee and lower leg are resting on the table or supported on a pillow.

POSITION OF THERAPIST AND HAND PLACEMENT

Stand behind the patient, placing one of your hands under the tibia to stabilize it. Place the base of your other hand posterior to the head of the fibula, wrapping your fingers anteriorly.

MOBILIZING FORCE

Comes from the heel of your hand against the posterior aspect of the fibular head, in an anterior-lateral direction.

4. **Distal tibiofibular articulation: anterior (ventral) or posterior (dorsal) glide (Fig. 6–57)**

INDICATION

To increase mobility of the mortise when it is restricting ankle dorsiflexion.

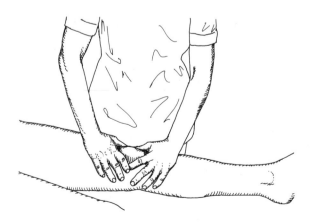

Figure 6–55. Medial-lateral glide of the patella.

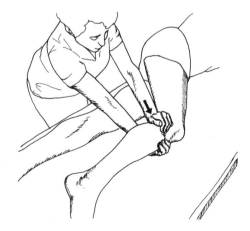

Figure 6–56. Anterior glide; fibular head.

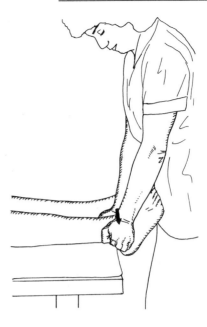

Figure 6–57. Posterior glide; distal tibiofibular articulation.

POSITION OF PATIENT
Supine or prone.

HAND PLACEMENT
Working from the end of the table, place the fingers of the more medial hand under the tibia and the thumb over the tibia to stabilize it. Place the base of your other hand over the lateral malleolus, with the fingers underneath.

MOBILIZING FORCE
Against the fibula in an anterior direction when prone and a posterior direction when supine.

G. Ankle and Tarsal Joints (Fig. 6–58)

1. Talocrural (upper ankle joint)

Convex talus articulates with the concave mortise made up of the tibia and fibula.

RESTING POSITION
Plantarflexion 10 degrees.

TREATMENT PLANE
In the mortise, in an anterior-posterior direction with respect to the leg.

STABILIZATION
Tibia strapped or held against the table.

a. **Joint traction (distraction)** (Fig. 6–59)

INDICATIONS
Testing; initial treatment; pain control; general mobility.

POSITION OF PATIENT
Supine, with the lower extremity extended and the ankle in resting position.

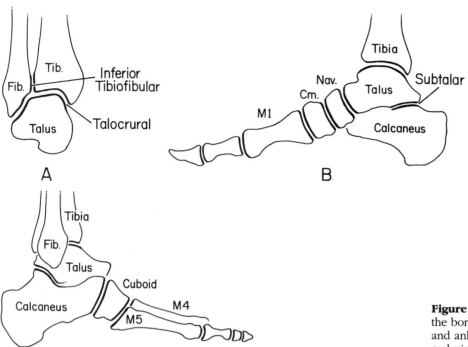

Figure 6–58. (A) Anterior view of the bones and joints of the lower leg and ankle. (B) Medial view. (C) Lateral view of the bones and joint relationships of the ankle and foot.

POSITION OF THERAPIST AND HAND PLACEMENT

Stand at the end of the table; wrap the fingers of both hands over the dorsum of the patient's foot, just distal to the mortise; place your thumbs on the plantar surface of the foot to hold it in resting position.

MOBILIZATION FORCE

Pull the foot away from the long axis of the leg in a distal direction by leaning backward.

b. **Dorsal (posterior) glide** (Fig. 6–60)

INDICATION

To increase dorsiflexion.

POSITION OF PATIENT

Supine, with the leg supported on the table and the heel over the edge.

POSITION OF THERAPIST AND HAND PLACEMENT

Stand to the side of the patient. Stabilize the leg with your cranial hand or use a belt to secure the leg to the table. Place the palmar aspect of the web space of your other hand over the talus just distal to the mortise. Wrap your fingers and thumb around the foot to maintain the ankle in resting position. A grade I distraction force is applied in a caudal direction.

MOBILIZING FORCE

Glide the talus posteriorly with respect to the tibia by pushing against the talus.

c. **Ventral (anterior) glide** (Fig. 6–61)

INDICATION

To increase plantarflexion.

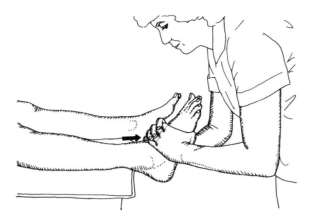

Figure 6–59. Joint traction; talocrural joint.

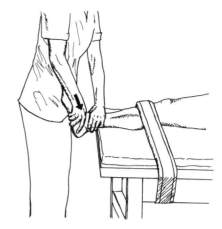

Figure 6–60. Posterior glide; talocrural joint.

POSITION OF PATIENT

Prone, with the foot over the edge of the table.

POSITION OF THERAPIST AND HAND PLACEMENT

Working from the end of the table, place your lateral hand across the dorsum of the foot to apply a grade I distraction. Place the web space of your other hand just distal to the mortise on the posterior aspect of the talus and calcaneus.

MOBILIZING FORCE

Push against the calcaneus in an anterior direction (with respect to the tibia); this glides the talus anteriorly.

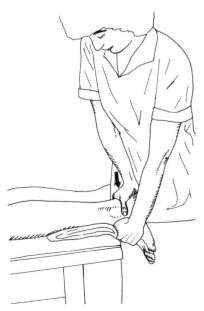

Figure 6–61. Anterior glide; talocrural joint.

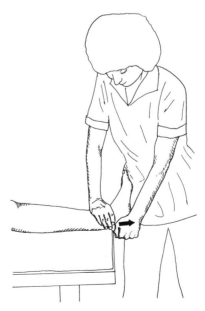

Figure 6–62. Joint traction; subtalar (talocalcaneal) joint.

ALTERNATE POSITION

Patient is supine. Stabilize the distal leg anterior to the mortise with your proximal hand. The distal hand cups under the calcaneus. When you push against the calcaneus in an anterior direction, the talus glides anteriorly.

2. Subtalar (talocalcaneal) joint, posterior compartment

The calcaneus is convex, articulating with a concave talus in the posterior compartment.

RESTING POSITION

Midway between inversion and eversion.

TREATMENT PLANE

In the talus, parallel to the sole of the foot.

a. Joint traction (distraction) (Fig. 6–62)

INDICATIONS

Testing; initial treatment; pain control; general mobility for inversion/eversion.

POSITION OF PATIENT

Supine, with the leg supported on the table and heel over the edge. The ankle is stabilized in dorsiflexion with pressure from the therapist's thigh.

HAND PLACEMENT

The distal hand grasps around the calcaneus from the posterior aspect of the foot. The other hand fixes the talus and malleoli against the table.

MOBILIZING FORCE

Pull the calcaneus distally with respect to the long axis of the leg.

b. Medial glide or lateral glide (Fig. 6–63)

INDICATION

Medial glide to increase eversion; lateral glide to increase inversion.

POSITION OF PATIENT

Side-lying or prone, with the leg supported on the table or with a towel roll.

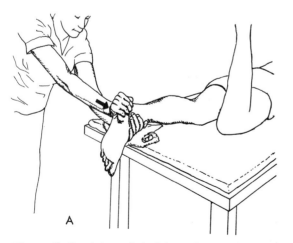
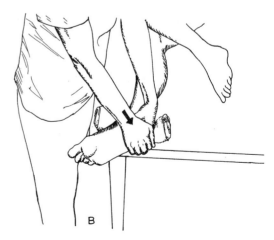

Figure 6–63. (*A*) Medial glide with patient prone to increase eversion. (*B*) Lateral glide with patient side-lying to increase inversion; subtalar joint.

POSITION OF THERAPIST AND HAND PLACEMENT

Align your shoulder and arm parallel to the bottom of the foot. Stabilize the talus with your proximal hand. Place the base of the distal hand on the side of the calcaneus, medially to cause a lateral glide and laterally to cause a medial glide, and wrap the fingers around the plantar surface.

MOBILIZING FORCE

Apply a grade I distraction force in a caudal direction, then push with the base of your hand against the side of the calcaneus parallel to the plantar surface of the heel.

ALTERNATE POSITION

Same as in Section a, moving the calcaneus in a medial direction with the fingers, or a lateral direction with the base of the hand.

3. Intertarsal joints and tarsometatarsal joints

When moving in a dorsal-plantar direction with respect to the foot, all of the articulating surfaces are concave and convex in the same direction; for example, the proximal articulating surface is convex and the distal articulating surface is concave. The technique for mobilizing each joint is the same; the hand placement is adjusted to stabilize the proximal bone partner so the distal bone partner can be moved.

a. **Plantar glide** (Fig. 6–64)

INDICATION

To increase plantarflexion accessory motions (necessary for supination).

POSITION OF PATIENT

Supine, with hip and knee flexed; or sitting, with knee flexed over the edge of the table and heel resting in the therapist's lap.

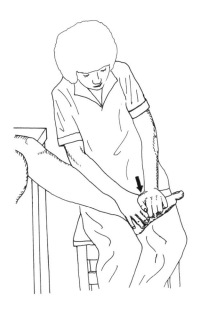

Figure 6–64. Plantar glide of a distal tarsal bone on a stabilized proximal bone; shown is the cuneiform bone on the navicular.

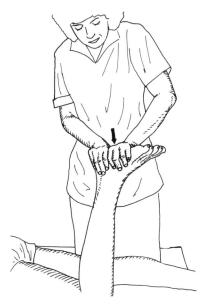

Figure 6–65. Dorsal gliding of a distal tarsal on a proximal tarsal; shown is the cuboid bone on the calcaneus.

STABILIZATION

Fixate the more proximal bone with your index finger on the plantar surface of the bone.

HAND PLACEMENT

To mobilize the medial tarsal joints, place the stabilizing hand on the dorsum of the foot with the fingers pointing medially, so that the index finger can be placed under the bone to be stabilized. Wrap the fingers of the other hand around the plantar surface of the tarsal joint to be moved and the base of the hand over the dorsal surface. To mobilize the lateral tarsal joints, position yourself medially and point your fingers laterally.

MOBILIZING FORCE

Push in a plantar direction from the dorsum of the foot.

b. **Dorsal glide** (Fig. 6–65)

INDICATION

To increase dorsal gliding accessory motion (necessary for pronation).

POSITION OF PATIENT

Prone, with knee flexed.

STABILIZATION

Fixate the more proximal bone.

HAND PLACEMENT

To mobilize the lateral tarsal joints (for example, cuboid on calcaneus), wrap your fingers around the lateral side of the foot (as in Fig. 6–65). To mobilize the medial bones (for example, navicular on talus), wrap your fingers around the medial aspect of the foot. Place your second metacarpophalangeal joint against the bone to be moved.

MOBILIZING FORCE

Push from the plantar surface in a dorsal direction.

ALTERNATE TECHNIQUE

Same as position of patient in Section a, except the distal bone is stabilized and the proximal bone is forced in a plantar direction. This is a relative motion of the distal bone moving in a dorsal direction.

H. The Intermetatarsal, Metatarsophalangeal, and Interphalangeal Joints

The intermetatarsal, metatarsophalangeal, and interphalangeal joints of the toes are stabilized and mobilized in the same manner as the fingers. In each case, the articulating surface of the proximal bone is convex, and the articulating surface of the distal bone is concave. (See Section D.)

VIII. Summary

Basic concepts of joint mobilization have been presented, including definitions of terminology, concepts of joint motion, and indications, limitations, and contraindications for the techniques. Basic procedures for applying the techniques have been described, from which adaptations can be made and other techniques developed as the skill of the therapist progresses.

References

1. Akeson, WH, et al: Effects of immobilization on joints. Clin Orthop Rel Res 219:28, 1987.
2. Cookson, JC, and Kent, BE: Orthopedic manual therapy an overview; Part I: The extremities. Phys Ther 59:136, 1979.
3. Cyriax, J: Textbook of Orthopaedic Medicine, Vol I: The Diagnosis of Soft Tissue Lesions, ed 8. Bailliere and Tindall, London, 1982.
4. Donatelli, R, and Owens-Burkhart, H: Effects of immobilization on the extensibility of periarticular connective tissue. Journal of Orthopaedic and Sports Physical Therapy 3:67, 1981.
5. Enneking, WF, and Horowitz, M: The intra-articular effects of immobilization on the human knee. J Bone Joint Surg Am 54:973, 1972.
6. Grieve, G: Manual mobilizing techniques in degenerative arthrosis of the hip. Bulletin of the Orthopaedic Section APTA 2/1:7, 1977.
7. Hoppenfield, S: Physical Examination of the Spine and Extremities. Appleton-Century-Crofts, New York, 1976.
8. Kaltenborn, FM: Manual Mobilization of the Extremity Joints: Basic Examination and Treatment Techniques, ed 4. Olaf Norlis Bokhandel, Universitetsgaten, Oslo, 1989.
9. Kessler, R, and Hertling, D: Management of Common Musculoskeletal Disorders. Harper & Row, Philadelphia, 1983.
10. Lehmkuhl, LD, and Smith, LM: Brunnstrom's Clinical Kinesiology, ed 4. FA Davis, Philadelphia, 1983.
11. Maitland, GD: Peripheral Manipulation, ed 2. Butterworth, Boston, 1977.
12. Norkin, C, and Levangie, P: Joint Structure and Function: A Comprehensive Analysis, ed 2. FA Davis, Philadelphia, 1992.
13. Paris, SV: Mobilization of the spine. Phys Ther 59:988, 1979.
14. Svendsen, B, Moe, K, and Merritt, R: Joint Mobilization Laboratory Manual: Extremity Joint Testing and Selected Treatment Techniques. Svendsen, B, Bryn Mawr, CA, 1981.
15. Warwick, R, and Williams, S (eds): Arthrology. In Gray's Anatomy, 35th British ed. WB Saunders, Philadelphia, 1973.
16. Wyke, B: The neurology of joints. Ann R Coll Surg 41:25, 1967.
17. Wyke, B: Articular neurology: A review. Physiotherapy March: 94, 1972.
18. Wyke, B: Neurological Aspects of Pain for the Physical Therapy Clinician. Physical Therapy Forum '82, Lecture, Columbus, 1982.
19. Magee, D: Orthopedic Physical Assessment, ed 2. WB Saunders, Philadelphia, 1992.
20. Wadsworth, C: Manual Examination of the Spine and Extremities. Williams & Wilkins, Baltimore, 1988.
21. Wegener, L: Static and dynamic balance responses in persons with bilateral knee osteoarthritis. Masters Thesis, The Ohio State University, Columbus, 1994.

Application of Therapeutic Exercise Techniques to Regions of the Body

Chapter

7

Principles of Treating Soft Tissue, Bony, and Postsurgical Problems

The proper use of therapeutic exercise in the treatment of musculoskeletal disorders depends on identifying the structure involved, recognizing its stage of recovery, and determining the functional limitations or disabilities. Evaluation is an important prerequisite for identifying the anatomic structure or structures that are causing the impairments and limiting function and also for determining whether the tissue is in the acute, subacute, or chronic stage of recovery. Information summarizing an orthopedic evaluation and suggested references for study are included in Chapter 1. This chapter and subsequent chapters in this section have been written with the assumption that the reader has a background in evaluation and assessment.

OBJECTIVES

After studying this chapter, the reader will be able to:

1 Identify examples of soft tissue lesions.
2 Identify characteristics of soft tissue repair during the stages of inflammation, healing, and restoration of function.
3 Identify special considerations, treatment goals, and plan of care for soft tissue lesions during the inflammatory and healing stages of tissue repair and during the restoration of function.
4 Identify special considerations, treatment goals, and a plan of care for specific joint disorders during exacerbation and remission of symptoms.
5 Identify special considerations, treatment goals, and a plan of care for recovery following fractures.
6 Identify special considerations, treatment goals, and a plan of care for presurgical and postsurgical management.

I. Soft Tissue Lesions

A. Examples of Soft Tissue Lesions

1. **Strain.** Overstretching, overexertion, overuse of soft tissue; tends to be less severe than a sprain. Occurs from slight trauma or unaccustomed repeated trauma of a minor degree.[5] This term is frequently used to refer specifically to some degree of disruption of the musculotendinous unit.[17]

2. **Sprain.** Severe stress, stretch, or tear of soft tissues such as joint capsule, ligament, tendon, or muscle. This term is frequently used to refer specifically to injury of a ligament and is graded as first- (mild), second- (moderate), or third- (severe) degree sprains.[17]

3. **Subluxation.** An incomplete or partial dislocation that often involves secondary trauma to surrounding soft tissue.

4. **Dislocation.** Displacement of a part, usually the bony partners within a joint, leading to soft tissue damage, inflammation, pain, and muscle spasm.

5. **Muscle/tendon rupture or tear.** If a rupture or tear is partial, pain is experienced in the region of the breach when the muscle is stretched or when it contracts against resistance. If a rupture or tear is complete, the muscle does not pull against the injury, so stretching or contraction of the muscle does not cause pain.[10]

6. **Tendinous lesions.**[4,12] **Tenosynovitis** is an inflammation of the synovial membrane covering a tendon. **Tendinitis** is an inflammation of a tendon; there may be resulting scarring or calcium deposits. **Tenovaginitis** is inflammation with thickening of a tendon sheath. **Tendinosis** is a degeneration of the tendon from repetitive microtrauma.

7. **Synovitis.** Inflammation of a synovial membrane; an excess of normal synovial fluid within a joint or tendon sheath from trauma or disease.[41]

8. **Hemarthrosis.** Bleeding into a joint, usually from severe trauma.[41]

9. **Ganglion.** Ballooning of the wall of a joint capsule or tendon sheath. Ganglia may arise following trauma; they sometimes occur with rheumatoid arthritis.

10. **Bursitis.** Inflammation of a bursa.

11. **Contusion.** Bruising from a direct blow, resulting in capillary rupture, bleeding, edema, and an inflammatory response.

12. **Overuse syndromes, cumulative trauma disorders, repetitive strain injury.** Repeated, submaximal overload and/or frictional wear to a muscle or tendon resulting in inflammation and pain.

B. Clinical Conditions Resulting from Trauma or Pathology

In many conditions involving soft tissue, the primary pathology is difficult to define, or the tissue has healed with limitations, resulting in a secondary loss of function. The following are examples of clinical manifestations resulting from a variety of causes, including those listed under the previous section:

1. **Dysfunction.** Loss of normal function of a tissue or region. The dysfunction may be due to adaptive shortening of the soft tissues, adhesions, muscle weakness, or any condition resulting in loss of normal mobility.

2. **Joint dysfunction.** Mechanical loss of normal joint play in synovial joints; commonly causes loss of function and pain. Precipitating factors may be trauma, immobilization, disuse, aging, or a serious pathologic condition.[40]

3. **Contractures.** Shortening or tightening of skin, fascia, muscle, or joint capsule that prevents normal mobility or flexibility of that structure.

4. **Adhesions.** Abnormal adherence of collagen fibers to surrounding structures during immobilization, following trauma, or as a complication of surgery, which restricts normal elasticity of the structures involved.

5. **Reflex muscle guarding.** The prolonged contraction of a muscle in response to a painful stimulus. The primary pain-causing lesion may be in nearby or underlying tissue or from a referred pain source. When not referred, the contracting muscle functionally splints the injured tissue against movement. Guarding ceases when the painful stimulus is relieved.

6. **Intrinsic muscle spasm.** The prolonged contraction of a muscle in response to the local circulatory and metabolic changes that occur when a muscle is in a continued state of contraction. Pain is a result of the altered circulatory and metabolic environment, so the muscle contraction becomes self-perpetuating regardless of whether the primary lesion that caused the initial guarding is still irritable (Fig. 7–1). Spasm may also be a response of muscle to viral infection, cold, prolonged periods of immobilization, emotional tension, or direct trauma to muscle.[40]

7. **Muscle weakness.** A decrease in the strength of contraction of muscle. Muscle weakness may be the result of a systemic, chemical, or local lesion of a nerve of the central or peripheral nervous system or the myoneural junction. It may also be the result of a direct insult to the muscle or may simply be due to inactivity.

C. Severity of Tissue Injury[17,18]

1. Grade 1 (first-degree)

Mild pain at the time of injury or within the first 24 hours; mild swelling, local tenderness, and pain occur when the tissue is stressed.

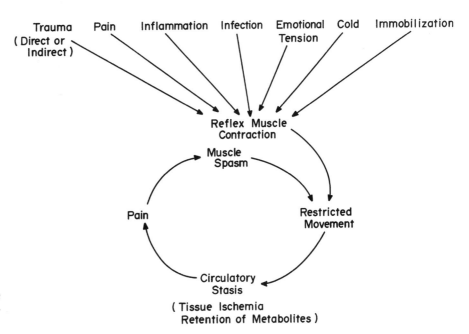

Figure 7–1. Schematic of the self-perpetuating cycle of muscle spasm.

2. Grade 2 (second-degree)

Moderate pain that requires stopping the activity. Stress and palpation of the tissue greatly increases the pain. When the injury is to ligaments, some of the fibers are torn, resulting in some increased joint mobility.

3. Grade 3 (third-degree)

Near-complete or complete tear or avulsion of the tissue (tendon or ligament) with severe pain. Stress to the tissue is usually painless; palpation may reveal the defect. A torn ligament results in instability of the joint.

II. Stages of Inflammation and Repair: General Descriptions

Following any insult to connective tissue, whether it is from mechanical injury (including surgery) or chemical irritant, the body responses and stages of healing are similar (Table 7–1). In the following outline, the number of days given for each stage is approximate, and the stages overlap. Differences in individual patients must also be taken into account. The response of the patient is the best guideline for determining when treatment should progress from one stage to the next.

A. Acute (Inflammatory Reaction) Stage

1. Characteristics

This stage involves both cellular and humoral responses. During the first 48 hours following insult to soft tissue, vascular changes predominate. Exudation of cells and solutes from the blood vessels takes place, and clot formation occurs. Within this period, neutralization of the chemical irritants or noxious stimuli, phagocytosis (cleaning up of dead tissue), early fibroblastic activity, and formation of new capillary beds begin. These physiologic processes serve as a protective mechanism as well as a stimulus for subsequent healing and repair.[36,38] Usually this stage lasts 4 to 6 days unless the insult is perpetuated.

2. Clinical signs

The signs of inflammation are present: swelling, redness, heat, pain, and loss of function. When testing the range of motion (ROM), the patient will experience pain, and there may be muscle guarding before completion of the range (Fig. 7–2A).

B. Subacute (Repair-Healing) Stage

As the inflammation decreases (during the second to fourth day), resolution of the clot and repair of the injured site begins. This usually lasts an additional 10 to 17 days (14 to 21 days after the onset of injury) but may last up to 6 weeks.

1. Characteristics

This stage is characterized by the synthesis and deposition of collagen. Noxious stimuli are removed, and growth of capillary beds into the area takes place. Fibroblastic activity, collagen formation, and granulation tissue development increase. Fibroblasts are in tremendous number by the 4th day after injury and continue in large number until about the 21st day.[6] The fibroblasts produce new collagen. The immature collagen replaces the exudate that originally formed the clot. Wound closure in muscle and skin usually takes 5 to 8 days; in tendons

TABLE 7–1. Characteristics and Clinical Signs of the Stages of Inflammation, Repair, and Maturation of Tissue

	Acute Stage, Inflammatory Reaction	Subacute Stage, Repair and Healing	Chronic Stage, Maturation and Remodeling
Characteristics	Vascular changes Exudation of cells and chemicals Clot formation Phagocytosis, neutralization of irritants Early fibroblastic activity	Removal of noxious stimuli Growth of capillary beds into area Collagen formation Granulation tissue Very fragile, easily injured tissue	Maturation of connective tissue Contracture of scar tissue Remodeling of scar Collagen aligns to stress
Clinical Signs	Inflammation Pain before tissue resistance	Decreasing inflammation Pain synchronous with tissue resistance	Absence of inflammation Pain after tissue resistance
Physical Therapy Intervention	PROTECTION PHASE Control effects of inflammation Modalities Selective rest/immobilization Promote early healing and prevent deleterious effects of rest Passive movement, massage and muscle setting with caution	CONTROLLED-MOTION PHASE Promote healing; develop mobile scar Nondestructive active, resistive, open and closed chain stabilization, and muscular endurance exercises, carefully progressed in intensity and range	RETURN-TO-FUNCTION PHASE Increase strength and alignment of scar; develop functional independence Progressive stretching, strengthening, endurance training, functional exercises, and specificity drills

241

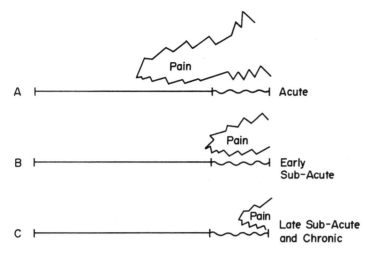

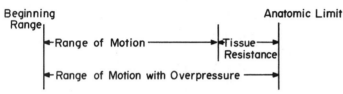

Figure 7–2. Pain experienced with range of motion when involved tissue is in the (*A*) acute stage, (*B*) early subacute stage, and (*C*) late subacute or chronic stage.

and ligaments, 3 to 5 weeks. During this stage, immature connective tissue is produced that is thin and unorganized. It is very fragile and easily injured if overstressed, yet proper growth and alignment can be stimulated by appropriate tensile loading in the line of normal stresses for that tissue. At the same time, adherence to surrounding tissues can be minimized.[8,9]

2. Clinical signs

The signs of inflammation progressively decrease and eventually are absent. When testing ROM, the patient experiences pain synchronous with encountering tissue resistance at the end of the available ROM (Fig. 7–2B).

C. Chronic (Maturation and Remodeling) Stage

1. The term *chronic* is used to describe either of the following:

a. That time during the late stages of tissue repair or recovery with no signs of inflammation, yet the patient has not gained full function (overlapping with the subacute stage around the 14th to 21st day after insult)

b. A condition that is long-standing with recurring episodes of pain from chronic inflammation or in which there are dysfunctions resulting from the healing process (see Section D)

2. Characteristics

There is maturation of the connective tissue as collagen fibers form from fibrils and scar tissue matures. Remodeling occurs as collagen fibers become thicker and reorient in response to stresses placed on the connective tissue. The scar begins to retract from activity of the myofibroblasts. The higher the density of the connective tissue, the longer the remodeling time.

a. Because of the way immature collagen molecules are held together (hydrogen bonding) and adhere to surrounding tissue, they can easily be remodeled with gentle and persistent treatment. This is possible for 8 to 10 weeks.[10] If not properly stressed, the fibers adhere to surrounding tissue and form a restricting scar.

b. As the structure of collagen changes (covalent bonding) and thickens, it becomes stronger and resistant to remodeling. At 14 weeks, the scar tissue is unresponsive to remodeling. An old scar has a poor response to stretch.[9] Treatment under these conditions requires either adaptive lengthening in the tissue surrounding the scar or surgical release.

3. Clinical signs

There are no signs of inflammation. When testing ROM, the patient does not feel pain until after resistance from the tissue is met and overpressure is applied to shortened or weakened structures. The patient may have decreased strength, decreased range of motion, and some loss of function. Restoration of function begins in this stage (Fig. 7–2C).

D. Chronic Inflammation

1. Characteristics

If excessive stresses or irritants are applied to the developing and remodeling scar tissue, the inflammatory process is perpetuated at low levels of intensity. Proliferation of fibroblasts with increased collagen production and degradation of mature collagen leads to a predominance of new, immature collagen. This has an overall weakening effect on the tissue. The myofibroblastic activity continues, which may lead to progressive limitation of motion. Efforts to stretch the tissue perpetuate the irritation and progressive limitation.

2. Clinical signs[8,9]

There are increased pain, swelling, and muscle guarding that last more than several hours after activity. There are an increased feeling of stiffness after rest, loss of range of motion 24 hours after activity, and progressive increased stiffness of the tissue as long as the irritation persists.

III. The Acute Stage: General Treatment Guidelines

A. Clinical Considerations During the Acute (Inflammatory) Stage of Soft Tissue Insult: The Protection Phase of Treatment

1. During the inflammatory stage pain and impaired movement are present from:
   a. Irritating chemicals
      The altered chemical state from the tissue reaction irritates the nerve endings.
   b. Edema
      Increased interstitial fluid from the altered circulatory pattern causes increased tension in the connective tissue, which restricts movement and causes pain.

   c. Muscle guarding and spasm

   The body's way of immobilizing an injured or painful area is with reflex muscle contraction. The spasm may be the result of direct muscle trauma but is usually in response to tissue injury in structures underlying the muscle.

   d. Joint swelling (effusion)

   This occurs if there is trauma to a joint or if there is an arthritic disease (see Sections VII and VIII). The increased effusion into the joint space distends the capsule and prevents normal movement of the bony partners. The joint assumes a position in which the capsule can distend to its maximum. This occurs only with joint trauma or joint disease.

2. To relieve the musculoskeletal pain and promote healing, *rest* and *protection* of the part affected by the inflammatory process are necessary during the first 24 hours, but complete immobilization can lead to the adherence of developing fibrils to surrounding tissue,[10] weakening of connective tissue,[41] and changes in articular cartilage.[20] The goals and methods of care at this stage are primarily to reduce the effects of inflammation, protect the area from further injury, and prevent the degrading effects of immobility.[31]

3. The *long-term goal of treatment* is the formation of a strong, mobile scar at the site of the lesion so that there is complete and painless restoration of function. Initially, the network of fibril formation is random. It acquires an organized arrangement according to the mechanical forces acting on the tissue. To influence the development of an organized scar, begin treatment during the acute stage, when tolerated, with carefully controlled *passive movements*.

   a. These movements should be specific to the structure involved to prevent abnormal adherence of the developing fibrils to surrounding tissue and thus avoid future disruption of the scar.

   b. The intensity (dosage) should be gentle enough so that the fibrils are not detached from the site of healing. Too much movement too soon will be painful and will reinjure the tissue. The dosage of passive movement depends on the severity of the lesion. Some patients tolerate no movement during the first 24 to 48 hours; others tolerate only a few degrees of gentle passive movement. Continuous passive movement (CPM; see Chapter 2) has been useful immediately following various types of surgery to joints; intra-articular, metaphyseal, and diaphyseal fractures; surgical release of extra-articular contractures and adhesions; as well as other selected conditions.[31] Any movement tolerated at this stage is beneficial, but it must *not* increase the inflammation or pain. Active movement is usually *contraindicated* at the site of an active pathologic process.

   c. Movement of structures in the same region should also be done in appropriate dosages to maintain functional integrity and mobility, but the movement should not be disruptive to the healing process of the involved tissue.

   d. Active movement is appropriate in neighboring regions to maintain integrity in uninjured tissue as well as to aid in circulation and lymphatic flow.

4. *Dosages and techniques specific to tissues* in a state of inflammation and to related structures in the same vicinity follow.

   Precaution: If the movement causes increased pain or increased inflammation, it is either of too great a dosage or it should not be done. Extreme care must be used with movement at this stage.

    a. *Joint and ligamentous pathology*
      (1) Passive range of motion, within the limit of pain, to maintain movement without stress. This range will probably be very small initially.[41]
      (2) Gentle passive joint traction or glides within the limit of pain; do not stretch the capsule or ligaments. Grade I or II distraction, glides, or oscillations performed in a pain-free position can be attempted; note the joint response before proceeding[16,19] (see Chapter 6). Besides maintaining mobility in the capsule and supporting ligaments and moving the synovial fluid to enhance cartilage nutrition and diffusion of waste products, these techniques may help to block the transmission of nociceptive stimuli to relieve pain via neurologic mechanisms.
      (3) Gentle massage to the injured site may benefit circulation and lymph flow to decrease edema and pain.[10,40]
      (4) Intermittent muscle setting benefits the related muscle and circulation without moving the joint.[41]

    b. *Muscle pathology*
      (1) Passive range of motion within the limit of pain to maintain movement without stress. Stretching at this stage is contraindicated.
      (2) Intermittent muscle setting, with the injured muscle in a relaxed or shortened position. This will cause the muscle to broaden and keep the developing scar mobile, yet will not cause separation of the healing breech.[10]
      (3) Electrical stimulation with the muscle in the shortened range will have the same benefit as muscle setting.
      (4) If tolerated, massage applied transverse to the injured fibers is advocated to keep the developing scar mobile but not separate the breach.[6,9,10] The dosage should be gentle in this early stage and should be followed with gentle muscle-setting contractions.
      (5) Gentle massage may benefit circulation and lymph flow to decrease edema and pain sensation.[40]
      (6) Passive joint-play movements (grade I or II) applied to related joints maintain normal motion while the muscle begins healing and cannot be moved through its full range of motion.[41]

    c. *Tendinous lesions*
      (1) Gentle dosage of massage applied transverse to the injured fibers is advocated to smooth roughened surfaces of a tendon. The tendon is kept taut during the massage.[10]
      (2) Passive ROM within the limit of pain and joint-play movements (grade I or II) maintain joint range without stressing the injured tissue.

    d. *Other connective tissue*
      (1) Passive range of motion within the limit of pain to maintain movement without stress. Stretching is contraindicated at this stage.
      (2) Muscle-setting exercises to assist with circulation and muscle function.
      (3) Passive joint-play movements (grade I or II) to maintain joint integrity.
      (5) Gentle massage to maintain mobility of the connective tissue and to assist lymph flow and circulation.[40]

5. During the protection phase maintain as normal a physiologic state as possible in related areas of the body. Include techniques to maintain or improve:
    a. Range of motion. These may be done actively or passively, depending on the proximity to and the effect on the injured tissue.
    b. Muscle strength. Resistance may be applied at an appropriate dosage to mus-

cles not directly related to the injured tissue to prepare the patient for use of assistive devices such as crutches or walkers and to improve functional activities.

c. Functional activities. Supportive or adaptive devices may be necessary depending on area of injury and necessary functional activities.

d. Circulation. It will be helped by doing the functional activities as well as by using supportive elastic wraps, by elevating the part, and by using appropriate massage and muscle-setting techniques.

B. Treatment Considerations: Acute Stage Protection Phase

1. Impairments/problems summarized

a. Inflammation, pain, edema, muscle spasm
b. Impaired movement
c. Joint effusion (if the joint is injured or if there is arthritis)
d. Decreased use of associated areas

2. General treatment goals and plan of care during the protection phase

Goals	*Plan of Care*
a. Control pain, edema, spasm.	a. Cold, compression, elevation, massage (48 hours). Immobilize the part (rest, splint, tape, cast). Avoid positions of stress to the part. Gentle (grade I) joint oscillations with joint in pain-free position.
b. Maintain soft tissue and joint integrity and mobility.	b. Appropriate dosage of passive movements within limit of pain, specific to structure involved. Appropriate dosage of intermittent muscle setting or electrical stimulation.
c. Reduce joint swelling if symptoms are present.	c. May require medical intervention if swelling is rapid (blood). Provide protection (splint, cast).
d. Maintain integrity and function of associated areas.	d. Active-assistive, free, resistive, and/or modified aerobic exercises, depending on proximity to and effect on the primary lesion. Adaptive or assistive devices as needed to protect the part during functional activities.
e. Educate the patient.	e. Inform patient of anticipated recovery time and how to protect the part while maintaining appropriate functional activities.

Precautions: The proper dosage of rest and movement must be used during the inflammatory stage. Signs of too much movement are increased pain or increased inflammation.

Contraindication: Active ROM, stretching activities, and resistance exercises are contraindicated at the site of inflammation.[41]

IV. The Subacute Stage: General Treatment Guidelines

A. Clinical Considerations During the Subacute Stage of Healing Following Soft Tissue Insult: The Controlled Motion Phase of Treatment

1. Pain and inflammation decrease as healing progresses. The new tissue being developed is fragile and easily interrupted. The patient often feels good and returns to normal activity too soon.

   a. Exercises progressed too vigorously or functional activities begun too early can be injurious to the fragile, newly developing tissue and therefore may delay recovery by perpetuating the inflammatory response.[38,41]

   b. If movement is not progressed, the new tissue adheres to surrounding structures and will become a source of pain and limited tissue mobility.

   c. Criteria for initiation of active exercises in the early subacute stage include decreased swelling, pain no longer constant, and pain not exacerbated with motion in the available range.

2. Because of the restricted use of the injured region, there will be muscle weakness even in the absence of muscle pathology. The subacute phase is a transition period during which *active* exercises within the pain-free range in the injured tissue can begin and be progressed with care, keeping within the tolerance of the healing tissues. If activity is kept within a safe dosage and frequency, symptoms of pain and swelling will progressively decrease each day. Patient response is the best guide to how quickly or vigorously to progress. Clinically, if signs of inflammation increase or the range of motion progressively decreases, then the intensity of the exercise and activity must decrease because a chronic inflammation has developed and a retracting scar will become more limiting.[8,9,41]

   a. *Multiple-angle, submaximal isometric exercises* are used in the early subacute stage to develop control of the muscles in the involved region in a nonstressful manner. They may also help the patient become aware of using the correct muscles. The intensity and angles for resistance are determined by the absence of pain.

      (1) To initiate isometric exercise in an injured, healing muscle, place it in the shortened or relaxed position so that the new scar is not pulled from the breached site.[9]

      (2) To initiate isometric exercises when there is joint pathology, the resting position for the joint may be the most comfortable position. The intensity of contraction should be kept below the perception of pain.

   b. *Active range of motion exercises in pain-free ranges* are used to develop control of the motion. Initially isolated, single plane motions are used. Emphasize control of the motion using light-resistive, concentric exercises of involved muscle and muscles needed for proper joint mechanics. Use of combined motions or diagonal patterns may facilitate contraction of the desired muscles, but care must be taken not to use patterns of motion dominated by stronger muscles with the weaker muscles not effectively participating at this early stage. Do not stress beyond the ability of the involved or weakened muscles to participate in the motion.

c. *Protected closed-chain exercises* may be used early to load the region in a controlled manner and stimulate stabilizing co-contractions in the muscles. Reinforcement from the therapist helps develop awareness of appropriate muscle contractions as well as help develop control while the patient shifts his or her weight in a side-to-side or anterior-to-posterior motion. As tolerated by the patient, progress by increasing the amplitude of movement or by decreasing the amount of support or protection. Resistance is added to progress strength in the stabilizing muscles.

d. *Eccentric exercises* may cause added trauma to muscle and are not used in the early subacute stage following muscle injury when the weak tensile quality of the healing tissue could be jeopardized.[27] For nonmuscular injuries, eccentrics may not reinjure the part, but the resistance should be limited to low intensity at this stage to avoid delayed-onset muscle soreness. This is in contrast to using eccentrics to facilitate and strengthen weak muscles when there has been no injury to take advantage of greater tension development with less energy in eccentric contractions (this is described in Chapter 3).

3. Restricted motion during the acute stage and adherence of the developing scar usually cause decreased flexibility in the healing tissue as well as related structures in the region. To increase mobility and stimulate proper alignment of the developing scar, stretching should be specific to the tissues involved. More than one technique may have to be used to regain the range of motion.

a. *Joint and ligament*

(1) Passive joint-play movements are continued within the limits of pain.

(a) If there is limited range with joint effusion, stretching of the capsule is contraindicated; continue use of grade I or II sustained or oscillating techniques.

(b) If there is limited range and decreased **joint play** with no joint effusion, stretching techniques to the capsule can begin; use sustained grade II techniques and note the joint response before proceeding (see Chapter 6).

(2) Increase the intensity of cross-fiber massage or soft tissue massage to keep the ligaments and surrounding soft tissue moving freely across the joint.

b. *Muscle*

(1) Progress lengthening of the muscle with gentle contract-relax techniques or electrical stimulation. Begin with the muscle in the shortened position; have the muscle contract isometrically against *minimal* resistance, then relax, then elongate it a short distance. Repeat with each new length. Do not elongate beyond the limit of pain; continue just to the point of discomfort.

(2) Progress the intensity of the cross-fiber massage with the patient's tolerance. The muscle is kept in the shortened position while applying the massage.

(3) Continue to maintain joint-play movements in associated joints until the muscle has regained full range of motion. Use sustained grade II glides.

c. *Tendon and tendon sheath*

(1) Increase the intensity of the cross-fiber massage at the site of the lesion.

(2) Maintain joint play with sustained grade II traction or glide techniques.

d. *Other connective tissue*

(1) Cross-fiber friction or soft tissue massage can be applied to specific sites

that have been injured. Begin gently and progress as the patient tolerates the massage.

(2) Continue to maintain joint-play movements (sustained grade II) in associated joints until soft tissue flexibility has been restored.

4. Continue to maintain or develop as normal a physiologic and functional state as possible in related areas of the body. Correct for postural stability problems or muscle length and strength imbalances that could have contributed to the problem. Resume low-intensity functional activities as the patient tolerates without exacerbating symptoms. Continue to reassess the patient's progress and understanding of the controlled activities.

B. Treatment Considerations: Subacute Stage—Controlled Motion Phase

1. Impairments/problems summarized

a. Pain when end of available range of motion is reached
b. Decreasing soft tissue edema
c. Decreasing joint effusion (if joints are involved)
d. Developing soft tissue, muscle, and/or joint contractures
e. Developing muscle weakness from reduced usage
f. Decreased functional use of the part and associated areas

2. General treatment goals and plan of care during the controlled motion phase

Goals	*Plan of Care*
a. Promote healing of injured tissues.	a. Monitor response of tissue to exercise progression; decrease intensity if inflammation increases.
	Protect healing tissue with assistive devices, splints, tape, or wrap; progressively increase amount of time the joint is free to move each day and decrease use of assistive device as strength in supporting muscles increases.
b. Progressively restore soft tissue, muscle, and/or joint mobility.	b. Progress from passive to active-assistive to active ROM within limits of pain.
	Gradually increase mobility of scar, specific to structure involved (see Section IV.A.3).
	Progressively increase mobility of related structures if they are tight; use techniques specific to tight structure.
c. Progressively strengthen involved and related muscles.	c. Initially, progress multiple-angle isometric exercises within patient's tolerance; begin cautiously with mild resistance.

Goals	*Plan of Care*
	Initiate protected closed-chain stabilization exercises.
	As range of motion, joint play, and healing improve, progress open- and closed-chain isotonic exercises with resistance progressing as tolerated. Emphasize control and proper mechanics.
d. Maintain integrity and function of associated areas.	d. Apply progressive strengthening and stabilizing exercises, monitoring effect on the primary lesion.
	Resume low-intensity functional activities involving the healing tissue that do not exacerbate the symptoms.
e. Educate the patient.	e. Instruct patient in proper home program and monitor effects.

Precautions: The signs of inflammation or joint swelling normally decrease early in this stage. Some discomfort will occur as the activity level is progressed, but it should not last longer than a couple of hours. Signs of too much motion or activity are resting pain, fatigue, increased weakness, and spasm.[41]

V. The Chronic Stage: General Treatment Guidelines

A. Clinical Considerations During the Chronic-Remodeling Stage: Return to Function Phase

1. The primary differences in the state of the healing tissue between the late subacute and chronic stages are the improvement in quality (orientation and tensile strength) of the collagen and the reduction in size of the wound during the chronic stages.[8,9,18] The quantity of collagen stabilizes; there is a balance between the synthesis and degradation. Because remodeling of the maturing collagen occurs in response to the stresses placed on it, it is important to use controlled forces that duplicate normal stresses on the tissue. Maximal strength of the collagen will develop in the direction of the imposed forces. Excessive or abnormal stresses will lead to reinjury and chronic inflammation, which can be detrimental to the return of function.

2. If mobility has been maintained in the injured tissue as well as the related structures, progression of activity and function continues but with greater intensity and complexity.

3. Pain that the patient now experiences arises only when stress is placed on contractures or adhesions beyond the available range of motion. This is often the case if a patient is first seen for therapy in this stage of recovery. Usually no pain is felt within the available range. To avoid chronic or recurring pain, the contractures need to be stretched or the adhesions need to be broken up. Stretching of the tissues should be selective, using techniques appropriate to the tissue involved.

4. For progression of exercises, two considerations are important.[41]
   a. Free joint play within a useful (or functional) range of motion is necessary to avoid joint trauma. If joint play is restricted, joint mobilizing techniques should be used. These stretching techniques can be vigorous as long as no signs of increased irritation result.
   b. Joint motion without adequate muscle support will cause trauma to that joint as functional activities are attempted. Zohn and Mennell[41] recommend that the criterion for strength be a muscle test grade of "good" in lower extremity musculature before discontinuing use of supportive or assistive devices for ambulation.
      (1) To increase strength when there is a loss of joint play, multiple-angle isometric exercises are recommended.
      (2) Once joint play within the available ROM is restored, resistive isotonic exercises are recommended for that available range. This does not imply that normal ROM needs to be present before initiating isotonic exercises but that joint play, within the available range, be present (see Chapter 6 for information on joint play).
   c. In summary, both joint dynamics and muscle strength and flexibility should be balanced as the injured part is progressed to functional exercises.
5. Any adhesions in the fascia, skin, or other soft tissue such as ligaments will restrict motion and should be mobilized with soft tissue stretching techniques specific to the tissue.
6. Depending on the size of the structure or degree of injury or pathology, healing, with progressively increasing tensile quality in the injured tissue, will continue for 12 to 18 months. The principles of treatment that follow should be continued until the part is pain free with normal range of motion and good strength.
7. As the patient progresses in the late subacute and chronic stages, not only does treatment progress to stimulate proper healing in the injured tissue, but also emphasis is placed on controlled progressive exercises designed to prepare the patient to meet the functional outcome goal(s).
   a. Exercises progress from isolated, unidirectional, simple movements to complex patterns and multidirectional movements requiring coordination with all muscles functioning for the desired activity.[39]
   b. The strengthening exercises progress to simulate specific demands including both closed and open chain using both eccentric and concentric contractions.
   c. Progression of controlled stabilization of the trunk and proximal segments continues for effective extremity motions.[39]
   d. Safe mechanics are taught and practiced.
   e. Often overlooked but of importance in preventing injury associated with fatigue is developing muscular endurance in the prime mover muscles and stabilizing muscles as well as cardiovascular endurance.
8. Patients who must return to activities with greater-than-normal demand such as is required in sports participation and heavy-work settings are progressed further to more intense exercises including plyometrics, agility training, and skill development. Exercise drills are developed to simulate the work[14] or sport[1,39] activities in a controlled environment with specific, **progressive resistance.** As the patient demonstrates capabilities, increased repetition and speed are added. Continued progression involves changing the environment and introducing surprise and uncontrolled events into the activity.[1,39]
9. The importance of proper education to teach safe progression of exercises and

how to avoid damaging stresses cannot be overemphasized. To return to the activity that caused the injury prior to regaining functional pain-free motion, strength, endurance, and skill to match the demands of the task will probably result in recurring injury and pain.

B. Treatment Considerations: Chronic Stage—Return to Function Phase

1. Impairments/problems summarized

(All, some, or none of the problems are present.)

a. Pain is experienced only when stress is applied to structures in dysfunction (pain after tissue resistance is met).

b. Soft tissue, and/or joint contractures or adhesions limit normal range of motion or joint play.

c. Muscle weakness.

d. Decreased functional usage of the involved part.

e. Unable to function normally in a described activity.

2. General treatment goals and plan of care during the return to function phase

Goals

a. Decrease pain from stress on contractures or adhesions.

b. Increase soft tissue, muscle, and/or joint mobility.

c. Strengthen supporting and related muscles; develop biomechanical balance between muscle groups.

d. Develop muscular endurance in prime mover and stabilizer muscles.

e. Progress functional independence.

Plan of Care

a. Stretch limiting structures.
Develop control and stabilization.
Biomechanical counseling.

b. Select stretching techniques specific to the tight tissue: soft tissue (passive stretch and massage); joints, capsules, and selected ligaments (joint mobilization); ligaments, tendons, and soft tissue adhesions (cross-fiber massage); muscles (active inhibition or flexibility techniques).

c. Progress:
Submaximal to maximal resistance.
Specificity of exercise using resisted concentric and eccentric, open and closed chain.
Single plane to multiplane motions.
Simple to complex motions.
Controlled proximal stability, superimpose distal motion.
Safe biomechanics.

d. Increase time at slow speed; progress complexity and time; progress speed and time.

e. Continue using supportive and/or assistive devices until the range of motion is functional with good joint play, and the results of sup-

Goals	*Plan of Care*
	porting muscle strength tests are good.
	Progress functional training with simulated activities from protected and controlled to unprotected and variable.
	Continue progressive strengthening exercises and advanced training activities until the muscles are strong enough and able to respond to the required functional demands.
f. Educate the patient.	f. Instruct patient in safe progressions. Monitor understanding and compliance. Teach prevention.

Precautions: There should be no signs of inflammation. Some discomfort will occur as the activity level is progressed, but it should not last longer than a couple of hours. Signs that activities are progressing too quickly or with too great a dosage are joint swelling, pain that lasts longer than 4 hours or that requires medication for relief, a decrease in strength, or fatiguing more easily.[41]

VI. Chronic Recurring Pain—Chronic Inflammation—General Treatment Guidelines

A. Mechanisms for Prolonged or Recurring Pain

1. **Overuse syndromes, cumulative trauma disorders, repetitive strain injury**[11] are terms descriptive of the repetitive nature of the precipitating event. Repetitive microtrauma or repeated strain overload over time results in structural weakening, or fatigue breakdown of connective tissue with collagen fiber cross-link breakdown and inflammation. Initially, the inflammatory response from the microtrauma is subthreshold but eventually builds to the point of perceived pain and resulting dysfunction

2. **Trauma** followed by superimposed repetitive trauma results in a condition that never completely heals. This may be the result of too early return to high-demand functional activities before proper healing of the original injury has occurred. The continued reinjury leads to the symptoms of chronic inflammation and dysfunction.

3. **Reinjury of an "old scar."** Scar tissue is not as compliant as surrounding, undamaged tissue. If the scar adheres to the surrounding tissues or is not properly aligned to the stresses imposed on the tissue, there is an alteration in the force transmission and energy absorption. This region becomes more susceptible to injury with stresses that normal, healthy tissue could sustain.

4. **Contractures or poor mobility** in tissues from faulty postural habits or prolonged immobility may be stressed with repeated or vigorous activity that the tissues are not prepared for.

B. Contributing Factors

By nature of the condition, there is usually some factor that perpetuates the problem. Not only should the tissue at fault and its stage of pathology be identified, but the *mechanical cause* of the repetitive trauma needs to be defined. Evaluate for faulty mechanics or faulty habits that may be sustaining the irritation. Possibilities include:

1. **Imbalances between the length and strength** in the muscles around the joint, leading to faulty mechanics of joint motion or abnormal forces through the muscles.

2. **Rapid or excessive repeated eccentric demand** placed on muscles not prepared to withstand the load, leading to tissue failure, particularly at the musculotendinous region.[27]

3. **Muscle weakness** or inability to respond to excessive strength demands that results in muscle fatigue with decreased contractility and shock-absorbing capabilities and increased stress to supporting tissues.[27]

4. **Bone malalignment or poor structural support** that causes faulty joint mechanics of force transmission through the joints (poor joint stability as in flat foot).[28]

5. **Change in the usual intensity or demands** of an activity such as an increase or change in an exercise or a training routine or change in job demands.[29]

6. **Returning to an activity too soon after an injury** when the muscle-tendon unit is weakened and not ready for the stress of the activity.[27]

7. **Sustained awkward postures or motions** placing parts of the body at a mechanical disadvantage that lead to postural fatigue or injury.

8. **Environmental factors** such as a work station not ergonomically designed to the individual, excessive cold, continued vibration, or inappropriate weight-bearing surface (for standing, walking, or running), which may contribute to any of the previous factors.

9. **Aging factors** such that a person attempts activities that could be done when younger but tissues are no longer in condition to withstand the sustained stress.[29]

10. **Training errors,** such as using improper methods, intensity, amount, equipment, or condition of the participant, which lead to abnormal stresses.[28]

11. **A combination of several contributing factors** are frequently seen that cause the symptoms.

C. Clinical Considerations with Chronic Inflammation

1. Chronic inflammation = acute stage

When the inflammatory response is perpetuated because of continued tissue irritation, the inflammation must be controlled to avoid the negative effects of continued tissue breakdown and excessive scar formation.

a. Besides the use of modalities and rest to the part, it is imperative to identify and modify the mechanism of chronic irritation with appropriate biomechanical counseling. This will require cooperation from the patient. Describe to the patient how the tissue reacts and breaks down under the continued inflammation, and explain the strategy of intervention. Using illustrations such as what happens when a person repeatedly hits a thumbnail with a hammer or repeatedly scrapes a skin area before it heals helps the patient visualize the repeated trauma occurring in the musculoskeletal problem and understand the need to quit "hitting the sore."

b. Initially, allow only nonstressful activities.

c. Exercises are initiated at *nonstressful* intensities in the involved tissues, as with any acute lesion, and at appropriate corrective intensities in related regions without stressing the involved tissues.

2. **Subacute and chronic stages of healing the chronic condition**

Once the constant pain from the chronic inflammation has decreased, the patient is progressed through an exercise program with controlled stresses until the connective tissue in the involved region has developed the ability to withstand the functional stresses.

a. Locally if there is a chronic, contracted scar that limits range or continually becomes irritated with microruptures, the scar should be mobilized within the tissue with friction massage, soft tissue manipulation, or stretching techniques.

   (1) If inflammation occurs from the stretching maneuvers, treat it as an acute injury.

   (2) Because chronic inflammation can lead to proliferation of scar tissue and contraction of the scar, progressive loss of range is a warning sign that the intensity of stretching is too vigorous.

   (3) Muscle guarding could be a sign that the body is attempting to protect the part from excessive motion. In this case the emphasis should be on developing stabilization of the part and training in safe adaptive patterns of motion.

b. The cause of the faulty muscle and joint mechanics must be identified. Strengthening and stabilization exercises, in conjunction with working or recreational adaptations, are necessary to minimize the irritating patterns of motion.

c. Because chronic irritation problems frequently result from inability to sustain repetitive activities, endurance is an appropriate component of the muscle reeducation program. Consider endurance in the postural stabilizers as well as in the prime movers of the desired functional activity.

d. As when treating patients in the chronic stage of healing, exercises are progressed to develop functional independence. The exercises become specific to the demand and include timing, coordination, and skill. Work-conditioning and work-hardening programs may be used to prepare the person for return to work; training in sports-specific exercises are important in returning an individual to sports.

D. Treatment Considerations: Chronic Inflammation

1. Impairments/problems summarized

a. Pain in the involved tissue of varying degrees[29]

   (1) Only after doing repetitive activities

   (2) When doing repetitive activities as well as after

   (3) When attempting to do activities; completion of demands prevented

   (4) Continued and unremitting

b. Soft tissue, muscle, and/or joint contractures or adhesions that limit normal range of motion or joint play

c. Muscle weakness and poor muscular endurance in postural or stabilizing muscles as well as primary muscle at fault

d. Imbalance in length and strength between antagonistic muscles; biomechanical dysfunction

e. Decreased functional use of the region

f. Faulty position or movement pattern perpetuating the problem

2. General treatment goals and plan of care during the chronic inflammation period

Goals

a. Promote healing; decrease pain and inflammation.

b. Eliminate irritating factors; involve patient in program.

c. Maintain integrity and mobility of involved tissue.

d. Develop support in related regions.

Plan of Care

a. Cold, compression, massage. Rest to the part (rest, splint, tape, cast).

b. Patient education and counseling on biomechanics. Environmental adaptation.

c. Nonstressful passive movement, massage, and muscle setting within limits of pain.

d. Awareness training. Stabilization exercises.

3. General goals and plan of care: return to function phase

Goals

a. Develop strong, mobile scar.

b. Develop a balance in length and strength of the muscles.

c. Progress functional independence.

d. Correct environmental factors causing problem.

Plan of Care

a. Friction massage. Soft tissue mobilization.

b. Correct cause of faulty muscle and joint mechanics with appropriately graded stretching and strengthening exercises.

c. Train muscle to function according to demand; provide alternatives or support if it cannot. Train coordination and timing. Develop endurance. Patient education.

d. Job, activity analysis. Environmental adaptation. Patient education.

Precaution: If there is progressive loss of range of motion as the result of stretching, do not continue to stretch. Re-evaluate the condition and determine if there is still a chronic inflammation with contracting scar or if there is protective muscle guarding. If the part should not be stressed into increased range, emphasize stabilizing the part and training in safe adaptive patterns of motion.

NOTE: Specific overuse syndromes are covered in detail in the respective chapters associated with the involved region.

VII. Rheumatoid Arthritis: General Treatment Guidelines

A. Characteristics of Rheumatoid Arthritis (RA)[4]

1. RA is a connective tissue disease. The onset and progression vary from mild joint symptoms with aching and stiffness to abrupt swelling, stiffness, and progressive deformity. There are usually periods of exacerbation (flare) and remission.

2. Joints are characteristically involved with early inflammatory changes in the synovial membrane, peripheral portions of the articular cartilage, and subchondral marrow spaces. In response, granulation tissue (pannus) forms, covers, and erodes the articular cartilage. Adhesions may form, restricting joint mobility. With progression of the disease, cancellous bone becomes exposed. Fibrosis or ossific ankylosis may eventually result, causing deformity and disability.

3. Inflammatory changes may also occur in tendon sheaths (tenosynovitis), and if subjected to a lot of friction, they may fray or rupture.

4. Extra-articular pathologic changes sometimes occur; these include rheumatoid nodules, atrophy, and fibrosis of muscles and mild cardiac changes.

B. Clinical Considerations with RA

1. With synovial inflammation, there is effusion and swelling of the joints, which cause aching and limited motion. Usually there is pain on motion, and a slight increase in temperature can be detected over the joints.

2. Onset is usually in the smaller joints of the hands and feet, most commonly in the proximal interphalangeal joints. Usually symptoms are bilateral.

3. With progression, the joints become deformed and may ankylose or sublux.

4. Pain is often felt in adjoining muscles; eventually muscle atrophy and weakness occur. Asymmetry in muscle pull adds to the deforming forces.

5. The person fatigues easily and requires additional rest during periods of flare-up in order not to stress the joints.

6. Therapeutic exercises cannot positively alter the pathologic process of rheumatoid arthritis, but if administered carefully, they can help prevent, retard, or correct the mechanical limitations that occur. (See precautions and contraindications in Section C.)

C. Treatment Considerations During the Active Disease Period of RA

1. Impairments/problems summarized

a. Tenderness and warmth over the involved joints with joint swelling

b. Muscle guarding and pain on motion

c. Joint stiffness and limited motion

d. Muscle weakness and atrophy

e. Potential deformity and ankylosis from the degenerative process and asymmetric muscle pull

2. General treatment goals and plan of care during the active disease period

Goals	*Plan of Care*
a. Relieve pain and muscle guarding and promote relaxation.	a. Modalities. Gentle massage. Immobilize in splint. Relaxation techniques.
b. Minimize joint stiffness and maintain available motion.	b. Passive or active-assistive ROM within limits of pain, gradual progression as tolerated. Gentle joint techniques using grade I or II oscillations.
c. Minimize muscle atrophy.	c. Gentle muscle setting.
d. Prevent deformity and protect the joint structures.	d. Use of supportive and assistive equipment for all pathologically active joints. Good bed positioning while resting. Avoidance of activities that stress the joints. Patient education.

Precautions during the active inflammatory period: The patient fatigues easily and therefore requires more rest than usual. He or she should be cautioned to avoid stress and fatigue and should be taught methods of energy conservation during daily activities.

Secondary effects of medications and steroids may include osteoporosis and ligamentous laxity, so exercises should not cause excessive stress to bones or joints.

If medication controls the swelling and secondary pain, exercise can be progressed carefully.

Contraindications during the active inflammatory period: Maximum resistive exercise should not be performed. Even though muscles tend to weaken, vigorous strengthening exercises will cause joint compression and increase the irritability of the joint, potentially increasing damage to the joint surfaces.

Stretching techniques should not be performed. The limited motion in a swollen joint is caused by excessive fluid in the joint space, not from adhesions. To force motion on the distended capsule will overstretch it with subsequent hypermobility (or subluxation) when the swelling abates. It may also increase the irritability of the joint and prolong the joint reaction.

D. Treatment Considerations During the Remission Period of RA

1. Potential impairments/problems summarized

a. Pain when stress is applied to mechanical restrictions
b. Limited range of motion and joint play from soft tissue, muscle, and/or joint contractures or adhesions
c. Secondary muscle weakness
d. Postural changes or joint deformities
e. Decreased functional use of the part and related regions

2. Goals and plan of care during the remission period

The treatment approach is the same as with any subacute and chronic musculoskeletal disorder, except appropriate precautions must be taken because the pathologic changes from the disease process make the parts more susceptible to damage. Nonimpact or low-impact conditioning exercises such as swimming and bicycling, performed within the tolerance of the individual with arthritis, improve aerobic capacity and physical activity and decrease depression and anxiety.[24]

Precautions: The joint capsule, ligaments, and tendons may be structurally weakened by the rheumatic process (also as a result of using steroids), so the dosage of stretching techniques used to counter any contractures or adhesions must be carefully graded.

Contraindications: Vigorous stretching or manipulative techniques.

VIII. Osteoarthritis: General Treatment Guidelines

A. Characteristics of Osteoarthritis or Degenerative Joint Disease (DJD)[4,32,35]

1. DJD is a chronic degenerative disorder primarily affecting the articular cartilage of synovial joints, with eventual bony remodeling and overgrowth at the margins of the joints (spurs and lipping). There is also a progression of synovial and capsular thickening and joint effusion. With degeneration, there may be capsular laxity as a result of bone remodeling and capsule distention, resulting in hypermobility or instability in some ranges. With pain and decreased willingness to move, contractures eventually develop in portions of the capsule and overlying muscle, so that as the disease progresses, motion becomes more limited.

2. Causes may be due to mechanical injury, from either a major stress or repeated minor stresses, or due to poor movement of synovial fluid when the joint is immobilized. Rapid destruction of articular cartilage occurs with immobilization, because the cartilage is not being bathed by moving synovial fluid and is thus deprived of its nutritional supply.

3. The cartilage loses its ability to withstand stress; it splits and thins out. Eventually the bone becomes exposed. There is increased density of the bone along the joint line, with cystic bone loss and osteoporosis in the adjacent metaphysis. In the early stages, the joint is usually asymptomatic because the cartilage is avascular and aneural.

B. Clinical Considerations

1. Pain usually occurs because of compressive stresses on or excessive activity of the involved joint and is relieved with rest. In the late stages of the disease, pain is often present at rest. The pain is probably from secondary involvement of subchondral bone, synovium, and the joint capsule. In the spine, if bony growth encroaches on the nerve root, there may be radicular pain.

2. Usually there are brief periods of stiffness in the morning or following periods of rest. Movement relieves the stiffness.

3. Affected joints may become enlarged. Heberden's nodes (enlargement of the distal interphalangeal joint of the fingers) are common.

4. Most commonly involved are weight-bearing joints (hips and knees), the cervical and lumbar spine, and the distal interphalangeal joints of the fingers and carpometacarpal joint of the thumb.

5. Crepitation or loose bodies may occur within the joint.

6. Stiffness occurs with inactivity, but increased pain occurs with excessive mechanical stress or activity. Therefore, moderation of activity and correction of the biomechanical stresses can prevent, retard, or correct the mechanical limitations.

7. With progression of the disease, the bony remodeling, swelling, and contractures alter the transmission of forces through the joint, which further perpetuates the deforming forces and creates joint deformity.

8. Progressive weakening in the muscle occurs either from inactivity or from inhibition of the neuronal pools.

9. Impairment of joint position sense may occur.

C. Treatment Considerations for Osteoarthritis

1. Impairments/problems summarized

a. Stiffness following inactivity
b. Pain with mechanical stress or excessive activity
c. Limitation of motion (as the condition progresses)
d. Pain at rest (in the advanced stages)
e. Potential deformity

2. General treatment goals and plan of care

Goals	Plan of Care
a. Decrease effects of stiffness from inactivity.	a. Patient education. Active range of motion. Joint-play techniques.
b. Decrease pain from mechanical stress.	b. Supportive and/or assistive equipment to minimize stress or to correct faulty biomechanics. Increase strength in supporting muscles. Alternate activity with periods of rest.
c. Increase range of motion.	c. Stretch muscle, joint, or soft tissue restrictions with specific techniques.
d. Decrease pain at rest if present.	d. Modalities. Grade I or II joint oscillations.
e. Prevent deformities.	e. Patient education in the above plan of care. Splinting.
f. Improve physical conditioning.	f. Nonimpact or low-impact aerobic exercise.

Precautions: When strengthening supporting muscles, increased pain in the joint during or following resistive exercises probably means that too great a weight is being used or stress is being placed at an inappropriate part of the range of motion. Analyze the joint mechanics and at what point during the range the greatest compressive forces are occurring. Maximum resistance exercise should not be performed through that range of the motion.

IX. Fractures: General Treatment Guidelines

Reduction, alignment, and immobilization for healing of a fracture are medical procedures and are not discussed in this text.

A. Clinical Considerations During the Period of Immobilization

1. With immobilization, there is connective tissue weakening, articular cartilage degeneration, muscle atrophy, and contracture development as well as sluggish circulation.[21] In addition, because of the fracture there is also soft tissue injury with bleeding and scar formation. Because immobilization is necessary for bone healing, the soft tissue scar cannot become organized along lines of stress as it develops. Early nondestructive motion, within the tolerance of the fracture site, is ideal. Structures in the related area should be kept in a state as near to normal as possible by using appropriate exercises without jeopardizing alignment of the fracture site.

2. If bed rest or immobilization in bed is required, as with skeletal traction, secondary physiologic changes will occur systematically throughout the body. General exercises for the uninvolved portions of the body can minimize these problems.

3. If there is a lower extremity fracture, alternate modes of ambulation need to be taught to the patient who is allowed out of bed, such as use of crutches or walker. The choice of device and gait pattern will depend on the fracture site, the type of immobilization, and the functional capabilities of the patient.

B. Treatment Considerations During the Period of Immobilization

1. Impairments/problems summarized

a. Initially, inflammation and swelling
b. In the immobilized area, progressive muscle atrophy, contracture formation, cartilage degeneration, and decreased circulation
c. Potential overall body weakening if confined to bed
d. Functional limitations imposed by the fracture site and method of immobilization used

2. General treatment goals and plan of care during the period of immobilization

Goals	Plan of Care
a. Decrease effects of inflammation during acute period.	a. Ice, elevation. Intermittent muscle setting.
b. Decrease effects of immobilization.	b. Intermittent muscle setting. Active ROM to joints above and below immobilized region.
c. If patient is confined to bed, maintain strength and ROM in major muscle groups.	c. Resistive ROM to major muscle groups not immobilized, especially in preparation for future ambulation.
d. Teach functional adaptations.	d. Use of assistive or supportive devices for ambulation or bed mobility.

C. Clinical Considerations After the Period of Immobilization

1. There will be decreased ROM, muscle atrophy, and joint pain in the structures that have been immobilized. Activities should be initiated carefully in order not to traumatize the weakened structures (muscle, cartilage, bone, and connective tissue).

2. Initially, the patient will experience pain as movement begins, but it should progressively decrease as joint movement, muscle strength, and range of motion progressively improve.

3. If there was soft tissue damage at the time of fracture, an inelastic scar will form, leading to decreased ROM or pain when stretch is placed on the scar. The scar tissue will have to be mobilized to gain pain-free movement. Choice of technique will depend on the tissue involved.

4. To determine if there is clinical or radiologic healing, consult with the referring physician. Until the fracture site is radiologically healed, use care any time stress is placed distal to the fracture site (for example, resistance, stretch force, or weight bearing). Once radiologically healed, the bone has normal structural integrity and can withstand normal stress.

5. Evaluate to determine the degree and ranges of motion lost, the strength available, and the tissues that are in dysfunction. When progressing stretching and strengthening exercises and functional activities, use the guidelines, goals, and plans of care presented in the sections in this chapter on subacute and chronic stages (see Sections IV and V).

X. Surgery

Many disorders of the musculoskeletal system that affect muscles, tendons, ligaments, cartilage, joints, capsules, or bones of the upper and lower extremities are treated successfully through surgical intervention. A well-planned, individualized therapeutic exercise program is an integral part of the preoperative and postoperative care of the surgical patient and significantly contributes to the success of the surgical procedure.

Acute, traumatic, soft tissue injuries, such as ruptures of muscles and tendons and severe lesions of cartilage and ligaments, often must be repaired surgically. Severe chronic joint dysfunction due to rheumatoid arthritis, osteoarthritis, or traumatic arthritis may also require surgical intervention. To effectively establish an exercise program for a patient, the therapist must understand the indications and rationale for surgery, must become familiar with the procedure itself, and must be aware of the overall postoperative management of the patient.[12,22,33,37] An overview of specific surgical procedures for the upper and lower extremities and guidelines for postoperative care are found in Chapters 8 through 13.

A. Indications for Surgery[4,26,33,37]

1. Severe pain due to trauma to soft tissue or deterioration of articular surfaces
2. Chronic joint swelling
3. Marked limitation of active or passive joint motion
4. Gross instability of a joint or bony segment that leads to limitation of function
5. Joint deformity and abnormal joint alignment
6. Overall decrease or loss of function needed to maintain independence in daily activities and personal care

B. Complications of Surgery[2-4,7,33,37]

1. Postoperative infection or poor wound healing
2. Postoperative vascular disorders, such as thrombophlebitis and pulmonary embolism
3. Delayed healing of soft tissue or bone
4. Adhesions and contractures of soft tissue and joints
5. Loosening of prosthetic implants leading to instability and pain
6. Biomechanical breakdown of implants
7. Increased pulmonary secretions and risk of pneumonia and atelectasis

C. General Considerations for Preoperative Therapeutic Management

Whenever possible, preoperative contact with the patient can be extremely valuable for the patient and the therapist. A specific evaluation of the patient's status should be made prior to elective surgery. This evaluation of the patient will help to determine the likelihood or extent of success of the proposed surgical procedure.[12] Patient education can also be initiated more easily before surgery.

1. Evaluation procedures

a. Determine the primary impairments such as the amount and type of joint pain, swelling, or crepitation the patient is experiencing.
b. Measure the active and passive range of motion of the involved joint or extremity.
c. Check the range of motion of all other joints.
d. Grade the strength of the affected extremity.
e. Estimate the strength of the unaffected joints or extremities as a basis for postoperative ambulation, transfers, and activities of daily living (ADL).
f. Determine the level of functional independence or functional limitations that the patient has preoperatively and the level of function that he or she expects postoperatively.
g. Evaluate the gait characteristics, type of assistive devices, and degree of weight bearing used during ambulation. Note any inequalities in leg lengths.

2. Early patient education

a. Explain the general plan of care the patient can expect during the postoperative period.
b. Advise the patient of any precautions or contraindications to movement or weight bearing that must be followed postoperatively.
c. Teach the patient any exercises that will be started in the very early postoperative period. These often include:
   (1) Deep-breathing exercises
   (2) Active ankle exercises, if possible, to prevent venous stasis
   (3) Gentle muscle-setting exercises of immobilized joints
d. Teach the patient bed mobility.
e. Teach the patient how to use any assistive devices, such as crutches or canes, that may be needed after surgery.

D. Postoperative Goals and Guidelines for Exercise

1. Impairments/problems summarized

a. Postoperative pain because of disruption of soft tissue
b. Postoperative edema
c. Postoperative circulatory and pulmonary complications
d. Joint stiffness or limitation of motion because of injury to soft tissue and necessary postoperative immobilization
e. Muscle atrophy because of immobilization
f. Loss of strength for functional activities
g. Limitation of weight bearing
h. Potential loss of strength and mobility in unoperated joints

2. General postoperative treatment goals and plan of care during the maximum-protection phase

Goals

a. Decrease postoperative pain, muscle guarding, or spasm.

b. Decrease or minimize postoperative edema.

c. Prevent circulatory and pulmonary complications such as thrombophlebitis, pulmonary embolus, or pneumonia.

d. Prevent unnecessary, residual joint stiffness or soft tissue contractures.

e. Decrease muscle atrophy across immobilized joints.

f. Maintain motion and strength in areas above and below the operative site.

g. Maintain functional mobility while protecting the operative site.

h. Educate the patient.

Plan of Care

a. Relaxation exercises.
   Use of modalities such as transcutaneous nerve stimulation (TNS), cold, or heat.
   Continuous passive motion (CPM) during the early postoperative period.

b. Elevation of the operated extremity.
   Active pumping exercises at the distal joints.
   Distal-to-proximal massage.[40]

c. Active exercises to distal musculature.
   Deep-breathing exercises.

d. CPM or passive ROM initiated in the immediate postoperative period.

e. Muscle-setting exercises begun immediately after surgery.

f. Active and resistive ROM exercises to unoperated areas.

g. Adaptive equipment and assistive devices.

h. Instruction in positions and movements to avoid during ADL.

3. General postoperative treatment goals and plan of care during the controlled motion/moderate-protection phase

Goals

a. Gradually restore soft tissue and joint mobility.
b. Strengthen involved tissues and improve joint stability.

Plan of Care

a. Active-assistive and active ROM exercises within limits of pain.
b. Multiple-angle isometrics using progressively increasing resistance.

Goals	*Plan of Care*
	Light isotonic resistance exercise in open and closed chain.
c. Continue to maintain functional integrity of unoperated areas.	c. Progressive strengthening of unoperated areas using resistive exercises in an open or closed kinematic chain.
d. Educate the patient.	d. Teach the patient to monitor the effects of the exercise program and make adjustments if swelling or pain increases.

4. General postoperative treatment goals and plan of care during the minimum-protection/return-to-function phase

The goals and plan of care in this final stage of rehabilitation are the same as the treatment plan discussed earlier in this chapter under Treatment Considerations: Chronic Stage (Section V.B). Because surgical intervention usually occurs with the more serious injuries, severe deformities, or late-stage joint diseases, the progression of exercise may be more gradual, and the return to a full functional activity level may take more time for postoperative patients than for patients who do not require surgery. Some patients may need to adapt or avoid recreational or occupational activities that could cause reinjury to joints or soft tissues or contribute to failure of the surgical repair or reconstruction.

5. General postoperative precautions

a. Avoid specific joint motions or weight bearing consistent with the surgical procedure.

b. Progress exercise gradually during the early postoperative period. Soft tissues disturbed during surgery will be inflamed. Allow adequate time for healing to occur.

c. Avoid vigorous/high-intensity stretching or resistance exercise to muscles or tendons that have been incised and reattached during surgery for at least 6 weeks to ensure adequate healing and stability.

d. Continually note the level of swelling, pain, and wound drainage. If a marked increase is noted, report immediately and discontinue exercise to that area until further notice.

e. Modify or avoid any recreational, occupational, or daily living activities that could contribute to eventual failure of the surgical repair or reconstruction.

E. Overview of Common Orthopedic Surgical Procedures and Guidelines for Postoperative Care

NOTE: The length of immobilization and the initiation, progression, and intensity of exercise may vary according to differences in surgical techniques and the philosophy of the surgeon. A patient's health status, age, and use of medications will also affect the rate of healing and subsequent progression in a postoperative exercise program.

1. Open versus arthroscopic procedures[23,33,37]

a. An open surgical procedure involves an incision of adequate length and depth through superficial and deep layers of skin, fascia, muscles, and joint capsule so that the operative field can be fully visualized by the surgeon during the procedure. The term **arthrotomy** is used to describe an open procedure in which the joint capsule is incised and joint structures are exposed. Some open approaches are necessary for surgeries such as joint replacement, arthrodeses, and internal fixation of fractures and for some soft tissue repairs such as muscle or tendon ruptures. There is extensive disturbance of soft tissues during an open procedure that requires a lengthy period of rehabilitation while soft tissues heal.

b. Arthoscopic procedures involve several very small incisions (punctures) in the skin, muscle, and joint capsule for insertion of an endoscope into the joint for visualization of the interior of the joint by means of a camera. The small incisions are called *portals*. Miniature, motorized surgical tools are inserted through the portals and used to repair soft tissues within or around the joint, remove loose bodies, or débride the joint surfaces. Arthroscopic techniques are most commonly used at the shoulder and knee. Procedures include ligament and tendon repairs or reconstruction, débridement of joints, and occasionally synovectomy. Because the incisions for the portals are very small, there is minimal disturbance of soft tissues during arthroscopic procedures. Therefore, rehabilitation can proceed more quickly than after an open procedure.

2. Repair of soft tissue lesions[4,15,17]

In general, at least 6 weeks are needed for soft tissues to heal after surgical repair.

a. *Complete rupture of a muscle*

(1) This is not common, but it may occur when a muscle that is already contracted takes a direct blow or is forcibly stretched.

(2) Procedure

The muscle is surgically resutured and immobilized so that muscle is in a shortened position for 10 to 21 days.

(3) Exercise

(a) Muscle-setting exercises of the sutured muscle may be started immediately after surgery.

(b) At 10 to 14 days postoperatively, the immobilization is removed and active exercise emphasizing controlled motion may be started to regain joint motion.

(c) Weight bearing is restricted until the patient achieves normal strength and mobility.

(d) Stretching, and return to full functional activities are contraindicated until soft tissue healing is complete—as long as 6 to 8 weeks postoperatively.

b. *Rupture of a tendon*

(1) A tendon usually ruptures from severe trauma in a young person or with a sudden, unusual motion in an elderly person with a history of chronic impingement and progressive deterioration of the tendon. Tendons usually rupture at musculotendinous or tendo-osseous junctions. It is most often seen in the bicipital tendon at the shoulder or the Achilles tendon.

(2) Procedure

The tendon is sutured, and the muscle and tendon are put in a shortened position, as with complete tears of a muscle. A longer immobilization period is required (usually 3 to 4 weeks) for a repaired tendon than for a repaired muscle, because the vascular supply to tendons is poor.

    (3) Exercise

        (a) Muscle setting is begun immediately after surgery during the protective phase of rehabilitation to prevent adhesions of the tendon to the sheath and to promote alignment of healing tissue.

        (b) Gentle active ROM exercise is allowed after approximately 4 weeks when the immobilization device can be safely removed.

        (c) In a lower extremity repair, weight bearing may be restricted for as long as 6 to 8 weeks.

        (d) Vigorous resistance exercise may be initiated after about 8 weeks, when complete healing of the tendon has occurred.

  c. *Ligamentous tears*[4,15]

    (1) When ligaments cannot be approximated for healing through closed reduction, surgical repair is indicated. Reconstruction of a ligament with tissue taken from a donor site may also be necessary. The knee and ankle joints are commonly affected.

    (2) Procedure

The torn ligament is repaired, or reconstructed, and the joint is immobilized in a position that places limited tension on the sutured ligament. Immobilization may be required for at least 10 to 21 days and in many cases a much longer period. After some ligament repairs or reconstruction, early passive or assisted motion in a limited portion of the range may be permissible shortly after surgery.

    (3) Exercise

The same guidelines may be followed as with repaired tendons. Early postoperative passive and assisted motion may be initiated early after some surgical repairs if motion can be controlled and the healing tissue can be protected. Support should be worn, and weight bearing should be restricted when the repair is at a potentially unstable joint, such as the knee, until muscle power can adequately protect the joint.

3. Soft tissue releases: tenotomy, myotomy, and lengthening[4,26]

  a. To improve range of motion in joints with severe contractures, surgical release of soft tissue may be indicated. This may be performed in young patients with severe arthritis in whom joint replacement is not advisable or as a preliminary procedure in adults prior to joint replacement. Releases are also performed in patients with myopathic and neuropathic diseases such as cerebral palsy and muscular dystrophy. Some form of splinting or bracing in the corrected position in conjunction with exercise is always used postoperatively to maintain the gained range of motion.

  b. Procedure

The muscle or tendon is surgically sectioned and any fibrous contractures of all involved periarticular structures are released.

  c. Exercise

    (1) Active-assistive motion may be initiated within 3 to 4 days after surgery. This is followed by active exercise through the gained range as soft tissue healing progresses.

    (2) Strengthening to the antagonists of the released muscle should also be started early to maintain active joint motion.

4. Synovectomy[12,26,33]

a. Procedure

Removal of the synovium (lining of the joint) in patients with chronic joint swelling. It is occasionally performed in patients who have rheumatoid arthritis with chronic proliferative synovitis but with minimal articular changes. The most common joints on which synovectomy is performed are the knee, wrist, elbow, and metacarpophalangeal joints.

b. Postoperative management

(1) Immobilization

A soft, bulky compression dressing is applied at the time of surgery and worn for several days.

(2) Elevation

The operated extremity is elevated to reduce edema.

(3) Exercise

(a) During the brief period of immobilization the patient may begin gentle setting exercises to the muscles around the affected joint.

(b) CPM, active-assistive, and active exercises are begun as soon as the dressing is removed. These exercises are gradually progressed to mild resistive exercise over 6 to 12 weeks.

(c) Full weight bearing or lifting heavy objects is restricted for 6 to 8 weeks.

5. Osteotomy[2,4,33]

a. Procedure

The surgical cutting and realignment of bone, undertaken in cases of severe arthritis to correct joint deformity and reduce pain. It is most often performed in osteoarthritis of the knee or hip. An osteotomy is primarily performed to reduce pain by realignment and modification of the loads placed on joint surfaces before significant deterioration of the joint occurs. Osteotomy of the hip is performed in young patients with severe hip pain secondary to hip problems such as Legg-Calvé-Perthes disease or congenital dislocation of the hip.

b. Postoperative management

(1) Immobilization

Either the osteotomy site is immobilized with internal fixation, which allows early joint motion and protected weight bearing, or the involved joint is placed in a cast until bony healing occurs, which may take as long as 8 to 12 weeks.[2,4]

(2) Exercise

(a) During immobilization in a cast the patient should be encouraged to actively move the joints above and below the site of the osteotomy to prevent joint stiffness and undue weakness.

(b) When motion and weight bearing are allowed or when the cast is removed, active-assistive, active, and mild-resistive exercise may be started to restore joint range of motion and strength. (See discussion of the chronic stage of soft tissue healing earlier in this chapter.)

(c) If chronic stiffness persists because of the long-term immobilization, joint mobilization and soft tissue stretching may also be necessary.

6. Arthrodesis

a. Procedure[2,4,33]

Fusion of bony surfaces of a joint with internal fixation such as pins, nails, plates, and bone grafts. This is usually performed in cases of severe joint pain and instability in which mobility of the joint is a lesser concern. It is commonly performed at the wrist, thumb, and ankle. Arthrodesis may be the only salvage procedure left for a patient with a failed joint arthroplasty.

b. Postoperative management

(1) Immobilization

The joint is immobilized in a cast in the desired position for maximum function for 8 to 12 weeks to ensure bony fusion.

(2) Exercise

Since no movement will be possible in the fused joint, range of motion and strength must be maintained above and below the operated joint.

(3) Weight bearing is restricted until x-ray studies show evidence of bony healing.

c. Optimum positions for arthrodesis[2]

(1) Shoulder: in a position so that the hand can reach the mouth.

(2) Wrist: in slight extension. If the patient has bilateral wrist joint disease, one joint may be fused and the other replaced.

(3) Thumb: MCP joint is usually fused in 20 degrees of flexion.

(4) Hip: in 15 to 20 degrees of flexion to allow ambulation and comfortable sitting.

(5) Ankle: in neutral position (90 degrees) or slight equinus for women who wear low heels. The subtalar joint is fused in neutral so there is no varus or valgus.

7. Arthroplasty

a. General definition

Any reconstructive joint procedure, with or without joint implant, designed to relieve pain and/or restore joint motion.

b. Types of procedures[3,4,7,12,22,26,34]

(1) *Excision arthroplasty*

Removal of periarticular bone from one or both articular surfaces. A space is left where fibrotic (scar) tissue is allowed to be laid down during the healing process. This is sometimes called *resectional arthroplasty.* This procedure may be performed in a variety of joints such as the hip, elbow, wrist, and foot to reduce pain and increase joint motion. Disadvantages of these procedures are:

(a) Possible joint instability

(b) A poor cosmetic result due to shortening of the operated extremity

(c) Persistent muscular imbalance and weakness

Excision arthroplasty, although an old procedure, is still appropriate in selected cases.

(2) *Excision arthroplasty with implant*

After removal of the articular surface, an artificial implant is fixed in place to help in the remodeling of a new joint. This is sometimes called *implant resection arthroplasty.* The implant usually is made of a flexible silicone material and becomes encapsulated by fibrous tissue as the joint reforms.[34]

(3) *Interpostional arthroplasty*[34]

Débridement of the joint is performed initially, and a foreign material is placed between (interposed) the two joint surfaces. A variety of materials may be used to cover the joint surface such as fascia, Silastic material, or metal.

Some examples of interpositional arthroplasties are Smith-Petersen cup arthroplasty of the hip (rarely performed now, with the advent of the total hip replacement), condylar replacement of the knee, and humeral replacement of the shoulder.

(4) *Total joint replacement arthroplasty*

Removal of both affected joint surfaces and replacement with an artificial joint. Implants can be held in place with an acrylic cement (methyl methacrylate); may be stabilized with bolts, pins, screws, or nails; or most recently may be secured without cement using either a press-fit (a very tight fit between bone and implant) or biologic fixation (microscopic ingrowth of bone into a porous-coated prosthesis).[7,25,26,37] The bone-cement interface is the portion of the joint replacement in which loosening occurs and is the primary source of mechanical failure of total joint replacements.[25,30,37]

Prosthetic replacements for almost every joint of the extremities have been developed and refined. A more complete description of those implants will be reviewed joint by joint in Chapters 8 through 13. Overall, total joint replacement arthroplasty has been most successful in the large joints, such as the hip and knee, rather than in the smaller joints of the foot and hand.[2,3] Total joint implants generally require less postoperative immobilization and less supervised graded exercise than excision arthroplasty (with or without implant) or interpositional arthroplasty, because the success of the procedure is less dependent on the encapsulation process during soft tissue healing.

c. Types of materials used in arthroplasty[2,3,25,26]

Many different materials have been used in the developing years in reconstructive surgery. Materials used today may be classified into three broad areas.

(1) Rigid

Inert metal, usually a cobalt-chrome alloy, stainless steel, or ceramic materials.

(2) Semirigid

Plastic, high-density polymers such as polyethylene.

(3) Flexible

Elastic polymers such as Silastic or silicone implants.

In general, flexible implants are used in conjunction with excision arthroplasty, and semirigid plastics and rigid metals or ceramics are used in total joint replacements.

d. Postoperative management

A detailed description of postoperative management and exercises for specific total joint replacements will be covered in Chapters 8 through 13.

XI. Summary

Chapter 7 has provided background information necessary to design therapeutic exercise programs based on a patient's level of orthopedic involvement during the acute, subacute, or chronic stage of soft tissue and joint healing. This approach is used whether the problem involves injury from trauma, insult from overuse, disease, or surgical intervention.

Soft tissue lesions and clinical conditions have been defined; the stages of inflammation and repair have been described with emphasis on how to manage soft tissues and joints with therapeutic exercise during each stage. Special considerations and therapeutic exercise management for repetitive trauma syndromes, rheumatoid arthritis, osteoarthritis, postfracture dysfunctions, and postsurgical conditions also have been described.

A problem list with goals and plan of care has been outlined to summarize each clinical situation. A list of clinical problems is used as the foundation for designing exercise programs for each region of the body as described in Chapters 8 through 13.

References

1. Bandy, WD: Functional rehabilitation of the athlete. Orthopaedic Physical Therapy Clinics of North America 1:269, 1992.
2. Benke, GJ: Osteotomy, arthrodesis and girdlestone arthroplasty. In Downie, PA (ed): Cash's Textbook of Orthopedics and Rheumatology for Physiotherapists. JB Lippincott, Philadelphia, 1984.
3. Bentley, JA: Physiotherapy following joint replacement. In Downie, PA (ed): Cash's Textbook of Orthopedics and Rheumatology for Physiotherapists. JB Lippincott, Philadelphia, 1984.
4. Braschear, R, and Raney, RB (eds): Shands' Handbook of Orthopaedic Surgery, ed 9. CV Mosby, St Louis, 1978.
5. Cailliet, R: Soft Tissue Pain and Disability, ed 2. FA Davis, Philadelphia, 1988.
6. Chamberlain, G: Cyriax's friction massage: A review. Journal of Orthopaedic and Sports Physical Therapy 4:16, 1982.
7. Cofield, R, Morrey, B, and Bryan, R: Total shoulder and total elbow arthroplasties: The current state of development—Part I. J Contin Educ Orthopedics 6:14, 1978.
8. Cummings, G, Crutchfield, C, and Barnes, MR: Soft-Tissue Changes in Contractures. Orthopedic Physical Therapy Series, Vol 1. Stokesville, Atlanta, 1983.
9. Cummings, GS, and Tillman, LJ: Remodeling of dense connective tissue in normal adult tissues. In Currier, DP, and Nelson, RM (eds): Dynamics of Human Biologic Tissues. FA Davis, Philadelphia, 1992.
10. Cyriax, J: Textbook of Orthopaedic Medicine, Vol 1. Diagnosis of Soft Tissue Lesions, ed 8. Bailliere and Tindall, London, 1982.
11. Guidotti, TL: Occupational repetitive strain injury. Am Fam Physician 45:585, 1992.
12. Hyde, SA: Physiotherapy in Rheumatology. Blackwell Scientific, Oxford, 1980.
13. Inglis, AE (ed): Symposium on Total Joint Replacement of the Upper Extremity (1979). American Academy of Orthopaedic Surgeons, CV Mosby, St Louis, 1982.
14. Isernhagen, SJ: Exercise technologies for work rehabilitation programs. Orthopaedic Physical Therapy Clinics of North America 1:361, 1992.
15. Iversen, LD, and Clawson, DK: Manual of Acute Orthopedic Therapeutics, ed 2. Little, Brown & Company, Boston, 1982.
16. Kaltenborn, F: Manual Mobilization of the Extremity Joints: Basic Examination and Treatment Techniques, ed 4. Olaf Norlis Bokhandel Norway, 1989.
17. Keene, J: Ligament and muscle-tendon unit injuries.

In Gould, J, and Davies, GJ (eds): Orthopaedic and Sports Physical Therapy, ed 2. CV Mosby, St Louis, 1990.
18. Kellet, J: Acute soft-tissue injuries: A review of the literature. Med Sci Sports Exerc 18:489, 1986.
19. Maitland, GD: Peripheral Manipulation, ed 2. Butterworth, Boston, 1977.
20. Maitland, GD: Vertebral Manipulation, ed 4. Butterworth, Boston, 1977.
21. McDonough, A: Effect of immobilization and exercise on articular cartilage: A review of literature. Journal of Orthopaedic and Sports Physical Therapy 3:2, 1981.
22. Melvin, J: Rheumatic Disease: Occupational Therapy and Rehabilitation, ed 2. FA Davis, Philadelphia, 1982.
23. Metcalf, RW: Arthroscopy. In Sledge, CB, et al (eds): Arthritis Surgery. WB Saunders, Philadelphia, 1994.
24. Minor, MA, et al: Efficacy of physical conditioning exercise in patients with rheumatoid arthritis and osteoarthritis. Arthritis Rheum 32:1396, 1989.
25. Morrey, BF, and Kavanaugh, BF: Cementless joint replacement: Current status and future. Bull Rheum Dis 37:1, 1987.
26. Nickel, VL (ed): Orthopedic Rehabilitation. Churchill-Livingstone, New York, 1982.
27. Noonan, TJ, and Garrett, WE: Injuries at the myotendinous junction. Clin Sports Med 11:783, 1992.
28. Pease, BJ: Biomechanical assessment of the lower extremity. Orthopaedic Physical Therapy Clinics of North America 3:291, 1994.
29. Puffer, JC, and Zachazewski, JE: Management of overuse injuries. Am Fam Physician 38:225, 1988.
30. Rand, JA, et al: A comparison of cemented vs cementless porous-coated anatomic total knee arthroplasty. In Rand, JA (ed): Total Arthroplasty of the Knee. Aspen, Rockville, MD, 1987.
31. Salter, RB, et al: Clinical application of basic research on continuous passive motion for disorders and injuries of synovial joints: A preliminary of a feasibility study. J Orthop Res 1:325, 1984.
32. Schrier, RW (ed): Clinical Internal Medicine in the Aged. WB Saunders, Philadelphia, 1982.
33. Sledge, CB: Introduction to surgical management. In Sledge, CB, et al (eds): Arthritis Surgery. WB Saunders, Philadelphia, 1994.
34. Swanson, AB: Flexible Implant Resection Arthroplasty in the Hand and Extremities. CV Mosby, St Louis, 1973.
35. Threlkeld, JA, and Currier, DP: Osteoarthritis: Effects on synovial joint tissues. Phys Ther 68:346, 1988.

36. van der Meulen, JCH: Present state of knowledge on processes of healing in collagen structures. Int J Sports Med 3:4, 1982.

37. Waugh, T: Arthroplasty rehabilitation. In Gouldgold, J (ed): Rehabilitation Medicine. CV Mosby, St Louis, 1988.

38. Wilhelm, DL: Inflammation and healing. In Anderson, WAD (ed): Pathology, CV Mosby, St Louis, 1971.

39. Wilk, KE, and Arrigo, C: An integrated approach to upper extremity exercises. Orthopaedic Physical Therapy Clinics of North America 1:337, 1992.

40. Woolf, CJ: Generation of acute pain: Central mechanisms. British Medical Bulletin 47:523, 1991.

41. Zohn, D, and Mennell, J: Musculoskeletal Pain: Principles of Physical Diagnosis and Physical Treatment. Little, Brown & Company, Boston, 1976.

The Shoulder and Shoulder Girdle

The design of the shoulder girdle allows for mobility of the upper extremity. As a result, the hand can be placed almost anywhere within a sphere of movement, being limited primarily by the length of the arm and the space taken up by the body. The combined mechanics of its joints and muscles provide for and control the mobility. When establishing a therapeutic exercise program for problems in the shoulder region, as with any other region of the body, the unique anatomic and kinesiologic features must be taken into consideration as well as the state of pathology and functional limitations imposed by the problems. The first section of this chapter briefly reviews anatomic and kinesiologic information on the shoulder complex; the reader is referred to several textbooks for in-depth study of the material.[16,24,46,53,56,76] The reader is also referred to Chapter 7 for review of principles of management. The following sections then describe common problems and guidelines for conservative and postsurgical management. The last two sections describe exercise techniques commonly used to meet the goals of treatment during the acute stage and during the healing and rehabilitative stages.

OBJECTIVES

After studying this chapter, the reader will be able to:

1 Identify important aspects of shoulder girdle structure and function for review.
2 Establish a therapeutic exercise program to manage soft tissue and joint lesions in the shoulder girdle region related to stages of recovery following an inflammatory insult to the tissues.
3 Establish a therapeutic exercise program to manage common musculoskeletal lesions, recognizing unique circumstances for their management.
4 Establish a therapeutic exercise program to manage patients following common surgical procedures.

I. Review of the Structure and Function of the Shoulder and Shoulder Girdle

A. Bony Parts Include the Proximal Humerus, Scapula, and Clavicle and Its Attachment to the Sternum (see Fig. 6–13)

B. Synovial Joints

1. Glenohumeral (GH) joint

a. Characteristics. This joint is an incongruous, ball-and-socket (spheroidal) tri-axial joint with a lax joint capsule. It is supported by the tendons of the rotator cuff and the glenohumeral (superior, middle, and inferior) and coracohumeral ligaments. The concave bony partner, the glenoid fossa, is located on the superior-lateral margin of the scapula. It faces anteriorly, laterally, and upward, which provides some stability to the joint. A fibrocartilage lip, the glenoid labrum, deepens the fossa for greater congruity and serves as the attachment site for the capsule. The convex bony partner is the head of the humerus. Only a small portion of the head comes in contact with the fossa at any one time, allowing for considerable humeral movement and potential instability.[78]

b. Arthrokinematics. With motions of the humerus (physiologic motions), the convex head slides in the opposite direction of the humerus.

Physiologic Motions of the Humerus	Direction of Slide of Humeral Head
Flexion	Posterior
Extension	Anterior
Abduction	Inferior
Adduction	Superior
Internal rotation	Posterior
External rotation	Anterior
Horizontal abduction	Anterior
Horizontal adduction	Posterior

If the humerus is stabilized and the scapula moves, the concave glenoid fossa slides in the same direction that the scapula moves.

c. Stability. Static and dynamic restraints provide joint stability.[17,23,89,105] The structural relationship of the bony anatomy, ligaments, and glenoid labrum and the adhesive and cohesive forces within the joint provide static stability. The tendons of the rotator cuff blend with the ligaments and glenoid labrum at the sites of attachment so that when the muscles contract they provide dynamic stability by tightening the static restraints. The coordinated response of the muscles of the cuff and tension in the ligaments provide varying degrees of support depending on the position and motion of the humerus.[86,89,100] In addition, the long head of the biceps and long head of the triceps brachii reinforce the capsule with their attachments and provide superior and inferior shoulder joint support respectively when functioning with elbow motions.[55] The long head of the biceps in particular stabilizes against humeral elevation[55] as well as contributes to anterior stability of the glenohumeral joint by resisting torsional forces when the shoulder is abducted and externally rotated.[7,86] Neuromuscular control, including movement awareness and motor response, underlies coordination of the dynamic restraints.[105]

2. Acromioclavicular (AC) joint

a. Characteristics. This joint is a plane, gliding triaxial joint, which may or may not have a disk. The weak capsule is reinforced by the superior and inferior acromioclavicular ligaments. The convex bony partner is a facet on the lateral end of the clavicle. The concave bony partner is a facet on the acromion of the scapula.

b. Arthrokinematics. With motions of the scapula, the acromial surface slides in the same direction in which the scapula moves, because the surface is concave. Motions affecting this joint include upward rotation (the scapula turns so that the glenoid fossa rotates upward), downward rotation, winging of the vertebral border, and tipping of the inferior angle.

c. Stability. The acromioclavicular ligaments are supported by the strong coracoclavicular ligament. No muscles directly cross this joint for dynamic support.

3. Sternoclavicular (SC) joint

a. Characteristics. This joint is an incongruent, triaxial, saddle-shaped joint with a disk. The joint is supported by the anterior and posterior sternoclavicular ligaments and the interclavicular and costoclavicular ligaments. The medial end of the clavicle is convex superior to inferior and concave anterior to posterior. The joint disk attaches to the upper end. The superior-lateral portion of the manubrium and first costal cartilage is concave superior to inferior and convex anterior to posterior.

b. Arthrokinematics. With anterior-posterior motions of the clavicle, the articulating surface slides in the same direction. With superior-inferior motions of the clavicle, the articulating surface slides opposite.

Physiologic Motions of the Clavicle	*Direction of Slide of the Clavicle*
Elevation	Inferior
Depression	Superior
Protraction	Anterior
Retraction	Posterior
Rotation	Spin

The motions of the clavicle occur as a result of the scapular motions of elevation, depression, protraction (abduction), and retraction (adduction), respectively. Rotation of the clavicle occurs as an accessory motion when the humerus is elevated above the horizontal position and the scapula upwardly rotates; it cannot occur as an isolated voluntary motion.

c. Stability. The ligaments crossing the joint provide static stability. There are no muscles crossing the joint for dynamic stability.

C. Functional Articulations

1. Scapulothoracic

a. Motions of the scapula require sliding of the scapula along the thorax. Normally there is considerable soft tissue flexibility, allowing the scapula to participate in all upper extremity motions. Motions of the scapula are:

(1) Elevation, depression, protraction (abduction), and retraction (adduction), seen with clavicular motions at the SC joint.

(2) Upward and downward rotation, seen with clavicular motions at the SC joint and rotation at the AC joint, concurrently with motions of the

humerus. Upward rotation of the scapula is a necessary component motion for full range of motion of flexion and abduction of the humerus.

(3) Winging of the medial border and tipping of the inferior angle, seen with motion at the AC joint concurrently with motions of the humerus. Tipping of the scapula is necessary to reach the hand behind the back in conjunction with internal rotation and extension of the humerus. Winging is an accessory motion with horizontal adduction of the humerus.

b. Scapular stability

(1) In the dependent position, the scapula is stabilized primarily through a balance of forces between the upper trapezius, levator scapulae, and the weight of the arm in the frontal plane and between the pectoralis minor and rhomboids and serratus anterior in the transverse and sagittal planes.

(2) With active arm motions the muscles of the scapula function in synchrony to control the position and stabilize the scapula so that the scapulohumeral muscles can maintain a good length-tension relationship as they function to stabilize to move the humerus. Without the positional control of the scapula, the efficiency of the humeral muscles decreases. The upper and lower trapezius with the serratus anterior upwardly rotate the scapula whenever the arm abducts or flexes, and the serratus anterior abducts (protracts) the scapula on the thorax to align the scapula during flexion or pushing activities. During arm extension or during pulling activities, the rhomboids function to downwardly rotate and adduct (retract) the scapula in synchrony with the latissimus dorsi, teres major, and rotator cuff muscles. These stabilizing muscles also eccentrically control acceleration motions of the scapula in the opposite directions.[80]

(3) With a faulty scapular posture from muscle imbalances, muscle length and strength imbalances also occur in the humeral muscles, altering the mechanics of the glenohumeral joint. A forward tilt of the scapula is associated with a tight pectoralis minor muscle and possibly weak serratus anterior or trapezius. This scapular posture changes the posture of the humerus in the glenoid, assuming a relatively abducted and internally rotated position. This results in tight glenohumeral internal rotators and stretched or weakened lateral rotators.

2. Suprahumeral

a. Coracoacromial arch, composed of the acromion and coracoacromial ligament, overlies the subacromial/subdeltoid bursa, the supraspinatus tendon, and a portion of the muscle.[76]

b. These structures allow for and participate in normal shoulder function. Compromise of this space from faulty muscle function, faulty joint mechanics, or injury to the soft tissue in this region leads to impingement syndromes.[14,16,91] Following a rotator cuff tear, the bursa may communicate with the glenohumeral joint cavity.[23]

D. Shoulder Girdle Function[23,56,76]

1. Scapulohumeral rhythm

a. Motion of the scapula, synchronous with motions of the humerus, allows for 150 to 180 degrees of shoulder range of motion into flexion or abduction with elevation. The ratio has considerable variation among individuals but is commonly accepted to be 2:1 (2 degrees of glenohumeral motion to 1 degree of scapular rotation) overall motion. During the setting phase (0 to 30 degrees abduction, 0 to 60 degrees flexion), motion is primarily at the gleno-humeral joint, whereas the scapula seeks a stable position. During the mid-range, the scapula has greater motion, approaching a 1:1 ratio with the humerus; later in the range, the glenohumeral joint again dominates the motion.

b. The synchronous motion of the scapula allows the muscles moving the humerus to maintain a good length-tension relationship throughout the activity as well as helps maintain good congruency between the humeral head and fossa while decreasing shear forces.

c. Muscles causing the upward rotation of the scapula are the upper and lower trapezius and serratus anterior. Weakness or complete paralysis of these muscles results in the scapula's being rotated downward by the contracting deltoid and supraspinatus as abduction or flexion is attempted. These two muscles then reach active insufficiency, and functional elevation of the arm cannot be reached, even though there may be normal passive ROM and normal strength in the shoulder abductor and flexor muscles.

2. Clavicular elevation and rotation with humeral motion

a. Initially, with upward rotation of the scapula, 30 degrees of elevation of the clavicle occurs at the SC joint. Then, as the coracoclavicular ligament becomes taut, the clavicle rotates 38 to 50 degrees about its longitudinal axis, which elevates its acromial end (because it is crank shaped). The scapula then rotates an additional 30 degrees at the AC joint.

b. Loss of any of these functional components will decrease the amount of scapular rotation and thus the range of motion of the upper extremity.

3. External rotation of the humerus with full elevation through abduction

a. For the greater tubercle of the humerus to clear the coracoacromial arch, the humerus must externally rotate as it is elevated above the horizontal while abducting the arm in the frontal plane.

b. Weak or inadequate external rotation will result in impingement of the soft tissues in the suprahumeral space, causing pain, inflammation, and eventually loss of function.

4. Internal rotation of the humerus with full elevation through flexion[10,11,81]

a. Medial rotation begins around 50 degrees of passive shoulder flexion when all structures are intact.[81] With full range of shoulder flexion and elevation, the humerus medially rotates 90 degrees and the medial epicondyle faces anteriorly.[81]

b. Most of the shoulder flexor muscles are also medial rotators of the humerus.[56]

c. As the arm elevates above the horizontal position in the sagittal plane, the anterior capsule and ligaments become taut, causing the humerus to medially rotate.

d. The bony configuration of the posterior aspect of the glenoid fossa contributes to the inward rotation motion of the humerus as the shoulder flexes.[56]

e. The infraspinatus and teres minor stabilize the humeral head against the inward rotating forces, helping to maintain alignment and stability of the head in the fossa. Weakness in these muscles may contribute to excessive anterior translation and instability.[17]

5. Elevation of the humerus through the plane of the scapula

    a. The plane of the scapula is described as 30 degrees anterior to the frontal plane. Motion of the humerus in this plane is popularly called **scaption**,[99,104] or scapular plane abduction.[23]

    b. In this range there is less tension on the capsule and greater elevation is possible than with pure frontal or sagittal plane elevation. Neither internal nor external rotation of the humerus is necessary to prevent greater tubercle impingement in elevation through scaption.[23,99] Many functional activities occur with the shoulder oriented in this plane.

6. Deltoid–short rotator cuff and supraspinatus mechanisms

    a. The majority of the force of the deltoid muscle causes upward translation of the humerus; if unopposed, it leads to impingement of the soft tissues within the suprahumeral space between the humeral head and the coracoacromial arch.

    b. The combined effect of the short rotator muscles (infraspinatus, teres minor, and subscapularis) causes a stabilizing compression and a downward translation of the humerus in the glenoid.

    c. The actions of the deltoid and short rotators result in a force couple that is necessary for abduction of the humerus.

    d. The supraspinatus muscle has a significant stabilizing compressive and slight upward translation effect on the humerus; these effects, combined with the effect of gravity, lead to abduction of the arm.

    e. Interruption of function leading to fatigue or poor coordination of any of these muscles can lead to microtrauma and eventual dysfunction in the shoulder region.

E. Referred Pain: Common Sources Referring Pain Into the Shoulder Region

1. Cervical spine

    a. Vertebral joints between C-3 and C-4 or between C-4 and C-5

    b. Nerve roots C-4 or C-5

2. Dermatomal references from related tissues

    a. Dermatome C-4 is over the trapezius to the tip of the shoulder.

    b. Dermatome C-5 is over the deltoid region and lateral arm.

3. Diaphragm: upper trapezius region

4. Heart: axilla and left pectoral region

5. Gallbladder irritation: tip of shoulder and posterior scapular region

6. Myofascial pain patterns: in the supraspinatus, infraspinatus, and trapezius.

II. Joint Problems: Nonoperative Management

A. Glenohumeral (GH) Joint

1. Related diagnoses and etiology of symptoms

    a. Joint problems may occur with *rheumatoid arthritis* or *osteoarthritis* and follow the clinical picture described in Chapter 7.

b. *Traumatic arthritis* occurs in response to a fall or blow to the shoulder or to microtrauma from faulty mechanics or overuse.

c. *Postimmobilization arthritis* or stiff shoulder occurs as a result of lack of movement or secondary effects from conditions such as heart disease, stroke, or diabetes mellitus.

d. *Idiopathic frozen shoulder* (also called adhesive capsulitis or periarthritis[33,36,69,72,87,101]) is characterized by the development of dense adhesions and capsular restrictions, especially in the dependent fold of the capsule, rather than arthritic changes in the cartilage and bone, as seen with rheumatoid arthritis or osteoarthritis. The insidious onset usually occurs between the ages of 40 and 60, without a known cause (primary frozen shoulder), although problems already mentioned, in which there is a period of pain and/or restricted motion such as with rheumatoid arthritis, osteoarthritis, trauma, or immobilization, may lead to a frozen shoulder (secondary frozen shoulder). In primary frozen shoulder, the pathogenesis may be from a provoking chronic inflammation in a musculotendinous or synovial tissue such as the rotator cuff, biceps tendon, or joint capsule that results in formation of capsular thickening and adhesions, particularly in the folds of the inferior capsule.[36,69,72] Consistent with this is a faulty posture and muscle imbalances predisposing the suprahumeral space to impingement and overuse syndromes (see Section IV).

2. **Symptoms**

a. Clinical picture: *acute joint problems*
Pain and muscle guarding limiting motion, usually preventing external rotation and abduction. Pain is frequently experienced radiating below the elbow and may disturb sleep.

b. Clinical picture: *subacute joint problems*
If the patient can be treated as the acute condition begins to subside by gradually increasing the shoulder motion and activity, the complication of joint and soft tissue contractures can usually be minimized.[69,74]

c. Clinical picture: *chronic joint problems*
If motion becomes restricted or if the patient is not treated until there is limited motion, capsular tightness develops, with pain felt as the capsule is stretched. Often, because of the pain, the person does not use the arm normally, and the joint progressively becomes more limited. Usually, external rotation and abduction are most limited, and internal rotation least limited. There may be aching, localized to the deltoid region.

d. Clinical picture: *idiopathic frozen shoulder*[33,36,69,72,87,101]
This clinical entity follows a classic pattern.
   (1) "Freezing." Characterized by intense pain even at rest and limitation of motion by 2 to 3 weeks following onset. These acute symptoms may last 10 to 36 weeks.
   (2) "Frozen." Characterized by pain only with movement, significant adhesions, and limited glenohumeral motions with substitute motions in the scapula. Atrophy of the deltoid, rotator cuff, biceps, and triceps brachii muscles occurs. This stage lasts 4 to 12 months.
   (3) "Thawing." Characterized by no pain and no synovitis but significant capsular restrictions from adhesions. This stage lasts 2 to 24 months or longer. Some patients never regain normal range of motion.
Spontaneous recovery occurs on the average of 2 years from onset.[33,36] Inap-

propriately aggressive therapy at the wrong time may prolong the symptoms.[9] Treatment guidelines are the same as acute for freezing stage, and subacute and chronic for the frozen and thawing stages, respectively.

3. **Common impairments/problems**

   a. Night pain and disturbed sleep during acute flairs
   b. Pain on motion and often at rest during acute flairs
   c. Decreased joint play and range of motion, usually limiting external rotation and abduction with some limitation of internal rotation and elevation in flexion
   d. Possible faulty postural compensations with protracted and anteriorly tipped scapula, rounded shoulders, and elevated and protected shoulder
   e. Poor arm swing during gait
   f. General muscle weakness and poor endurance in the glenohumeral muscles with overuse of the scapular muscles leading to pain in trapezius and posterior cervical muscles
   g. Guarded shoulder motions with substitute scapular motions

4. **Common functional limitations/disabilities**

   a. Unable to reach overhead, behind head, and behind back; thus has difficulty with dressing (such as putting on a jacket or coat or women fastening undergarments behind their back), with reaching hand into back pocket of pants (to retrieve wallet), with self-grooming (such as combing hair, brushing teeth, washing face), and with bringing eating utensils to the mouth
   b. Unable to lift weighted objects such as dishes into a cupboard
   c. Unable to sustain repetitive activities

5. **Management of acute joint lesions**

   a. See guidelines for management in Chapter 7, Section III.
   b. To control the pain, edema, and muscle guarding
      (1) Immobilization in a sling provides rest to the part, but complete immobilization can lead to contractures and limited motion.
      (2) Gentle joint oscillation techniques of small amplitude (grade I) may be used with the joint in a pain-free position (see Chapter 6).

      Precaution: During the first 2 days following trauma, this technique may not be tolerated by some people. Use with extreme care and use only if it decreases the pain.

   c. To maintain soft tissue and joint integrity and mobility
      (1) Passive range of motion (ROM) to all ranges of pain-free motion (see Chapter 2). As pain decreases, the patient should be able to progress to active ROM with or without assistance, depending on severity of the injury.
      (2) Passive joint traction and glides, with the joint placed in a pain-free position as it is treated (see Chapter 6). Begin with grade I; progress to grade II as symptoms improve.

      Precaution: If there is increased pain or irritability in the joint following use of these techniques, either the dosage was too strong or the techniques should not be used at this time.

      Contraindication: Stretching (grade III) techniques. If there are mechanical restrictions causing limited motion, appropriate stretching can be initiated *after* the inflammation subsides.

(3) Gentle muscle setting to all muscle groups of the shoulder. Also include scapular and elbow muscles because of their close association with the shoulder. Instruct the patient to gently contract a group of muscles while you apply slight resistance—just enough to stimulate a muscle contraction. It should not provoke pain. The emphasis is on rhythmic contracting and relaxing of the muscles to help stimulate blood flow and prevent circulatory stasis.

d. To maintain integrity and function of associated areas

(1) Either the therapist or the patient should perform ROM to the elbow, forearm, wrist, and fingers several times each day while the shoulder is immobilized. If tolerated, active or gentle resistive ROM is preferred to passive for a greater effect on circulation and muscle integrity.

(2) Shoulder-hand syndrome is a potential complication following shoulder injury or immobility; special attention should be given to the hand with additional exercises, such as repetitively squeezing a ball or other soft object (see Section VII).

(3) If edema is noted in the hand, the hand should be elevated, whenever possible, above the level of the heart.

(4) Instruct the patient in the importance of keeping the joints distal to the injured site as active and mobile as possible.

6. **Management of subacute and chronic joint limitations**

a. Follow the guidelines as described in Chapter 7, Sections IV and V, emphasizing joint mobility.

b. To control pain, edema, and joint effusion.
Carefully monitor increasing activities. If the joint was splinted, progressively increase the amount of time that the shoulder is free to move each day.

c. To decrease the effect of contracture formation and progressively increase soft tissue and/or joint mobility.[50,74]

(1) Passive joint mobilization techniques (see Chapter 6)

NOTE: A grade I distraction is used with all gliding techniques.
Begin with sustained grade II traction and gliding techniques with the joint placed in a pain-free position; as the joint responds, gradually progress to grade III.

If the joint is highly irritable and gliding in the direction of restriction is not tolerated, glide in the opposite direction. As pain and irritability decrease, begin to glide in the direction of restriction.[50]

(a) To increase abduction, caudal glide humeral head (see Figs. 6–15 to 6–17).

(b) To increase flexion or internal rotation, posterior glide humeral head (see Figs. 6–18 and 6–19).

(c) To increase extension or external rotation, anterior glide humeral head (see Fig. 6–20).

(d) As joint pain decreases and the available range reaches a plateau, progress by taking the shoulder to the limits of its motion and apply the appropriate glide.

Precaution: Vigorous stretching should not be undertaken until the chronic stage.

NOTE: For normal joint mechanics, there must be good scapular mobility and control and the humerus must be able to externally rotate. Increasing abduction beyond 90 degrees should not occur until adequate external rotation is available and the scapula has unrestricted motion. With a traumatic injury also involving the AC or SC joints, these joints tend to become hypermobile. Care should be taken not to stretch them when mobilizing the glenohumeral joint by providing good stabilization to the scapula.

(2) Early joint mobility exercises; **pendulum (Codman's) exercises**[20] (Fig. 8–1)

These are self-mobilization techniques that use the effects of gravity to distract the humerus from the glenoid fossa.[16,20] They help relieve pain through gentle traction and oscillating movements (grade II) and provide early motion of joint structures and synovial fluid. No weight is used initially. When the patient tolerates stretching, a weight is added to the hand or as wrist cuffs to cause a grade III joint distraction force. To direct the stretch force to the glenohumeral joint, stabilize the scapula against the thorax manually or with a belt.

POSITION OF PATIENT

Standing, with the trunk flexed at the hips about 90 degrees or prone on a treatment table, with the involved shoulder over the edge. The arm hangs loosely downward in a position between 60 and 90 degrees flexion or scaption.

TECHNIQUE

A pendulum or swinging motion of the arm is initiated by having the patient move the trunk slightly back and forth. Motions of flexion, extension, and horizontal abduction, adduction, and circumduction can be done. Increase the arc of motion as tolerated. This technique should not cause pain.

Precautions: Some patients may get dizzy when standing upright after being bent over; if so, have them sit and rest.

If patients cannot balance themselves leaning over, have them hold on to a solid object or lie prone on a table.

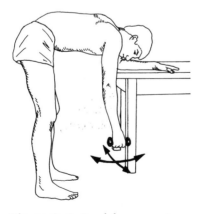

Figure 8–1. Pendulum exercises. For gentle distraction, no weight is used. Use of a weight causes a grade III (stretching) distraction force.

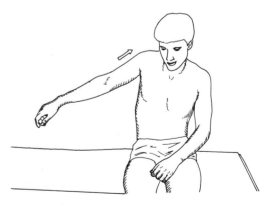

Figure 8–2. Poor mechanics with patient hiking the shoulder while trying to abduct the shoulder, thus elevating rather than depressing the humeral head.

If the patient experiences back pain from bending over, use the prone position.

Adding a weight to the hand or using wrist cuffs causes a greater distraction force on the glenohumeral joint. This should be performed only when joint stretching maneuvers are indicated late in the sub-acute and chronic stages—and then only if the scapula is stabilized by the therapist or a belt is placed around the thorax and scapula, so that the stretch force is directed to the joint, not the soft tissue of the scapulothoracic region.

With increased pain or decreased ROM, the technique may be an inappropriate choice.

(3) Range of motion
   (a) Begin with active ROM up to the point of pain, including all shoulder and scapular motions (see Chapter 2).
   (b) Use self-assistive ROM techniques, such as the shoulder wheel, overhead pulleys, or wand exercises (see Chapter 2).
   (c) When the patient can tolerate stretching, the patient takes the extremity to the limit of the range and holds it 10 to 15 seconds or longer if tolerated, relaxes; then repeats.

   Precaution: With increased pain or decreased motion, the activity may be too intense or the patient may be using faulty mechanics. Reassess the technique and modify it if faulty joint mechanics exist.

(4) Control of muscle spasm and rotator cuff stabilization
   Muscle spasm may lead to a faulty deltoid-rotator cuff mechanism when the patient attempts abduction. The head of the humerus may be held in a cranial position within the joint, making it difficult and/or painful to abduct the shoulder because the greater tuberosity impinges on the coracoacromial arch. In this case, repositioning the head of the humerus with a caudal glide is necessary before proceeding with any other form of shoulder exercise.
   (a) Gentle oscillations will help decrease the muscle spasm (grade I or II).
   (b) Sustained caudal glides will help reposition the humeral head in the glenoid fossa.
   (c) Closed chain with protected weight bearing, such as leaning hands against a wall or on a table, will stimulate co-contraction of the rotator cuff and scapular stabilizing muscles. If tolerated, gentle rocking forward/backward and side to side requires the muscles to begin controlling motion. Because weight bearing causes joint compression, progress within the tolerance of the joint.
   (d) Training the external rotators of the shoulder will help to depress the humeral head as the arm abducts. This needs to be accomplished if the patient tends to hike the shoulder while abducting, thus elevating rather than depressing the humeral head (Fig. 8–2).
       Teach the patient active and progress to resistive external rotation exercises (see Fig. 8–24).
       Teach voluntary humeral depression. Have the patient attempt to push the arm caudally; provide slight resistance against the elbow

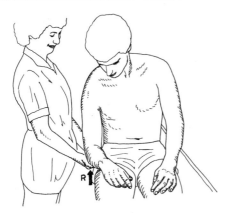

Figure 8–3. Resisting humeral depression.

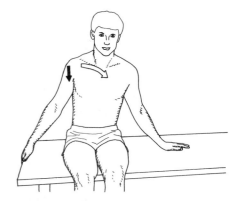

Figure 8–4. Self-mobilization; caudal glide of the humerus occurs as the person leans away from the fixed arm.

for proprioceptive feedback (there will also be some scapular depression). Give verbal reinforcement any time the patient causes caudal glide of the humerus (Fig. 8–3).

Progress by having the patient attempt active abduction while maintaining the caudal glide.

(5) Self-stretching exercises[28,53]

As the joint reaction becomes predictable and the patient begins to tolerate stretching, he or she can be taught self-stretching using techniques in which the body is moved in relation to the stabilized arm (see Figs. 8–14 through 8–17).

(6) Self-mobilization techniques for a home program

(a) Caudal glide

The patient sits on a firm surface and grasps the fingers under the edge. He or she then leans the trunk away from the stabilized arm (Fig. 8–4).

(b) Anterior glide

The patient sits and places both arms behind him or her, fixing both hands on a solid surface. He or she then leans the body weight between the arms (Fig. 8–5).

(c) Posterior glide

The patient lies prone, propped up on both elbows. The body weight shifts downward between the arms (Fig. 8–6).

d. Determine any faulty mechanics in the shoulder girdle or faulty posture. Stretch the tight and strengthen the weak components, then retrain the muscles to function within normal patterns of movement. If the patient returns to normal functional activities before normal mechanics are restored, the problem may be perpetuated. Frequently, problems are related to a faulty deltoid–rotator cuff mechanism with muscle flexibility and strength imbalances. If the joint restriction has been long standing, the person usually has compensated with excessive scapular mobility and has developed faulty patterns of scapular movement. Scapular stabilization and control exercises will be needed.

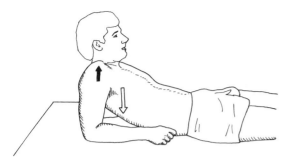

Figure 8–5. Self-mobilization; anterior glide of the humerus occurs as the person leans between the fixed arms.

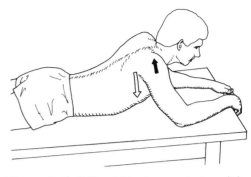

Figure 8–6. Self-mobilization; posterior glide of the humerus occurs as the person shifts his weight downward between the fixed arms.

e. Once proper mechanics are restored, the patient should perform active ROM of all shoulder motions daily and return to functional activities as much as tolerated.

7. **Management postmanipulation under anesthesia**

Occasionally, no progress is made, and the physician chooses to perform manipulation under anesthesia. Following this procedure, there is an inflammatory reaction and the joint is treated as though there were an acute lesion. Begin joint-play and passive ROM techniques while the patient is still in the recovery room.

a. The arm is kept elevated overhead in abduction and external rotation during the inflammatory-reaction stage; treatment principles progress as with any joint lesion.

b. Therapeutic exercise begins the same day while the patient is still in the recovery room, with emphasis on internal and external rotation in the 90-degree (or higher) abducted position.

c. Joint mobilization procedures, particularly caudal glide, are used to prevent readherence of the inferior capsular fold.

d. When sleeping, the patient may be required to position the arm abducted for up to 3 weeks postmanipulation.[72]

e. Surgical intervention with incision of the dependent capsular fold may be used if the adhesions are not broken with the manipulation. Postoperative treatment is the same.[72]

B. Joint Problems: Acromioclavicular (AC) and Sternoclavicular (SC) joints

1. **Related diagnoses and etiology of symptoms**

a. *Overuse syndromes*

Overuse syndromes of the AC joint are frequently arthritic or posttraumatic conditions. The causes may be from repeated stressful movement of the joint with the arm at waist level, such as with grinding, packing assembly, and construction work,[37] or repeated diagonal extension, adduction, and internal rotation motions, as with spiking a volleyball or serving in tennis.

b. *Subluxations or dislocations*

Subluxations or dislocations of either joint are usually caused by falling against the shoulder or against an outstretched arm. In the AC joint the distal end of the clavicle displaces posteriorly and superiorly on the acromion; the ligaments supporting the AC joint may rupture.[71] Clavicular fractures may result from the fall.[71] Following trauma with overstretching of the capsules and ligaments of either joint, hypermobility is usually permanent because there is no muscle support to restrict movement.

c. *Hypomobility*

Decreased clavicular mobility may occur with sustained faulty postures involving clavicular and scapular depression or retraction. Complications from this may contribute to a thoracic outlet syndrome (TOS) with compromise of space for the neuromuscular bundle as it courses between the clavicle and first rib (see Section VI).

2. Common impairments/problems

a. Pain localized to the involved joint or ligament
b. Painful arc with shoulder elevation
c. Pain with shoulder horizontal adduction or abduction
d. Hypermobility in the joints if trauma or overuse is involved
e. Hypomobility in the joints if sustained posture or immobility is involved
f. Neurologic or vascular symptoms if TOS is present

3. Common functional limitations/disabilities

a. Unable to sustain repeated loaded movements related to forward/backward motions of the arm such as with grinding, packing, assembly, and construction work.[37]
b. Unable to effectively serve at tennis or spike a volley ball.
c. See also limitations/disabilities from TOS if involved (Section VII).

4. Nonoperative management if hypermobile

a. Rest the joint by putting the arm in a sling to support the weight of the arm.
b. Cross-fiber massage to the capsule or ligaments.
c. ROM to the shoulder and grade II traction and glides to the glenohumeral joint to prevent glenohumeral restriction.
d. Teach the patient how to apply cross-fiber massage if joint symptoms occur following excessive activity.

5. Nonoperative management if hypomobile

a. Sternoclavicular joint
   (1) To increase elevation, caudal glide proximal clavicle (see Fig. 6–23B).
   (2) To increase depression, superior glide proximal clavicle (see Fig. 6–22).
   (3) To increase protraction, anterior glide proximal clavicle (see Fig. 6–23A).
   (4) To increase retraction, posterior glide proximal clavicle (see Fig. 6–22).
b. Acromioclavicular joint
   To increase motion, anterior glide distal clavicle (see Fig. 6–21).

6. Operative management of clavicular problems

Surgical resection of the distal clavicle is sometimes used when AC joint pain is unrelenting and causes disability.[37] Grade III instabilities, in which the clavicle has been traumatically dislocated on the acromion, may be surgically reduced and stabilized with a variety of techniques.[71] Postsurgical management usually involves immobilization in a sling or strapping. Exercise intervention should be directed at functional recovery as the signs of healing allow. No specific muscles cross the AC and SC joints, so scapular and glenohumeral strength is developed to provide indirect control.

III. Glenohumeral Joint Surgery and Postoperative Management

Surgical intervention and postoperative rehabilitation for severe glenohumeral joint arthritis are often indicated to achieve the following goals: (1) relieve pain, (2) correct deformity, (3) improve mobility or stability, and (4) restore functional use of the upper extremity. The most common form of surgical intervention used to treat severe arthritis and restore upper extremity function is *glenohumeral joint arthroplasty* (total shoulder replacement). In some instances *hemireplacement* of the GH joint is indicated. In rare situations arthrodesis (surgical anklyosis) of the glenohumeral joint is used as a salvage procedure.

A. Glenohumeral (Total Shoulder) Joint Replacement

1. Indications for surgery[2,21,63,68,97]

a. Intractable pain (at rest or with motion) secondary to severe glenohumeral joint destruction associated with rheumatoid or traumatic arthritis or degenerative joint disease (osteoarthritis)
b. Severe loss of upper extremity strength and function secondary to pain
c. Inability to perform functional tasks with the involved upper extremity
d. Decreased range of motion

2. Procedures[6,21,63,68,96,97]

a. Many types of total shoulder replacements (TSRs) have been developed, ranging from *unconstrained* (resurfacing) to *constrained* designs that provide varying amounts of glenohumeral joint stability. The most commonly used design is unconstrained, was developed by Neer,[63,68] and is referred to as a *resurfacing* prosthesis. Many variations of the Neer total shoulder replacement are available. These unconstrained designs provide the greatest freedom of movement but are indicated only when the rotator cuff mechanism is intact or can be adequately repaired to provide dynamic stability to the glenohumeral joint. Partially constrained and constrained replacements have stability built into the design and are used only when the rotator cuff musculature functions insufficiently and cannot be adequately repaired.[21,27,63]
b. All total shoulder replacements are composed of a high-density polyethylene (plastic) glenoid component (some with metal backing) and a two-piece stainless steel humeral prosthesis. The glenoid component is usually cemented in place, although bioingrowth fixation has also been used. The humeral stem component is usually press fit for fixation but can also be cemented in the humeral canal.
c. The procedure involves an anterior approach with a deltopectoral incision that extends from the AC joint to the deltoid insertion. The pectoralis major is released, an anterior capsulotomy is performed, the GH joint is dislocated, a humeral osteotomy is performed, and the head of the humerus is removed. Deltoid reflection is not required. The glenoid fossa is also débrided.

d. A concomitant rotator cuff repair and, occasionally, an anterior acromioplasty may also be necessary if the patient has a history of impingement or rotator cuff deficiency.

3. Postoperative management[79,96]

a. *Immobilization*

(1) The operated shoulder is immobilized with the arm at the patient's side in adduction, internal rotation, and slight forward flexion. The elbow is flexed and supported in a sling or soft (Velpeau) dressing. When the patient is lying supine, the arm remains in the Velpeau dressing, and a pillow is placed under the humerus to maintain the shoulder in 10 to 20 degrees of flexion. If, in addition to the TSR, a rotator cuff repair has been performed, the arm is often supported in an abduction splint or on an abduction pillow. Immobilization is necessary after any type of TSR to protect the anterior incision and capsule and the reattached rotator cuff musculature.

(2) The immobilization may be maintained for a few days or for as long as several weeks if the rotator cuff has been surgically repaired. (See Section V.G for additional information on surgical repair of the rotator cuff.)

b. *Exercise*

The progression and types of exercise performed will vary depending on the surgical procedure and philosophy of the surgeon. Descriptions of the exercises are in Sections VIII and IX of this chapter.

MAXIMUM-PROTECTION PHASE

(1) While the shoulder is immobilized, encourage the patient to keep the shoulder, neck, and upper trunk musculature as relaxed as possible. Use gentle massage to these areas and have the patient perform active movements of the neck and scapula to maintain normal motion and minimize muscle guarding and spasm.

(2) To maintain normal hand, wrist, and forearm function, begin active exercises to these areas immediately after surgery.

(3) Continuous passive motion (CPM). CPM to the shoulder within a limited and safe range of forward flexion may be initiated as early as 1 to 3 days after surgery.

(4) Passive and active-assistive ROM. Remove the shoulder immobilization during the first week to initiate passive and active-assistive shoulder motions, emphasizing flexion, scaption, and abduction to 90 degrees, with the arm internally rotated and elbow flexed, as well as external rotation to neutral with the arm at the patient's side. Active elbow flexion and extension can also be performed out of the immobilization or sling.

(5) Initiate gentle pendulum exercises without a weight (See Fig. 8–1) and "gearshift" exercises (See Fig. 8–9) as the patient progresses through the maximum-protection phase.

(6) Generally the maximum-protection phase is approximately 1 to 3 weeks. If the patient has a deficient rotator cuff that was surgically repaired, maximum protection may last as long as 4 to 6 weeks.

MODERATE-PROTECTION PHASE

(1) To regain control of shoulder girdle musculature, emphasize transition from active-assistive to active shoulder motions.

(a) Have the patient perform open-chain active exercises in supine side-lying, prone, sitting, and standing.

(b) Use wand, overhead pulley, or wall-climbing exercises, emphasizing active or self-assisted movements in the diagonal and anatomic planes of motion.

Precaution: continue to perform external rotation with the arm at the side. (See Fig. 8–8.)

(2) To improve strength of shoulder girdle, begin isometric exercises against gentle resistance at multiple points in the ROM with the arm at the side. (See Figs. 8–10 through 8–13A.) Emphasize rotator cuff, deltoid, and scapular musculature.

(3) The moderate-protection phase may begin as early as 2 to 4 weeks postoperatively and continue to 4 to 6 weeks. If the rotator cuff is deficient or has been surgically repaired, moderate protection may be necessary for 6 to 8 weeks.

MINIMUM-PROTECTION PHASE

(1) To strengthen the shoulder girdle, begin progressive resistive exercise (PRE) against light resistance through the available active ROM. Use TheraBand or elastic tubing or hand-held weights. Emphasize low loads and high repetitions. (See Figs. 8–24A, 8–25, and 8–28.)

(2) To develop stability in the shoulder girdle, begin closed-chain upper extremity exercise such as rhythmic stabilization (see Figs. 8–29A and B) and bilateral push-ups against a wall performed in a standing position.

(3) To improve ROM, initiate gentle stretching exercises using hold-relax techniques or a low-load, prolonged stretch. Follow up with gentle self-stretching procedures (see Figs. 8–14 and 8–16).

(4) To improve functional use of the upper extremity, emphasize specificity of exercise with respect to speed and direction of motions. Replicate functional movements when performing resistance exercises.

(5) Although the minimum protection phase of rehabilitation may begin as early as 4 to 6 weeks postoperatively, the patient may need to continue a home program of progressive exercises for up to 6 months to a year to attain optimal function.

4. Long-term results[2,6,21,68,96]

a. Almost all patients report total relief or a substantial decrease in shoulder pain and therefore an improvement in function.

b. Active ROM and strength may be partially limited on a permanent basis or for an extended period of time.

c. If the rotator cuff and deltoid muscles are functioning well, a patient can expect to regain 70 percent normal strength and motion by 1 year postoperatively.

d. Long-term follow-up studies indicate that active ROM often improves 30 to 60 percent postoperatively. Active pain-free shoulder flexion after 1 year may range from 100 to 115 degrees, which provides adequate movement for most functional activities.[2,6]

B. Hemireplacement of the Shoulder (Humeral Head Replacement)[63,65-67,79,96]

1. Indications for surgery

a. Fracture dislocations of the proximal humerus

b. Severe pain due to traumatic arthritis or osteoarthritis of the head of the humerus

2. Procedure

a. The head of the humerus is surgically excised and replaced with a stainless steel intramedullary-stemmed prosthesis.

b. The prosthesis is press fit or held in place with methyl methacrylate, an acrylic cement.

c. The rotator cuff mechanism is repaired if indicated.

d. The shoulder is immobilized in an abduction splint if a rotator cuff repair has been performed. If no cuff repair was necessary, the patient's arm is immobilized and supported at the side in a sling.

3. Postoperative management[63,79]

a. If a surgical repair of the rotator cuff was performed, follow the postoperative exercise plan discussed later in this chapter on repair of the rotator cuff (see Section IV.G).

b. If no cuff repair was necessary, follow the guidelines for exercise after total shoulder replacement just outlined in this section of Chapter 8.

C. Arthrodesis of the Shoulder[27,79,102]

1. Indications for surgery

a. Severe pain

b. Gross instability of the glenohumeral joint

c. Complete paralysis of the deltoid and rotator cuff muscles

d. Good compensatory scapular motion and strength of the serratus anterior and trapezius muscles

2. Procedure

a. The glenohumeral joint is fused with pins and bone grafts in a position of 15 to 20 degrees of flexion, 20 to 40 degrees of abduction, and neutral to internal rotation.

b. The shoulder is immobilized in a shoulder spica cast or brace that extends across the elbow joint for approximately 3 to 5 months.

3. Postoperative management[79]

a. While the shoulder is immobilized, the patient should be encouraged to maintain mobility in the wrist and hand.

b. If a brace with a hinged elbow is used, active elbow flexion and extension through the full range may be initiated the day after surgery.

c. After the brace or cast has been removed, active and active-resistive scapulothoracic motion may be started.

4. Long-term results

a. A patient may expect to achieve approximately 90 degrees of active elevation of the arm because of scapulothoracic motion.

b. The shoulder will be stable and pain free for all activities that require strength or weight bearing at the shoulder. The patient will be able to bring the hand to the mouth and touch the hand behind the head.

IV. Painful Shoulder Syndromes: Repetitive Trauma (Overuse) Syndromes, Impingement Syndromes, Shoulder Instabilities, and Rotator Cuff Tears

A. Related Diagnoses

1. **Supraspinatus tendinitis**

   The lesion is usually near the musculotendinous junction and results in a painful arc with overhead reaching; pain occurs with the impingement test (forced humeral elevation in the plane of the scapula while the scapula is passively stabilized so that the greater tuberosity impacts against the acromion[38,62]; may also be performed with the arm in internal rotation while flexing the humerus[38] and on palpation of the tendon just inferior to the anterior aspect of the acromion when the patient's hand is placed behind the back). It is difficult to differentiate from partial tears or from subdeltoid bursitis because of the anatomic proximity.

2. **Infraspinatus tendinitis**

   The lesion is usually near the musculotendinous junction and results in a painful arc with overhead or forward motions. Pain occurs on palpation of the tendon just inferior to the posterior corner of the acromion when the patient horizontally adducts and laterally rotates the humerus.

3. **Bicipital tendinitis[73]**

   The lesion involves the long tendon in the bicipital groove beneath or just distal to the transverse humeral ligament. Swelling in the bony groove is restrictive and compounds and perpetuates the problem. Pain occurs with exertion of the forearm in a supinated position while the shoulder is flexing (Speed's sign) and on palpation of the bicipital groove. A rupture or dislocation of this humeral depressor may escalate impingement of tissues in the suprahumeral space.[62]

4. **Other musculotendinous problems**

   Injury, overuse, or repetitive trauma can occur in any muscle being subjected to stress. Pain will occur when the involved muscle is placed on a stretch or when contracting against resistance. Palpation of the site of the lesion will cause the familiar pain.

5. **Bursitis (subdeltoid or subacromial)**

   When acute, symptoms are the same as supraspinatus tendinitis. Once the inflammation is under control, there are no symptoms with resistance.

6. **Postural imbalance/muscle length-strength imbalance**

   This describes the proposed etiology leading to the faulty mechanics in the region and the development of the painful syndrome, in which the postural components demonstrate tight anterior and stretched and weak posterior structures in the shoulder girdle complex. It may also involve faulty spinal posture.

7. Shoulder instability/subluxation

Instability is becoming recognized as a clinical entity that may be the result of joint laxity, but it is usually related to rotator cuff fatigue and inadequate dynamic stabilizing mechanisms of the rotator cuff and long head of the biceps. The tissues in the subacromial space may then become impinged or a tendinitis may develop. Shoulder instability may be diagnosed by its frequency (acute/recurrent), degree of trauma involved (macrotrauma, microtrauma, involuntary, voluntary), the direction (anterior, posterior, inferior, multidirectional), and amount of instability (dislocation, subluxation).[78]

8. Rotator cuff tears

Rotator cuff tears can be classified as acute, chronic, degenerative, partial- or full-thickness tears. Neer has identified rotator cuff tears as a stage III impingement syndrome, a condition that typically occurs over the age of 40 following repetitive microtrauma to the rotator cuff or long head of the biceps.[62] With aging, the distal portion of the supraspinatus tendon is particularly vulnerable to impingement or stress from overuse strain. With degenerative changes, calcification and eventual tendon rupture may occur.[32,77,91] Chronic ischemia caused by tension on the tendon and decreased healing in the elderly are possible explanations,[53,91] although Neer states that, in his experience, 95 percent of tears are initiated by impingement wear rather than by impaired circulation or trauma.[62]

Partial-thickness tears may occur in the elderly as the result of a fall on an outstretched arm. In young patients tears are usually caused by violent injury. The tears may be partial or complete and may occur with or without dislocation or a displaced fracture of the tuberosity.[70] Tears are associated with pain and most commonly weakness of shoulder abduction and external rotation.

B. Etiology of Symptoms

Continued repetitive use of the upper extremity, particularly with forward, overhead, or swinging activities, may lead to stress breakdown of the tissues.[14] Symptoms occur from two possible interrelated mechanisms:

1. *Repetitive eccentric strain* to a contracting musculotendinous unit will cause microtrauma and inflammation if the strain exceeds the tissue strength. Progressive damage continues if the repetitive stress exceeds the tissue repair. Muscle weakness and fatigue lend the tissue vulnerable to this type of injury.[61,75]

   a. Frequently the structures of the rotator cuff and long head of the biceps are involved due to the nature of their stabilizing function in overhead and forward motion activities.

   b. Other musculotendinous units such as the pectoralis minor, short head of the biceps, and coracobrachialis are subject to microtrauma, particularly in racket sports requiring a controlled backward then rapid forward swinging of the arm, and also the scapular stabilizers as they function to control forward motion of the scapula.[57]

   c. The long head of the triceps and scapular stabilizers are often injured in motor vehicle accidents as the driver holds firmly to the steering wheel on impact. Falls on an outstretched hand or against the shoulder may also cause trauma to the scapular stabilizers, which, if not properly healed, will continue to have symptoms whenever using the arm or when sustaining shoulder posture.

2. *Impingement* of the rotator cuff and subacromial bursa between the humeral head and coracoacromial arch occurs from repetitive compressive loads.

   a. Mechanisms such as inadequate caudal glide of the humeral head when elevating the humerus above the horizontal or inadequate lateral rotation during elevation of the humerus cause the greater tubercle to impinge against the acromion, compressing the tissue between.

   b. A faulty scapular posture during humeral motions alters the mechanics of the rotator cuff and decreases its effective stabilizing actions, leading to mechanical impingement.

   c. Structural variations in the acromion,[32,85] hypertrophic degeneration changes of the AC joint, or other trophic changes in the arch can decrease the suprahumeral space with resulting repetitive trauma when elevating the arm.[45]

   d. Many individuals, particularly those involved in overhand throwing or lifting activities, have some inherent laxity of the capsule and instability from continually subjecting the joint to stretch forces.[32,49] With strong rotator cuff muscles a hypermobile joint is satisfactorily supported, but once they fatigue, poor humeral head stabilization leads to faulty humeral mechanics, trauma, and inflammation to the suprahumeral tissues.[49,61] This trauma is magnified with the rapidity of control demanded in the overhead throwing action.[32] Similarly, in individuals with poor rotator cuff muscle strength and function, the ligaments become stressed with repetitive use and hypermobility and impingement result. With instability, the impingement of tissue in the suprahumeral space is the secondary effect.[32]

   e. Neer identified impingement lesions of the rotator cuff and long head of the biceps in three progressive stages:

      Stage I: edema and hemorrhage, typically occurring below the age of 25 years

      Stage II: fibrosis and tendinitis (the bursa may also become fibrotic and thickened), seen typically between 25 and 40 years

      Stage III: bone spurs, rotator cuff tears, and biceps rupture, typically seen in persons over age 40 years[62]

   Other authors have identified chronic inflammation, possibly from repetitive microtraumas in the joint region, as a stimulus for the development of frozen shoulder (Section II).[36,69,72]

C. Common Impairments/Problems Summarized

1. Pain at the musculotendinous junction of involved muscle on palpation, on resisted muscle contraction, and when stretched.
2. Irritated, adhered, or contracted scar tissue.
3. Faulty scapular and shoulder posture with anteriorly tilted or protracted scapula and internally rotated shoulder, which may also be associated with faulty forward head posture and round thoracic spine.
4. Tight pectoralis major and minor, tight anterior thorax, tight shoulder internal rotators.
5. Weak scapular retractors and humeral lateral rotators.
6. Weakness or poor endurance in the scapular stabilizers and rotator cuff muscles.
7. Uncoordinated scapulohumeral rhythm.

8. Painful arc on humeral elevation.

9. With a complete rotator cuff tear, inability to abduct the humerus against gravity.

10. When acute, pain is referred to the C-5 and C-6 reference zones.

D. Common Functional Limitations/Disabilities

1. When acute, pain may interfere with sleep, particularly when rolling onto involved shoulder.

2. Pain with overhead reaching, pushing, or pulling.

3. Pain with lifting loads.

4. Inability to sustain repetitive shoulder activities (such as reaching, lifting, throwing, pushing, pulling, or swinging the arm).

5. Pain with dressing, particularly putting a shirt on overhead.

E. Nonoperative Management*

NOTE: Even through the symptoms may be "chronic" or recurring, if there is inflammation, the initial treatment approach is to get the inflammation under control.

1. Acute or chronic inflammation phase of treatment

a. To control inflammation and promote healing, use modalities and low-intensity cross-fiber massage to the site of the lesion by positioning the extremity to maximally expose the involved region.[25] Support the arm in a sling for rest.

b. To reduce the repetitive trauma causing the problem, patient education and cooperation are necessary. The environment and habits that provoke the symptoms must be modified (or avoided completely during this stage).

c. To maintain integrity and mobility of the tissues, initiate early motion.

(1) Utilize the early exercise intervention described in Section VIII. Include passive, active-assistive, or self-assisted ROM, multiple-angle muscle setting, and protected closed-chain and co-contraction exercises. Of particular importance in the shoulder is to stimulate the stabilizing function of the rotator cuff, biceps brachii, and scapular muscles at an intensity tolerated by the patient.

(2) To control pain and maintain joint integrity, use pendulum exercises without weights to cause pain-inhibiting grade II joint distraction and oscillation motions (see Fig. 8–1).

(3) The caution with exercises in this stage is to avoid the impingement positions, which are often in the mid-range of abduction or end-range position when the involved muscle is on a stretch.

d. To develop support in related regions, begin to teach the patient postural awareness and correction techniques. Initiate training of scapular and thoracic posture using shoulder strapping or scapular taping, tactile cues, and use of mirrors for reinforcement. Repetitive practice of correct posture is necessary throughout the day. Forward head posture is often related to forward shoulder posture (see Chapter 15 for additional suggestions if this dysfunction is present).

*Refs. 15, 26, 48, 52, 89, 99, 104, 105.

2. Subacute/healing phase of treatment

NOTE: Once the acute symptoms are under control, the main emphasis becomes use of the involved region in progressive nondestructive movement using proper mechanics while the tissues heal. The components of the desired function are analyzed and initiated in a controlled exercise program. When the components can be controlled in a safe, nonprovoking manner, the person is progressed to the rehabilitation phase for return to full activity. Patient education for compliance with the program throughout their daily activities is necessary. The exercise techniques are described in Section IX.

a. To develop a strong, mobile scar and regain flexibility in the region of the contracted scar, position the part on a stretch if it is a tendon or in the shortened position if it is in the muscle belly and apply cross-fiber or friction massage to the tolerance of the individual. This should be followed by isometric contraction of the muscle in several positions of the range and at an intensity that does not cause pain.

b. To improve postural awareness, continue to reinforce proper postural habits. Every time an exercise is performed, make the patient aware of scapular and cervical posture with tactile and verbal reinforcement such as touching the scapular adductors and chin and reminding the person to "pull the shoulders back" and "straighten the head" while doing the shoulder exercises.

c. To regain balance in length and strength of shoulder girdle muscles, design a program that specifically addresses the patient's limitations. Typical goals in the shoulder girdle include but are not limited to:

   (1) Stretch tight muscles. These typically include the pectoralis major, pectoralis minor, latissimus dorsi and teres major, subscapularis, and levator scapulae.

   (2) Isolate, strengthen, and train contraction of scapular stabilizers, particularly for scapular retraction and upward rotation.

   (3) Isolate, strengthen, and train the rotator cuff muscles, especially the shoulder lateral rotators.

   (4) Isolate and strengthen any weak muscles.

d. To develop co-contraction, stabilization, and endurance in the muscles of the scapula and shoulder:

   (1) Increase loads on closed-chain exercises for the upper extremity and progress as the patient tolerates by increasing the amount of time performing the activity, then adding resistance in a progressive manner and increasing the time at that level.

   (2) Progress open-chain rhythmic stabilization exercises. Increase endurance by increasing the amount of time the stabilization is held.

e. To progress shoulder function, as the patient develops strength in the weakened muscles, develop a balance in strength of all shoulder and scapular muscles within the range and tolerance of each muscle.

f. To increase coordination between scapular and arm motions, dynamically load the upper extremity within tolerance of the synergy with submaximal resistance. The goal is to develop control from 1 to 3 minutes.

3. Rehabilitation during chronic phase

NOTE: As soon as the patient has developed control of posture and the basic components of the desired activities without exacerbating the symptoms, initiate specificity of training toward the desired functional outcome.

a. To increase endurance, increase repetitive loading of defined patterns from 3 to 5 minutes.
b. To increase speed, superimpose stresses at faster speeds to tolerance.
c. To develop function, progress to specificity of training; emphasize timing and sequencing of events.
   (1) Progress eccentric training to maximum load.
   (2) Simulate desired functional activity, first under controlled conditions, then under progressively challenged situations using acceleration/deceleration drills.
   (3) Assess the total-body function while doing the desired activity and modify any component that causes faulty patterning.
d. To educate the patient, instruct the patient on how to progress the program when discharged as well as how to prevent recurrences. Prevention should include:
   (1) Prior to exercise or work, massage the involved tendon or muscle; follow with isometric resistance and then with full range of motion and stretching of the muscle.
   (2) Take breaks from the activity if repetitive in nature. If possible, alternate the stressful provoking activity with other activities or patterns or motion.
   (3) Maintain good postural alignment; adapt seating or work station to minimize stress. If sport related, seek coaching in proper techniques or adapt equipment for safe mechanics.
   (4) Prior to initiating a new activity or returning to an activity not conditioned for, begin a strengthening and training program.

F. Postoperative Management of Impingement Syndromes

1. Indications for surgery[12,29,39,60,63,64,85]

a. Insufficient subacromial joint space leading to impingement at the anterior edge and undersurface of the acromium
b. Stage II (Neer classification) impingement with nonreversible fibrosis or bony alterations (degenerative spurring) of the subacromial compartment
c. Intact or minor tears of the rotator cuff; calcific deposits in the cuff tendons
d. Unsuccessful conservative (nonoperative) rehabilitation program of 3 to 6 months

2. Procedure

a. Anterior acromioplasty (subacromial decompression) involves removal of the anterior prominence of the acromium.[63] A modified (two-step) anterior acromioplasty with beveling of the inferior aspect of the remaining portion of the acromium to provide adequate gliding space for the inflamed tendons can also be done.[39,60,85]
   (1) Both are open surgical procedures involving an arthrotomy.
   (2) An incision is made at the lateral border of the acromium; the anterior and lateral origins of the deltoid are detached from the acromium and later repaired before closure.
   (3) The coracoacromial ligament is removed.
b. Arthroscopic subacromial decompression and débridement involve removal of a portion of the anterior acromium (arthroscopic acromioplasty) and/or arthroscopic removal of the coracoacromial ligament.[29,61]
c. Arthroscopic AC joint inferior osteophyte resection may also be performed.

3. Postoperative management[12,29,51,85]

NOTE: The position and duration of immobilization of the shoulder and initiation of exercise vary with the surgery. Rehabilitation after arthroscopic procedures is more rapid than after an arthrotomy, in which muscle insertions such as the deltoid have been detached for adequate exposure and then reattached.

a. *Immobilization*

The shoulder is usually positioned in adduction and internal rotation and the forearm is supported in a sling with the elbow flexed to 90 degrees.

b. *Exercise*

MAXIMUM-PROTECTION PHASE

(1) The sling is removed for exercise the day after surgery.

(2) Exercises, as performed with acute-phase nonoperative management, can also be performed after acromioplasty and decompression procedures.

(3) To maintain mobility of the GH joint:

   (a) Begin passive or active-assistive shoulder flexion in the plane of the scapula (scaption) within a pain-free range (usually to 90 to 120 degrees) the day after surgery.

   (b) Begin pendulum exercises without weights (see Fig. 8–1).

   (c) Begin "gear shift" exercises (see Fig. 8–9).

   (d) Begin wand exercises for assisted external rotation with the arm held at the side of the trunk (see Fig. 8–8) and assisted shoulder flexion with the patient sitting or supine.

   (e) Begin transition from passive to therapist or self-assisted ROM, which should be done as long as motions remain pain free.

   (f) If muscles (such as the deltoid) have been reflected and reattached, active free shoulder flexion should not be initiated for at least 2 or as much as 6 weeks to protect the healing tissues.

(4) To regain control and strength of shoulder girdle musculature, initiate (submaximal) pain-free multiple-angle isometric exercises, emphasizing the scapula, rotator cuff, and other GH joint musculature. (See Figs. 8–10 through 8–13.)

(5) To maintain strength in scapular stabilizing muscles, begin rhythmic stabilization exercises, emphasizing control of the upper, middle, and lower trapezius and serratus anterior muscles.

(6) Initiate postural training as early as possible to prevent forward shoulders and round back.

MODERATE-AND MINIMUM-PROTECTION PHASES

(1) Rehabilitation proceeds very quickly. Controlled, active ROM is emphasized while moderate protection of the area is necessary. By 6 weeks postoperatively a patient can achieve full active ROM of the shoulder. Active ROM is emphasized initially and then resistance is added. If dynamic exercises against resistance are painful, keep the exercise load low or perform multiple-angle isometrics against resistance. Shoulder motion is usually more comfortable in the scapular plane than in the anatomic planes of abduction or flexion. By 6 weeks postoperatively minimal protection is necessary as tissues are well healed by this time.

(2) As the need for protection of any incised or reattached tissues lessens, open- and closed-chain resistance exercises can be added using manual

resistance, elastic tubing, free weights, or isokinetics to strengthen the GH and scapulothoracic muscles. (See Figs. 8–24 through 8–32.)

(3) If full ROM is not achieved by 6 weeks, manual or self-stretching exercises and joint mobilization can be added. (See Figs. 8–4 through 8–7 and 8–14 through 8–20.) If horizontal adduction or forward flexion is limited, pay particular attention to stretching the posterior capsule.

(4) Progress to advanced strengthening and endurance activities with functional movement patterns by increasing the speed and intensity of exercise with stretch-shortening drills.[103]

G. Postoperative Management of Rotator Cuff Tears

1. Indications for surgery*

a. Partial- or full-thickness tears of the rotator cuff tendons associated with irreversible degenerative changes in soft tissues (stage II and III lesions of the rotator cuff) and failed conservative management. Tears are most common in the supraspinatus and infraspinatus tendons and are often associated with calcific changes in the tendons. Surgery is indicated in the elderly patient with chronic impingement and partial-thickness tears when weakness and atrophy in the external rotators are evident and there is significant loss of upper extremity function.

b. Acute, traumatic rupture (frank tears) of the rotator cuff tendons, which can also be associated with traumatic dislocation of the glenohumeral (GH) joint. Full-thickness, traumatic tears occur most often in young, active adults and require immediate surgical repair.

2. Procedures[27,43,61,83,92,98]

a. Repairs of the rotator cuff can be performed arthroscopically for small tears or by an open procedure with an anterolateral or posterolateral approach. The deltoid may be longitudinally split and the acromial insertion preserved or the deltoid may be detached and reflected.

b. Both procedures involve approximation and reattachment of the torn tendons to the head of the humerus with direct sutures. In an open procedure the deltoid muscle is reflected and later reattached.

c. If there is a history of impingement and bony alterations of the subacromial compartment, an anterior acromioplasty for decompression and débridement of the subacromial arch may also be performed.

d. If torn, the coracoacromial ligament is removed.

e. Excision of the subacromial bursa or capsular reconstruction may also be indicated.

3. Postoperative management†

NOTE: The rehabilitation program and its rate of progression are based on the size of the rotator cuff tear, the integrity of the surrounding tissues, and the status of the deltoid.

---

*Refs. 1, 8, 27, 40, 43, 47, 83–85, 98.
†Refs. 1, 8, 16, 40, 41, 43, 54, 64, 83, 92, 98.

a. *Immobilization*

As with impingement syndromes, the position and duration of immobilization vary with the surgical procedures. The size of the tear and operative procedure also dictate the position and duration of immobilization. For most massive tears the shoulder is often immobilized in abduction and internal rotation with the arm supported in an abduction splint for as long as 4 to 6 weeks. The abducted position places no excessive stretch on the repaired tendons and maximizes the blood supply to the cuff muscles.

b. *Exercise*

MAXIMUM-PROTECTION PHASE

(1) The most important priority in this phase of rehabilitation is protection of the surgically repaired tissues. Exercises are consistent with nonoperative or operative management of impingement syndromes discussed earlier in this section.

(2) To protect healing tissues but maintain mobility, perform passive or active-assisted ROM of the GH joint through the pain-free ranges, usually to 90 to 120 degrees. In some cases, continuous passive motion (CPM) may be used to maintain mobility after surgery. Other passive or active-assisted exercises such as pendulum, gear shift, pulley, and wand exercises and scapular mobilization as discussed under nonoperative or operative rehabilitation of impingement syndromes are also appropriate.

(3) To initiate strengthening of the repaired musculature, when the arm is immobilized in abduction, begin submaximal isometric exercises to the shoulder musculature with a small pillow or bolster under the axilla to protect the reattached tendons.

(4) Rhythmic stabilization exercises for scapular muscles can be initiated immediately after surgery against a pain-free level of resistance.

MODERATE- AND MINIMUM-PROTECTION PHASE

(1) Components of the exercise program are consistent with nonoperative and operative rehabilitation of impingement syndromes already discussed in this section of Chapter 8. The progression of exercises is usually slower after surgical repair of massive tears than repair of impingement problems.

(2) Since weakness and atrophy of the external rotators are usually present, restore adequate strength in the external rotators before adding forward flexion and abduction of the shoulder. Continue multiple-angle isometrics against resistance to shoulder girdle musculature until the patient has full, active, pain-free ROM.

(3) It is important to strengthen scapular muscles such as the serratus anterior and upper, middle, and lower trapezius muscles for appropriate stabilization of the scapula with active arm movement. (See Figs. 8–13 and 8–27 through 8–29.) It is equally important to strengthen the rhomboids for posture control. (See Figs. 8–31 and 8–32.)

(4) Full, active, overhead shoulder flexion should not be initiated for 6 weeks to allow adequate time for incised and reattached tissues to heal.

(5) When the patient has achieved full, active, pain-free overhead motion, begin isotonic strengthening of GH joint musculature with elastic resistance and weights (see Fig. 8–26).

(6) Progress strengthening activities in functional movement patterns, incorporating concentric and eccentric resistance exercises as well as closed-

and open-chain activities.

(7) Gradually increase the speed and intensity of exercises and functional activities in preparation for return to full activity (see Fig. 8–33).

V. Shoulder Dislocations

A. Related Diagnoses and Mechanisms of Injury

1. Traumatic anterior shoulder dislocation

There is complete separation of the articular surfaces of the glenohumeral joint caused by direct or indirect forces applied to the shoulder.[78] Anterior dislocation most frequently occurs when there is a blow to the humerus while it is in a position of external rotation and abduction. Stability normally is provided by the subscapularis, glenohumeral ligament, and long head of the biceps when in that position.[55,86,100] Instability from any of these structures can predispose the joint to dislocation, or a significant blow to the arm may damage them along with the glenoid labrum. When dislocated, the humeral head usually rests in the subcoracoid region, rarely subclavicular or intrathoracic. Traumatic anterior dislocation is usually associated with a complete rupture of the rotator cuff.

2. Traumatic posterior shoulder dislocation

Most posterior dislocations are subacromial, although subglenoid or subspinous posterior dislocations may occur. The mechanism of injury is usually a force applied to the humerus that combines flexion, adduction, and internal rotation such as a fall on an outstretched arm.[90]

3. Recurrent dislocation

With significant ligamentous and capsule laxity, unidirectional or multidirectional recurrent subluxations or dislocations may occur with any movement that reproduces the abduction and external rotation forces or the flexion, adduction, and internal rotation forces, causing significant pain and functional limitation. Some individuals can voluntarily dislocate their shoulder anteriorly or posteriorly without apprehension and with minimal discomfort.[78,90]

B. Etiology of Symptoms

If the dislocation is traumatic, symptoms are from tissue damage, bleeding, and resulting inflammation.

C. Common Impairments/Problems Summarized

1. Acute. Pain, muscle guarding, and effects of inflammation.
2. Muscle length-strength imbalances.
3. When a dislocation is associated with a complete rotator cuff tear, there is an inability to abduct the humerus against gravity, except the range provided by the scapulothoracic muscles.
4. Asymmetric joint restrictions/hypermobilities. In an anterior instability, the posterior capsule may be tight; in a posterior instability, the anterior capsule may be tight. Following healing, there may be adhesions.

D. Common Functional Limitations/Disabilities

1. With rotator cuff rupture, inability to reach or lift objects to the level of horizontal, thus interfering with all activities using humeral elevation
2. Possibility of recurrence when replicating the dislocating action
3. With anterior dislocation, restricted ability in sports activities such as pitching, swimming, serving (tennis, volleyball), spiking (volleyball)
4. Restricted ability, particularly when overhead or horizontal abduction movements are required in dressing, such as putting on a shirt or jacket, and with self-grooming, such as combing back of hair
5. Discomfort or pain when sleeping on the involved side in some cases
6. With posterior dislocation, restricted ability in sports activities such as follow-through in pitching; restricted ability in pushing activities, such as pushing open a heavy door or pushing self up out of a chair or out of a swimming pool

E. Nonoperative Management of Instabilities/Dislocations

1. **Acute phase of treatment following closed reduction of anterior dislocation**

   NOTE: Reduction manipulations should be undertaken only by someone specially trained in the maneuver.
   a. To protect the healing tissue, the part is immobilized for 3 to 4 weeks in a sling, which is removed only for exercise. The position of dislocation must be avoided when exercising, and the patient must be cautious when dressing or doing other daily activities.
   b. To initiate early movement for tissue health, use the exercises described in Section VIII, including protected range of motion, intermittent muscle setting of the rotator cuff and biceps brachii muscles, and grade II joint techniques with the following precautions in order not to disrupt healing of the capsule and other damaged tissues:
      (1) Following anterior dislocation, range of motion into external rotation is performed with the elbow at the patient's side, with the shoulder flexed in the sagittal plane, and with the shoulder in the resting position (in the plane of the scapula, abducted 55 degrees and horizontally adducted 30 degrees), but not in the abducted position. While healing, limit the range of external rotation to 50 degrees in all positions of humeral motion.
      (2) Maintain joint play by using sustained grade II distraction or gentle grade II oscillations with the glenohumeral joint at the side or in the resting position (Fig 6–13).

2. **Subacute and chronic rehabilitative phases of treatment following anterior shoulder dislocation[3,13]**

   a. To provide protection, the patient continues to wear the sling for 3 weeks, then increases the time the sling is off; the sling is used when the shoulder is tired or protection is needed.
   b. To increase limited ranges, begin mobilization techniques using all appropriate glides except the anterior glide.
      (1) Anterior glide is **contraindicated** even though external rotation is necessary for functional elevation of the humerus. To safely stretch for external rotation, place the shoulder in the resting position (abducted 55 degrees and horizontally adducted 30 degrees), then externally rotate it to the limit

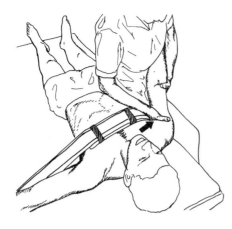

Figure 8–7. Mobilizing to increase external rotation when an anterior glide is contraindicated. Place the shoulder in resting position, externally rotate it, then apply a grade III distraction force.

of its range, and then apply a grade III distraction force perpendicular to the treatment plane in the glenoid fossa (Fig. 8–7).

(2) Passively stretch the posterior joint structures with horizontal adduction self-stretching techniques.

c. To increase strength and regain rotator cuff control for stability, both the internal and external rotators need to be strengthened as healing occurs. The internal rotators and adductors must be strong to support the anterior capsule. The external rotators must be strong to stabilize the humeral head against anterior translating forces and to participate in the deltoid–rotator cuff force couple when abducting and laterally rotating the humerus.

(1) Begin with *isometric resistance* exercises with the joint positioned at the side and progress to various pain-free positions within the available ranges.

(2) Progress to *isotonic resistance*, limiting external rotation to 50 degrees and avoiding the position of dislocation.

(3) At 3 weeks, begin supervised *isokinetic resistance* for internal rotation and adduction at speeds 180 degrees per second or higher.[3] Position the patient standing with the arm at the side and elbow flexed 90 degrees. The patient performs internal rotation beginning at the zero position with the hand pointing anteriorly and moving to across the front of the body. Progress to positioning the shoulder at 90 degrees flexion, then perform the exercise from zero to full internal rotation. Do not position in 90 degrees abduction.

(4) By 5 weeks, all shoulder motions are incorporated on isokinetic or other mechanical equipment except the position of 90 degrees abduction with external rotation.

(5) Initiate closed-chain partial-weight-bearing and rhythmic stabilization exercises.

d. To progress to functional activities, develop a balance in strength of all shoulder and scapular muscles, develop coordination between scapular and arm motions, and develop endurance for each exercise. As stability improves, progress eccentric training to maximum load, increase speed and control, and progress to simulating desired functional patterns for activity.

e. To return to maximum function, the person learns to recognize signs of fatigue and impingement and stay within the tolerance of the tissues. The patient can return to normal activities when there is no muscle imbalance, when good coordination of skill is present, and when the apprehension test is negative. Full rehabilitation takes 2 1/2 to 4 months.[3]

3. Treatment following posterior dislocation of the shoulder with closed reduction

The management approach is the same as anterior dislocation with the exception of avoiding the position of flexion with adduction and internal rotation during the acute and healing phases.

   a. To protect the part, the arm is immobilized. A sling may be uncomfortable because of the adducted and internally rotated position, particularly if the sling elevates the humerus so the head translates in a superior and posterior direction. The patient may be more comfortable with the arm hanging freely in a dependent position while kept immobile.

   b. To increase limited ranges, begin joint mobilization techniques using all appropriate glides except the posterior glide. Posterior glide is *contraindicated.* If adhesions develop, preventing internal rotation, mobility can safely be regained by placing the shoulder in the resting position (abducted 55 degrees and horizontally adducted 30 degrees), then internally rotating it to the limit of its range, and then applying a grade III distraction force perpendicular to the treatment plane in the glenoid fossa (same as Fig. 8–7 but with the arm internally rotated).

F. Postoperative Management of Recurrent Anterior Dislocation of the Shoulder

1. Indications for surgery[18,19,48,54,84]

   a. Recurrent dislocation requiring reduction
   b. Recurrent subluxation that does not have to be reduced by someone else
   c. Significant anterior joint laxity resulting in instability
   d. Significant compromise of functional use of the upper extremity as the result of fear of placing the arm in positions that will cause dislocation
   e. Tears of the rotator cuff musculature and detachment of the anterior glenoid labrum (Bankart lesion) or avulsion of the greater tuberosity
   f. Failure of nonoperative rehabilitation

2. Procedures[18,19,47–49,84]

   a. Glenohumeral stabilizing procedures for recurrent anterior dislocation include:

     (1) Anterior capsulolabral reconstruction involving a longitudinal split in the subscapularis and anterior capsule with inferior and superior flaps of the capsule attached to the glenoid with bony anchors.

     (2) Capsular shift or imbrication and resuturing of the anterior structures to stabilize and tighten a lax or stretched capsule (Bankart procedure).[88]

     (3) Lateral transfer of the subscapularis from the lesser to the greater tuberosity to shorten and advance the subscapularis and stabilize the anterior aspect of the joint (Putti-Platt or Manguson-Stack procedures).

     (4) Transfer of the tip of the coracoid process (with the short head of the bi-

ceps and coracobrachialis still attached) to the glenoid rim (Bristow procedures).

(5) Capsulorrhaphy (replacement of the torn shoulder capsule to the glenoid rim) with sutures or staples.[35]

(6) Other procedures may involve modification or a combination of the preceding procedures.

b. Stabilization procedures may be performed using an open surgical technique that requires a deltopectoral arthrotomy, or arthroscopically, and often involves repair of the rotator cuff and reattachment of the GH ligament to the glenoid rim.

3. Postoperative management[12,48,49,61,88,103]

NOTE: To achieve adequate anterior stability, some procedures may mechanically block full external rotation and horizontal abduction.

a. *Immobilization*

As with rotator cuff surgeries the shoulder will be immobilized in either abduction with the arm in a splint or adduction with the arm in a sling to protect healing tissues. The duration of complete immobilization is dependent upon the type of stabilization procedure chosen by the surgeon, the severity of the instability, and the characteristics of the patient with respect to pain, tissue type, and healing. In patients with unidirectional anterior dislocations the immobilization device is worn for as little as 1 week or up to 6 to 8 weeks for patients with multidirectional instabilities.

b. *Exercise*

MAXIMUM-PROTECTION PHASE

(1) To minimize the adverse effects of immobility and maintain mobility in healing tissues, the sling or splint is removed for passive or active assisted ROM within a limited, pain-free range immediately or within a few days after surgery. Include pendulum, gear shift, or pulley exercises. Avoid external rotation with abduction, the position of instability, which will place excessive stress on healing tissues.

(2) All other aspects of postoperative management during this phase of treatment are consistent with the rehabilitation procedures previously outlined for nonoperative management of anterior instabilities during the acute stage of healing.

MODERATE- AND MINIMUM-PROTECTION PHASES

(1) Follow the guidelines for nonoperative management of anterior dislocation (subacute and chronic rehabilitative phases) discussed earlier in this section of Chapter 8. Emphasis is placed on achieving full, pain-free ROM, if allowed by the specifics of the surgery, and strengthening the dynamic stabilizers of the GH joint (the rotator cuff musculature) and the scapula. Full active ROM may be attained as early as 6 weeks postoperatively or as late as 3 months if a bony procedure was performed.

(2) Some procedures will allow full ROM and return to activities that place the shoulder in the position of dislocation (abduction and external rotation) and others will not. Before initiating any stretching activities to obtain full ROM, be sure to have a clear understanding of any limitations of ROM intentionally imposed by the surgical procedure.

G. Postoperative Management for Recurrent Posterior Dislocation of the Shoulder

1. Indications for surgery[30,42,44,54]

a. Recurrent and painful dislocation or subluxation of the GH joint, particularly during activities that require full flexion or internal rotation, due to laxity of the posterior capsule and tears of the posterior rotator cuff and glenoid labrum

b. Pain and limited use of the upper extremity during overhead functional activities

c. Failed conservative management after initial dislocation

2. Procedures[42,44,84]

a. NOTE: Reconstruction is undertaken to provide stability to the posterior portion of the capsule and may limit full forward flexion and internal rotation.

b. Some procedures may involve an open approach (arthrotomy), whereas others are performed arthoscopically. The operative procedures may involve:

(1) Capsular plication and advancement of the infraspinatus

(2) Posterior capsulorrhaphy

(3) Biceps tendon transfer

(4) Posterior glenoid osteotomy

3. Postoperative management[30,44,54]

a. *Immobilization*
The shoulder is immobilized with the arm held at the side of the trunk in a splint in slight shoulder extension and neutral rotation or in external rotation in a reverse sling or spica cast for several days or weeks.

b. *Exercise*

MAXIMUM-PROTECTION PHASE

(1) The immobilization is removed for exercise in the early stages of healing for passive and active-assistive ROM. To maintain mobility in GH structures, follow the progression of exercises for anterior shoulder dislocation during the maximum-protection phase discussed in this section.

   Precaution: Avoid excessive and painful forward flexion with internal rotation or horizontal adduction across the chest.

(2) To maintain or develop strength in the scapulothoracic musculature, perform manual resistance in linear and diagonal planes and rhythmic stabilization.

(3) To maintain strength in the rotator cuff musculature, perform submaximal, pain-free multiple-angle isometrics.

MODERATE- AND MINIMUM-PROTECTION PHASES

(1) Progress exercises to increase strength and endurance, particularly in the infraspinatus/teres minor complex.

   NOTE: Particular care should be taken during active and resisted exercise in the 70- to 100-degree arc of forward flexion to note any posterior instability. When strengthening the external rotators, do not begin in full internal rotation. Adequate cuff strength should be present before proceeding to overhead flexion.

(2) Follow a progression of exercises and functional activities discussed previously in this section for nonoperative management of posterior and anterior instabilities.

VI. Thoracic Outlet Syndrome[22,31,58,82,93-95]

A. Related Diagnoses and Symptoms

In thoracic outlet syndrome (TOS), symptoms of pain, paresthesia, numbness, weakness, discoloration, swelling, ulceration, gangrene, or in some cases, Raynaud's phenomenon may be experienced in the related upper extremity.

B. Etiology of Symptoms

1. **Symptoms are evoked as blood vessels and nerves are compressed by structures in thoracic outlet region**

   a. The cervical nerve roots may be compressed in the foramina of the vertebrae. This is not a TOS, but it causes neurologic signs in the upper extremity and should be considered in the testing procedures.

   b. The proximal portion of the brachial plexus or the subclavian artery may be compressed as they course through the scalene muscles if the muscles are tight or hypertrophied or have anatomic variations.

   c. The brachial plexus and subclavian artery and vein may be compressed against the first rib or a cervical rib as they course under the clavicle, particularly if the clavicle is in a depressed position, as when carrying a heavy shoulder bag or in an extreme posture. A fractured clavicle or anomalies in the region can also lead to symptoms.

   d. The brachial plexus and axillary artery may be compressed against the ribs as they course under the pectoralis minor muscle if it is tight from faulty posture or if the person maintains an arm in a fully elevated position.

   e. A brachial plexus stretch may occur as the plexus is pulled around the coracoid process when the arm is held in a fully elevated position.

2. **Contributing factors**

   a. There is a wide latitude of motion in the various joints of the shoulder complex that may result in compression or impingement of the nerves or vessels.

   b. Postural variations such as a forward head or round shoulders lead to associated muscle tightness in the scalene, levator, subscapularis, and pectoralis minor muscles and a depressed clavicle.

   c. Respiratory patterns that continually use the action of the scalene muscles to elevate the upper ribs lead to hypertrophy of these muscles. Also, the elevated upper ribs decrease the space under the clavicle.

   d. Congenital factors such as an accessory rib, a long transverse process of the C-7 vertebra, or other anomaly in the region can reduce the space for the vessels. A traumatic or arteriosclerotic insult can also lead to TOS symptoms.

   e. Traumatic injuries such as clavicular fracture or subacromial dislocations of the humeral head can injure the plexus and vessels, leading to TOS symptoms.

   f. Hypertrophy or scarring in the pectoralis minor muscles.

C. Common Impairments/Problems Summarized

1. Intermittent brachial plexus and vascular symptoms of pain, paresthesia, numbness, weakness, discoloration, and swelling
2. Muscle length-strength imbalances in the shoulder girdle with tightness in anterior and medial structures and weakness in posterior and lateral structures
3. Faulty postural awareness in the upper quarter
4. Poor endurance in the postural muscles
5. Shallow respiratory pattern, characterized by upper thoracic breathing
6. Poor clavicular and anterior rib mobility

D. Common Functional Limitations/Disabilities

1. Sleep disturbances that could be from excessive pillow thickness or arm posture when sleeping
2. Inability to carry briefcase, suitcase, purse with shoulder strap, or other weighted objects on the involved side
3. Inability to maintain prolonged overhead reaching position
4. Symptoms with sustained desk work, cradling a telephone receiver between head and involved shoulder, and driving a car

E. Nonoperative Management[4]

The primary emphasis of management is to decrease the mechanical pressure by increasing mobility of tissues in the thoracic outlet region, preventing recurrence of the compression loads by correcting the postural alignment, and developing endurance to maintain the correct posture.

1. To increase flexibility in tight structures, use manual and self-stretching techniques. Common problems include but are not limited to the scalene, levator scapulae, pectoralis minor, pectoralis major, anterior portion of the intercostals, and short suboccipital muscles and to the sternoclavicular joint.
2. To train weak muscles, develop a program of strengthening, endurance, and postural awareness. Common weaknesses include but are not limited to scapular adductors and upward rotators, shoulder lateral rotators, short anterior throat cervical flexor muscles, and thoracic extensors. Techniques for cervical exercises and posture correction are discussed in Chapter 15.
3. To correct a faulty respiratory pattern (upper chest breathing) and elevated upper ribs, teach diaphragmatic breathing patterns and relaxation exercises to relax the upper thorax. (See Chapter 20.)
4. To progress to functional independence, determine activities that provoke the symptoms and involve the patient in adapting the environment and faulty habits to minimize the stress.

VII. Reflex Sympathetic Dystrophy[16,27,34]

A. Related Diagnoses

Common synonyms for reflex sympathetic dystrophy (RSD) include shoulder-hand syndrome, Sudeck's atrophy, sympathetically mediated pain syndrome, reflex neurovascular dystrophy, traumatic angiospasm or vasospasm, and sympathetically maintained pain (SMP).

B. Etiology of Symptoms

The underlying mechanism that stimulates onset of this condition is unclear. It develops in association with a persistent painful lesion such as a painful shoulder after a cardiovascular accident or myocardial infarction, cervical osteoarthritis, trauma such as a fracture or sprain, or after catheterization. The condition can last for months or years, but spontaneous recovery often occurs in 18 to 24 months. Three stages are identified.

1. Acute, or vasodilation stage, lasts 3 weeks to 6 months. Pain is the predominant feature, usually out of proportion to the severity of the injury.
2. Dystrophic, or vasoconstriction stage, lasts 3 to 6 months. It is characterized by sympathetic hyperactivity, burning pain, and hyperesthesia exacerbated by cold weather.
3. Atrophic stage is characterized by pain either decreasing or becoming worse. Muscle wasting and contractures may occur.

C. Common Impairments/Problems Summarized

1. Pain or hyperesthesia at the shoulder, wrist, or hand
2. Limitation of motion of the:
   a. Shoulder, with most restriction in lateral flexion and abduction
   b. Wrist, with most restriction in wrist extension
   c. Hand, with most restriction in metacarpophalangeal and proximal interphalangeal flexion secondary to shortened collateral ligaments
3. Edema of the hand and wrist secondary to circulatory impairment of the venous and lymphatic systems, which, in turn, precipitates stiffness in the hand
4. Vasomotor instability
5. Trophic changes in the skin
6. As the condition progresses:
   a. Pain subsides but limitation of motion persists.
   b. The skin becomes cyanotic and shiny.
   c. Intrinsic muscles of the hand atrophy.
   d. Subcutaneous tissue in the fingers and palmar fascia thicken.
   e. Nail changes occur.

D. Management

1. This is a progressive disorder unless vigorous intervention is used.
2. To increase ROM of the shoulder and hand, if limited, use techniques specific to the limiting structures and working within the pain-free range.
3. To facilitate active muscle contractions, use both isotonic and isometric exercise and controlled closed-chain activities.
4. To relieve pain and increase sensory input, use transcutaneous electrical nerve stimulation (TENS) or ice.
5. To control edema, apply intermittent pneumatic compression and massage. Elevate and use elastic compression when not receiving the pneumatic compression treatment.
6. To educate the patient, emphasize the importance of following the program of increased activity.

7. Medical intervention. The physician may choose to perform a stellate block or use oral steroids or intramuscular medication in conjunction with therapeutic exercise.

8. Prevention is the best therapy. When there is shoulder involvement or referred pain to the shoulder, the entire upper extremity should be moved as soon as allowed at an intensity safe for the condition.

VIII. Exercise Techniques for Management of Acute and Early Subacute Soft Tissue Lesions

If, on evaluation, it is determined that an inflammation is present, whether it is from an acute injury, repetitive trauma or overuse, an arthritic disease, or surgery, the approach to treatment is the same. General guidelines for management during the acute stage are listed in Chapter 7, Section III. Techniques other than the ones described as follows may be appropriate depending on the patient's individual problem.

A. Techniques to Inhibit Pain and Muscle Guarding and to Maintain Joint Integrity and Nutrition

1. *Gentle grade I or II joint distraction or oscillation* of the humeral head in the fossa. Place the joint in pain-free positions and glide the head anterior/posterior or in a caudal direction (see Figs. 6–14 and 6–15).

   NOTE: Stretching the joint capsule is contraindicated in the acute stage.

2. *Pendulum (Codman's) exercises.* When *no weight* is used, these techniques cause a grade II distraction from the weight of the arm and a grade II physiologic oscillation as the arm swings. (See Section II and Fig. 8–1.)

B. Techniques to Initiate Early Motion and Maintain Soft Tissue Integrity and Mobility in the Shoulder

1. Passive to active-assistive range of motion within the patient's pain-free range. These techniques are described in Chapter 2.

2. If the patient is able, teach *self-assisted motion* using a cane, wand, or T-bar. Patient position is supine. If scapular mobility is normal, these exercises, as well as pulley exercises, can be progressed in the subacute stage to sitting and/or standing as described in Chapter 2.

   a. *Shoulder flexion.* The patient begins with arms at the sides and grasps the cane with both hands and lifts the involved extremity through a nonstressful range.

   NOTE: Even though the shoulder naturally internally rotates during flexion,[10,81] if there is an instability with an impingement syndrome, it will be magnified with internal rotation, so the patient should perform shoulder flexion with lateral rotation, that is, grab the cane at the end so the thumb points up and back.

   b. *Shoulder rotation.* The patient's arm is resting at the side with elbows flexed to 90 degrees. The normal extremity rotates the involved extremity both internally and externally within the pain-free range (Fig. 8–8). If tolerated, rotation is also performed with the arm abducted 45 and 90 degrees.

3. *"Gear shift"* exercises can be used for assisted shoulder and scapular motions during the acute phase. While in a seated position with the arm at the side, the

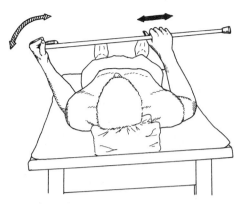

Figure 8–8. Assisted shoulder rotation using a cane, with the arm at the side.

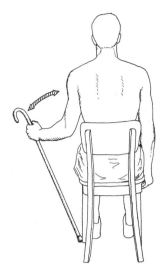

Figure 8–9. Gear shift exercise. Self-assisted shoulder rotation using a cane. Flexion/extension and diagonal patterns can also be done.

patient holds a pole or stick with the tip resting on the floor. He or she moves the pole forward and back, diagonally, or laterally and medially in a motion similar to shifting gears in a car with a floor shift (Fig. 8–9).

4. With a specific muscle injury, apply *intermittent muscle-setting techniques* with the involved muscle in its shortened position. Additional techniques are described in the following sections for specific muscle functions.

C. Techniques to Maintain Integrity and Function for Humeral Head Control

Frequently, the muscles of the rotator cuff are inhibited when there is trauma or surgery.[104]

1. *Muscle setting.* Perform multiple-angle, submaximal, intermittent isometrics against gentle resistance to the rotator cuff and biceps brachii actions in pain-free positions and at an intensity that does not cause symptoms. Initially, apply the gentle resistance manually so the position and intensity can be controlled while the patient learns the feel of the correct muscle contracting. Apply the resistance above the elbow to minimize shear forces within the glenohumeral joint. If pain from joint compression occurs, apply a slight traction to the joint as the resistance is given.

   Begin with the patient supine; as the condition improves, progress to sitting and standing.

   a. *Internal and external rotation.* Position the shoulder at the side and the arm in various positions of rotation such as at 0 and 30 degrees.

   b. *Abduction.* Position the arm at 0, 30, and 60 degrees if tolerated.

   c. *Scaption.* Abduction with the arm in the plane of the scapula at 0, 30, and 60 degrees, if tolerated (Fig. 8–10).

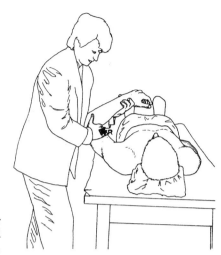

Figure 8–10. Isometric resistance in scaption. The shoulder is positioned between 30 and 60 degrees of scaption, and controlled manual resistance is applied against the humerus.

    d. *Elbow flexion with the forearm supinated.* The arm is kept at the side, neutral to rotation, while resistance is applied to the forearm, causing tension in the long head of the biceps (see Fig. 3–7). Change the position of shoulder rotation as the patient tolerates, and repeat the isometric resistance to elbow flexion.

2. Teach patients how to apply the isometric setting techniques to themselves using *self-resistance* (Fig. 8–11). These can be progressed to resistance against a stationary object such as a wall or door frame (Fig. 8–12).

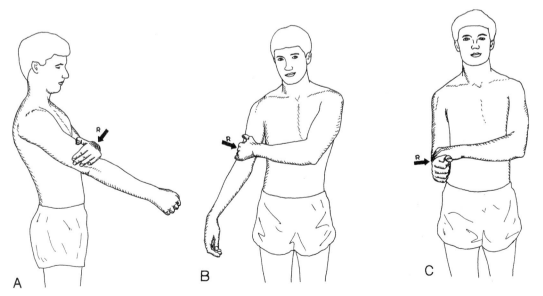

Figure 8–11. Self-resistance for isometric (*A*) shoulder flexion, (*B*) abduction, and (*C*) rotation.

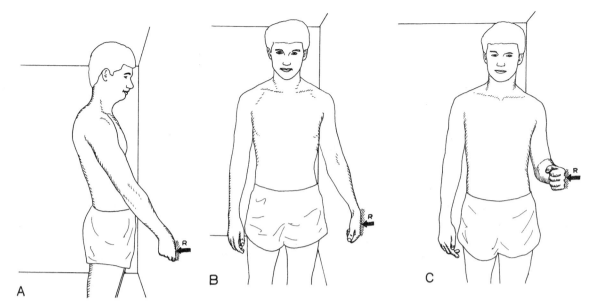

Figure 8–12. Using a wall to provide resistance for isometric (*A*) shoulder flexion, (*B*) abduction, or (*C*) rotation.

D. Techniques to Maintain Integrity and Function for Scapular Control

1. Initiate *intermittent isometrics* of the scapular muscles. If any of these muscles are injured, the intensity of resistance is very light; if not injured, the intensity should match the capability of the muscle.

2. Begin with the patient side-lying, with the affected extremity up. Drape the forearm of the involved extremity over your shoulder. The degree of shoulder flexion, scaption, or abduction can be controlled by your stance and the relative position of the patient.

   a. *Scapular elevation/depression.* Place your top hand superiorly and the other hand inferiorly around the scapula to provide manual resistance (Fig. 8–13A).

   b. *Scapular protraction/retraction.* Place one hand along the medial border and the other around the coracoid process to provide resistance.

   c. *Scapular upward and downward rotation.* Place one hand around the inferior angle and the other hand around the acromion and coracoid process to provide resistance.

3. Progress the patient to sitting with his or her arm draped over your shoulder; apply resistance to all scapular motions in the same manner as described previously (Fig. 8–13B).

4. These setting exercises can be progressed to active and manual-resistive as the patient tolerates.

E. Techniques to Stimulate the Co-contraction of the Shoulder Girdle Muscles

Protected weight-bearing exercises are introduced if tolerated to facilitate the stabilization function of the shoulder girdle.

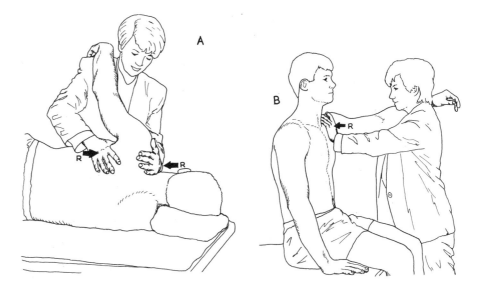

Figure 8–13. Manual resistance to scapular motions. (*A*) Resistance to elevation/depression. (*B*) Resistance to protraction/retraction. The patient reaches across the therapist's shoulder to protract the scapula while the therapist resists against the coracoid and acromion process; the other hand is placed behind the scapula to resist retraction.

1. Patient stands and places both elbows or both hands on a wall or a solid object such as a treatment table and places some body weight through the upper extremity. Initially, have the patient bear just enough weight so as not to provoke symptoms (see Fig. 20–3).
2. As tolerated, the patient gently shifts the weight forward and backward, side to side, then diagonally within a pain-free range.

IX. Exercise Techniques for Management of Muscle Strength and Flexibility Imbalances in Subacute and Chronic Shoulder Problems

Whether the cause is nerve injury, disuse, or faulty posture or whether dysfunction is the result of a traumatic insult, overuse, instability, or surgery, muscle imbalance and faulty shoulder mechanics will exist. Restoring the balance of muscle strength, flexibility, and coordination is necessary for full recovery. Once the acute symptoms from the impairment begin to diminish, exercises to regain a balance in length and strength of the musculoskeletal system and to train the neuromuscular system to respond appropriately are used to help restore the patient to the desired functional outcome. The exercise techniques in this section are suggestions for progressing the patient through the subacute healing and chronic rehabilitative phases of treatment.* The principles of exercise intervention during these phases are discussed in Chapter 7, Sections IV, V, and VI. When designing an exercise program, the intensity and type of exercises must not exceed the capability of the healing tissue. The following exercises are described from simplest or least stressful to more difficult. Choose exercises to challenge patients at a level they can meet so they can safely progress to more intense levels. (See also Chapter 15 for correction of cervical and thoracic postural problems that might underlie faulty shoulder girdle mechanics.)

---

*Refs. 5, 15, 26, 48, 52, 57, 59 ,89, 99, 104.

A. Techniques to Progressively Increase Range of Motion

1. **Inhibition techniques to lengthen tight muscles** are described in Chapter 5.
   a. If there was an inflammatory reaction and the region now is in the early subacute stage of healing, the muscle contraction should be submaximal and not cause increased pain. As healing continues and the response of the tissue becomes predictable, the intensity of contraction can be progressively increased until maximum effort is used.
   b. Conclude the lengthening procedure with active ROM through the available range.

2. **Self-stretching techniques.** The patient should be taught a low-intensity prolonged stretch.
   a. To increase *flexion and elevation* of the arm
      The patient sits with the side next to the table, the forearm resting along the table edge with the elbow slightly flexed (Fig. 8–14A). He or she then slides the forearm forward along the table while bending from the waist. Eventually the head should be level with the shoulder (Fig. 8–14B).
   b. To increase *external (lateral) rotation*
      The patient sits as with flexion (Fig. 8–14A). He or she then bends forward from the waist, bringing the head and shoulder level with the table (Fig. 8–15).
   c. Alternate position for *external rotation*
      The patient stands, facing the edge of a door frame with the palm of the hand against the frame and the elbow flexed 90 degrees. While keeping the arm against the side, the patient turns away from the fixed hand.
   d. To increase *abduction and elevation* of the arm
      The patient sits with the side next to the table, the forearm resting with palm up on the table and pointing toward the opposite side of the table (Fig. 8–16A). He or she then brings the head down toward the arm while moving the thorax away from the table (Fig. 8–16B).
   e. To increase *extension*
      The patient stands with the back to the table, both hands grasping the edge with the fingers facing forward (Fig. 8–17A). He or she then begins to squat while letting the elbows flex (Fig. 8–17B).

   Precaution: If a patient is prone to anterior subluxation or dislocation, this activity should not be performed.

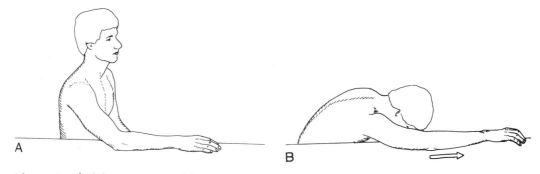

Figure 8–14. (*A*) Beginning and (*B*) end positions for self-stretching to increase shoulder flexion with elevation.

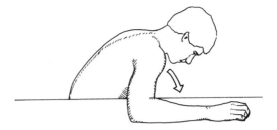

Figure 8–15. End position for self-stretching to increase shoulder external rotation.

3. **Additional manual and self-stretching exercises for specific muscles.**
   a. To stretch the *latissimus dorsi muscle*
      (1) Position of patient supine, with hips and knees flexed so the pelvis is stabilized in a posterior pelvic tilt. The therapist provides additional stabilization to the pelvis with one hand, if necessary; the other hand grasps the distal humerus (see Fig. 5–6) and flexes, laterally rotates, and partially abducts the humerus to the end of range of the latissimus. The patient is asked to contract into extension, adduction, and medial rotation while the therapist provides resistance for a hold-relax maneuver. During the relaxation phase, the patient or therapist elongates the muscle.
      (2) Self-stretching. The patient assumes the above position without help and reaches overhead as far as possible without allowing the back to arch. Or the patient stands with the back to a wall and feet forward enough to allow hips and knees to partially flex so the low back is flat against the wall and pelvis is stabilized. The patient actively flexes, externally rotates, and slightly abducts the arms as far as possible (thumbs pointing toward the floor if supine or toward the wall if standing) and attempts to reach the mat or wall with the arms while maintaining the back flat.
   b. To stretch the *pectoralis major muscles*
      (1) Patient position sitting on a treatment table or mat, with the hands behind the head. The therapist kneels behind the patient, grasping the patient's elbows (Fig. 8–18). Have the patient breathe in as he or she brings the elbows out to the side (horizontal abduction and scapular adduction). The therapist holds the elbows at this end-point as the patient breathes

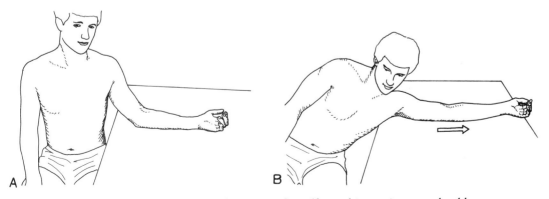

Figure 8–16. (*A*) Beginning and (*B*) end positions for self-stretching to increase shoulder abduction with elevation.

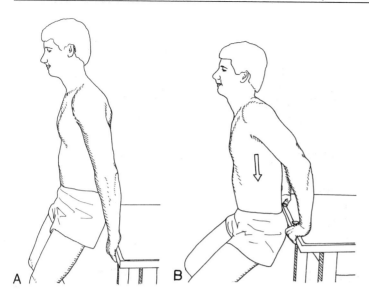

Figure 8–17. (*A*) Beginning and (*B*) end positions for self-stretching to increase shoulder extension.

out. No forceful stretch is needed against the elbows, because the rib cage is elongating the proximal attachment of the pectoralis major muscles bilaterally. As the patient repeats the inhalation, the therapist moves the elbows up and out to the end of the available range, then holds as the patient breathes out.

NOTE: Hyperventilation should not occur, because the breathing is slow and comfortable. If the patient does become dizzy, allow him or her to rest, then reinstruct for proper technique. Be sure the patient maintains the neck in the neutral position, not flexed.

(2) Self-stretching

Patient position standing, facing a corner or open door, with the arms in a reverse T or a V against the wall (Figs. 8–19A and B). The patient then

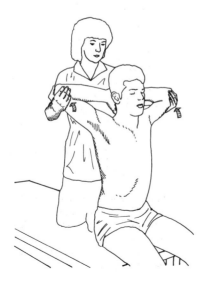

Figure 8–18. Active stretching of the pectoralis major muscle. The therapist holds the elbow at the end-point as the patient breathes out.

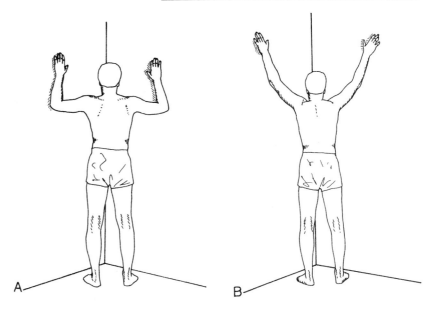

Figure 8–19. Self-stretching the pectoralis major muscle with the arms in a reverse **T** to stretch (*A*) the clavicular portion, and in a **V** to stretch (*B*) the sternal portion.

leans the entire body forward from the ankles (knees slightly bent). The degree of stretch can be adjusted by the amount of forward movement.

(3) Wand exercises for stretching

Patient position sitting or standing. The patient grasps the wand with the forearms pronated and elbows flexed 90 degrees. He or she then elevates the shoulders and brings the wand behind the head and shoulders (Fig. 8–20). The scapulae are adducted and elbows brought out to the side. Combine with breathing by having the patient inhale as he or she brings the wand into position behind the shoulders, then exhale while holding this stretched position.

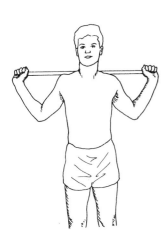

Figure 8–20. Wand exercises to stretch the pectoralis major muscle.

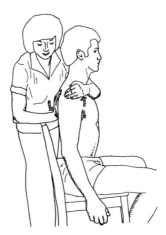

Figure 8–21. Active stretching of the pectoralis minor muscle. The therapist holds the scapular and coracoid process at the end-point as the patient breathes out.

c. To isolate stretch to the *pectoralis minor muscle*

Patient position sitting. The therapist places one hand posterior on the scapula, stabilizing it against the rib cage, and the other hand anterior on the shoulder, just above the coracoid process (Fig. 8–21). The patient breathes in; the therapist fixes the scapula at the end position; then the patient breathes out. Repeat, with the therapist readjusting the end-position with each inhalation, and stabilizing as the patient exhales.

d. To stretch the *levator scapulae muscle*

NOTE: The muscle attaches to the superior angle of the scapula and causes it to rotate downward and elevate; it also attaches to the transverse processes of the upper cervical vertebrae and causes them to backward bend and rotate to the ipsilateral side. Because the muscle is attached to two movable structures, both ends must be stabilized opposite to the pull of the muscle.

(1) Patient position sitting. The patient rotates the head opposite to the side of tightness (looks away from the tight side) and forward bends until a slight pull is felt in the posterior-lateral aspect of the neck (in the levator muscle). He or she then abducts the arm on the side of tightness, placing that hand behind the head to help stabilize it in the rotated position. The therapist stands behind and places one hand across the shoulder to stabilize the scapula and the elbow of the other arm anteriorly across the patient's rotated head. The therapist's hand can then help abduct the patient's arm (Fig. 8–22). With the muscle now in its stretched position, have the patient breathe in, then out. The therapist holds the shoulder and scapula down to maintain the stretch as the patient breathes in again (he or she contracts the muscle against the resistance of the fixating hand). To increase the stretch, increase the shoulder abduction. This is not a forceful stretch but a gentle contract-relax maneuver. Do not stretch the muscle by forcing rotation on the head and neck.

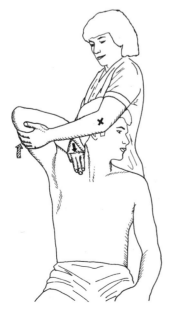

Figure 8–22. Active stretching of the levator scapulae muscle. The therapist stabilizes the head and scapula as the patient breathes in, contracting the muscle against the resistance. As the patient relaxes, the rib cage and scapula depress, which stretches the muscle.

(2) To perform the above maneuver in a home program as a self-stretching technique, the patient assumes the same head and arm position as in (1) and then stands with the bent elbow against the wall and, if necessary, the other hand across the forehead to stabilize the rotated head. He or she then inhales, exhales, and moves the elbow up the wall (Fig. 8–23A).

(3) Alternate self-stretching technique with the patient sitting. The head placement is the same; the head is rotated away from the side of tightness; then the patient looks down until a slight pull is felt in the levator. To stabilize the scapula, the patient reaches down and back with the hand on the side of tightness and holds on to the seat of the chair. The other hand is placed on the head to gently pull it forward and to the side in an oblique direction opposite the line of pull of the tight muscle (Fig. 8–23B).

e. To stretch the *long head of the biceps brachii*

Patient position, supine or standing. The shoulder and elbow are extended and forearm pronated (see Fig. 2–8). For self-stretching, the patient stands and places the tight arm behind the back as far as possible (back of hand against body) and grasps the wrist with the other hand and stretches it into extension and adduction.

f. To stretch the *long head of the triceps brachii*

Patient position, sitting or standing with the shoulder and elbow flexed as far as possible (see Fig. 2–9). For self-stretching, the patient flexes the elbow as far as possible, then flexes the shoulder and places the stretch force with the other hand against the distal humerus.

g. To self-stretch the *posterior deltoid and lateral rotators*

Patient position, supine, sitting, or standing. The patient horizontally adducts with the arm internally rotated by reaching as far as possible toward the op-

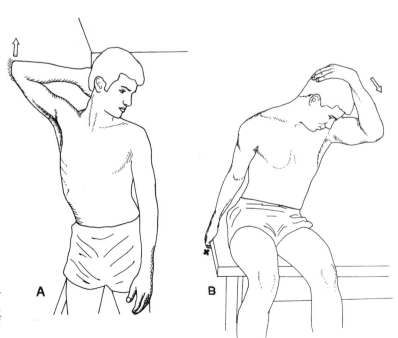

Figure 8–23. Self-stretching the levator scapulae muscle. (*A*) Using upward rotation of the scapula and (*B*) using depression of the scapula.

posite shoulder. The stretch force is applied by the other hand against the elbow, pressing it toward the uninvolved shoulder.

B. Techniques to Progressively Strengthen Muscles and Prepare for Functional Activities

NOTE: Chapter 3 describes principles and techniques of resistance exercises and Chapter 7 presents procedures for exercising muscles at various stages of inflammation and repair. Refer to these chapters for guidelines and precautions.

First isolate and strengthen weakened muscles with multiple-angle isometric, manual, and mechanical resistance and develop control within the mechanical limits of the involved tissues. Progress to combined patterns of motion and training for muscle groups to function in a coordinated sequence of control and motion, then progress to functional activities.

1. To progress isometric exercises

The multiple-angle, submaximal isometric exercises described in Section VIII are progressed in intensity of resistance at multiple angles to strengthen the muscles at different lengths and reinforce their stabilizing actions in various positions (see Figs. 8–11 and 8–12). If pain from joint compression occurs, place a small towel roll in the axilla to cause joint distraction or use manual resistance and apply a slight distraction to the joint as resistance is given.

2. To isolate and train awareness of the muscle action and strengthen key scapular and shoulder motions

   a. *External rotation (infraspinatus and teres minor)*. The arm can be positioned at the patient's side or in various positions of abduction, scaption, or flexion. The elbow is bent and the resistive force is applied through the hand at right angles to the forearm. Be sure the patient rotates the humerus and does not extend the elbow.

      (1) Patient position, sitting or standing using elastic resistance or wall pulley in front of the body at elbow level. He or she grasps the elastic material or the pulley handle and rotates his or her arm outward (Figs. 8–24A and C).

      (2) Patient position, side-lying on normal side with involved shoulder upright and arm resting on the side of the thorax. Using a hand-held weight, weight cuff, or elastic resistance, he or she rotates the weight through the desired range of motion.

      (3) Patient position, prone on a treatment table, upper arm resting on the table with shoulder at 90 degrees if possible, elbow flexed with forearm over the edge of the table. Lift the weight as far as possible by rotating the shoulder, not extending the elbow (Fig. 8–24B).

      (4) Patient position, sitting with elbow flexed 90 degrees and supported on a table so the shoulder is in the resting position. The patient lifts the weight from the table by rotating the shoulder.

   b. *Internal rotation (subscapularis)*. The arm is positioned at the patient's side or in various positions of flexion, scaption, or abduction. The elbow is bent and the resistive force is applied through the hand.

      (1) Patient is side-lying on involved side with arm forward in partial flexion. The patient lifts the weight upward into internal rotation (Fig. 8–25).

      (2) Patient is sitting or standing using an elastic material or pulley system

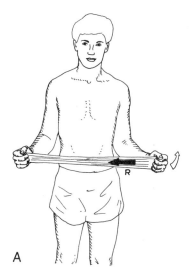

A

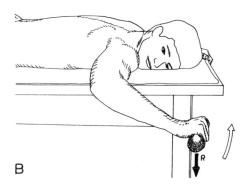

B

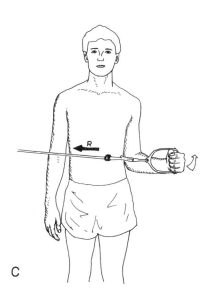

C

Figure 8–24. Resisting shoulder external rotation using (*A*) elasticized material, (*B*) hand-held weight, and (*C*) wall pulley.

with the line of force out to the side and at the level of the elbow. He or she pulls across the front of the trunk into internal rotation.

c. *Abduction and scaption (deltoid and supraspinatus)*. If the arm abducts beyond 90 degrees, it must externally rotate to avoid impingement of the greater tubercle against the acromion. These same exercises can be performed in the plane of the scapula.

(1) "Military press". Patient sitting, arm at the side in external rotation with elbow flexed and forearm supinated (thumb pointing posteriorly). The patient lifts the weight straight up overhead (Fig. 8–26).

(2) Patient is sitting or standing with weight in hand and abducts the arm to 90 degrees, then laterally rotates and elevates the arm through the rest of

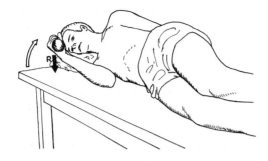

Figure 8–25. Resisted internal rotation of the shoulder using a hand-held weight. To resist external rotation, place the weight in the patient's upper hand.

the range. This same motion can be performed with an elastic resistance secured under the patient's foot, but be cautious in that the greater the elastic stretch, the greater the resistance. The patient may not be able to complete the range of motion because of the increased resistance.

(3) Patient is side-lying with involved arm uppermost. The patient lifts a weight up to 90 degrees. The greatest effect of the resistance is at the beginning of the range. At 90 degrees, all of the force is through the long axis of the bone.

(4) *Scaption* with internal rotation ("empty can"), neutral, and external rotation ("full can"). The patient stands with a weight in the hand and raises the arm away from the side in the plane of the scapula, halfway between abduction and flexion. Performing scaption with the humerus in various positions of rotation has the value of emphasizing each of the rotatory muscles of the cuff in their synergy with the supraspinatus and deltoid muscles.

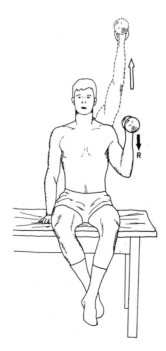

Figure 8–26. Military press-up. Beginning with the arm at the side in external rotation with elbow flexed and forearm supinated (thumb pointing posteriorward), the weight is lifted overhead.

NOTE: It is currently popular to emphasize the supraspinatus muscle by internally rotating the shoulder while in scaption,[104] the empty-can position, because this position supposedly isolates this muscle. A recent EMG study confirmed that the supraspinatus contracts strongly in this position but does not isolate it from other shoulder muscles such as the anterior and middle deltoid and subscapularis, which contract even more strongly.[99] The supraspinatus contracts more strongly when doing the military press.[99]

d. *Flexion (anterior deltoid)*. Patient is sitting, standing, or supine and elevates the weight through the range of motion. When supine, the greatest resistive force is at the beginning of the range; when standing, the greatest resistive force is when the shoulder is flexed 90 degrees (see Figs. 3–30 and 3–31). An elastic resistive force can be used while standing if secured under the patient's foot or solid object.

e. *Adduction (pectoralis major, teres major, and latissimus dorsi)* and *horizontal adduction (anterior deltoid)*
   (1) Patient is sitting or standing. The arm is abducted and the patient pulls down against a pulley force or elastic resistance tied overhead. The greatest resistance will be when the line of the resistive force is at right angles to the patient's arm.
   (2) Patient is supine, beginning with arms out to the side in horizontal abduction, then bringing the arms forward into horizontal adduction until the arms are vertical and the hands are touching in midline.

f. *Extension (posterior deltoid)*
   (1) Patient is prone with the arm over the side of the table in 90 degrees flexion. He or she lifts the weight backward into extension.
   (2) Patient sitting or standing. The arm is flexed and the patient pulls down against a pulley force or elastic resistance tied overhead.

g. *Manual resistance* to scapular motions. Patient is side-lying or sitting with the arm resting on the therapist's shoulder; progress manual resistance range of motion to the scapular motions as described for isometric setting (see Fig. 8–13).

h. *Scapular retraction (rhomboids and middle trapezius)*

   NOTE: Scapular retraction is a motion necessary for good scapulothoracic posture. Activities encompassing retraction are also discussed in Chapter 15 in combination with developing strength and in the region for functional control of posture.

   (1) Patient position, prone. Instruct the patient to grasp the hands together behind the low back. This activity should cause scapular adduction. Draw attention to the adducted scapulae and have the patient hold the adducted position of the scapulae while the arms are lowered to the sides. Have the patient repeat the activity without arm motion. This action is practiced supine, sitting, and standing.
   (2) Patient sits or stands with arms flexed 90 degrees and elbows extended. He or she grasps each end of an elastic resistance or a pulley and simply retracts the scapula against the resistance, keeping the arms aligned with the pulley. This same action can be resisted with the patient prone and arm hanging over the edge of the table with a weight in the hand (Fig. 8–27).

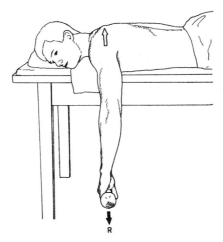

Figure 8–27. Scapular retraction against hand-held resistance in the prone position.

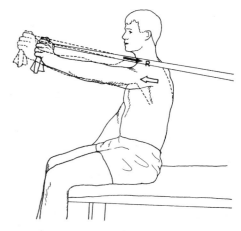

Figure 8–28. Scapular protraction; pushing against elastic resistance.

(3) Combining arm motions and resistance with scapular adduction further strengthens these muscles as described in the combined patterns section.

i. *Scapular upward rotation (upper and lower trapezius and serratus anterior).* This motion cannot be isolated from arm motions because it is part of the synergy for humeral elevation. Train awareness by passively placing the arm in elevation, then asking the patient to hold it there and drawing attention to scapular function through tactile cues.

Patient is prone with arm elevated above the head. The arm is picked up, causing the rotators to contract.

j. *Scapular protraction (serratus anterior)*
   (1) Patient is supine with arm flexed 90 degrees and elbow extended. The patient "pushes" the weight upward without rotating the body.
   (2) Patient is sitting or standing with arm flexed 90 degrees and elbow extended. An elastic resistance or pulley is behind the patient. The patient "pushes" against this resistance without rotating the body (Fig. 8–28).

k. *Scapular elevation (upper trapezius and levator scapulae).* Patient is sitting or standing, holding weights in the hands or ends of elastic resistance secured under the feet, and shrugs the shoulders.

3. To increase stabilization and control of proximal muscles

a. Increase loads during *closed-chain exercises*.
   (1) The patient stands and rests the hands on a wall, on the treatment table, or on the floor. The exercise load is added with pressure from the therapist or by resisting the motion as the patient rocks in various directions (Fig. 8–29A).
   (2) Progress by having the patient alternately lift one arm; this requires additional stabilization from the extremity holding the body weight. Increase the challenge by having the patient lift a weight with the free (non–weight-bearing) arm.
   (3) Initiate endurance by progressing length of time at each level of resis-

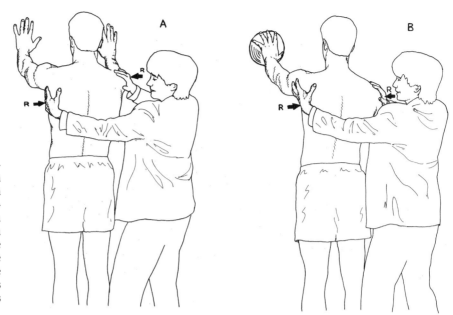

Figure 8–29. Closed-chain scapular and glenohumeral stabilization exercises. (*A*) Bilateral support in a minimum weight-bearing position with both hands against a wall. (*B*) Unilateral support on a less stable surface (ball). The therapist applies resistance while the patient stabilizes against the resistance or the therapist applies resistance as the patient moves from side to side.

tance before progressing. As the patient demonstrates good stability and endurance, progress to the hands and knees (all-fours) position.

   (4) Suggestions for additional challenges include placing a ball, a rocker board, or a wobble board under the hands to develop balance reactions on an unstable surface (Fig. 8–29B).

  b. Advanced *total-chain exercises* can also be performed by using a ProFitter (see Fig. 3–29) or Stairmaster while weight bearing bilaterally or unilaterally on the upper extremities. These mimic closed-chain exercises and require coordination and stabilization of the shoulder girdle muscles as the hand moves through an arc of motion.

  c. *Open-chain rhythmic stabilization exercises*

   (1) Patient lies supine, holding a rod at shoulder width, shoulders flexed to 90 degrees. Instruct the patient to hold against or match your resistance as you push and pull in various directions. Initially, tell the patient which direction you are pushing and gradually increase the resistance; indicate this each time you change directions and verbally reinforce what he or she should be feeling in the muscles (Fig. 8–30).

   (2) Progress these exercises by decreasing the verbal warnings, by increasing the intensity of the resistance, and by increasing the speed of shifting directions. The resistance can be applied unilaterally to just the involved extremity so that no assistance is provided by the normal shoulder. Increase endurance by increasing the amount of time the stabilization is held.

4. To progress shoulder girdle strengthening and develop coordination and control of combined patterns of motion between the scapula and arm

Dynamically load the upper extremity within tolerance of the synergy. Each exercise is continued until one of the components in the pattern cannot be con-

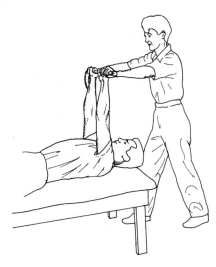

Figure 8–30. Rhythmic stabilization. The patient stabilizes with the shoulder girdle musculature (isometrically) against the resistance imposed by the therapist. Flexion/extension, abduction/adduction, and rotation resistance is applied in a rhythmic sequence.

trolled under the defined circumstance, so that the weakest link in the chain is being challenged but substitutions are not allowed to begin. Initially the goal is to develop control for 1 minute and progress to 3 minutes. In the described patterns, lying provides the greatest trunk support so that the patient has to concentrate only on the scapula and shoulder motions. When under control, progress to sitting, emphasizing to the patient to maintain good spinal posture; then progress to standing or whatever functional position is defined. In each position, progress by adding resistance or by increasing speed depending on the desired functional outcome. In the subacute phase, submaximal resistance is applied to the concentric phase of the activity. No additional resistance is added during the eccentric phase so eccentric resistance is not maximum. In the chronic rehabilitative phase, maximum resistance is applied based on the desired functional outcome.

a. *Scapular retraction with shoulder horizontal abduction*
   (1) Patient prone, pinches scapulae together and lifts elbow to the horizontal in a rowing motion; weight is added to progress resistance. Performing this exercise with the elbows extended also increases resistance (Fig. 8–31).
   (2) Patient sits or stands. He or she pulls against an elastic resistance that is secured at shoulder height, with horizontal abduction of the arms while adducting the scapulae, usually with the elbows flexed; greater strength and control are required if the elbows are extended.

b. *Scapular retraction with shoulder abduction and lateral rotation*
   (1) Patient is prone, with the arm over the edge of the table. He or she

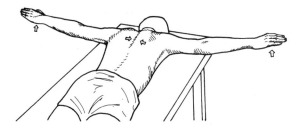

Figure 8–31. Scapular adduction exercises, with the arms positioned for maximum resistance from gravity. To progress the exercise further, weights can be placed in the patient's hands.

pinches the scapulae together, abducts the shoulder, and laterally rotates (thumb points toward ceiling); weight is added for resistance. (See Fig. 8–24B with scapular adduction emphasized.)

 (2) Patient is sitting or standing. He or she pulls against elastic resistance so that the end position is scapular retraction with shoulder abduction and lateral rotation (Fig. 8–32).

 (3) Diagonal patterns such as combined flexion, abduction, and lateral rotation can be initiated supine, progressed to sitting and then to standing, with resistance being applied manually, with free weights, or with elastic resistance.

 c. *Closed-chain scapular protraction and horizontal adduction.* Push-ups with an isometric hold at the end are performed in a position the patient can control. Begin with wall push-ups to develop control and strength if weak. To progress, increase the angle of the trunk by pushing up against a bar, end of a table, or a bench and eventually with the hands on the floor. Resistance can also be adjusted by using the knees as the fulcrum rather than the feet.

 d. *Closed-chain humeral adduction and scapular depression.* Sitting press-ups. The patient places both hands on the side of the chair and pushes down to lift the trunk up off the chair.

 e. Basic patterns that are part of the final desired outcome should be identified and progressed in a similar manner to that described.

C. Methods for Progressing to Functional Activities

As soon as the patient develops control of scapular and humeral motions and the basic components of the desired activities without exacerbating the symptoms, initiate specificity of training toward the desired functional outcome by progressing the strengthening exercises to maximum resistance concentrically and eccentrically. Use the actual patterns and type of contraction required in the desired outcome and progress to the desired speed first in a controlled manner, then with less control.

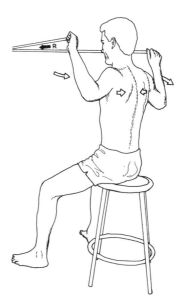

Figure 8–32. Combined scapular adduction with shoulder horizontal abduction and lateral rotation against resistance.

1. Increase *endurance* with repetitive loading from 3 to 5 minutes using the patterns of motion as described in the previous section.

2. Progress *eccentric training* to maximum load. Because eccentric contractions tolerate greater resistance than concentric, when loading resistance for eccentric training, the patient is taught to assist the arm to the end of the shortened range of the muscles to be stressed; then the muscles control the return motion. This can be performed with elastic resistance, pulleys, or free weights first in single-plane motions and then progressed to simulated patterns. Concentric/eccentric patterns on isokinetic machines may be used to simulate desired patterns.

3. Initiate *stretch-shortening drills* (plyometrics) in a safe, controlled pattern with light resistance; then progress speed and resistance as tolerated.

    Example: The therapist tosses a weighted ball such as a plyoball for the patient to reach and catch in various arm positions and immediately toss back using the reciprocal pattern (Fig. 8–33). Spring-loaded rebounders or elastic tubing is commercially available so the patient can do the activity on his or her own once the drills are learned.[103,104,105]

4. Increase *speed* with superimposed stresses to tolerance while simulating desired activity. Assess the total-body function while the desired activity is being carried out. Note timing and sequencing of events.

X. Summary

Treatment of common orthopedic conditions in the shoulder girdle using appropriate therapeutic exercise intervention has been described in this chapter following a brief review of anatomy and kinesiology of the region. The reader has been provided background information on etiology and typical impairments and common functional limitations of shoulder, clavicular, and scapular conditions including arthritis, hypomobility, instability, overuse syndromes, muscle imbalances, traumatic dislocation, reflex sympathetic dystrophy, and thoracic outlet syndrome. Background information on common surgical interventions for joint problems, impingement syndromes, and instabilities has

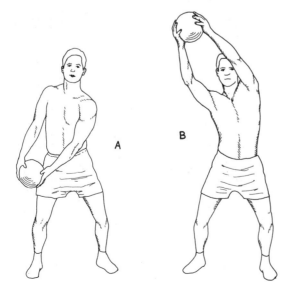

Figure 8–33. Catching a weighted plyoball in an (*A*) diagonal extension pattern and in a (*B*) diagonal flexion pattern.

also been described. Suggested guidelines to meet the goals and carry out the plan of care during each stage of recovery for the various conditions and surgical procedures have been described in a manner that provides a foundation for the therapist to design an individualized exercise program. The final sections of the chapter have described therapeutic exercise techniques for progressively stretching, strengthening, and developing functional use of the shoulder girdle complex.

References

1. Andrews, JR, and Angelo, RL: Shoulder arthroscopy for the throwing athlete. In Paulos, LE, and Tibone, JE (eds): Operative Technique in Shoulder Surgery. Aspen, Gaithersburg, MD, 1991.

2. Arntz, CT, and Jackins, S: Prosthetic replacement of the shoulder for the treatment of defects in the rotator cuff and the surface of the glenohumeral joint. J Bone Joint Surg Am 75:485–491, 1993.

3. Aronen, JG, and Regan, K: Decreasing the incidence of recurrence of first-time anterior dislocations with rehabilitation. Am J Sports Med 12:283, 1984.

4. Baker, CL, and Liu, SH: Neurovascular injuries to the shoulder. Journal of Orthopaedic and Sports Physical Therapy 18:361, 1993.

5. Ballantyne, BT, et al: Electromyographic activity of selected shoulder muscles in commonly used therapeutic exercises. Phys Ther 73:668, 1993.

6. Barrett, WP, and Frankin, JL: Total shoulder arthroplasty. J Bone Joint Surg Am 69:866–872, 1987.

7. Bassett, RW, et al: Glenohumeral muscle force and movement mechanics in a position of shoulder instability. J Biomech 23:405, 1990.

8. Bigliani, LV, et al: Repair of rotator cuff tears in tennis players. Am J Sports Med 20(2):112–117, 1992.

9. Binder, AI, et al: Frozen shoulder: A long-term prospective study. Ann Rheum Dis 43:361, 1984.

10. Blakely, RL, and Palmer, ML: Analysis of rotation accompanying shoulder flexion. Phys Ther 64:1214, 1984.

11. Blakely, RL, and Palmer, ML: Analysis of shoulder rotation accompanying a proprioceptive neuromuscular facilitation approach. Phys Ther 66:1224, 1986.

12. Brewster, C, and Schwar, DRM: Rehabilitation of the shoulder following rotator cuff injury or surgery. Journal of Orthopaedic and Sports Physical Therapy 18:422, 1993.

13. Brostrom, LA, et al: The effect of shoulder muscle training in patients with recurrent shoulder dislocations. Scand J Rehabil Med 24:11, 1992.

14. Brunet, ME, Haddad, RJ, and Porche, EB: Rotator cuff impingement syndrome in sports. The Physician and Sports Medicine 10:87, 1982.

15. Burkhead, WZ, and Rockwood, CA: Treatment of instability of the shoulder with an exercise program. J Bone Joint Surg Am 74:890, 1992.

16. Cailliet, R: Shoulder Pain, ed 3. FA Davis, Philadelphia, 1991.

17. Cain, PR, et al: Anterior stability of the glenohumeral joint. Am J Sports Med 15:144, 1987.

18. Cash, JD: Recent advances and perspectives on arthroscopic stabilization of the shoulder. Clin Sports Med 10(4):871–886, 1991.

19. Caspari, RB: Arthroscopic reconstruction for anterior shoulder instability. In Paulos, LE, and Tibone, JE (eds); Operative Techniques in Shoulder Surgery. Aspen, Gaithersburg, MD, 1991.

20. Codman, EA: The Shoulder. Thomas Todd Company, Boston, 1934.

21. Cofield, R, Morrey, B, and Bryan, R: Total shoulder and total elbow arthroplasties: The current state of development—Part I. Journal of Continuing Education Orthopedics 6:14, 1978.

22. Cuetter, AC, and Bartoszek, DM: The thoracic outlet syndrome: Controversies, overdiagnosis, overtreatment, and recommendations for management. Muscle Nerve 12:410, 1989.

23. Culhan, E, and Peat, M: Functional anatomy of the shoulder complex. Journal of Orthopaedic and Sports Physical Therapy 18:342, 1993.

24. Cyriax, J: Textbook of Orthopaedic Medicine, Vol. 1. Diagnosis of Soft Tissue Lesions, ed 8. Baillière Tendall, London, 1982.

25. Cyriax, J: Textbook of Orthopaedic Medicine, Vol. 2. Treatment by Manipulation, Massage and Injection, ed 10. Baillière Tendall, London, 1980.

26. Davies, GJ, and Dickoff-Hoffman, S: Neuromuscular testing and rehabilitation of the shoulder complex. Journal of Orthopaedic and Sports Physical Therapy 18:449, 1993.

27. DePalma, AF: Surgery of the Shoulder, ed 3. JB Lippincott, Philadelphia, 1983.

28. Dontigny, R: Passive shoulder exercises. Phys Ther 50:1707, 1970.

29. Ellman, H: Arthroscopic subacromial decompression. In Welsh, RP, and Shephard, RJ (eds): Current Therapy in Sports Medicine, Vol. 2. BC Decker, Toronto, 1990.

30. Engle, RP, and Canner, GC: Posterior shoulder instability: Approach to rehabilitation. Journal of Orthopaedic and Sports Physical Therapy 10(12): 70–78, 1989.

31. Fahey, VA: Thoracic outlet syndrome. J Cardiovasc Nurs 1:12, 1987.

32. Fu, FH, Harner, CD, and Klein, AH: Shoulder impingement syndrome: a critical review. Clin Orthop 269:162, 1991.

33. Grey, RG: The natural history of idiopathic frozen shoulder. J Bone Joint Surg Am 60:564, 1978.

34. Griffin, JW: Hemiplegic shoulder pain. Phys Ther 66:1884, 1986.

35. Gross, RM: Arthroscopic shoulder capsulorrhaphy: Does it work? Am J Sports Med 17:495, 1989.

36. Grubbs, N: Frozen shoulder syndrome: A review of literature. Journal of Orthopaedic and Sports Physical Therapy 18:479, 1993.

37. Guidotti, TL: Occupational repetitive strain injury. Am Fam Physician 45:585, 1992.
38. Hawkins, RJ, and Abrams, JS: Impingement syndrome in the absence of rotator cuff tear (stages 1 and 2). Orthop Clin North Am 18:373, 1987.
39. Hawkins, RJ, et al: Acromioplasty for impingement with an intact rotator cuff. J Bone Joint Surg Br 70 (5):795–797, 1988.
40. Hawkins, RJ, and Kunkel, SS: Rotator cuff tears. In: Welsh, RP, and Shepherd, RJ (eds): Current Therapy in Sports Medicine, Vol 2. BC Decker, Toronto, 1990.
41. Hawkins, RJ, Misamore, GW, and Hobeika, PE: Surgery of full thickness rotator cuff tears. J Bone Joint Surg Am 67(9):1349–1355, 1985.
42. Hawkins, RJ, Koppert, G, and Johnston, G: Recurrent posterior instability (subluxation) of the shoulder. J Bone Joint Surg Am 66:169, 1984.
43. Hawkins, RJ, Misamore, GW, and Hobeika, PE: Surgery for full-thickness rotator cuff tears. J Bone Joint Surg Am 67:1349, 1985.
44. Hernandez, A, and Drez, D: Operative treatment of posterior shoulder dislocation by posterior glenoidplasty, capsulorrhapy and infraspinatus advancement. Am J Sports Med 14:187, 1986.
45. Ho, CP: Applied MRI anatomy of the shoulder. Journal of Orthopaedic and Sports Physical Therapy 18:351, 1993.
46. Hoppenfeld, S: Physical Examination of the Spine and Extremities. Appleton-Century-Crofts, New York, 1976.
47. Jobe, FW, and Glousman, RE: Anterior capsulolaboral reconstruction. Techniques in orthopedics: The Shoulder, Vol 3. Aspen, Rockville, MD, 1989.
48. Jobe, FW, Moynes, DR, and Brewster, CE: Rehabilitation of shoulder joint instabilities. Orthop Clin North Am 18:473, 1987.
49. Jobe, FW, and Pink, M: Classification and treatment of shoulder dysfunction in the overhead athlete. Journal of Orthopaedic and Sports Physical Therapy 18:427, 1993.
50. Kaltenborn, F: Manual Mobilization of the Extremity Joints, ed 4. Olaf Norlis Bokhandel, Oslo, 1989.
51. Kamkar, A, Irrgang, JJ, and Whitney, SI: Nonoperative management of secondary shoulder impingement syndrome. Journal of Orthopaedic and Sports Physical Therapy 17(5):212–224, 1993.
52. Kennedy, K; Rehabilitation of the unstable shoulder. Sportsmedicine Performance and Research Center, WB Saunders, 1993.
53. Kessler, R, and Hertling, D: Management of Common Musculoskeletal Disorders. Harper & Row, Philadelphia, 1983.
54. Kuland, DN: The Injured Athlete, ed 2. JB Lippincott, Philadelphia, 1988.
55. Kumar, VP, Satku, K, and Balasubramaniam, P: The role of the long head of the biceps brachii in the stabilization in the head of the humerus. Clin Orthop 244:172, 1989.
56. Lehmkuhl, LD, and Smith, LK: Brunnstrom's Clinical Kinesiology, ed 4. FA Davis, Philadelphia, 1983.
57. Litchfield, R, et al: Rehabilitation for the overhead athlete. Journal of Orthopaedic and Sports Physical Therapy 18:433, 1993.
58. Lord, J, and Rosati, JM: Thoracic outlet syndromes, Vol 23. CIBA Pharmaceutical Co, Summit, NJ, 1971.
59. Malone, TR: Principles of rehabilitation and prehabilitation. Sports Injury Management 1:42, 1988.
60. Matzen, FA, and Arntz, CT: Subacromial impingements. In Rockwood, CA, and Matzen, FA (eds): The Shoulder, Vol 2. WB Saunders, Philadelphia, 1990.
61. Meister, K, and Andrews, JR: Classification and treatment of rotator cuff injuries in the overhand athlete. Journal of Orthopaedic and Sports Physical Therapy 18:413, 1993.
62. Neer, CS: Impingement lesions. Clin Orthop 173:70, 1983.
63. Neer, CS: Shoulder Reconstruction. WB Saunders, Philadelphia, 1990.
64. Neer, CS: Anterior acromioplasty for the chronic impingement syndrome in the shoulder. A preliminary report. J Bone Joint Surg Am 54:41, 1972.
65. Neer, CS: Articular replacement of the humeral head. J Bone Joint Surg Am 37:215, 1955.
66. Neer, CS: Displaced proximal humeral fractures. J Bone Joint Surg Am 52:1077, 1970.
67. Neer, CS: Prosthetic replacement of the humeral head: Indications and operative technique. Surg Clin North Am 43:158, 1963.
68. Neer, CS: Replacement arthroplasty for glenohumeral osteoarthritis. J Bone Joint Surg Am 56:1, 1974.
69. Nevaiser, RJ, and Nevaiser, TJ: The frozen shoulder: Diagnosis and management. Clin Orthop 223:59, 1987.
70. Nevaiser, RJ: Ruptures of the rotator cuff. Orthop Clin North Am 18:387, 1987.
71. Nevaiser, RJ: Injuries to the clavicle and acromioclavicular joint. Orthop Clin North Am 18:433, 1987.
72. Nevaiser, TJ: Adhesive capsulitis. Orthop Clin North Am 18:439, 1987.
73. Nevaiser, TJ: The role of the biceps tendon in the impingement syndrome. Orthop Clin North Am 18:383, 1987.
74. Nicholson, GG: The effects of passive joint mobilization on pain and hypomobility associated with adhesive capsulitis of the shoulder. Journal of Orthopaedic and Sports Physical Therapy 6:238, 1985.
75. Noonan, TJ, and Garrett, WE: Injuries at the myotendinous junction. Clin Sports Med 11:783, 1992.
76. Norkin, C, and Levangie, P: Joint Structure and Function: A Comprehensive Analysis, ed 2. FA Davis, Philadelphia, 1992.
77. O'Brien, M: Functional anatomy and physiology of tendons. Clin Sports Med 11:505, 1992.
78. O'Brien, SJ, Warren, RF, and Schwartz, E: Anterior shoulder instability. Orthop Clin North Am 18:385, 1987.
79. Occupational Therapy Staff: Upper Extremity Surgeries for Patients with Arthritis: A Pre and Postoperative Occupational Therapy Treatment Guide. Rancho Los Amigos Hospital, California, 1979.
80. Paine, RM, and Voight, M: The role of the scapula. Journal of Orthopaedic and Sports Physical Therapy 18:386, 1993.
81. Palmer, ML, and Blakely, RL: Documentation of medial rotation accompanying shoulder flexion: A case report. Phys Ther 66:55, 1986.
82. Pang, D, and Wessel, HB: Thoracic outlet syndrome. Neurosurgery 22:105, 1988.
83. Penny, JW, and Welsh, MB: Shoulder impingement

syndromes in athletes and their surgical management. Am J Sports Med 9:11, 1981.

84. Post, M, Morrey, BE, and Hawkins, RJ (eds): Surgery of the Shoulder. Mosby Year-Book, St Louis, 1990.

85. Rockwood, CA, and Lyons, FR: Shoulder impingement syndrome: Diagnosis, radiographic evaluation, and treatment with a modified Neer acromioplasty. J Bone Joint Surg Am 75:409, 1993.

86. Rodosky, MW, and Harner, CD: The role of the long head of the biceps muscle and superior glenoid labrum in anterior stability of the shoulder. Am J Sports Med 22:121, 1994.

87. Rose, BS: Frozen shoulder. N Z Med J 98(792):1039, 1985.

88. Rowe, CR: Anterior glenohumeral subluxation/dislocation: The Bankart procedure. In Welsh, RP, and Shephard, RJ (eds): Current Therapy in Sports Medicine, Vol 2. BC Decker, Toronto, 1990.

89. Schieb, JS: Diagnosis and rehabilitation of the shoulder impingement syndrome in the overhand and throwing athlete. Rheum Dis Clin North Am, 16:971, 1990.

90. Schwartz, E, et al: Posterior shoulder instability. Orthop Clin North Am 18:409, 1987.

91. Simkin, PA: Tendinitis and bursitis of the shoulder, anatomy and therapy. Postgrad Med J 73:177, 1983.

92. Simon, ER, and Hill, JA: Rotator cuff Injuries: An update. Journal of Orthopaedic and Sports Physical Therapy 10(10):394–398, 1989.

93. Smith, K: The thoracic outlet syndrome: A protocol of treatment. Journal of Orthopaedic and Sports Physical Therapy 1:89, 1979.

94. Sucher, BM: Thoracic outlet syndrome: A myofascial variant: Part 1. Pathology and diagnosis. J Am Osteopath Assoc 90:686, 1990.

95. Sucher, BM: Thoracic outlet syndrome: A myofascial variant: Part 2. Treatment, J Am Osteopath Assoc 90:810, 1990.

96. Swanson, AB, et al: Upper limb joint replacement. In Nickel, VL (ed): Orthopedic Rehabilitation. Churchill-Livingstone, New York, 1982.

97. Thomas, BJ, and Amstuts, HC: Shoulder arthroplasty for rheumatoid arthritis. Clin Orthop 269:125, 1991.

98. Tibone, JE, et al: Surgical treatment of tears of the rotator cuff in athletes. J Bone Joint Surg Am 68:887, 1986.

99. Townsend, H, et al: Electromyographic analysis of the glenohumeral muscles during a baseball rehabilitation program. Am J Sports Med 19:264, 1991.

100. Turkel, SJ, et al: Stabilizing Mechanisms Preventing Anterior Dislocation of the Glenohumeral Joint. J Bone Joint Surg Am 61:1208, 1981.

101. Wadsworth, CT: Frozen shoulder. Phys Ther 66: 1878, 1986.

102. Wilde, AH, Brems, JJ, Bounphrey, FRS: Artrodesis of the Shoulder: Current indications and operative technique. Orthop Clin North Am 18:463–472, 1987.

103. Wilk, KE, et al: Stretch-shortening drills for the upper extremities: Theory and clinical application. Journal of Orthopaedic and Sports Physical Therapy 17(5):225–239, 1993.

104. Wilk, KE, and Arrigo C: An integrated approach to upper extremity exercises. Orthopaedic Physical Therapy Clinics of North America 1:337, 1992.

105. Wilk, KE, and Arrigo, C: Current concepts in the rehabilitation of the athletic shoulder. Journal of Orthopaedic and Sports Physical Therapy 18:365, 1993.

Chapter

9

The Elbow and Forearm Complex

The design of the elbow and forearm adds to the mobility of the hand in space by shortening and lengthening the upper extremity and by rotating the forearm. The muscles provide control and stability to the region as the hand is used for various activities from eating, pushing, and pulling to coordinated use of tools and machines.[22]

The anatomic and kinesiologic relationships of the elbow and forearm are outlined in the first section of this chapter; the reader is also referred to several textbooks for in-depth study of the background material.[3,5,7,9,10,13] Chapter 7 presents information on principles of management; the reader should be familiar with that material before proceeding with establishing a therapeutic exercise program for the elbow and forearm.

OBJECTIVES

After studying this chapter, the reader will be able to:

1 Identify important aspects of elbow and forearm structure and function for review.
2 Establish a therapeutic exercise program to manage soft tissue and joint lesions in the elbow and forearm region related to stages of recovery following an inflammatory insult to the tissues, recognizing unique circumstances for their management.
3 Establish a therapeutic exercise program to manage patients following common surgical procedures.

I. Review of the Structure and Function of the Elbow and Forearm

A. Bony Parts Are the Distal Humerus, Radius, and Ulna (see Fig. 6–25)

B. Joints and Their Movements

1. The capsule of the elbow encloses three joints

a. The humeroulnar, which is the primary joint for flexion and extension

b. The humeroradial, which moves with flexion and extension but primarily affects pronation and supination

c. The proximal radioulnar, which participates in pronation and supination

2. The distal radioulnar joint

This joint is structurally separate from the elbow complex but moves with the proximal radioulnar joint as a functional unit for pronation and supination.

3. Elbow joint characteristics

The elbow is a compound joint with a lax joint capsule, supported by two major ligaments: the medial (ulnar) and lateral (radial) collateral.

a. Humeroulnar articulation

(1) This is a modified hinge joint. The medially placed hourglass-shaped trochlea at the distal end of the humerus is convex. It faces anteriorly and downward 45 degrees from the shaft of the humerus. The concave trochlear fossa, on the proximal ulna, faces upward and anteriorly 45 degrees from the ulna[9] (see Fig. 6–26).

(2) The primary motion is flexion and extension; the concave fossa slides in the same direction in which the ulna moves.

(3) There is also slight medial and lateral sliding of the ulna, allowing for full elbow ROM; it results in a valgus angulation of the joint with elbow extension and a varus angulation with elbow flexion. When the bone moves in a medial/lateral direction, the trochlear ridge provides a convex surface, and the trochlear groove provides a concave surface, so the sliding of the ulna is opposite the bone motion.

Physiologic Motion of Ulna	Direction of Slide of Ulna on Trochlea
Flexion	Distal/anterior
Varus angulation	Lateral
Extension	Proximal/posterior
Valgus angulation	Medial

b. The humeroradial joint

(1) This is a hinge-pivot joint. The laterally placed, spherical capitulum at the distal end of the humerus is convex. The concave bony partner, the head of the radius, is at the proximal end of the radius.

(2) As the elbow flexes and extends, the concave radial head slides in the same direction as the bone motion. With pronation and supination of the forearm, the radial head spins on the capitulum.

Physiologic Motion of Radius	Direction of Slide of Radius on Capitulum
Flexion	Anterior
Extension	Posterior

4. Forearm joint characteristics

Both the proximal and distal radioulnar joints are uniaxial pivot joints that function as one joint to produce pronation and supination (rotation) of the forearm.

a. The proximal (superior) radioulnar joint

(1) It is within the capsule of the elbow joint but is a distinct articulation.

(2) The convex rim of the radial head articulates with the concave radial notch on the ulna so that, with rotation of the radius, the convex rim moves opposite to the bone motion.

Physiologic Motion of Radius	*Direction of Slide of Proximal Radius on Ulna*
Pronation	Posterior (dorsal)
Supination	Anterior (volar)

(3) With rotation of the radial head, it spins in the annular ligament and against the capitulum of the humerus.

b. The distal (inferior) radioulnar joint

(1) The concave ulnar notch on the distal radius articulates with the convex portion of the head of the ulna.

(2) With physiologic movements, the articulating surface of the radius slides in the same direction.

Physiologic Motion of Radius	*Direction of Slide of Distal Radius on Ulna*
Pronation	Anterior (volar)
Supination	Posterior (dorsal)

C. Muscle Function at the Elbow and Forearm

1. Elbow flexor muscles

a. Brachialis

The brachialis is a one-joint muscle that inserts close to the axis of motion on the ulna, so it is unaffected by the position of the forearm or the shoulder; it participates in all flexion activities of the elbow.

b. Biceps brachii

The biceps is a two-joint muscle that crosses both the shoulder and elbow and inserts close to the axis of motion on the radius, so it also acts as a supinator of the forearm. It functions most effectively as a flexor of the elbow between 80 and 100 degrees of flexion. For optimal length-tension relationship, the shoulder extends to lengthen the muscle when it contracts forcefully for elbow and forearm function.

c. Brachioradialis

With its insertion a great distance from the elbow on the distal radius, the bracioradialis mainly functions to provide stability to the joint, but it also participates as the speed of flexion motion increases and a load is applied with the forearm from midsupination to full pronation.[22]

2. Elbow extensor muscles

a. Triceps brachii

The long head crosses both the shoulder and elbow; the other two heads are uniaxial. The long head functions most effectively as an elbow extensor if the shoulder simultaneously flexes; this maintains an optimal length-tension relationship in the muscle.

    b. Anconeus

    This muscle stabilizes the elbow during supination and pronation and assists in elbow extension.

3. Forearm supinator muscles

    a. Biceps brachii

    See Section 1.a.

    b. Supinator

    The proximal attachment of the supinator at the annular and lateral collateral ligaments may function to stabilize the lateral aspect of the elbow. Its effectiveness as a supinator is not affected by the elbow position as is the biceps brachii.[27]

4. Forearm pronator muscles

    a. Pronator teres

    This muscle pronates as well as stabilizes the proximal radioulnar joint and helps approximate the humeroradial articulation.[22]

    b. Pronator quadratus

    The pronator quadratus is a one-joint muscle and is active during all pronation activities.

D. Wrist and Hand Muscles

Many muscles that act on the wrist and hand are attached on the distal portion (epicondyles) of the humerus. This allows for movement of the fingers and wrist, whether the forearm is in pronation or supination.

1. Originating on the medial epicondyle are the flexor carpi radialis, flexor carpi ulnaris, palmaris longus, and flexor digitorum superficialis and profundus.
2. Originating on the lateral epicondyle are the extensor carpi radialis longus and brevis, extensor carpi ulnaris, and extensor digitorum.
3. The muscles provide stability to the elbow but contribute little to motion at the elbow. The position of the elbow will affect the length-tension relationship of the muscles during their actions on the wrist and hand.[22]

E. Major Nerves Subject to Pressure and Trauma Around the Elbow[11]

1. Ulnar nerve

The nerve is superficial to the olecranon fossa, posterior to the medial epicondyle, and covered by a fibrous sheath, which forms the cubital tunnel; it then passes between the heads of the flexor carpi ulnaris. Pressure or injury to the nerve at these sites will cause sensory changes in the cutaneous distribution of the nerve (ulnar border of the hand, little finger, and ulnar half of the ring finger), with progressive weakness in the muscles innervated distal to the site of injury (flexor carpi ulnaris, ulnar half of the flexor digitorum profundus, hypothenar eminence, interossei, lumbricals III and IV, flexor pollicis brevis, and adductor pollicis).

2. Radial nerve

The nerve pierces the lateral muscular septum anterior to the lateral epicondyle and passes under the origin of the extensor carpi radialis brevis and then divides.

   a. The deep branch may become entrapped as it passes under the edge of the extensor carpi radialis brevis and the fibrous slit in the supinator, causing progressive weakness in the wrist and finger extensor and supinator muscles (except the extensor carpi radialis longus, which is innervated proximal to the bifurcation).

   b. The deep branch may also be injured with a radial head fracture.

   c. The superficial radial nerve may receive direct trauma that causes sensory changes in the lateral aspect of the forearm to the anatomic snuffbox, and the radial side of the dorsum of the wrist and hand and radial three and one-half digits.

3. Median nerve

The nerve courses deep in the cubital fossa, medial to the tendon of the biceps and brachial artery, then progresses between the ulnar and humeral heads of the pronator teres and dips under the flexor digitorum sublimis muscle. Entrapment may occur between the heads of the pronator muscle, causing sensory changes duplicating carpal tunnel syndrome (palmar aspect of the thumb, index, middle, and half of the ring finger, and dorsal aspect of distal phalanges of index and ring fingers). Motor changes include the pronator teres, wrist flexors, extrinsic finger flexors, and the intrinsic thenar and lumbricals I and II. (Carpal tunnel syndrome involves just the intrinsic muscles of the thenar eminence and lumbricals I and II; see Chapter 10.)

II. Joint Problems: Nonoperative Management

A. Related Diagnoses and Etiology of Symptoms

Pathologies such as rheumatoid arthritis (RA) and degenerative joint disease (DJD) as well as acute joint reactions following trauma, dislocations, or fractures affect this joint complex. Postimmobilization tightness develops in the joint and surrounding tissues any time the joint is splinted or casted, most commonly following dislocations and fractures of the humerus, radius, or ulna.

B. Common Impairments/Problems[4]

1. When symptoms are acute, the joint effusion, muscle guarding, and pain restrict elbow flexion and extension, and there is usually pain at rest. If pronation and/or supination are restricted following an acute injury, other conditions such as fracture, subluxation, or dislocation may be present.

2. When subacute or chronic, elbow flexion is usually more restricted than extension with a firm end-feel.

3. In long-standing arthritis and radial head involvement, pronation and supination also become restricted with a firm end-feel.

4. Arthritis in the distal radioulnar joint results in pain on overpressure.

C. Common Functional Limitations/Disabilities

1. Unable to turn a door knob or key in the ignition

2. Difficulty or pain with pushing and pulling activities such as opening and closing doors

3. Restricted hand to mouth activities for eating and drinking, and hand to head activities for personal grooming and using a telephone

4. Difficulty or pain with pushing self up from a chair
5. Unable to carry objects with a straight arm

D. Management of Acute Joint Lesions

See guidelines for management in Chapter 7, Section III.

1. To control pain effusion and muscle guarding
   a. Immobilization in a sling provides rest to the part, but complete immobilization can lead to contractures and limited motion, so frequent periods of controlled movement within a pain-free range should be performed.
   b. Gentle grade I or II distraction and oscillation techniques in the resting position may inhibit pain and move synovial fluid for nutrition in the involved joints (see Chapter 6 for techniques).

2. To maintain soft tissue mobility
   a. Passive or active assistive ROM within limits of pain; include flexion/extension and pronation/supination.
   b. Multiple-angle muscle setting to elbow flexors, extensors, pronators and supinators, and to wrist flexors and extensors in pain-free positions.

3. To maintain integrity and function to related areas
   a. Shoulder, wrist, and hand range of motion and activities should be encouraged within the tolerance of the individual.
   b. If edema develops in the hand, the arms should be elevated whenever possible and distal to proximal massage techniques applied.

E. Management of Subacute and Chronic Joint Restrictions

Precaution: Following trauma, if the brachialis muscle is injured, ossification of the injured tissue is a potential complication; therefore, evaluate for signs of myositis ossificans (see Section C to follow). If myositis ossificans is not present, progress stretching carefully.

1. To increase joint play in the humeroulnar joint
   a. To increase flexion
      Sustained distraction of the ulna (see Figure 5–27A).
      Sustained distraction with distal glide of the ulna (see Figure 5–27B).
      Sustained lateral glide or varus angulation of the ulna is used to gain the terminal degrees of flexion.
   b. To increase extension
      (1) Sustained distraction of the ulna (see Fig. 6–27A).
      (2) Medial glide or valgus angulation of the ulna is used to gain the terminal degrees of extension.

2. To increase joint play of the humeroradial joint

Precaution: If flexion and extension are limited as well as rotation following trauma, there may be a fracture of the radial head.[5] This must be ruled out before proceeding with treatment. Or there may be a subluxation of the radial head, which requires special procedures depending of the type of subluxation. (See Sections 3 and 4 following.)

   a. To increase flexion
      (1) Sustained distraction of the radial head (see Fig. 6–28)
      (2) Sustained volar glide head of radius (see Fig. 6–29)

b. To increase extension
   (1) Sustained distraction of the radial head
   (2) Sustained dorsal glide head of radius (see Fig. 6–29)
c. See also Sections 5 and 6 below to increase pronation and supination.

3. To treat a proximal subluxation of the radial head (pushed elbow)

a. Clinical picture
   There may be limited flexion or extension of the elbow, limited wrist flexion, and limited pronation. It often occurs from falling on an outstretched hand.[31] The radial head is pushed proximally in the annular ligament and impinges against the capitulum. This sometimes accompanies a fracture of the distal radius (Colles' fracture) or scaphoid and is not considered a clinical problem until after healing of the fracture and removal of the cast. It is often overlooked because there is considerable soft tissue and joint restriction caused by the period of immobilization. Bilateral palpation of the joint spaces will reveal the decreased space on the involved side.

b. Management
   If acute (and no fracture), a distal traction of the radius will reposition the radial head. If chronic, it will require repetitive stretching with sustained grade III distal traction to the radius (see Fig. 6–28), in addition to the soft tissue stretching and strengthening techniques needed for increasing motion.

4. To treat a distal subluxation of the radial head (pulled elbow)

a. Clinical picture
   There is limited supination with pain in the elbow region following a forceful traction to the forearm. This is usually seen as an acute injury in children and is sometimes labeled "tennis elbow" when it occurs in adults.[31]

b. Management
   A quick compressive manipulation with supination to the radius (see Fig. 6–30) will usually reposition the head. If it is an initial injury, there may be soft tissue trauma from the injury, which is treated with cold and compression.

5. To increase joint play of the proximal radioulnar joint

a. To increase pronation
   Dorsal glide radial head (see Fig. 6–31)
b. To increase supination
   Volar glide radial head (see Fig. 6–31)

6. To increase joint play of the distal radioulnar joint

a. To increase pronation
   Sustained volar glide distal radius (see Fig. 6–32)
b. To increase supination
   Sustained dorsal glide distal radius (see Fig. 6–32)
c. To treat for pain
   Grade I or II oscillations, dorsal-volar glides

NOTE: Following healing of fractures in the forearm, malunion is not unusual, preventing full range of pronation or supination. A bony block end-feel or an abnormal appearance of the forearm should alert the therapist. X-ray films are helpful in verifying the problem. No amount of stretching or mobilizing will change the patient's range. Indiscriminate stretching may lead to hypermobility of related joints, which could cause additional trauma and pain.

7. To progress functional exercises

    a. Use muscle inhibition techniques to gain muscle flexibility if necessary.

    b. Progress strengthening exercises as described in Section VI. Use care to stay within the tolerance of the joints.

III. Joint Surgery and Postoperative Management

Surgical intervention at the elbow is often necessary following a variety of fractures or dislocations that affect the joint and require open reduction, possible excision of bone fragments or portions of the radial head, and internal fixation. The most common fracture in the elbow region is a fracture of the head of the radius. If displacement occurs or if the fracture is comminuted, a *radial head excision (resection)* is indicated. Fracture dislocation at the elbow that involves the radial head will also have to be treated surgically. In general, open reduction with internal fixation is more often indicated for adults than for children.

Another indication for surgery is long-standing rheumatoid arthritis or osteoarthritis leading to synovial proliferation and destruction of articular surfaces of the elbow joints, which result in pain, limitation of motion, and loss of upper extremity function. In early-stage rheumatoid arthritis in which synovial proliferation is present but joint surfaces are still in good condition, *arthroscopic synovectomy* is the procedure of choice if medications have not controlled the disease. Late-stage arthritis may need to be treated surgically by resection of the radial head with or without joint implant and concurrent synovectomy or by *total elbow arthroplasty.*

The goals of surgery and postoperative rehabilitation of the elbow joint[4,16,19,28] can include (1) relief of pain, (2) restoration of bony alignment and joint stability, and (3) sufficient strength and range of motion to allow functional use of the elbow and upper extremity. Procedures done to relieve pain and improve elbow stability tend to be more successful than procedures done solely to increase range of motion. Heterotopic bone formation, which leads to joint stiffness, is often a complication of elbow fractures and elbow joint surgery.[8] Therefore, the single goal of improving range of motion is rarely an indication for surgery.[19,20]

In the postoperative period, as with any other surgical procedure of the extremities, it is important to maintain range of motion and strength in all unoperated joints. Special attention should be given to the shoulder, wrist, and hand after elbow surgery. Elevation of the operated extremity and active range of motion of the shoulder and hand, as soon after surgery as possible, will prevent dysfunction in these unoperated regions.

A. Excision of the Radial Head

1. Indications for surgery[19,20]

    a. Severe comminuted fractures or fracture dislocations of the head of the radius often as the result of a fall on an outstretched arm

    b. Chronic synovitis and mild deterioration of the articular surfaces associated with arthritis of the humeroradial and proximal radioulnar joints resulting in joint pain at rest or with motion, possible subluxation of the head of the radius, and significant loss of upper extremity function

2. Procedure[19,20]

    a. A lateral incision at the elbow and forearm is made (arthrotomy); the radial head is resected.

b. For the patient with synovitis a synovectomy precedes the removal of the head of the radius. The head of the radius may or may not be replaced with a prosthetic implant.

3. Postoperative management[17,24]

a. *Immobilization*

The elbow is immobilized in a posterior splint or compression bandage for up to 3 to 5 days for maximum protection of the area. The elbow is held in a position of 90 degrees of flexion and the forearm is held in mid-position. The arm is elevated for comfort and to prevent or minimize edema distally. The splint is removed for exercise but is replaced after exercise and worn at night for several weeks.

b. *Exercise*

MAXIMUM-PROTECTION PHASE

(1) To maintain mobility and prevent stiffness in the shoulder, hand, and wrist, initiate active ROM to the regions immediately.

(2) To maintain mobility of the elbow, remove the splint several times daily and begin passive or active-assisted ROM within the pain-free ranges as soon as possible after surgery. Continuous passive motion (CPM) may also be used in the first few postoperative days.

(3) To minimize atrophy, submaximal pain-free multiple-angle isometrics of elbow musculature are also indicated.

MODERATE- AND MINIMUM-PROTECTION PHASES

(1) Progress from active-assistive to active exercise over the next 3 to 6 weeks. During this time the patient must avoid lifting heavy objects with the operated arm and hand.

(2) By 6 weeks postoperatively full joint activity is allowed.

(a) Progressive resistance exercises (open- and closed-chain and eccentric and concentric isotonic resistance training) may be implemented slowly and cautiously. Emphasis is placed on improving strength and endurance.

(b) Gentle stretching using inhibition/elongation techniques or joint mobilizations (see Chapters 5 and 6) may be necessary to increase ROM.

(3) A more aggressive exercise program is appropriate for the patient who has undergone excision of the radial head for a comminuted fracture or fracture dislocation than for the patient with arthritis of the elbow. High-intensity, high-speed training activities in functional movement patterns are indicated for the individual wishing to return to high-demand recreational or occupational activities. The rehabilitation program for the patient with polyarticular rheumatoid arthritis is less strenuous. A good result in these patients is relief of pain and adequate strength for ADL even if some degree of limitation of motion persists.

B. Total Elbow Arthroplasty

1. Indications for surgery[4,19,20,25,28]

a. Pain and articular destruction of the humeroulnar and humeroradial joints, resulting in loss of functional use of the upper extremity

b. Marked limitation of motion at the elbow, particularly in patients with bilateral ankylosis of the elbow

c. Gross instability of the elbow

d. Bone stock loss from trauma or tumors

2. Procedure

a. *General background*[4,18–20,25,28]

Several humeroulnar joint replacements have been developed over the years. The early designs were *hinged (constrained) metal prostheses,* allowing only flexion and extension of the elbow joint. These implants eventually failed because no allowances for normal varus and valgus and rotational movements of the elbow were incorporated into these early designs and, hence, the prosthesis loosened. More recent implants now build in all appropriate elbow motions. The majority of total elbow replacements done today are either *semiconstrained* or *unconstrained (resurfacing) replacements.* The unconstrained designs do not provide additional elbow joint stability. If significant joint instability is present, semiconstrained designs are used.

b. *Overview of the procedure*[4,14,19,20,28,29]

(1) A longitudinal incision is made at the posterior aspect of the elbow.

(2) The triceps muscle is incised (split), reflected, and later reattached, and small portions of the distal humerus and proximal ulna are resected.

(3) A stainless steel humeral replacement and a polyethylene ulnar component are cemented in place with methyl methacrylate. Other designs are composed of stainless steel humeral and ulnar components. More recent implants, designed to minimize loosening, include an intramedullary cemented stem and extramedullary flange for osseous ingrowth. In the future, cementless elbow components may minimize prosthetic loosening at the bone-cement interface, which continues to be the most common cause of failure of elbow arthroplasty.

(4) If the head of the radius is removed, it may or may not be replaced with a prosthetic implant.

3. Postoperative management[2,17,24,28]

a. *Immobilization*

Immediately after surgery a soft compression dressing and posterior splint are applied to immobilize the elbow in approximately 60 to 90 degrees of flexion and a neutral position of the forearm

b. *Exercise*

MAXIMUM-PROTECTION PHASE

(1) During the period (3 to 5 days) of immobilization of the elbow

    (a) The arm is elevated in bed or supported with a sling when the patient is upright.

    (b) Active finger, wrist, and shoulder exercises are performed to minimize edema in the hand and maintain normal motion in the joints proximal and distal to the elbow.

(2) Between 3 and 5 days postoperatively the splint is removed, and active-assistive range of motion of the elbow is started with the patient in a supine position and the patient's arm at the side. The exercises include:

(a) Active-assistive flexion and passive extension of the elbow with the forearm in supination, pronation, and mid-position.

> **Precaution:** Avoid any *antigravity* elbow extension or stretch to the triceps to protect the reattachment of the triceps mechanism.

(b) Active supination and pronation of the forearm with the elbow in 90 degrees of flexion.

(c) The splint should be worn for the next 4 to 6 weeks when the patient is not exercising.

MODERATE- AND MINIMUM-PROTECTION PHASES

(1) Between 8 and 10 days, a new splint is fabricated with the elbow in maximum comfortable extension. The patient alternates wearing the extension and the flexion splints to maintain as much range of motion as possible.

(2) At 3 to 4 weeks, active anti-gravity elbow extension may be added to the patient's exercises.

(3) By 6 weeks postoperatively, when the triceps mechanism is secure, gentle isotonic resistance exercise and partial weight-bearing closed-chain activities may be started. This is continued until the patient is using the arm in all normal activities of daily living.

4. Long-term results[2,4,19,28]

a. A good functional result gives the patient at least a 90-degree arc of pain-free elbow flexion and extension. The patient should strive for at least 110 degrees of flexion and full extension, but elbow flexion contractures often persist. Forearm pronation and supination usually correlate with preoperative ROM, averaging a total of 60 degrees.

b. **Precaution:** The patient should avoid using the operated arm for lifting and carrying heavy objects, as this may result in loosening of the components.

IV. Myositis Ossificans

A. Etiology of Symptoms

The brachialis muscle may be affected following trauma in the elbow region. Myositis ossificans is most commonly seen with a supracondylar fracture and posterior dislocation[12] or with a tear of the brachialis tendon.[5] It may also develop as the result of aggressive stretching of the elbow flexors after injury and a period of immobilization. It is distinguished from traumatic arthritis of the humeroulnar joint in that passive extension is more limited than flexion, resisted elbow flexion causes pain, flexion is limited and painful when the inflamed muscle is pinched between the humerus and ulna, and resisted flexion in mid-range causes pain in the brachialis muscle. Palpation of the distal brachialis muscle is tender. After the acute inflammatory period, heterotopic bone formation is laid down in muscle, which can permanently restrict elbow extension and make the muscle extremely firm to touch.

B. Management

If the brachialis muscle is implicated following trauma, massage, passive stretching, and exercise should *not* be undertaken. The elbow should be kept at rest.

V. Overuse Syndromes: Repetitive Trauma Syndromes

A. Related Diagnoses

1. Lateral epicondylitis or tennis elbow

There is pain in the common wrist extensor tendons along the lateral epicondyle and radiohumeral joint. Activities such as the backhand stroke in tennis, requiring firm wrist stability, or pulling weeds in a garden, which requires repeated wrist extension, can inflame the musculotendinous unit and cause symptoms. The highest incidence is in the musculotendinous junction of the extensor carpi radialis brevis.[5,10,23] Symptoms also occur when the annular ligament is stressed.

NOTE: Pulled elbow, pushed elbow, rotated elbow, radial head fracture, pinched synovial fringe, meniscal lock, radial tunnel syndrome, and periosteal bruise are also possible sources of pain at the elbow and are sometimes erroneously called tennis elbow.[15,31]

2. Medial epicondylitis, or golfer's elbow

This involves the common flexor/pronator tendon at the tenoperiosteal junction near the medial epicondyle and is associated with repetitive movements into wrist flexion such as swinging a golf club, pitching a ball, or work-related grasping, shuffling papers, and lifting heavy objects.

3. Other

Overuse can occur in any muscle in the elbow region including the flexors and extensors of the elbow.

B. Etiology of Symptoms

1. With epicondylitis the most common cause is repetitive or excessive use of the wrist or forearm, causing microdamage and partial tears, usually near the musculotendinous junction when the strain exceeds the strength of the tissues and when the demand exceeds the repair process. The inflammation becomes a chronic inflammation with continued irritation.
2. Inflammation of the periosteum may develop with formation of granulation tissue and adhesions.[23]
3. Recurring problems are seen because the resulting immobile or immature scar is redamaged when returning to activities before sufficient healing occurs.
4. Causes of problems anterior or posterior to the elbow are frequently from excessive extension or flexion strain in sporting activities.[1]

C. Common Impairments/Problems

1. There is gradually increasing pain in the elbow region following excessive activity of the wrist and hand.
2. Pain is experienced when the involved muscle is stretched or when it contracts against resistance while the elbow is extended.
3. Decreased muscle strength and endurance for the demand.
4. Decreased grip strength, limited by pain.
5. Tenderness with palpation at the site of inflammation, such as over the lateral or medial epicondyle, head of the radius, or within the muscle belly.

D. Common Functional Limitations/Disabilities

1. Inability to participate in provoking activity such as racket sports, throwing, or golf.
2. Difficulty with repetitive forearm/wrist tasks such as sorting or assembling small parts, gripping activities, using a hammer, turning a screwdriver, shuffling papers, or playing a percussion instrument.

E. Management: Acute Stage

1. To control pain, edema, or spasm
  a. Rest the muscles in a splint. If the extensor muscles are involved, immobilize the wrist in a cock-up splint, while keeping the elbow free to move.
  b. Instruct the patient to not perform strong or repetitive gripping activities.
  c. Utilize cryotherapy to help control edema and swelling.

2. To maintain soft tissue and joint mobility
  a. Remove the splint several times a day and perform nonstressful motion. Apply gentle multiple-angle setting techniques to the involved muscle followed by pain-free range of motion. Begin with the muscle in the shortened position.
    (1) Position of the patient and technique for extensor tendons
       The patient sits with the elbow flexed and forearm resting on a table. With the wrist in extension, provide a gentle resistance to the wrist extensor muscles; hold the contraction to the count of six, then slowly move the wrist toward flexion, just to the point at which pain begins. No forcing is attempted when pain is acute. When full wrist flexion is obtained progress by placing the elbow in greater degrees of extension until it is fully extended. The patient can be taught to apply gentle resistance with his other hand.
    (2) Position and technique for flexor tendons
       Begin with the elbow flexed and wrist flexed. Gently resist the wrist flexors. After several contractions, slowly move the wrist toward extension and repeat the gentle setting contractions. When full extension is obtained, progress by placing the elbow in greater degrees of extension until it is fully extended. The intensity of contractions and range must be controlled so that no pain occurs.
  b. Electrical stimulation to the muscle may also keep it mobile.[12]
  c. Gentle cross-fiber massage within tolerance to the site of the lesion.

3. To maintain integrity in upper extremity function
  a. Active ROM should be performed in all other elbow, forearm, and wrist motions, and functional integrity of the rest of the upper extremity should be maintained.
  b. Resistive shoulder and scapular ROM are performed with the resistance applied proximal to the elbow.

F. Management: Subacute or Chronic Stage

NOTE: If there is chronic inflammation, treat the inflammation first as was described.

1. To gradually increase the flexibility of the muscle and create a mobile scar
  a. Active inhibition technique for the extensor carpi radialis brevis
     The patient begins with the elbow extended and forearm pronated. While

holding this position, he or she ulnarly deviates the wrist and flexes the wrist and fingers. Pain should not increase; just a stretching sensation should be felt.[10] Gentle contract-relax techniques can also be used.

b. Self-stretching technique for the extensor muscle group

The patient places the back of the hand against the wall, fingers pointed down. Keeping the elbow in extension and forearm in pronation, he or she moves the back of the hand up the wall[26] (Fig. 9–1). When a pulling sensation in the extensors is felt, the position is maintained. Active inhibition can then be added by maintaining the position and having the patient flex the fingers.

c. Self-stretching technique for the flexor muscle group

Elongate the muscles by placing the palm of the hand against the wall, fingers pointed down, then moving the hand up the wall in the same manner as was described in b, keeping the elbow extended.[26]

d. The intensity of the cross-fiber massage at the site of the scar formation is increased.

2. To strengthen the muscle

a. Progress the isometric exercises in various pain-free positions. When there is no pain through the range of motion, progress to concentric resistance at an appropriate dosage.

b. Progressive resistance exercises (PREs) using a hand-held weight are used for flexion, extension (Fig. 9–2), pronation, and supination (Figs. 9–3A and B). Elastic resistance is used for wrist flexion and extension by placing a loop of elastic material under the foot and holding the other end in the hand; the arm is held or supported in a horizontal position. When the forearm is pronated, resistance is against the wrist extensors; when supinated, the resistance is against the wrist flexors.

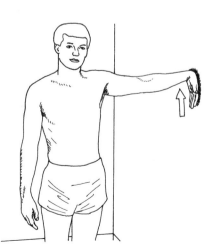

Figure 9–1. Self-stretching of the muscles of the lateral epicondyle.

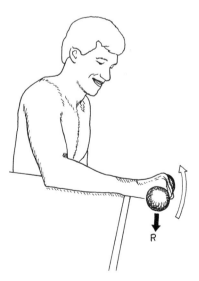

Figure 9–2. Mechanical resistance exercise using a hand-held weight for strengthening the muscles of the lateral epicondyle (wrist extensors).

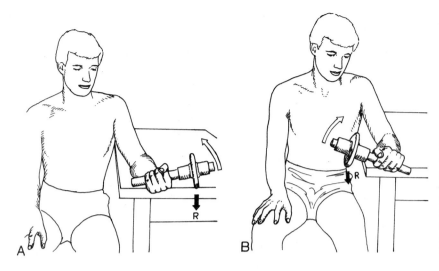

Figure 9–3. Mechanical resistance exercise using a small bar with asymmetrically placed weights for strengthening (*A*) forearm pronators and (*B*) supinators. The bar can also be rotated through a downward arc to affect the other half of the range for each muscle by placing the weight on the ulnar side of the hand.

    c. Initiate eccentric loading, first with light weights, and develop pain-free control. Increase the time for each exercise from 1 to 3 minutes to develop endurance; then increase the load or speed, depending on the desired outcome.

3. To strengthen and develop endurance in combined patterns of motion

Simulate the desired activity. For example use wall pulleys or elastic resistance to simulate tennis swings (Figs. 9–4A, B, and C).[12]

4. To determine if there are faulty components contributing to the overuse at the elbow

Assess the pattern of motion of the entire upper quarter and trunk control.

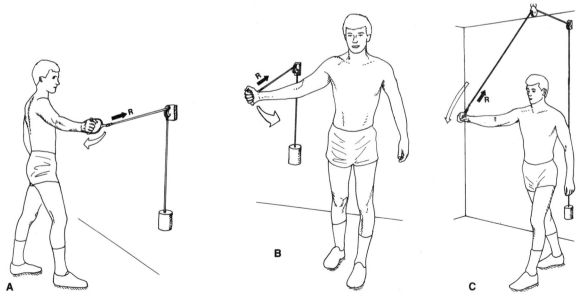

Figure 9–4. Mechanical resistance exercise using wall pulleys to simulate tennis swings. (*A*) Backhand stroke. (*B*) Forehand stroke. (*C*) Serve.

5. To progress to functional training and conditioning

Include strength, endurance, power, and flexibility exercises in the upper quarter with controlled loading of forces. Of equal importance is reducing the overload forces that caused the problem and retraining for proper technique.[10,11,21]

a. Instruct the patient to apply friction massage and to stretch the involved muscle prior to using it.

b. Begin strength and power training sessions with warm-up exercises that include general flexibility exercises for the shoulder, elbow, wrist, and trunk.

c. Increase repetitions in the defined pattern from 3 to 5 minutes to develop muscular endurance.

d. Attain general strengthening and conditioning of any unused or underused part of the extremity or trunk before returning to the stressful activity.

e. Include exercises simulating the desired activity at high speeds with low resistance to improve timing.

f. Assess the patient's technique and advise him or her on how to modify it before returning to the stressful activity. (This may require taking tennis lessons to correct improper tennis techniques.) If equipment is used (as in tennis or with a hammer), it should also be analyzed and modified to reduce stress.[10,21,23]

VI. Exercises for Muscle Strength and Flexibility Imbalances

In addition to the conditions already described in this chapter, imbalances in length and strength of muscles crossing the elbow and forearm can result from a variety of causes such as nerve injury or following surgery, trauma, disuse, or immobilization. Selections of appropriate exercises following biomechanical evaluation can be made from the following exercises as well as the stretching and strengthening techniques described in the previous sections and in Chapters 3 and 5. For patients with elbow problems, exercises to the joints above (shoulder) and below (wrist and hand) should also be incorporated into the therapeutic program to prevent complications, aid in healing, and restore proper function in the entire upper quarter. The general principles for treating any acute soft tissue lesion are discussed in Chapter 7. The exercises described in this section are for use during the healing and rehabilitation phases.

A. To Stretch Tight Muscles

NOTE: Prior to initiating a muscle-stretching program, be sure the joint capsule is not restricting motion. If joint play is limited, use joint mobilization techniques in conjunction with muscle-stretching techniques. (See Chapter 6.)

1. Elbow flexors

Precaution: When stretching tight elbow flexors, it is important to differentiate between the biceps and brachialis muscles by elongating the biceps muscle across the shoulder while maintaining the elbow in extension and pronation. If the brachialis is the limiting muscle and is tender over the distal muscle belly, stretching is *contraindicated* because stretching may precipitate myositis ossificans.[5] See Section IV.

a. If the biceps are tight, use active inhibition, passive, or self-stretching techniques (see Fig. 2–8).

b. To self-stretch the biceps, the individual places the arm behind the back with the elbow extended and forearm pronated and pulls the arm back with the other hand.

   c. Low-intensity long-duration stretching with dynamic splinting may be used to reduce elbow flexion contractures.[6]

   d. For mild contractures, use a light weight held in the hand or a band around the distal forearm for 5 to 7 minutes. Place a towel under the distal humerus as a fulcrum.[30]

2. Elbow extensors

   a. If the triceps is tight, use inhibition, passive stretching, and self-stretching techniques; include shoulder flexion to stretch the long head (see Figs. 2–7 and 2–9).

   b. For self-stretching, the individual flexes the elbow and shoulder as far as possible, then pushes against the humerus with the other hand.

   c. To self-stretch to increase elbow flexion, the patient lies in a prone-propped position with elbows flexed and forearms resting on the table. The patient lowers the chest as far as the elbow flexion allows and maintains the position as long as tolerated.

3. Supinators and pronators

   a. If pronation or supination is limited, stretch with the patient's elbow flexed to stabilize the humerus against rotational forces (see Fig. 2–10).

   b. To self-stretch into pronation, the patient grasps the back of the involved forearm with the normal hand so that the base is against the posterior radius and fingers are wrapped around the ulna.

   c. To self-stretch into supination, the heel of the normal hand is placed on the volar side of the radius. The force is applied against the radius so that there is no trauma to the wrist.

B. To Strengthen Weak Muscles

1. Elbow flexion

   a. To most efficiently use the long head of the biceps, allow the shoulder to extend while flexing the elbow. The patient sits or stands with weight in the hand and flexes the elbow, keeping the forearm supinated while the hand moves up toward the waist (Fig. 9–5). This can also be performed with an elastic resistance secured under the feet.

   b. Elbow flexors are also strengthened with the humerus maintained at the side or stabilized in flexion or abduction and the forearm pronated to de-emphasize the biceps.

2. Elbow extension

   a. To most efficiently use the long head of the triceps, the shoulder flexes while extending the elbow. Patient sits or stands with the elbow flexed and with a weight in the hand at the level of the shoulder. The weight is lifted straight overhead. Caution: good shoulder girdle muscle function is needed to effectively perform this exercise (see Fig. 8–26).

   b. Patient position sitting or standing. Begin with the long head on a stretch by positioning the humerus in flexion with the elbow flexed, then extending the elbow against a hand-held or elastic resistance (Fig. 9–6).

   c. Patient position supine with the shoulder flexed 90 degrees and the elbow flexed, with the hand either beginning by the same shoulder or middle of the

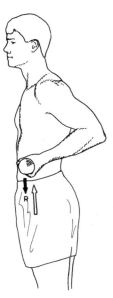

Figure 9–5. Resisting elbow flexion with emphasis on the biceps brachii. The shoulder extends as the elbow flexes with the forearm in supination. This combined action lengthens the proximal portion of the musculotendinous unit across the shoulder while it contracts to move the elbow, thus maintaining a more optimal length-tension relationship through a greater range of motion.

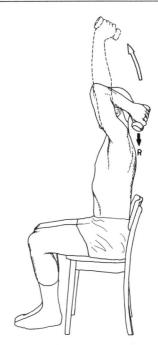

Figure 9–6. Resisting elbow extension, beginning with the long head of the triceps brachii on a stretch.

sternum (external or internal rotation of the shoulder). Extend the elbow against a hand-held weight or elastic resistance.

    d. Patient position prone with the arm abducted 90 degrees and the elbow flexed over the side of the table. Extend the elbow against a hand-held weight or elastic resistance.

3. Pronation and supination

    a. When using a free weight to strengthen the pronators and supinators, the weight must be placed to one side or the other of the hand. If a person holds a dumbbell with weight equal on each side of the hand, one side of the weight will be assistive while the other will be resistive, in essence cancelling out the resistive force. See Fig. 9–3A and B. Note also the position of the thumb in each exercise so that it is not lifting the bar. The weight can also be turned through a downward arc by placing the resistance on the ulnar side of the hand.

    b. Stand facing a door knob with the arm kept at the side to avoid substituting with shoulder rotation and turn the knob.

4. Combined patterns of motion. The elbow functions in activities of the shoulder and hand. Resistance to diagonal and combined patterns of motion should be incorporated into the rehabilitation program, being careful that substitute motions do not develop to compensate for a weak link in the chain.

   5. **Closed-chain exercises.** Upper extremity closed-chain exercises are described in Chapter 8. Utilize exercises that emphasize elbow control in flexion and extension.

   6. **Functional training and conditioning.** Increase resistance and speed, increase repetitions, and progress eccentric control. Progress patterns of motion to simulate the desired activity and impose controlled forces to challenge the patient.[30] A graded program of stretch-shortening drills such as throwing and catching weighted balls or practicing specific occupational or sports-related tasks that include pushing, pulling, lifting, or swinging may be appropriate in the late stages of rehabilitation.

VII. Summary

Following a brief review of anatomy and kinesiology of the elbow and forearm region, common musculoskeletal conditions that can be treated with therapeutic exercise have been described. Suggestions and guidelines for treatment and proper application of mobilization, stretching, and strengthening exercises have been outlined. The reader again is encouraged to use the information provided in Chapter 7 as the foundation for designing appropriate therapeutic exercise programs.

Common surgical procedures of the elbow and the use of therapeutic exercises during the postoperative rehabilitation period have been described. Guidelines for the progression of exercise during the maximum-, moderate-, and minimum-protection postoperative phases have been described.

References

1. Andrews, JR, and Whiteside, JA: Common elbow problems in the athlete. Journal of Orthopaedic and Sports Physical Therapy 17:289, 1993.
2. Bentley, JA: Physiotherapy following joint replacements. In Downie, PA: Cash's Textbook of Orthopedics and Rheumatology for Physiotherapists. JB Lippincott, Philadelphia, 1984.
3. Cailliet, R: Soft Tissue Pain and Disability, ed 2. FA Davis, Philadelphia, 1988.
4. Cofield, RH, Morrey, BF, and Bryan, RS: Total shoulder and total elbow arthroplasties: The current state of development. Part II. Journal of Continuing Education Orthopedics, Jan. 1979, p 17.
5. Cyriax, J: Textbook of Orthopaedic Medicine, Vol. 1. Diagnosis of Soft Tissue Lesions, ed 8. Bailliere Tindall, London, 1982.
6. Hepburn, G, and Crivelli, K: Use of elbow dynasplint for reduction of elbow flexion contractures: A case study. Journal of Orthopaedic and Sports Physical Therapy 5:259, 1984.
7. Hoppenfeld, S: Physical Examination of the Spine and Extremities. Appleton-Century-Crofts, New York, 1976.
8. Iversen, LD, and Clawson, DK: Manual of Acute Orthopedic Therapeutics, ed 2. Little, Brown & Company, Boston, 1982.
9. Kapadji, IA: The Physiology of the Joints, Vol. I. Churchill-Livingstone, Edinburgh, 1970.
10. Kessler, R, and Hertling, D: Management of Common Musculoskeletal Disorders. Harper & Row, Philadelphia, 1983.
11. Kopell, H, and Thompson, W: Peripheral Entrapment Neuropathies, ed 2. Robert E Krieger, Huntington, NY, 1976.
12. LaFreniere, J: Tennis elbow: Evaluation, treatment and prevention. Phys Ther 59:742, 1979.
13. Lehmkuhl, LD, and Smith, LK: Brunnstrom's Clinical Kinesiology, ed 4. FA Davis, Philadelphia, 1983.
14. Lowe, LW, et al: The development of an unconstrained elbow arthroplasty: A clinical review. J Bone Joint Surg Br 66:243, 1984.
15. Lutz, FR: Radial tunnel syndrome: An etiology of chronic lateral elbow pain. Journal of Orthopaedic and Sports Physical Therapy 14:14, 1991.
16. Marmor, L: Surgery of the rheumatoid elbow. J Bone Joint Surg Am 54:573, 1972.
17. Melvin, J: Rheumatic Disease: Occupational Therapy and Rehabilitation. FA Davis, Philadelphia, 1977.
18. Morrey, BF, and Kavanagh, BF: Cementless joint replacement: Current status and future. Bull Rheum Dis 37:1, 1987.
19. Morrey, BF: Surgery of the elbow. In Sledge, CB, et al (eds): Arthritis Surgery. WB Saunders, Philadelphia, 1994.
20. Morrey, BF (ed): The Elbow and Its Disorders. WB Saunders, Philadelphia, 1985.

21. Nerschl, R, and Sobel, J: Conservative treatment of tennis elbow. The Physician and Sportsmedicine 9.6:43, 1981.
22. Norkin, C, and Levangie, P: Joint Structure and Function: A Comprehensive Analysis, ed 2. FA Davis, Philadelphia, 1992.
23. Noteboom, T, et al: Tennis elbow: A review. Journal of Orthopaedic and Sports Physical Therapy 19:357, 1994.
24. Occupational Therapy Staff: Upper Extremity Surgeries for Patients with Arthritis: A Pre and Post-operative Occupational Therapy Treatment Guide. Rancho Los Amigos Hospital, California, 1979.
25. Pritchard, RW: Semiconstrained elbow prosthesis: A clinical review of five years' experience. Orthop Rev 8:33, 1979.
26. Sheon, R, Moskowitz R, and Goldberg, V: Soft Tissue Rheumatic Pain: Recognition, Management, Prevention. Lea & Febiger, Philadelphia, 1982.
27. Stroyan, M, and Wilk, KE: The functional anatomy of the elbow complex. Journal of Orthopaedic and Sports Physical Therapy 17:179, 1993.
28. Waugh, T: Arthroplasty rehabilitation. In Goodgold, J (ed): Rehabilitation Medicine, CV Mosby, St Louis, 1988.
29. Weiland, AJ, et al: Capitellocondylar total elbow replacement. J Bone Joint Surg Am 71:217, 1989.
30. Wilk, KE, Arrigo, C, and Andrews, JR: Rehabilitation of the elbow in the throwing athlete. Journal of Orthopaedic and Sports Physical Therapy 17:305, 1993.
31. Zohn, D, and Mennell, J: Musculoskeletal Pain: Principles of Physical Diagnosis and Physical Treatment. Little, Brown, Boston, 1976.

The Wrist and Hand

The wrist is the final link of joints that position the hand. It has the significant function of controlling the length-tension relationship of the multiarticular muscles of the hand as they adjust to various activities and grips.[26] The hand is a valuable tool through which we control our environment and express ideas and talents. It also has an important sensory function of providing feedback to the brain.

The anatomy and kinesiology of the wrist and hand are rather complex but are important to know to effectively treat hand problems. The first section of this chapter reviews highlights of the anatomy and function of those areas that the reader should know and understand. The reader is also referred to several texts for study of the material.[5,16,17,20,26] Chapter 7 presents information on principles of management; the reader should be familiar with that material before proceeding with establishing a therapeutic exercise program for the wrist or hand. The remaining sections describe common wrist and hand problems, their conservative or surgical management, and exercise techniques and progressions.

OBJECTIVES

After studying this chapter, the reader will be able to:

1 Identify important aspects of wrist and hand structure and function for review.
2 Establish a therapeutic exercise program based on the desired functional outcome to manage soft tissue and joint lesions in the wrist and hand related to stages of recovery following an inflammatory insult to the tissues, recognizing unique circumstances in the wrist and hand for their management.
3 Establish a therapeutic exercise program to manage patients following common surgical procedures in the wrist and hand.

I. Review of the Structure and Function of the Wrist and Hand

A. Bony Parts (see Fig. 6-33)

1. Wrist

Distal radius, scaphoid (S), lunate (L), triquetrum (Tri), pisiform (P), trapezium (Tm), trapezoid (Tz), capitate (C), and hamate (H).

2. Hand

Five metacarpals and 14 phalanges make up the hand and five digits.

B. Joints of the Wrist Complex and Their Movements

1. The wrist complex

The wrist complex is multiarticular and is made up of two compound joints. It is biaxial, allowing for flexion (volar flexion), extension (dorsiflexion), radial deviation (abduction), and ulnar deviation (adduction).

2. The radiocarpal joint

a. It is enclosed in a loose but strong capsule, reinforced by ligaments also shared with the midcarpal joint.

b. The biconcave articulating surface is the distal end of the radius and radio-ulnar disk (discus articularis); it is angled slightly volarly and ulnarly.

c. The biconvex articulating surface is the combined proximal surface of the scaphoid, lunate, and triquetrum. The triquetrum primarily articulates with the disk. These three carpals are bound together with numerous interosseous ligaments.

d. With motions of the wrist, the convex proximal row of carpals slides in the direction opposite the physiologic motion of the hand.

Physiologic Motion of Wrist	Direction of Slide of Carpals on Radius or Disk
Flexion*	Dorsal
Extension	Volar
Radial deviation	Ulnar
Ulnar deviation*	Radial

3. The midcarpal joint

a. This is a compound joint between the two rows of carpals. It has a capsule that is also continuous with the intercarpal articulations.

b. The combined distal surfaces of the scaphoid, lunate, and triquetrum articulate with the combined proximal surfaces of the trapezium, trapezoid, capitate, and hamate.

(1) The articulating surfaces of the capitate and hamate are in essence convex and slide on the concave articulating surfaces of a portion of the scaphoid, lunate, and triquetrum.

(2) The articulating surfaces of the trapezium and trapezoid are concave and slide on the convex distal surface of the scaphoid.

---

*Greater movement in flexion and ulnar deviation than the other two motions occurs at this joint.[42]

c. With physiologic motions of the wrist, a complex of motions occurs between the carpals. In summary:

Physiologic Motion of the Wrist	Direction of Slide of Distal Carpal Bones With Respect to the Proximal Carpal Bones
Flexion	C and H—dorsal
	Tm and Tz—volar
Extension*	C and H—volar
	Tm and Tz—dorsal
Radial deviation*	C and H—ulnar
	Tm and Tz—dorsal
Ulnar deviation	C and H—radial
	Tm and Tz—volar

4. The pisiform

The pisiform is categorized as a carpal and is aligned volar to the triquetrum in the proximal row of carpals. It is not part of the wrist joint but functions as a sesamoid bone in the flexor carpi ulnaris tendon.

5. The ligaments

Stability and some passive movement of the wrist complex are provided by numerous ligaments: the ulnar and radial collateral, the dorsal and volar (palmar) radiocarpal, the ulnocarpal, and the intercarpal.

C. Joints of the Hand Complex and Their Movements

1. Carpometacarpal (CMC) joints of digits 2 through 5

a. The joints are enclosed in a common joint cavity and include the articulations of each metacarpal with the distal row of carpals and the articulations between the bases of each metacarpal.

b. The joints of digits 2, 3, and 4 are plane uniaxial joints; the joint of digit 5 is biaxial. They are supported by transverse and longitudinal ligaments. The fifth metacarpal is most mobile, with the fourth being the next mobile.

c. The flexion of the metacarpals and additional adduction of the fifth contribute to the cupping (arching) of the hand, which improves prehension.

Physiologic Motions of the Metacarpals	Direction of Slide of Metacarpals on Carpals
Flexion (cupping)	Volar
Extension (flattening)	Dorsal

2. Carpometacarpal joint of the thumb (digit 1)

a. This joint is a saddle-shaped (sellar) biaxial joint between the trapezium and base of the first metacarpal. It has a lax capsule and wide ROM, which allows the thumb to move away from the palm of the hand for opposition in prehension activities.

b. For flexion-extension of the thumb (components of opposition-reposition, respectively) occurring in the frontal plane, the trapezium surface is convex and the base of the metacarpal is concave; therefore, its surface slides in the same direction as the angulating bone.

---

*Greater movement in extension and radial deviation than the other two motions occurs at this joint.[42]

c. For abduction-adduction, occurring in the sagittal plane, the trapezium surface is concave and the metacarpal is convex; therefore, its surface slides in the opposite direction of the angulating bone.

Physiologic Motion of the First Metacarpal	Direction of Slide of Base of Metacarpal
Flexion	Ulnar
Extension	Radial
Abduction	Dorsal
Adduction	Volar

3. Metacarpophalangeal (MCP) joints

a. They are biaxial condyloid joints with the distal end of each metacarpal convex and proximal phalanx concave, supported by a volar and two collateral ligaments. The collaterals become taut in full flexion and prevent abduction and adduction in this position.

b. The MCP of the thumb differs in that it is reinforced by two sesamoid bones and has minimal abduction and adduction even in extension.

Physiologic Motion of the First Phalanx	Direction of Slide of First Phalanx
Flexion	Volar
Extension	Dorsal
Abduction	Away from center of hand
Adduction	Toward center of hand

4. Interphalangeal (IP) joints

a. There is a proximal (PIP) and distal (DIP) interphalangeal joint for each digit, 2 through 5; the thumb has only one interphalangeal joint. Each is a uniaxial hinge joint. The articulating surface at the distal end of each phalanx is convex; the articulating surface at the proximal end of each phalanx is concave.

b. Each capsule is reinforced with collateral ligaments.

c. Going radial to ulnar, there is increasing flexion-extension range in the joints. This allows for greater opposition of the ulnar fingers to the thumb and also causes a potentially tighter grip on the ulnar side.

Physiologic Motion of Each Phalanx	Direction of Slide of Base of Phalanx
Flexion	Volar
Extension	Dorsal

D. Hand Function

1. Length-tension relationships

The wrist position controls the length of the extrinsic muscles to the digits.

a. As the fingers or thumb flex, the wrist must be stabilized by the wrist extensor muscles to prevent the flexor digitorum profundus and flexor digitorum superficialis or flexor pollicis longus from simultaneously flexing the wrist. As the grip becomes stronger, synchronous wrist extension lengthens the extrinsic flexor tendons across the wrist and maintains a more favorable overall length of the musculotendinous unit for a stronger contraction.

b. For strong finger or thumb extension, the wrist flexor muscles stabilize or flex the wrist so the extensor digitorum communis, extensor indicis, extensor digiti minimi, or extensor pollicis longus muscles can function more efficiently. In addition, there is ulnar deviation; the flexor and extensor carpi ulnaris muscles are both active as the hand opens.[22]

2. Cupping and flattening

Cupping of the hand occurs with finger flexion, and flattening of the hand occurs with extension. Cupping improves the mobility of the hand for functional usage and flattening for release of objects.

3. Extensor mechanism

Structurally, the extensor hood is made up of the extensor digitorum communis tendon, its connective tissue expansion, and fibers from the tendons of the dorsal and volar interossei and lumbricals.[26] Each structure has an effect on the extensor mechanism.

   a. An isolated contraction of the extensor digitorum produces clawing of the fingers (MCP hyperextension with IP flexion from passive pull of the extrinsic flexor tendons).

   b. PIP and DIP extensions occur concurrently and can be caused by the interossei or lumbrical muscles through their pull on the extensor hood.

   c. There must be tension in the extensor digitorum communis tendon for there to be interphalangeal extension. This occurs by active contraction of the muscle, causing MCP extension concurrently as the intrinsic muscles contract, or by stretch of the tendon, which occurs with MCP flexion.

4. Grips and prehension patterns

The nature of the intended activity dictates the type of grip used.[21,22,25]

   a. *Power grips* involve clamping an object with partially flexed fingers against the palm of the hand, with counterpressure from the adducted thumb. Power grips are primarily isometric functions. The fingers are flexed, laterally rotated, and ulnarly deviated. The amount of flexion varies with the object held. The thumb reinforces the fingers and helps make small adjustments to control the direction of the force. Varieties include cylindrical grip, spherical grip, hook grip, and lateral prehension.

   b. *Precision patterns* involve manipulating an object that is not in contact with the palm of the hand between the opposing abducted thumb and fingers. The muscles primarily function isotonically. The sensory surface of the digits is used for maximum sensory input to influence delicate adjustments. With small objects, precise handling occurs primarily between the thumb and index finger. Varieties include pad-to-pad, tip-to-tip, and pad-to-side prehension.

   c. *Combined grips* involve digits 1 and 2 (and sometimes 3) performing precision activities, whereas digits 3 through 5 supplement with power.

E. Hand Control[22]

1. Control of the unloaded (free) hand

Involves anatomic factors, muscular contraction, and viscoelastic properties of the muscles.

   a. Clawing motions occur with only extrinsic muscle contractions.

   b. Closing motions can occur only with extrinsic muscle contraction but also require the viscoelastic force of the biarticular interossei.

    c. Opening motions require the synergistic contraction of the extrinsic extensor and the lumbrical muscles.

    d. Reciprocal motion of MCP flexion and IP extension is caused by the interossei. The lumbrical removes the viscoelastic tension from the profundus tendon and assists IP extension.

2. Power grip

    a. Extrinsic flexors provide the major gripping force.

    b. Extrinsic extensor provides a compressive force preventing subluxation of the finger joints.

    c. Interossei rotate the first phalanx for positioning to compress the external object and also flex the MCP joint.

    d. Lumbricals do not participate in the power grip (except the fourth).

    e. The thenar muscles and adductor pollicis provide compressive forces against the object being gripped.

3. Precision handling

    a. Extrinsic muscles provide the compressive force to hold the objects between the fingers and thumb.

    b. For manipulation of an object the interossei abduct and adduct the fingers, the thenar muscles control movement of the thumb, and the lumbricals help move the object away from the palm of the hand. The amount of participation of each muscle varies with the amount and direction of motion.

4. Pinch

Compression between the thumb and fingers is provided by the thenar eminence muscles, the adductor pollicis, the interossei, and extrinsic flexors. The lumbricals also participate.

F. Major Nerves Subject to Pressure and Trauma at the Wrist and Hand[7,19]

1. Median nerve

To enter the hand, this nerve passes through the carpal tunnel at the wrist with the flexor tendons. The carpal tunnel is covered by the thick, relatively inelastic transverse carpal ligament. Entrapment in the tunnel causes sensory changes (over the radial two-thirds of the palm, the palmar surfaces of the first three and one-half digits, and the dorsum of the distal phalanges) and progressive weakness in the muscles innervated distal to the wrist (opponens pollicis, abductor pollicis brevis, superficial head of the flexor pollicis brevis, and lumbricals I and II), resulting in ape-hand deformity (thenar atrophy and thumb in plane of hand). The branch innervating the opponens muscle hooks over the carpal ligament two-thirds of the way up the thenar eminence and can be entrapped separately.

2. Ulnar nerve

This nerve enters the hand through a trough formed by the pisiform bone and hook of the hamate bone and is covered by the volar carpal ligament and palmaris brevis muscle. Trauma or entrapment causes sensory changes (ulnar third of the hand, entire fifth digit, and ulnar side of the fourth digit) and progressive weakness to muscles innervated distal to the site (palmaris brevis, muscles of the hypothenar eminence, lumbricals III and IV, interossei, adductor pollicis, and deep head of the flexor pollicis brevis), resulting in partial claw-hand (benediction hand) deformity. Injury to the nerve after it bifurcates leads to partial involvement, depending on the site of injury.

3. Radial nerve

This nerve enters the hand on the dorsal surface as the superficial radial nerve, which is sensory only. Injury to it in the wrist or hand causes sensory changes only (over the radial two-thirds of the dorsum of the hand and thumb and the proximal phalanx of the second, third, and half of the fourth digit). Influence of the radial nerve on hand musculature is entirely proximal to the wrist. It innervates extrinsic wrist and hand muscles (see Chapter 9). Injury near the elbow results in wrist drop.

G. Referred Pain and Nerve Injury Patterns

The hand is the terminal point for several major nerves. Injury or entrapment of these nerves may occur anywhere along their course, from the cervical spine to their termination. What the patient perceives as pain or sensory disturbance in the hand may be from injury of the nerve anywhere along its course, or the pain may be from irritation of tissue of common segmental origin. For treatment to be effective, it must be directed to the source of the problem, not to the site where the patient perceives the pain or sensory changes. Therefore, a thorough history is taken and a selective tension examination done when referred pain patterns or sensory changes are reported by the patient.[8]

1. Common sources of segmental sensory reference in the hand
   a. Cervical spine
      (1) Vertebral joints between C-5 and C-6, between C-6 and C-7, or between C-7 and T-1 vertebrae
      (2) C-6, C-7, or C-8 nerve roots
   b. Tissue derived from the same spinal segments as C-6, C-7, or C-8

2. Common sources of extrasegmental sensory reference in the hand
   a. Peripheral nerves
      Median, ulnar, or radial nerve entrapments
   b. Brachial plexus
      Thoracic outlet syndrome

II. Joint Problems: Nonoperative Management
A. Related Diagnoses and Etiology of Symptoms

Pathologies such as rheumatoid arthritis (RA) and degenerative joint disease (DJD), as well as acute joint trauma, affect the joints of the wrist and hand. Tightness and adhesions from immobilization develop in the joints, tendon sheaths, muscles, and surrounding tissues any time the joints are splinted or casted. Chapter 7 describes the etiology of these arthritic and joint symptoms.

B. Common Impairments/Problems

1. Rheumatoid arthritis[29,41]

a. Synovial inflammation (synovitis) and tissue proliferation with bilateral swelling, pain, limitation, and warmth in joints of the wrists and hands, most commonly the MCP, PIP, and wrist joints.

b. Extrinsic tendon and sheath inflammation (tenosynovitis) and synovial proliferation, with pain, progressive muscle weakness, and imbalances in length and strength between antagonists.

c. Carpal tunnel syndrome may occur in conjunction with tenosynovitis due to compression of the median nerve from the swollen tissue.

d. Fatigue.

e. Advanced stages: joint capsule weakening, cartilage destruction, bone erosion, and tendon rupture lead to subluxations and deformities, including:

    (1) Volar subluxation of the triquetrum on the articular disk and ulna with the extensor carpi ulnaris tendon displaced volarly, causing a flexor force at the wrist joint

    (2) Ulnar subluxation of the carpals resulting in radial deviation of the wrist

    (3) Ulnar drift of the fingers at the MCP joints and volar subluxation of the proximal phalanx

    (4) Swan-neck deformity (PIP hyperextension with DIP flexion)

    (5) Boutonnière deformity (PIP flexion with DIP extension)

2. DJD and joint trauma

a. When acute, there is swelling with restricted and painful motion.

b. When chronic, flexion and extension are both limited in the affected joints with a firm capsular end-feel.

c. General muscle weakness, weak grip strength, and poor muscular endurance.

Precaution: Following trauma, the therapist must be alert to signs of a fracture in the wrist or hand because small bone fractures may not show on x ray for up to 2 weeks. Signs include swelling, muscle spasm when passive motion is attempted, increased pain when the involved bone is stressed (such as deviation toward the involved bone), and tenderness on palpation over the fracture site.[8]

3. Postimmobilization stiffness

a. Decreased range of motion, joint-play stiffness, and tendon adhesions

b. Muscle weakness, weak grip strength, decreased flexibility, and poor endurance

C. Common Functional Limitations/Disabilities

1. When acute, all prehension activities will be painful, interfering with ADL such as dressing, eating, grooming, and toileting or almost any functional activity, including writing and typing.

2. Depending on which joints are involved, the amount of restricted movement and residual weakness, fatigue or dexterity loss, and type of grip or amount of precision handling required, functional loss may be minor or significant.

D. Management of Acute Joint Lesions

General guidelines for managing acute joint lesions are described in Chapter 7.

1. To control pain

a. The physician may prescribe medication.
b. Modalities.
c. Rest with brief periods of nonstressful motion, intermittently throughout the day.

2. To protect the joint

a. Proper positioning to prevent contractures. Splint or tape the joint when in situations that may stress it; otherwise, remove the restraint and allow nonstressful, nonpainful motion.
b. Adaption of ADL with assistive devices, if necessary.

3. To maintain joint motion, joint nutrition, and tissue health

a. Grade I or II distraction and joint oscillation techniques.
b. Passive to active-assistive range of motion. It is important to move the joints as tolerated because immobility in the hand quickly leads to muscle imbalance and contracture formation or further articular deterioration.

4. To maintain muscle and tendon mobility

a. Multiple-angle muscle-setting techniques.
b. Passive, active-assistive, or active ROM. Full range of motion in uninvolved joints as well as nonstressful ranges in involved joints should be performed to maintain the gliding of the long tendons in their synovial sheaths across the involved joints and prevents adhesions.[11]

E. Management of Subacute and Chronic Joint Restrictions

1. To increase mobility in the articulations of the wrist

The main emphasis is on joint mobilization techniques.[30] The distal radioulnar (RU) joint may be painful just proximal to the wrist and be described as wrist pain by the patient. Restrictions affect the forearm functions of pronation and supination. See Chapter 9 for discussion of this joint and its treatment.

a. *To increase flexion*
   (1) Traction on the carpals (see Fig. 6–34)
   (2) General dorsal glide of the carpals (see Fig. 6–35)
   (3) Specific carpal glides as indicated
       Stabilize the bone that has the convex articulating surface, and apply the mobilizing force against the bone with the concave articulating surface. The force is in a volar direction.
       (a) Stabilize lunate, volar glide radius (see Fig. 6–38).
       (b) Stabilize capitate, volar glide lunate (see Fig. 6–38).
       (c) Stabilize scaphoid, volar glide radius (see Fig. 6–38).
       (d) Stabilize scaphoid, volar glide trapezium (see Fig. 6–39).

b. *To increase extension*
    (1) Traction on the carpals (see Fig. 6–34)
    (2) General volar glide of the carpals (see Fig. 6–36)
    (3) Specific carpal glides as indicated
        Stabilize the bone that has the concave articulating surface, and apply the mobilizing force against the dorsal surface of the bone with the convex articulating surface. The force is in a volar direction.
        (a) Stabilize radius, volar glide lunate (see Fig. 6–39).
        (b) Stabilize radius, volar glide scaphoid (see Fig. 6–39).
        (c) Stabilize trapezium, volar glide scaphoid (see Fig. 6–38).
        (d) Stabilize lunate, volar glide capitate (see Fig. 6–39).
        (e) Stabilize scaphoid, volar glide capitate (see Fig. 6–39).

c. *To increase radial deviation*
    (1) Traction on the carpals (see Fig. 6–34)
    (2) General ulnar glide (see Fig. 6–37)
    (3) Specific carpal glides as indicated
        (a) Stabilize trapezius, volar glide scaphoid (see Fig. 6–38).
        (b) Stabilize radius, volar glide scaphoid (see Fig. 6–39).

d. *To increase ulnar deviation*
    (1) Traction on the carpals (see Fig. 6–34)
    (2) General radial glide (opposite of Fig. 6–37)

e. *To unlock the subluxed ulnomeniscal-triquetral (UMT) joint* to allow for supination and wrist function.
    Volar glide the ulna on a stabilized triquetrum (similar to Fig. 6–38).

f. *To teach the patient UMT self-mobilization*
    The patient grasps the distal ulna with the fingers of the opposite hand and places the thumb on the palmar surface of the triquetrum just medial to the pisiform. He or she then presses with the thumb, causing a dorsal glide of the triquetrum on the radioulnar disk and ulna (Fig. 10–1).

2. To increase mobility in the joints of the hand and fingers

a. *To increase mobility of the CMC joint of the thumb*
    (1) Joint traction

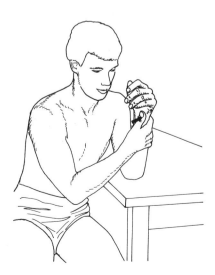

Figure 10–1. Self-mobilization of the ulnomeniscal-triquetral (UMT) joint.

    (2) To increase flexion
        Ulnar glide of first metacarpal on stabilized trapezium (see Fig. 6–41A).
    (3) To increase extension
        Radial glide first metacarpal (see Fig. 6–41B).
    (4) To increase abduction
        Dorsal glide first metacarpal (see Fig. 6–41C).
    (5) To increase adduction
        Palmar glide first metacarpal (see Fig. 6–41D).

b. *To increase the arch of the hand*
    (1) Joint traction of the carpometacarpal joints of the hand (see Fig. 6–40).
    (2) Palmar glide base of each metacarpal on its fixated carpal.

c. *To increase mobility of the MCP and IP joints of the digits*
    (1) Joint traction (see Fig. 6–42).
    (2) Rotation with traction (see Fig. 6–44).
    (3) To increase flexion
        Volar glide base of phalanx (see Fig. 6–43).
    (4) To increase extension
        Dorsal glide base of phalanx.
    (5) To increase abduction or adduction
        Glide radially or ulnarly, depending on digit and direction of limitation.

3. To develop mobility and control in the tendons and muscles

Carefully evaluate for flexibility imbalances in the multijoint and intrinsic muscles. See Section VI for a description of the techniques and special precautions.

a. *Passive and active inhibition stretching* techniques are used to selectively elongate tight muscles.

b. If adhesions are present, apply *friction massage* with the involved tendon placed on a stretch.

c. Teach *self-stretching* techniques, emphasizing protection of joints when stretching multijoint muscles.

d. Teach the patient *ROM* to each of the extrinsic muscles to maintain free gliding between the tendons and the tendons and bones.[33] This is particularly important when there has been immobilization following trauma or a fracture and scar tissue and adhesions as well as contractures restrict motion. Include:
    (1) *Claw fist.* Flexion of the DIP and PIP while maintaining MP extension to emphasize the flexor digitorum profundus gliding on the bone as well as gliding of the extensor digitorum communis tendons.
    (2) *Sublimis fist.* Flexion of the MP and PIP while maintaining DIP extension to emphasize flexor digitorum superficialis gliding on the profundus tendon.
    (3) *Full fist.* Flexion of the MP, PIP, and DIP simultaneously to promote gliding of the profundus and superficialis tendons on each other.
    (4) *Long horn sign.* Extension of the second and fourth digits to promote isolated motion of the extensor indices and extensor digiti quinti tendons on the extensor digitorum communis tendons.

e. Promote *coordination* between the intrinsic and extrinsic muscles by moving from the claw hand position to the intrinsic position (see Fig. 10–5).

f. Develop *control* of all thumb motions including flexion and extension as described for the other digits as well as abduction and opposition.

g. Promote abduction and adduction of all the MP joints.

4. **To develop strength and function**

Progress exercises with controlled and nondestructive forces to increase strength and muscle balance between antagonists, and progress endurance training. With pathologic joints use caution when applying weights so as not to stress the joints beyond the capability of the stabilizing tissues.

F. Nonoperative Management of RA in the Wrist and Hand

Because of the systemic and progressive nature of this disease, special care and precautions are necessary to protect the joints and minimize progression of deformities.

1. **Acute stage**

In addition to the guidelines presented in Section D, not only are rest and proper positioning critical, but also nonstressful ROM is critical to prevent joint stiffness. Careful monitoring of activities is done to reduce increased inflammation. Use of aquatic therapy for exercises reduces stiffness and promotes comfort.

2. **Subacute stage**

As pain and swelling begin to subside, emphasize joint protection and energy conservation while increasing activities.[29]

a. In addition to the use of splints, the patient should avoid using strong grasping activities when the joints are reactive or when the muscles are weak, because they facilitate the deforming forces of radial deviation and extension at the wrist and ulnar drift and volar subluxation of the MP joints. Use the hand in nonprehensile functional ways or in motions opposite to those of the deforming forces such as opening jars with the left hand, cutting food with the blade of the knife protruding from the ulnar side of the hand, or stirring food with the spoon on the ulnar side of the hand.[41]

b. Look for early signs of muscle tightness in the intrinsic muscles. If tight, elongate them, because one cause of swan-neck deformity is tight interossei muscles pulling on the extensor tendon, leading to hyperextension of the hypermobile PIP joints.[41]

3. **Chronic stage**

a. Once the inflammation is controlled with medication or the disease is in remission, mobilization techniques are used to stretch the mechanical restrictions in the joints. Do not stretch vigorously because the disease process and use of steroid therapy weaken the tensile quality of the connective tissue.

b. Resistive exercises are used to increase strength. The patient is taught to monitor activities and be alert to signs of increased inflammation, indicating excessive stress, and to modify exercises to reduce the stress.[29] When motion causes increased pain, the patient should perform multiple-angle isometrics at an intensity that does not provoke symptoms.

c. Physical conditioning exercises are initiated, using activities that do not provoke joint symptoms, such as exercising in a pool or cycling.

III. Joint Surgery and Postoperative Management

Long-standing RA or DJD that affects the joints and soft tissues of the wrist and hand can lead to chronic pain, instability and deformity of joints, and restricted ROM, as well as loss of strength in the hand and functional use of the upper extremity. When nonoperative management fails, surgical intervention with careful postoperative rehabilitation is used to restore function to the hand and wrist.

Surgical options include soft tissue procedures such as *tenosynovectomy* for chronic tenosynovitis of the extensor and flexor tendons of the wrist, *repair of ruptured tendons*, and *synovectomy* of the wrist or finger joints. These procedures are employed independently when articular surfaces of the involved joints remain intact. If joint deterioration is significant, arthrodesis, resection arthroplasty, or implant arthroplasty, often performed in conjunction with soft tissue surgery, are the procedures of choice. Some procedures are elected to minimize or delay further deformity. For example, if medical management fails, **tenosynovectomy** is performed to remove proliferated synovium from tendon sheaths and prevent erosion or rupture of tendons before significant deformity and loss of active control of the wrist and fingers occur. If rupture occurs, tendon repairs and transfers can improve function of the hand and delay or prevent the development of fixed deformities or subluxation and dislocation of joints. Arthrodesis is still the procedure of choice to correct deformity of the wrist or individual finger joints because it gives the patient a stable and pain-free joint with little compromise of function. If fusion is inappropriate and pain-free mobility is necessary, several types of *joint arthroplasty* are available. In most situations a combination of surgeries is often most appropriate.

The goals of surgery and postoperative management of chronic arthritis and associated deformities include[24,35]: (1) restoration of normal or adequate function to the wrist and hand, (2) relief of pain, (3) correction of instability or deformity, (4) restoration of ROM, and (5) improved strength of the wrist and fingers for functional grasp and pinch.

A discussion of postoperative management of several types of arthroplasty follows. Information on surgical management and postoperative rehabilitation of tendon repairs and transfers associated with chronic arthritis is then outlined.

A. Total Wrist Arthroplasty (Radiocarpal Implant Arthroplasty)

1. Indications for surgery[1,14,35,38,40]

a. Severe instability of the wrist joint and deterioration of the distal radius, carpals, and distal ulna as a result of chronic arthritis
b. Marked limitation of motion of the wrist
c. Subluxation or dislocation of the radiocarpal joint
d. Severe pain at the wrist that compromises hand strength and function
e. Appropriate for patients with bilateral wrist involvement in which arthrodesis of both wrists would limit rather than improve hand function

2. Procedures[1,14,35,38,40]

a. The total wrist replacement arthroplasty is an alternative to arthrodesis of the wrist. A successful total wrist replacement provides a balance of functional wrist motion combined with adequate joint stability.
b. There are two general types of radiocarpal implant arthroplasties. Both require a dorsal incision of the wrist.
  (1) The flexible-implant arthroplasty is a double-stemmed unit of silicone rubber. After removal of the proximal row of carpals and resection of the distal aspect of the radius and the base of the capitate, the proximal stem of the prosthesis is placed in the intramedullary canal of the distal radius. The distal stem is placed through the capitate and into the intramedullary canal of the third metacarpal. The prosthesis does not require cement but rather becomes encapsulated over time by a new fibrous capsule.

This procedure is often combined with synovectomy of the wrist, **dorsal clearance** of the extensor tendons, and repair of ruptured extensor tendons.

   (2) Various rigid (metal and high-density plastic), hinged total wrist prostheses have also been developed.[14] These prostheses are all cemented in place with methyl methacrylate. In most procedures, the distal radius, possibly the distal ulna, and adequate carpal bones are resected. The implant inserts proximally into the intramedullary canal of the distal radius and distally into the third and possibly second or fourth metacarpals.

  c. In both types of procedures, the hand and wrist are placed in a bulky dressing for 3 to 6 days postoperatively and elevated to reduce edema.

3. Postoperative management[13,27,41]

  a. *Immobilization*

    (1) Flexible implant arthroplasty requires approximately 2 to 4 weeks of immobilization in a short arm cast with the wrist in neutral or 20 degrees of extension. No wrist exercise is begun until there is adequate joint stability.[13,27,41]

    (2) Hinged implants of rigid plastic and metal that are cemented in place require a shorter period of immobilization, usually 1 to 2 weeks, before wrist exercise is begun.

  b. *Exercise*[27,41]

MAXIMUM-PROTECTION PHASE

    (1) During the period of immobilization, the patient is encouraged to carry out frequent active finger flexion and extension exercises in the splint or cast to maintain finger mobility and reduce edema in the hand.

    (2) When wrist motion is allowed, the splint is removed and the patient begins:

      (a) Active pronation and supination of the forearm

      (b) Active radial and ulnar deviation of the wrist

      (c) Active or active-assistive wrist extension with the fingers relaxed and flexed

      (d) Active or active-assistive wrist flexion with the fingers relaxed and extended

      (e) Active finger flexion and extension with the wrist in neutral

      (f) Active opposition of the thumb to each of the digits

MODERATE- AND MINIMUM-PROTECTION PHASES

    (1) The wrist splint is worn between exercise sessions during the day for at least 6 to 8 weeks. Light functional activities may be begun at 8 weeks without the splint. The splint is worn at night for up to 12 weeks.

    (2) Active exercises are continued until functional range of motion of the wrist is achieved.

    (3) Gentle resistance exercises may be begun at 6 to 8 weeks to improve grip strength.

    (4) Full use of the hand and wrist for light activities is permissible by 12 weeks postoperatively.

  c. *Precautions*

    (1) If a repair of extensor tendons has also been done, follow the precautions for tendon repair discussed in Section III.E of this chapter.

(2) The patient must be advised that heavy lifting or excessive weight bearing on the hand is contraindicated postoperatively to minimize the risk of loosening of the implant.

B. Metacarpophalangeal (MCP) Implant Arthroplasty

1. Indications for surgery[3,4,13,14,24]

a. Pain at the MCP joint(s) of the hand and deterioration of the joint, usually because of rheumatoid arthritis
b. Instability and deformity (ulnar drift) of the fingers that cannot be corrected with soft tissue releases alone
c. Stiffness and decreased range of motion at the MCP joints
d. Possible subluxation of the MCP joints

2. Procedure[3,4,13,14,24]

a. Prerequisites
For this implant arthroplasty to be successful, a patient must have an intact extensor digitorum communis, or repair of these tendons must be accomplished prior to or at the time of surgery.
b. Dorsal clearance (removal of diseased synovium along the extensor tendon sheaths) or an arthrodesis of the wrist may be performed at the same time as the implant arthroplasty.
c. Overview of the procedure.

NOTE: The majority of implant arthroplasties performed for the digits are one-piece, flexible, stemmed prostheses made of silicone. The implant acts as a dynamic spacer as the joint heals. Flexible implant arthroplasty was an improvement over the hinged metal prosthesis. Newer designs that are still less commonly used than the flexible silicone implant include a two-piece, plastic-to-metal articulated implant that is cemented in place and, most recently, a cementless, nonconstrained implant made of pyrolite carbon.[34]

(1) A transverse incision is made over the dorsal aspect of the MCP joint, and the joint capsules are incised.
(2) The thick, proliferated synovium is removed.
(3) Release of soft tissue contractures (at the volar capsule or collateral ligaments) and repair of the extensor tendons are performed if necessary.
(4) The heads of the involved metacarpals are excised and the intramedullary canals of the metacarpal and proximal phalanx are widened.
(5) The prosthesis is implanted in the intramedullary canal of each involved metacarpal and proximal phalanx. Each joint capsule is then repaired.
(6) The wound is closed and a bulky compression dressing is placed around the hand; the MCP joints are held in extension and the distal joints in some flexion.

3. Postoperative management[13,23,27,34,39]

a. *Immobilization*[39]
For the first 2 to 3 days postoperatively, the hand is elevated to control edema and remains in the bulky compression dressing. Immobilization after either flexible implant arthroplasty or cemented or cementless plastic and metal implant arthroplasty is not lengthy.
(1) If only an MCP implant has been performed, the hand remains immobilized for approximately 3 days.

(2) If, in addition to the MCP arthroplasty, a reconstruction of ruptured extensor tendons has also been performed, the hand remains immobilized longer to protect the repaired or transferred tendons.

(3) Between 2 and 3 days postoperatively the compression dressing is removed, and the hand is placed in a dynamic extension splint with an outrigger.

   (a) The dynamic splint keeps the MCP joints in extension. During the day, the patient wears the dynamic splint except when it is removed for exercise. At night the patient wears a static wrist and finger extension splint.

   (b) The dynamic splint is worn to protect healing structures, to prevent recurrent deformity, such as ulnar drift of the fingers, and to control and guide joint motion during healing. The dynamic splint holds the MCP joints in extension but does not control motion in the IP joints.

b. *Exercise*

MAXIMUM-PROTECTION PHASE

From a few days to 3 weeks postoperatively the focus of management is to protect healing structures but apply a safe level of stress to soft tissues to influence organized scar tissue formation by means of controlled motion.

(1) To maintain adequate joint ROM and gliding of tendons within their sheaths

   (a) While in the dynamic splint, have the patient begin:

      — Active, pain-free PIP and DIP flexion and extension with the MCP joints held in extension.

      — Active, pain-free MCP flexion with the IP joints held in extension. Manually stabilize the IP joints in extension or temporarily splint them with tape and a tongue depressor.

      — Active, pain-free MCP extension with the IP joints flexed (the intrinsic minus position of the hand) to minimize activation of the intrinsics and promote gliding of the extrinsic extensor tendons in the tendon sheaths.

      — Active wrist and forearm movements with the fingers relaxed.

      — Active opposition of the thumb to each digit.

   (b) While the hand is out of the splint, the therapist begins passive, pain-free full MCP ROM while being sure to avoid any ulnar or radial deviation of the digits. The goal is 70 degrees of MCP flexion.

      Precaution: During the first few postoperative weeks do not apply any stretch or resistance to the extensors, particularly if an extensor tendon reconstruction or transfer has been performed.

(2) Gentle mobilization of the incision can be initiated within a week or two to maintain mobility of the scar and prevent restrictions in motion.

(3) Massage and heat can also be applied for edema control and to relieve postoperative pain and stiffness.

MODERATE-PROTECTION PHASE

(1) By 3 to 4 weeks initiate active ROM out of the splint. The goal is full active flexion of the MCP joints with a minimum of active extensor lag.

(2) If no tendon repair was made, gentle passive stretching of the intrinsic muscles can be initiated.

(3) It is important to achieve full active ROM early.

(a) If an extension lag of the MCP joints is a persistent problem, place greater emphasis on active extension exercises.

(b) By 3 weeks, if at least 60 to 70 degrees of MCP flexion have not been achieved, a flexor outrigger may be added to the splint or a flexor cuff may be worn 1 to 2 hours per day.

NOTE: MCP flexion is most important in the third, fourth, and fifth digits for a good functional grasp.

(4) Active radial deviation of the digits is also added. Have the patient place the hand on a table, palm down, stabilize the dorsum of the hand, and practice sliding or walking the fingers radially.

(5) The dynamic splint is still worn when the patient is not exercising, and the static splint is still worn at night.

MINIMUM-PROTECTION AND RETURN-TO-ACTIVITY PHASES

(1) By 6 to 8 weeks the dynamic splint is discontinued. The night splint is worn until at least 12 weeks or longer if an extensor lag persists.

(2) Stretching is continued if contractures of the digits are present.

(3) Isometric strengthening activities are initiated at 6 weeks and for optimal results should be continued until at least 12 weeks postoperatively. Gentle dynamic resistance activities with small spring-loaded hand exercisers to improve grip strength may also be added.

C. Proximal Interphalangeal (PIP) Implant Arthroplasty

1. Indications for surgery[13,14,24,35,39]

a. Pain at the PIP joint(s) of the fingers and deterioration of the joint surfaces because of synovitis, usually associated with RA

b. Decreased range of motion at the PIP joints

c. Deformity of the fingers
 (1) Swan-neck deformity
 (2) Boutonnière deformity

2. Procedure[13,14,23,24,35,39]

a. The joint surface of the involved proximal phalanx and middle phalanx are excised and replaced with a flexible silicone implant.

b. The joint is realigned.

c. Repair may also be performed to the extensor tendon mechanism if necessary.

d. If either swan-neck or boutonnière deformities exist, they are corrected at this time.

e. The joint capsule is repaired, the wound is closed, and a bulky compression dressing is placed on the hand.
 (1) If a swan-neck deformity existed prior to surgery, the PIP joints are held in 10 to 20 degrees of flexion.
 (2) If a boutonnière deformity existed, the PIP joints are held in extension.

3. Postoperative management[13,27,34,39,40]

a. *Immobilization*

The period of time required for immobilization will vary, depending on whether or not extensor tendon reconstruction of the fingers was part of the procedure.

(1) If no tendon repair was done, only 2 to 3 days of immobilization of the PIP joints will be necessary before exercises can be started.

(2) If the extensor tendons have been repaired, a longer period of immobilization will be required to protect the extensor mechanism.

(3) The PIP joints are immobilized in extension with a small foam-covered aluminum or plastic resting splint between exercise sessions and at night.

b. *Exercise*

MAXIMUM-PROTECTION PHASE

NOTE: The postoperative exercise program differs based on the original impairments present, that is, tendon rupture, swan-neck deformity, or boutonnière deformity.

(1) If no tendon reconstruction was performed, the bulky compression dressing is removed in 3 to 4 days, and active exercise of the fingers, thumb, and wrist is started. These include:

(a) Active flexion and extension of the PIP joints with the MCP and DIP joints stabilized in neutral to direct the movement to the PIP joints

(b) Active flexion and extension of the MCP and DIP joints of the fingers

(c) Active exercises of the thumb

(d) Active range of motion of the wrist and forearm

(2) If a swan-neck deformity was corrected at the time the joint implant was performed, it is extremely important to avoid hyperextension of the PIP joint.

(a) Active flexion and extension exercise of the PIP joints is begun at approximately 10 to 14 days postoperatively. Be sure to stabilize the DIP joints in neutral during exercise.

(b) It may be appropriate to allow the patient to develop a slight (10 degree) flexion contracture at the PIP joint. This will protect the volar aspect of the joint capsule and lessen the possibility that a recurrent hyperextension deformity will develop.

(c) The PIP joint is immobilized in a splint in 10 to 20 degrees of flexion between exercises and at night.

(3) If a boutonnière deformity has been repaired at the time the joint arthroplasty was performed, it is important to maintain as much extension at the PIP joint as possible. Because the extensor tendons are repaired as a part of the procedure, stretching or heavy resistance to the extensor mechanism must be avoided for 6 to 8 weeks postoperatively.

(a) At 14 to 21 days postoperatively, active flexion and extension exercises to the PIP joints may be started.

(b) During active motion of the PIP joints, the MCP joints should be stabilized in neutral at the edge of a table or book.

(c) After exercise, the PIP joints are held in full extension in an aluminum splint.

MODERATE-PROTECTION PHASE

(1) By 3 weeks if PIP flexion is not sufficient (the goal is 70 degrees of flexion and full extension), initiate use of a dynamic flexion splint during the day. Continue use of a resting (static) extension splint at night, particularly if the patient also has an extension lag.

(2) Begin gentle stretching to increase flexion at the PIP joints.

MINIMUM-PROTECTION AND RETURN-TO-ACTIVITY PHASES

(1) In all variations of the PIP implant arthroplasty, active exercises are continued for 6 to 8 weeks postoperatively or until functional range of motion of the PIP joints (0 degrees of extension and 70 degrees of flexion) is attained.

(2) Gentle isometric strengthening or low-intensity dynamic resistance of the finger musculature can be achieved with a variety of exercise equipment designed for hand rehabilitation.

(3) If no tendon reconstruction was performed, discontinue use of static or dynamic splints by 6 to 8 weeks.

(4) Use the hand for light functional activities by 6 to 8 weeks postoperatively, but continue to employ principles of joint protection.

(5) Gentle manual stretching exercises should be continued for about 3 months to avoid recurrence of stiffness and contractures.

D. Carpometacarpal (CMC) Joint Replacement of the Thumb

1. Indications for surgery[13,14,35]

a. Pain at the carpometacarpal (trapeziometacarpal) joint of the thumb because of osteoarthritis or traumatic or rheumatoid arthritis. The majority of CMC arthroplasties are performed for pain and instability associated with degenerative joint disease.

b. Dorsoradial subluxation or dislocation of the first metacarpal, leading to a hyperextension deformity at the MCP joint of the thumb.

c. Limited range of motion, often an adduction contracture of the thumb.

d. Decreased pinch and grip strength because of pain in or subluxation of the CMC joint.

e. When arthrodesis of the CMC joint is inappropriate.

2. Procedures[13,14,35,40]

A number of procedures have been developed to replace the carpometacarpal joint. They may be classified into three broad categories:

a. Resection of the trapezium with autogenous tissue interposition (procedure of choice)

b. Replacement of the trapezium with a silicone prosthesis (hemiarthroplasty)

c. Replacement of the CMC joint with a metal-to-plastic ball-and-socket prosthesis held in place with methyl methacrylate

3. Postoperative management[14,35,40]

a. *Immobilization*

In all procedures the thumb and hand are immobilized postoperatively in a bulky compression dressing and elevated for several days to a week to control edema. The length of time the CMC joint is immobilized is dependent on the surgery.

b. *Exercise*

The progression of exercise varies with the type of implant.

MAXIMUM-PROTECTION PHASE

(1) When the bulky dressing is removed but while CMC immobilization continues, begin active motion of the fingers and wrist.

(2) As soon as the CMC immobilization can be removed for daily exercise, ini-

tiate gentle active motion of the thumb (abduction, flexion, extension, opposition, and circumdirection) in pain-free ranges.

(3) A protective splint is worn between exercise sessions and at night.

> ***Precaution:*** Avoid hyperextension of the CMC joint.

MODERATE- AND MINIMUM-PROTECTION PHASES

(1) Progress active exercises gradually.

(2) Between 6 and 12 weeks, if limitations in functional range persist, add gentle self-stretching without compromising joint stability.

(3) Initiate gentle grasp-and-pinch activities in functional patterns to increase strength of thumb musculature.

(4) Unrestricted use of the thumb for functional activities is permissible by 12 weeks postoperatively.

E. Repair of Ruptured Extensor Tendons Associated with RA

1. Background of the problem and indications for surgery[23,35,40,41]

a. Patients with chronic rheumatoid arthritis of the hand may experience rupture of one or more of the extensor digitorum communis or extensor pollicis longus tendons. The most common ruptures occur in the fourth and fifth fingers.

b. This may be caused by:

(1) Chronic tenosynovitis that infiltrates and weakens the tendons

(2) Pressure on the tendons from extensive proliferative synovitis at the MCP and PIP joints

(3) Progressive deterioration of a tendon at the distal ulna because the tendon rubs against an irregular bony surface

c. Rupture of extensor tendons leads to lack of active MCP joint extension (extensor lag). Multiple extensor tendon ruptures cause loss of functional use of the hand.

2. Procedure[35,40]

(1) If the patient has good passive range of motion of the fingers, repair of the extensor tendons can restore active extension to the MCP joints of the hand. This procedure may also be performed prior to or in conjunction with a flexible implant arthroplasty of an MCP joint or a wrist arthrodesis.

(2) A *tendon anastomosis* to an adjoining, intact extensor tendon is one method of repair. The ruptured extensor tendon is rewoven into the remaining extensor tendons.

(3) A *tendon graft* or a *tendon transfer*, rather than a tendon anastomosis to restore hand function, is another option. The most common techniques involve transfer of the extensor indicis proprius to the extensor digitorum communis at the MCP joints.

(4) Dorsal clearance (extensor tendon synovectomy) of the proliferated synovium along the extensor tendon sheaths of the wrist is also performed.

3. Postoperative management

a. *Immobilization*[23,35,41]

(1) The wrist and hand are immobilized in a short arm cast or splint for at least 4 weeks. All motion of the MCP joints must be avoided to protect the repaired tendon.

(2) The wrist is held in slight extension, and the MCP joints are held in 45 degrees of flexion to full extension.

(3) The hand is elevated and placed in a bulky surgical dressing for several days to minimize edema. When the surgical dressing is removed, the hand and wrist are held in extension in a volar splint.

b. *Exercise*

MAXIMUM-PROTECTION PHASE

(1) At 4 weeks the splint is removed for exercise. Gentle active exercises of the fingers are initiated with emphasis on MCP joint extension while the wrist and PIP joints are stabilized in neutral.

(2) Active wrist and forearm exercises are also begun.

MODERATE- AND MINIMUM-PROTECTION PHASE

(1) At 5 weeks gentle active flexion of the fingers is added.

(2) Submaximal isometric exercises of the finger flexors and extensors may be cautiously added.

(3) The splint is removed during the day at 6 weeks, and the patient may use the hand for light functional activities.

> ***Precaution:*** If the patient must use the hands for transfer activities, have him or her avoid putting pressure on the dorsum of the hand.

(4) Gentle stretching and dynamic resistance exercises may be added at 6 to 8 weeks to increase range of motion and strength.

IV. Repetitive Trauma Syndromes/Overuse Syndromes

A. Carpal Tunnel Syndrome

1. Etiology of symptoms

Irritation, inflammation, and swelling of the long flexor tendons from repetitive wrist motions, wrist joint swelling from trauma (such as falling on an outstretched hand), postfracture, arthritis, tenosynovitis and synovial tissue hypertrophy, and sometimes swelling from pregnancy result in compromise of the confined space in the carpal tunnel, leading to *compression of the median nerve* and resulting neurologic symptoms distal to that site.

2. Common impairments/problems

a. Increasing pain in the hand with repetitive use

b. Weakness or atrophy in the thenar muscles and first two lumbricals: ape hand deformity

c. Tightness in the adductor pollices and extrinsic extensors of the thumb and digits II and III

d. Sensory loss in the median nerve distribution

e. Possible decreased joint mobility in the wrist and MP joints of the thumb and digits II and III

3. Common functional limitations/disabilities

a. Decreased prehension in tip-to-tip, tip-to-pad, and pad-to-pad activities requiring fine control with opposition of the thumb

b. Inability to perform provoking sustained or repetitive wrist motion such as cashier checkout scanning, assembly line work, fine tool manipulation, or typing

4. **Nonoperative management**

The intervention is directed to the causative factor. Considerations include:

a. Splint to support the wrist or rest from the provoking activity.

b. Biomechanical analysis to identify faulty wrist or upper extremity motions. Adapt the environment if possible to reduce need for faulty motion, and strengthen and increase endurance in stabilizing muscles.

c. Mobilization of the carpals (specifically the capitate) for increased carpal tunnel space.

5. **Postoperative management**

Frequently, surgical release of the transverse carpal ligament is performed to relieve the compressive forces on the median nerve. Therapy may be initiated postsurgery if there are restrictions or muscle weakness. Exercises and mobilization techniques are used based on the functional loss. Suggestions include:

a. Mobilization of restricted joints as described in Section II.

b. Massage to restrictive scar tissue.

c. Stretching and strengthening exercises to weak muscles as described in Section VI. Functional strengthening may include activities such as pinching a spring-loaded clothespin using the type of prehension grip most needed by the patient.

d. Strengthening and endurance training in shoulder, elbow, and forearm stabilizing muscles.

B. Compression in Tunnel of Guyon

1. **Etiology of symptoms**

Swelling from injury or irritation of the *ulnar nerve* in the tunnel between the hook of the hamate and pisiform. This can occur from sustained pressure such as prolonged handwriting or leaning forward onto extended wrists while biking, from repetitive use of the gripping action of the fourth and fifth fingers, as with knitting or tying knots, or from trauma such as falling on the ulnar border of the wrist.

2. **Common impairments/problems**

a. Pain and paresthesia along the ulnar side of the palm of the hand and digits in the distribution of the ulnar nerve

b. Weakness or atrophy in the hypothenar, interossei, ulnar two lumbricals, adductor pollicis, and deep head of the flexor pollicis brevis muscles: bishop's or benediction hand deformity

c. Tightness in the extrinsic finger flexor and extensor muscles

d. Possible restricted mobility of the pisiform

3. **Common functional limitations/disabilities**

a. Decreased grip strength

b. Decreased ability to perform provoking activity

4. **Nonoperative management**

Management is basically the same as with carpal tunnel syndrome, with emphasis on modifying the provoking activity, avoiding pressure to the base of the palm, and use of a cock-up resting splint.

5. Postoperative management

Following release of the ulnar tunnel the wrist is immobilized 3 to 5 days; then treatment begins with gentle ROM. Follow the same guidelines as with carpal tunnel surgery.

C. Tenosynovitis, Tendinitis

1. Etiology of symptoms

Inflammation from continued or repetitive use of the involved muscle, from the effects of RA, from a stress overload to the contracting muscle, or from roughening of the surface of the tendon or its sheath.

2. Common impairments/problems

a. Pain whenever the related muscle contracts or whenever there is movement of another joint that causes gliding of the tendon through the sheath.
b. Warmth and tenderness to palpation in the region of inflammation.
c. In RA, synovial proliferation and swelling in affected tendon sheaths such as over the dorsum of the wrist or in the flexor tendons in the carpal tunnel.[29]
d. Frequently there is an imbalance in muscle length and strength or poor endurance in the stabilizing muscles. The fault may be more proximal in the elbow or shoulder, thus causing excessive load and substitute motions at the distal end of the chain.

3. Common functional limitations/disabilities

Pain that worsens with the provoking activity of the fingers, thumb, or wrist, which may affect the grip or repetitive hand motions.

4. Management of acute symptoms

Follow the guidelines for acute muscle lesions described in Chapter 7, with special emphasis on relieving the stress in the involved muscle and maintaining a healthy environment for healing with nondestructive forces.
a. Splint the related joints to rest the involved tendon.
b. If the tendon is in a sheath, apply cross-fiber massage while the tendon is in an elongated position so mobility is developed between the tendon and sheath.
c. Perform multi-angle muscle setting techniques in pain-free positions followed by pain-free range of motion.

5. Management in the subacute and chronic phases

a. Progress the intensity of massage, exercises, and stretching techniques.
b. Assess the biomechanics of the functional activity provoking the symptoms and design a program to regain a balance in length and strength and endurance of the muscles. Frequently problems may occur from poor stabilization or endurance in the shoulder or elbow.

V. Traumatic Lesions in the Hand

A. Simple Sprain: Nonoperative Management

1. Etiology of symptoms

Following trauma from a blow or a fall, an excessive stretch force may strain the supporting ligamentous tissue. There may be a related fracture, subluxation, or dislocation.

2. Common impairments/problems

a. Pain at the involved site whenever a stretch force is placed on the ligament.

b. There may be hypermobility or instability in the related joint.

3. Common functional limitations/disabilities

a. With a simple sprain, pain may interfere with functional use of the hand for a couple of weeks if the joint is stressed. There will be no limitation of function if a splint or taping can be worn to protect the ligament and the splint does not interfere with the task.

b. With significant tears there will be instability and the joint may subluxate or dislocate with provoking activities requiring surgery.

4. Nonoperative management

a. Follow the guidelines in Chapter 7 for treating acute lesions with emphasis on maintaining mobility while minimizing stress to the healing tissue. If immobilization is necessary to protect the part, only the involved joint should be immobilized. Joints above and below should be free to move. This will maintain mobility of the long tendons in their sheaths that cross the involved joint.[11]

b. Cross-fiber massage to the site of the lesion may help to prevent the developing scar from adhering and restricting motion.

c. Avoid positions of stress and activities that provoke the symptoms while healing.

B. Repair of Lacerated Flexor Tendons of the Hand

1. Background of the problem and indications for surgery[1,31,36,37]

a. Lacerations of the flexor tendons of the hand are common and can occur in various areas (zones) along the volar surface of the fingers, palm, and wrist. The musculotendinous structures damaged will depend upon the depth and location of the wound.

b. The volar surface of the wrist and hand is divided into five zones; the thumb is divided into three zones (Fig. 10–2). Repair and rehabilitation of a laceration in zone 2 (no-man's land), which extends between the distal insertion of the flexor digitorum superficialis (FDS) tendon of the middle phalanx to the metacarpals, are a particular challenge. Because of the confined space in which tendons lie and the limited vascular supply of tendons in zone 2, healing tissues in this area are particularly prone to adhesions. Scar tissue formation interrupts normal gliding of tendons and restricts ROM.

c. Laceration and severance of one or more tendons may also be accompanied by vascular, nerve, and skeletal injuries that will complicate the management of tendon repairs.

2. Procedures[12,18,31,37]

a. Simple flexor tendon lacerations are managed with *direct primary repair* or *delayed primary repair* within the first 24 hours to several days after injury. The severed tendon is reopposed and sutured. Nonreactive sutures are placed in the volar aspect of the tendon so as not to disturb the dorsal aspect of the tendon in which the blood supply lies. The tendon sheath is also repaired to

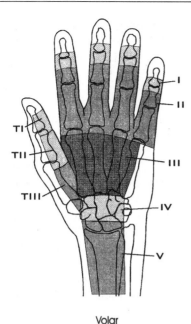

Volar

Figure 10–2. Flexor tendon zones; volar aspect of the hand and wrist.

maintain circulation or synovium within the sheath for extrinsic nutrition to the tendon.

   b. An alternative procedure is a *two-stage tendon reconstruction with graft*. Depending on the severity of injury to other structures of the hand, débridement of the wound, repair of nerves or vascular structures, and stabilization of skeletal injuries must be managed before tendons can be repaired. Placement of a tendon spacer may be necessary with a tendon graft reconstruction delayed for several months. When the graft is surgically implanted, it is sutured to the proximal and distal portions of the severed tendon.

3. Postoperative management[6,10,36]

   a. *Immobilization*

     (1) The involved fingers and hand are immobilized in a bulky surgical dressing for several days and elevated to control edema.

     (2) The fingers and wrist are immobilized in flexion to initially keep the repaired tendons or graft site on a slack.

   b. *Exercise*

   NOTE: The progression of exercises throughout the rehabilitation program is more conservative after graft reconstruction than after direct repair to allow time for vascularization of the graft.

   MAXIMUM-PROTECTION PHASE

   (1) After the surgical dressing is removed, the most conservative method of management is to place the involved fingers and wrist in a static splint and immobilize the hand in flexion 24 hours per day for 3 weeks. This provides maximum protection to the healing structures but leads to severe adhesions and irreversible flexion contractures of the digits.

(2) A more commonly used postoperative approach today is to allow *early controlled motion* to prevent contractures. Motion is performed while the wrist and fingers are held in flexion in a dorsal blocking splint, a dynamic splint with rubber band traction, or a combination of both types of splint.[6,10,12,18]

    (a) A *static* blocking splint placed on the dorsal surface of the wrist and fingers holds the wrist in approximately 20 degrees of flexion, the MCP joints in 70 degrees of flexion, and the IP joints in neutral. The splint is loosened or removed for exercise.

    (b) A *dynamic* splint with rubber-band traction passively holds the wrist in neutral and the fingers in flexion but allows active extension of the fingers through a protected portion of the ROM against the resistance of rubber bands. When the patient relaxes the finger extensors, the rubber bands *passively* flex the fingers.

(3) To control edema, initiate gentle massage when the bulky dressing is removed.

(4) To prevent contractures and maintain differential tendon gliding in the sheath but protect the sutured tendon, begin early controlled motion with the following exercises and continue for the first 3 to 4 weeks postoperatively:

    (a) In a dynamic (rubber-band) splint begin active finger extension; passive finger flexion by means of the rubber bands will occur when the extensors relax.

    (b) In a static dorsal blocking splint (no rubber bands) with the stabilizing straps temporarily loosened, begin passive flexion and extension of the fingers applied manually by a therapist or by the patient. Extend or flex one joint at a time while stabilizing the others.

(5) Begin scar mobilization with friction massage to prevent adhesions.

(6) By 3½ to 4 weeks or as late as 5 weeks the splint is modified or a wrist cuff is fabricated to allow wrist motion and greater finger motion. The following exercises are performed:

    (a) Active finger flexion with the wrist in extension

    (b) Active wrist extension with finger flexion

    (c) Active finger extension with wrist flexion

MODERATE-PROTECTION PHASE

(1) At 6 weeks discontinue protective splinting.

(2) If the patient has not achieved full finger extension, begin very gentle stretching of the finger flexors with the wrist stabilized in neutral.

(3) Add light resistance activities with therapeutic putty or manual resistance.

(4) Allow the patient to use the hand for light functional activities.

MINIMUM PROTECTION AND RETURN TO ACTIVITY

(1) By 8 to 10 weeks emphasize progressive grip-strengthening activities.

(2) Improve endurance with sustained grasp exercises and activities.

(3) Incorporate work or leisure time activities into hand exercises.

(4) If finger flexion contractures exist, use dynamic splinting for a prolonged stretch, more vigorous manual stretching, and joint mobilization techniques.

(5) The patient should return to full functional use of the hand by 12 weeks postoperatively.

C. Repair of Lacerated Extensor Tendons of the Hand

1. Background of the problem and indications for surgery[31,37]

   a. Lacerations and traumatic rupture of the extensor tendons of the fingers, thumb, or wrist are more common than flexor tendon lacerations because the extensor tendons lie just below the skin and are more superficial than the flexor tendons.

   b. The extensor surface of the fingers and wrist are divided into seven zones, and the extensor surface of the thumb is divided into four zones (Fig. 10–3). The location of a laceration to the extensor tendons determines which structures of the extensor mechanism will be injured. For example, a laceration of the extensor surface of the DIP joint and distal phalanx (zone 1) will disrupt terminal extension of a digit. A laceration across the MCP joints (zone 5) will disrupt the common extensor tendons and MCP extension.

   c. The mechanism of injury can be a laceration, fracture dislocation, or extensive trauma resulting in multiple fractures and disruption of the nerve or blood supply to the hand.

2. Procedures[1,31,37]

   a. The ends of the lacerated tendons are reopposed (approximated) and sutured together.

   b. If an associated fracture or fracture/dislocation has occurred, a K-wire is used to stabilize involved bones or joints.

   c. After the incision is closed, a bulky dressing and volar blocking splint are placed on the hand and involved digits.

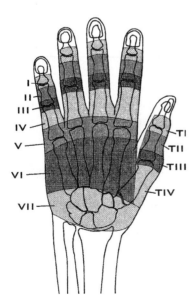

Dorsal

Figure 10–3. Extensor tendon zones; dorsal aspect of the hand and wrist.

3. Postoperative management[1,36]

a. *Immobilization*

   (1) The position of immobilization, regardless of the zone of injury, is extension. The bulky dressing and volar blocking splint prevent wrist and finger flexion.

   (2) The length of immobilization depends upon the zone in which the injury occurred and the type of surgical repair that was chosen. Repair of tendons in zones 1 to 4 across the digits usually requires 4 to 6 weeks of immobilization in an extension splint. Repairs in zones 5 to 7 require a less extensive period of complete immobilization. In zone 7 only the wrist and MP joints are immobilized. Early controlled motion in a protected range is permissible several days after surgery.

b. *Exercise*

   (1) In general, the maximum-, moderate-, and minimum-protection phases of an exercise program after extensor tendon repairs are longer and exercises are progressed more conservatively than after flexor tendon repairs. Extensor tendons require a longer time to heal than flexor tendons because of differences in vascularity and because the synovial tendon sheath, which provides nutrition to the extensor tendons, is found only at the wrist. Because the extensor tendons are enclosed by a synovial sheath only at the wrist, they are less likely than the flexor tendons to develop adhesions that restrict motion.

   (2) The initiation and progression of exercises depend on where (in what zone) the repair was made, as previously noted.

   (3) The movements emphasized and points of stabilization depend on the zone of injury.

      (a) In zones 1 and 2 emphasize active DIP flexion while stabilizing the proximal joints.

      (b) In zones 3 and 4 emphasize active PIP flexion with the MCP joints in extension and PIP extension with the MCP joints in flexion. Be sure to stabilize the DIP joints.

      (c) In zones 5 and 6 earlier motion is allowable within a protected range than in zones 1 to 4. Begin active blocked MCP flexion and passive extension of the involved digits at 4 days after surgery. Active PIP and DIP flexion with the wrist and MCP joints held in extension are also appropriate. At 4 weeks, add active MCP extension with the PIP and DIP joints semiflexed (the intrinsic minus position of the hand) to emphasize action of the extensor digitorum communis.

      (d) In zone 7 initiate PIP and DIP motions immediately with the MCP joints and wrist held in extension. After approximately 3 weeks of immobilization in extension of the wrist and MCP joints, gradually increase wrist and MCP flexion. Then add gentle active MCP and wrist extension with the fingers extended as well as radial and ulnar deviation of the wrist.

   (4) *Remember:* The flexors are a much stronger muscle group than are the extensors, so active flexion must be gentle and controlled to avoid a stretch to the repaired extensor tendons. A dynamic extension splint to assist extension and resist flexion sometimes is used for the first few weeks after the immobilization device is removed to protect the repaired extensor tendons.

(5) Exercises and splinting are continued for approximately 8 to 10 weeks. During the moderate- and minimum-protection phases, gentle resistive exercises can be added as healing progresses. The hand is used for progressively more vigorous daily functional activities in the later stages of rehabilitation.

VI. Exercises for Muscle Strength or Flexibility Imbalance

NOTE: No matter what the cause, muscle strength or flexibility imbalance can lead to poor hand mechanics. If there is nerve damage with motor loss or faulty mechanics from progressive joint degeneration, splinting is necessary to prevent contracture formation and to provide stabilization for the functioning of remaining muscles. (Techniques of functional splinting are beyond the scope of this textbook.) The general principles for treating acute lesions have been described in the preceding sections. The reader is also referred to Chapter 7. Exercises described in this section are for use during the subacute and chronic phases of healing and should be progressed at the patient's tolerance.

A. Techniques to Stretch Tight Muscles

Precautions: Before initiating stretching techniques to muscle or inert tissue, there should be normal gliding of the joint surfaces to avoid joint damage; if normal gliding is not present, joint-play techniques should be initiated first.

Because there are many multijoint muscles in the hand, stabilization and specific stretching techniques are critical to avoid joint damage or hypermobility.

1. **Active inhibition and passive stretching**
   These techniques for increasing flexibility of the muscles and soft tissues of the wrist and hand are described in Chapter 5.

2. **Self-stretching of tight lumbricale and interossei muscles**
   The patient actively extends the MCP joints and flexes the IP joints. For reciprocal inhibition, manual resistance is applied against the fingertips with the fingers of the patient's other hand as finger flexion is performed (see Fig. 10–6).

3. **Self-stretching interossei muscles**
   The patient places the hand flat on a table with the palm down and the MP joints extended. He or she abducts or adducts the appropriate digit with the force applied to the distal end of the proximal phalanx. Stabilization is provided by fixating against the adjacent digit.

4. **Self-stretching adductor pollicis**
   The patient rests the ulnar border of the hand on a table. He or she applies the stretch force with the other hand against the metacarpal heads, attempting to increase the web space.

5. **To stretch the extrinsic muscles**
   Because they are multijoint muscles, the final step is to elongate each tendon over all the joints simultaneously, but *do not* initiate stretching procedures in this manner because joint compression and damage can occur to the smaller or less stable joints. Begin by allowing the wrist and more proximal finger joints to relax; stretch the tendon unit over the most distal joint first. Stabilize the distal joint at the end of the range, then stretch the tendon unit over the next joint. Then stabilize the two joints as you stretch the tendon over the next joint and progress in this manner until the desired length is reached.

Precaution: Do not let the PIP and MCP joints hyperextend as you stretch the tendons over the wrist.

6. **Self-stretching of the flexor digitorum profundus and superficialis**

    Have the patient begin by resting the palm of the involved hand on a table. He or she first extends the DIP joint, using the other hand to straighten the joint; keeping it extended, he or she then straightens the PIP and MCP joints in succession. If the patient can actively extend the finger joints to this point, the motion should be performed unassisted. He or she firmly fixates the hand on the table with the other hand and then begins to extend the wrist by actively bringing the arm up over the hand. The patient goes just to the point of feeling discomfort, holds the position, then progresses as the length improves (Fig. 10–4).

7. **Self-stretching of the extensor communis**

    The fingers are flexed to the maximum range, beginning with the distalmost joint first and progressing until the wrist is simultaneously flexed. The patient should accomplish this actively if possible.

8. **Stretching techniques for wrist flexors and extensors**

    These were described in the section on medial and lateral epicondylitis (Chapter 9, Sections V.D and V.E).

9. **Selective stretching**

    Patients with C-6 quadriplegia are able to use tendon action to flex their fingers for functional grasp if the extrinsic flexor muscles (profundus and superficialis) are allowed to tighten. This action is called tenodesis; it is the passive movement of the finger joints caused by the multijoint muscles as they are stretched over the wrist. The fingers close as the wrist is actively extended and open as the wrist flexes.[20]

B. Techniques to Strengthen Weak Muscles

If musculature is weak, progressive strengthening exercises are used to gain muscle balance (see Chapter 3 for descriptions of resistive exercise programs).

1. **To strengthen wrist musculature**

    a. Allow the fingers to relax. The wrist muscles can be exercised as a group if their strength is similar. If one muscle is weaker, the wrist should be guided through the range desired to minimize the action of the stronger muscles. For

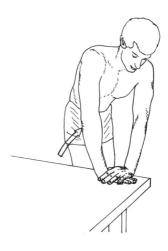

Figure 10–4. Self-stretching of the extrinsic finger flexor muscles, showing stabilization of the small distal joints.

example, with wrist flexion, if the flexor carpi radialis is stronger than the flexor carpi ulnaris, instruct the patient to attempt to flex the wrist toward the ulnar side as you guide the wrist into flexion and ulnar deviation. If the muscle is strong enough to tolerate resistance, place your manual resistance over the fourth and fifth metacarpals (similar to Fig. 3–10).

b. Mechanical resistance with a hand-held weight or elastic resistance. The patient's forearm rests on a table with the forearm pronated to resist extension (See Fig. 9–2), mid-range to resist radial deviation, or supinated to resist flexion.

c. Progress to controlled patterns of motion requiring stabilization of the wrist for functional hand activities. Develop endurance and progress to the desired functional pattern by loading the upper extremity to the tolerance of the wrist stabilizers. When the stabilization begins to fatigue, stop the activity.

2. **To strengthen weak intrinsic musculature**

   NOTE: Imbalance from weak intrinsic muscles leads to a claw hand.

   a. *MCP joint flexion with IP joint extension*
      (1) Begin with the MP joints stabilized in flexion. Have the patient actively extend the DIP joint against a resistive force on the middle phalanx. Progress the resistive force to the distal phalanx. The resistance may be applied manually or with rubber bands.
      (2) Have the patient start with the MCP joints extended and the PIP joints flexed; then actively push the fingertips outward, performing the desired combined motion (Fig. 10–5A and B). If he or she tolerates resistance, have the patient push the fingers into the palm of the other hand (Fig. 10–5C).

   b. *Isolated or combined abduction/adduction of each finger*
      (1) Have the patient rest the palm of the hand on a table. Give resistance at the distal end of the first phalanx, one finger at a time, for either abduction or adduction.
      (2) To resist adduction, the patient interlaces the fingers of both hands (or with your hand) and pinches the fingers together.
      (3) Place a rubber band around two digits and have the patient spread them apart.

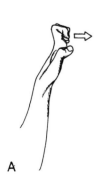

A

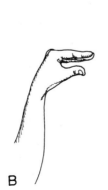

B

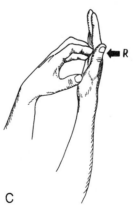

C

Figure 10–5. To strengthen intrinsic muscle function for combined MCP flexion and IP extension, the patient begins with (*A*) MCP extension and IP flexion and (*B*) pushes his fingertips outward. The same motion is resisted by (*C*) pushing the fingertips against the palm of the other hand.

c. *Abduction of the thumb*
(1) The patient rests the dorsum of the hand on a table, and resistance is applied at the base of the first phalanx of the thumb as the patient lifts the thumb away from the palm of the hand.
(2) Place a rubber band around the thumb and index finger. The patient abducts the thumb against the resistance.

d. *Opposition of the thumb*
For manual resistance, see Fig. 3–12.

3. **To strengthen weak extrinsic musculature of the fingers**

NOTE: The wrist must be stabilized for the action of the extrinsic hand musculature to be effective. With inadequate wrist strength for stabilization, manually stabilize it during exercises and splint it for functional usage.

a. *Metacarpophalangeal extension*
(1) Manual resistance is applied at the distal end of the proximal phalanx; the wrist is neutral or partially flexed.
(2) For mechanical resistance, the hand rests on a table with the palm down and digits over the edge. Place a loop over the distal end of the proximal phalanx with the weight hanging down from it.
See also mechanical resistance techniques in the next section.

b. *Interphalangeal flexion*
(1) The profundus and superficialis actions can be isolated for manual resistance, as is done with manual muscle testing procedures.[9] This may be necessary following isolated tendon injuries when retraining of the injured tendon is necessary.[11] Or the muscles can be resisted together if their strength is similar. The wrist must be stabilized in mid-position or partially extended.
(2) Self-resistance: With the hands pointing in opposite directions, the patient places the pads of each finger on one hand against the pads of each finger of the other hand (or against your hand). He or she then curls the fingers against the resistance provided by the other hand (Fig. 10–6). The same technique is used to resist thumb flexion.

4. **Mechanical resistance techniques requiring intrinsic and extrinsic muscle function**

NOTE: Proper stabilization is important; either the patient's stabilizing muscles must be strong enough or the weakened areas must be supported manually. If a weight causes stress because the patient cannot control it, the exercise will be detrimental rather than beneficial.

a. Spread a towel out on a table. The patient places the palm of the hand down at one end of the towel. While maintaining contact with the heel of the hand,

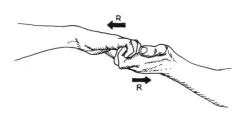

Figure 10–6. Self-resistance to strengthen extrinsic finger flexor muscles.

he or she crumples the towel into the hand. The same exercise can be carried out by placing a stack of newspapers under the hand. The patient crumples the top sheet into a ball (and tosses it into a basket for coordination and skill practice), then repeats it with each sheet in succession.

   b. Using a disk weight as tolerated

     (1) Grasp the disk with the tips of all five digits spread around the outer edge. Lift with the forearm pronated and palm down. Hold the position for isometric resistance to grasp and wrist extension. Increase the effect of the resistance by extending one finger.

     (2) Pick up the side of the disk weight, either with fingertips or between the pads of the distal phalanx of thumb and individual fingers.

     (3) The hand is placed palm down on the table; place a weight on the dorsum of the fingers; the patient hyperextends the fingers by lifting the weight.

   c. Other resistance aids such as putty, spring-loaded hand resistance, and various grades and sizes of soft balls can be used for general strengthening. Observe the pattern used by the patient and be sure he or she does not substitute or develop damaging forces.

5. Progress to specific patterns of activity needed for ADL, job activation, or recreational function.

To develop muscular endurance, resist the pattern with light resistance until fatigued. Progress intensity and duration of exercises as required by the functional activity.

VII. Summary

The anatomy and kinesiology of the wrist and hand have been outlined in this chapter. Clinical application of this information has included a discussion of hand control, grasp, and pinch. Guidelines for therapeutic exercise management of specific musculoskeletal problems and reconstructive surgical procedures of the wrist and hand have been outlined. These guidelines include nonoperative and postoperative management of problems of the wrist, fingers, and thumb secondary to arthritis, overuse syndromes, and traumatic lesions. The chapter has concluded with a description of stretching, strengthening, and functional exercises appropriate for rehabilitation of the wrist and hand.

References

1. Beasley, RW: Basic Considerations for Tendon Transfer Operations in the Upper Extremity. In AAOS Symposium on Tendon Surgery of the Hand. CV Mosby, St Louis, 1975.
2. Bentley, JA: Physiotherapy following joint replacements. In Downie, PA (ed): Cash's Textbook of Orthopedics and Rheumatology for Physiotherapist. JB Lippincott, Philadelphia, 1984.
3. Bieber, EJ, Wieland, AJ, and Volenec-Dowling, S: Silicone-rubber implant arthroplasty of the metacarpophalangeal joints for rheumatoid arthritis. J Bone Joint Surg Am 68:206, 1986.
4. Blair, WF, Schurr, DG, and Buckwalter, JA: Metacarpophalangeal joint implant arthroplasty with Silastic spacer. J Bone Joint Surg Am 66:365, 1984.
5. Cailliet, R: Hand Pain and Impairment, ed 4. FA Davis, Philadelphia, 1994.

6. Chow, JA, et al: A combined regimen of controlled motion following flexor tendon repair in "no man's land." Plast Reconstr Surg 79(3):447, 1987.
7. Chusid, J, and McDonald, J: Correlative Neuroanatomy and Functional Neurology, ed 17. Land, Medical Publications, Los Altos, CA, 1979.
8. Cyriax, J: Textbook of Orthopaedic Medicine, Vol 1. Diagnosis of Soft Tissue Lesions, ed 8. Bailliere Tindall, London, 1982.
9. Daniels, L, and Worthingham, C: Muscle Testing: Techniques of Manual Examination, ed 5. WB Saunders, Philadelphia, 1986.
10. Duran, RJ, and Houser, RC: Controlled passive motion following flexor tendon repair in zones II and III. In AAOS Symposium on Tendon Surgery in the Hand. CV Mosby, St Louis, 1975.
11. Foreman, S, and Gieck, J: Rehabilitative manage-

ment of injuries to the hand. Clin Sports Med 11:239, 1992.

12. Hunter, JM: Two stage flexor tendon reconstruction: A technique using a tendon prosthesis before tendon grafting. In Hunter, JM (ed): Rehabilitation of the Hand, ed 2. CV Mosby, St Louis, 1984.

13. Hyde, SA: Physiotherapy in Rheumatology. Blackwell Scientific, Oxford, 1980.

14. Inglis, AE (ed): Symposium on Total Joint Replacement of the Upper Extremity (1979). American Academy of Orthopedic Surgeons, CV Mosby, St Louis, 1982.

15. Iversen, LD, and Clawson, DK: Manual of Acute Orthopedic Therapeutics, ed 2. Little, Brown, Boston, 1982.

16. Kapandji, IA: The Physiology of the Joints, Vol I. Churchill-Livingstone, Edinburgh, 1970.

17. Kessler, R, and Hertling, D: Management of Common Musculoskeletal Disorders. Harper & Row, Philadelphia, 1983.

18. Kleinert, HE, and Cash, SL: Current guidelines for flexor tendon repair within the fibro-osseus tunnel: Indications timing and techniques. In Hunter, JM, Schneider, LH, and Mackin, EJ (eds): Tendon Surgery in the Hand. CV Mosby, St Louis, 1987.

19. Kopell, H, and Thompson, W: Peripheral Entrapment Neuropathies, ed 2. Robert E Krieger, Huntington, NY, 1976.

20. Lehmkuhl, LD, and Smith, LK: Brunnstrom's Clinical Kinesiology, ed 4. FA Davis, Philadelphia, 1983.

21. Long, R, et al: Intrinsic-extrinsic muscle control of the hand in power grip and precision handling. J Bone Joint Surg Am 52:853, 1970.

22. Long, C: Normal and Abnormal Motor Control in the Upper Extremities. Final Report, Case Western Reserve University, Cleveland, OH, 1970.

23. Melvin, J: Rheumatic Disease in the Adult and Child: Occupational Therapy and Rehabilitation, ed 3. FA Davis, Philadelphia, 1989.

24. Nalebuff, E, Feldon, P, and Millender, L: Rheumatoid arthritis in the hand and wrist. In Green, DP (ed): Operative Hand Surgery, ed 2. Churchill-Livingstone, New York, 1988.

25. Napier, JR: The prehensile movements of the human hand. J Bone Joint Surg Br 38:902, 1956.

26. Norkin, C, and Levangie, P: Joint Structure and Function: A Comprehensive Analysis, ed 2. FA Davis, Philadelphia, 1992.

27. Occupational Therapy Staff: Upper Extremity Surgeries for Patients with Arthritis; A Pre and Post-Operative Occupational Therapy Treatment Guide. Rancho Los Amigos Hospital, Downey, CA, 1979.

28. Omer, GE: Tendon transfers for reconstruction of the forearm and hand following peripheral nerve injuries. In Omer, GE, and Spinner, M (eds): Management of Peripheral Nerve Problems. WB Saunders, Philadelphia, 1980.

29. Phillips, CA: Rehabilitation of the patient with rheumatoid hand involvement. Phys Ther 69:1091, 1989.

30. Randall, T, Portney, L, and Harris, BA: Effects of joint mobilization on joint stiffness and active moxtion of the metacarpal-phalangeal joint. Journal of Orthopaedic and Sports Physical Therapy 16:30, 1992.

31. Rosenblum, NI, and Robinson, SJ: Advances in flexor and extensor tendon management. In Moran, CA (ed): Hand Rehabilitation. Churchill-Livingstone, New York, 1986.

32. Rosenthal, EA: The extensor tendons. In Hunter, JM (ed): Rehabilitation of the Hand. CV Mosby, St Louis, 1980.

32. Rosenthal, EA: The extensor tendons. In Hunter, JM (ed): Rehabilitation of the Hand. CV Mosby, St Louis, 1980.

33. Saunders, SR: Physical therapy management of hand fractures. Phys Ther 69:1065, 1989.

34. Shurr, DG: The therapist's role in finger joint arthroplasty. In Moran, CA (ed): Hand Rehabilitation. Churchill-Livingstone, New York, 1986.

35. Simmons, BP, Millender, LH, and Nalebuff, EA: Surgery of the hand. In Sledge, CB, et al (eds): Arthritis Surgery. WB Saunders, Philadelphia, 1994.

36. Stewart, KM: Review and comparisons in the postoperative management of tendon repair. Hand Clin 7(3):447–460, 1991.

37. Stewart, KM: Tendon injuries. In Stanley, BG, and Tribuzi, SM (eds): Concepts in Hand Rehabilitation. FA Davis, Philadelphia, 1992.

38. Swanson, AB, Swanson, GD, and Maupin, BK: Flexible implant arthroplasty of the radiocarpal joint. Surgical techniques and long-term study. Clin Orthop 187:94, 1984.

39. Swanson, AB, et al: Postoperative rehabilitation program in flexible implant arthroplasty of the digits. In Hunter, JM, et al (eds): Rehabilitation of the Hand, ed 3 CV Mosby, St Louis, 1990.

40. Swanson, AB, et al: Upper limb joint replacement. In Nickel, VL (ed): Orthopedic Rehabilitation. Churchill-Livingstone, New York, 1982.

41. Trombly, CA: Occupational Therapy for Physical Dysfunction, ed 2. Williams & Wilkins, Baltimore, MD, 1983.

42. Zohn, D, and Mennell, J: Musculoskeletal Pain: Principles of Physical Diagnosis and Physical Treatment. Little, Brown, Boston, 1976.

The Hip

The hip is often compared with the shoulder in that it is a triaxial joint, able to function in all three planes, and is also the proximal link to its extremity. In contrast to the shoulder, which is constructed for mobility, the hip is a stable joint, constructed for weight bearing. Forces from the lower extremities are transmitted upward through the hips to the pelvis and trunk during gait and other lower extremity activities. The hips also support the weight of the head, trunk, and upper extremities.

The initial section of this chapter reviews highlights of the anatomy and function of the hip and its relation to the pelvis and lumbar spine. The reader is referred to several texts for study of the material.[9,32,38] Chapter 7 presents information on principles of management; the reader should be familiar with that material as well as the components of an effective, objective evaluation of the hip and pelvis before determining a diagnosis and proceeding with establishing a therapeutic exercise program.

OBJECTIVES

After studying this chapter, the reader will be able to:

1 Identify important aspects of the hip structure and function for review.
2 Establish a therapeutic exercise program to manage soft tissue and joint lesions in the hip that are related to stages of recovery following an inflammatory insult to the tissues, recognizing unique circumstances in the hip and pelvis for their management.
3 Establish a therapeutic exercise program to manage patients following common surgical procedures for the hip.

I. Review of the Structure and Function of the Hip

A. Bony Parts Are the Proximal Femur and the Pelvis (see Fig. 6-45).

B. Hip Joint

1. Characteristics

The hip is a ball-and-socket (spheroidal) triaxial joint; supported by a strong articular capsule that is reinforced by the iliofemoral, pubofemoral, and ischiofemoral ligaments. The two hip joints are linked to each other through the bony pelvis and to the vertebral column through the sacrum and lumbosacral joint.

2. The acetabulum

The concave bony partner, the acetabulum, is made up of the fusion of the ilium, ischium, and pubic bones and is deepened by a ring of fibrocartilage, the acetabulum labrum. It is located in the lateral aspect of the pelvis and faces laterally, anteriorly, and inferiorly. The articular cartilage is horseshoe-shaped, being thicker in the lateral region. The central portion of the acetabular surface is nonarticular.

3. The femoral head

The convex bony partner is the spherical head of the femur, which is attached to the femoral neck. It projects anteriorly, medially, and superiorly.

4. Motions of the femur

The convex head slides in the direction opposite the physiologic motion of the femur.

Physiologic Motions of the Femur	Direction of Slide of the Femoral Head
Flexion	Posterior
Extension	Anterior
Abduction	Inferior
Adduction	Superior
Internal rotation	Posterior
External rotation	Anterior

5. Motions of the pelvis

When the lower extremity is fixated, as in standing or during the stance phase of gait, the concave acetabulum moves on the convex femoral head, so the acetabulum slides in the same direction as the pelvis. (See Section C following.)

Physiologic Motions of the Pelvis	Direction of Slide of of the Acetabulum
Anterior pelvic tilt	Anterior
Posterior pelvic tilt	Posterior
Lateral pelvic tilt	
Pelvis elevated	Inferior
Pelvis dropped	Superior
Forward pelvic rotation	Anterior
Backward pelvic rotation	Posterior

NOTE: When the pelvis moves, it affects both hip joints, but the motion is not necessarily the same on the contralateral side.

6. Angle of inclination

The angle between the axis of the femoral neck and shaft of the femur is normally 125 degrees. A pathological larger angle is called coxa valga, and a pathologically smaller angle is called coxa vara. Unilateral coxa valga results in a relatively longer leg on that side and associated genu varum. Unilateral coxa vara leads to a relatively shorter leg with associated genu valgum on that side. Compensations with unilateral differences usually occur in the pelvis, foot, and ankle.

7. Torsion

The angle formed by the transverse axis of the femoral condyles and the axis of the neck of the femur ranges from 8 to 25 degrees, with a normal angle of 12 degrees. An increase in the angle is called anteversion and causes the shaft of the femur to be rotated medially; a decrease in the angle is called retroversion and causes the shaft of the femur to be rotated laterally. Anteversion often results in genu valgum and pes planus. Unilateral anteversion results in a relatively shorter leg on that side with compensations in the position of the pelvis. Retroversion causes the opposite effects.

C. Functional Relationships of the Hips and Pelvis in the Kinematic Chain

1. Changes in the angle of the hip and lumbar spine with pelvic motion

a. *Anterior pelvic tilt (PT)*

The anterior superior iliac spines of the pelvis move anteriorly and inferiorly and thus closer to the anterior aspect of the femur as the pelvis rotates forward around the transverse axis of the hip joints. This results in hip flexion and increased lumbar spine extension (hyperextension).

(1) Muscles causing this motion are the hip flexors and back extensors.

(2) When standing, with the line of gravity of the trunk falling anteriorly to the axis of the hip joints, the effect is an anterior PT. Stability is provided by the abdominals and hip extensor muscles.

b. *Posterior PT*

The posterior superior iliac spines of the pelvis move posteriorly and inferiorly, thus closer to the posterior aspect of the femur as the pelvis rotates backward around the axis of the hip joints. This results in hip extension and lumbar spine flexion.

(1) Muscles causing this motion are the hip extensors and trunk flexors.

(2) When standing and the line of gravity of the trunk falls posteriorly to the axis of the hip joints, the effect is a posterior pelvic tilt. Stability may be provided by the hip flexors and back extensors.

c. *Pelvic shifting*

When standing, a forward translatory shifting of the pelvis results in extension of the hip and extension of the lower lumbar spinal segments. There is a compensatory posterior shifting of the thorax on the upper lumbar spine with increased flexion of these spinal segments. This is often seen with slouched or relaxed postures (see Chapter 15). Little muscle action is required; the posture is maintained by the iliofemoral ligaments at the hip, anterior longitudinal ligament of the lower lumbar spine, and posterior ligaments of the upper lumbar and thoracic spine.

d. *Lumbopelvic rhythm*[9]

A coordinated movement between the lumbar spine and pelvis occurs for maximal forward bending of the trunk as when reaching toward the floor or the toes. As the head and upper trunk initiate flexion, the pelvis shifts posteriorly to maintain the center of gravity balanced over the base of support. The trunk continues to forward bend, being controlled by the extensor muscles of the spine, until approximately 45 degrees. The ligaments are then taut and the facets oriented in the frontal plane approximated, both providing stability for the vertebrae, and the muscles relax.[46] Once all of the vertebral segments are at the end of the range and stabilized by the posterior ligaments and facets, the pelvis begins to rotate forward (anterior pelvic tilt), being controlled by the gluteus maximus and hamstring muscles. The pelvis continues to rotate forward until the full length of the muscles is reached. Final range of motion (ROM) in forward bending is dictated by the flexibility in the various back extensor muscles and fasciae as well as hip extensor muscles. The return to the upright position begins with the hip extensor muscles rotating the pelvis posteriorly through reverse muscle action (posterior pelvic tilt), then back extensor muscles extending the spine from the lumbar region upward. Variations in the normal synchronization of this activity occur because of faulty habits, restricted muscle or fascia length, or injury and faulty proprioception.

e. *Lateral pelvic tilt*

Frontal plane pelvic motion results in opposite motions at each hip joint. On the side that is elevated (hip hiking), there is hip adduction; on the side that is lowered (hip drop), there is hip abduction. When standing, the lumbar spine laterally flexes toward the side of the elevated pelvis (convexity of the lateral curve is toward the lowered side).

(1) Muscles causing lateral pelvic tilting include the quadratus lumborum on the side of the elevated pelvis and reverse muscle pull of the gluteus medius on the side of the lowered pelvis.

(2) With an asymmetric slouched posture, the person shifts the trunk weight onto one lower extremity and allows the pelvis to drop on the other side. Passive support comes from the iliofemoral ligament and iliotibial band on the elevated side (stance leg).

f. *Pelvic rotation*

Rotation occurs around one lower extremity that is fixed on the ground. The unsupported lower extremity swings forward or backward along with the pelvis. When the unsupported side of the pelvis moves forward, it is called forward rotation of the pelvis. The trunk concurrently rotates opposite, and the femur on the stabilized side concurrently rotates internally. When the unsupported side of the pelvis moves backward, it is called posterior rotation; the femur on the stabilized side concurrently rotates externally, and the trunk rotates opposite.

2. Motions and postures of the lower extremity that affect the pelvis and spine

a. *Active hip flexion* will result in anterior pelvic tilt and increased lumbar extension unless the pelvis is stabilized by the abdominal musculature. The opposite occurs with active hip extension.

b. *Tight hip muscles or joints* will cause weight-bearing forces and movement to be transmitted to the spine rather than absorbed in the pelvis. Tight hip extensors will cause increased lumbar flexion when the thigh is flexed. Tight hip flexors will cause increased lumbar extension as the thigh extends. Hip flexion contractures with incomplete hip extension on weight bearing will also place added stresses on the knee because the knee cannot lock while the hip is in flexion unless the trunk is bent forward. Tight adductors cause lateral pelvic tilt opposite and side bending of the trunk toward the side of tightness when weight bearing. The opposite occurs with tight abductors.

c. *A unilateral short leg* will cause lateral pelvic tilting (drop on the short side) and side bending of the trunk away from the short side (convexity of lateral lumbar curve toward side of short leg). This may lead to a functional or eventually a structural scoliosis. Causes of a short leg could be unilateral lower extremity asymmetries such as flat foot, genu valgum, coxa vara, tight hip muscles, anterior rotated innominate bone, poor standing posture, or asymmetry in bone growth.

3. **The hip and gait**

a. During the normal gait cycle, the hip goes through a range of motion of 40 degrees (10 degrees extension at terminal stance to 30 degrees flexion at midswing and initial contact). There is also some lateral pelvic tilt and rotation (about 8 degrees) that require hip abduction/adduction and hip internal/external rotation. Loss of any of these motions will affect the smoothness of the gait pattern.

b. Muscle control during gait

(1) *Hip flexors* control hip extension at the end of stance, then contract concentrically to initiate swing. With loss of flexor function, a posterior lurch of the trunk to initiate swing is seen. Contractures in the hip flexors will prevent complete extension during the second half of stance; the stride is shortened. The person increases the lumbar lordosis or walks with the trunk bent forward.

(2) *Hip extensors* control the flexor moment at initial foot contact; then the gluteus maximus initiates hip extension. With loss of extensor function, a posterior lurch of the trunk occurs at foot contact to shift the center of gravity of the trunk posterior to the hip. With contractures in the gluteus maximus, some decrease occurs in the terminal swing as the femur comes forward, or the person may compensate by rotating the pelvis more forward. The lower extremity may rotate outward because of the external rotation component of the muscle or place greater tension on the iliotibial band through its attachment, leading to irritation along the lateral knee with excessive activity.

(3) *Hip abductors* control the lateral pelvic tilt during swinging of the opposite leg. With loss of function of the gluteus medius, lateral shifting of the trunk occurs over the weak side during stance when the opposite leg swings. This lateral shifting also occurs with a painful hip, because it minimizes the torque at the hip joint during weight bearing. The tensor fasciae latae also functions as an abductor and may become tight and affect gait with faulty use.

c. **Orthopedic problems**
Bony and joint deformities will change alignment of the lower extremity and therefore the mechanics of gait. Painful conditions cause antalgic gait patterns,

which are characterized by minimum stance on the painful side to avoid the stress of weight bearing.

4. **Hip muscle imbalances and their effect**[43]

Muscles function through habit. Faulty mechanics from inadequate or excessive length and imbalanced strength cause hip, knee, or back pain. Overuse syndromes, soft tissue stress, and joint pain develop in response to continued abnormal stresses.

a. *Tight iliotibial (IT) band with tight tensor fasciae latae (TFL) or tight gluteus maximus*

Often there are associated postural dysfunctions of an anterior pelvic tilt posture, slouched posture, or flat back posture (see Chapter 15).

(1) Anterior pelvic tilt posture; hip musculature imbalances
 (a) Tight TFL and IT band
 (b) General limitation of hip external rotation
 (c) Weak, stretched posterior portion of the gluteus medius and piriformis
 (d) Excessive medial rotation of femur during first half of stance with increased stresses on the medial structures of the knee
 (e) Associated lower extremity compensations including medial rotation of the femur, genu valgum, lateral tibial torsion, pes planus, and hallux valgus

(2) Slouched posture; hip musculature imbalances
 (a) Tight rectus femoris and hamstrings
 (b) General limitation of hip rotators
 (c) Weak, stretched iliopsoas
 (d) Weak and tight posterior portion of the gluteus medius
 (e) Weak, poorly developed gluteus maximus
 (f) Associated lower extremity compensations including hip extension, sometimes medial rotation of femur, genu recurvatum, genu varum, and pes valgus

(3) Flat back posture; hip musculature imbalances
 (a) Tightness in the rectus femoris, IT band, and gluteus maximus
 (b) Variations of the above two postures

b. *Overuse of the two-joint hip flexor muscles (TFL, rectus femoris, and sartorius) rather than iliopsoas*

This may cause faulty hip mechanics or knee pain from overuse of these muscles as they cross the knee.

c. *Overuse of the TFL rather than gluteus medius*

This leads to lateral knee pain from IT band tension or medial rotation of the femur with medial knee stresses from increased bowstring effect.

d. *Overuse of hamstring muscles rather than gluteus maximus*

The gluteus maximus becomes tight and range of hip flexion decreases; compensation occurs with excessive lumbar spine flexion whenever the thigh is flexed. Tightness in the gluteus maximus also causes increased tension on the IT band with associated lateral knee pain. Overuse of the hamstring muscles causes muscle tightness as well as muscle imbalances with the quadriceps femoris muscle at the knee. The hamstrings dominate the stabilizing function by pulling posteriorly on the tibia to extend the knee in closed-chain activities. This alters the mechanics at the knee and may lead to overuse syndromes in the hamstring tendons or anterior knee pain from imbalances in quadriceps pull.

e. *Lateral trunk muscles for hip abductors.* This results in excessive trunk motion and increased stress in the lumbar spine.

D. Equilibrium and Posture Control

The joint capsule is richly supplied with mechanoreceptors that respond to variations in position, stress, and movement for control of posture, balance, and movement. Reflex muscle contractions of the entire kinematic chain, known as balance strategies, occur in a predictable sequence when standing balance is disturbed and regained. Joint pathologies, restricted motion, or muscle weakness can impair balance and postural control.[14,23]

E. Nerves in the Hip and Buttock Region[31]

1. Major nerves subject to entrapment

a. *Sciatic nerve*

Forms in the posterior region of the pelvis from the sacral plexus (L-4, L-5, S-1, S-2, and S-3 nerve roots) and leaves the pelvis across the lower edge of the greater sciatic notch. It then passes deep to the piriformis muscle. (Occasionally, it passes over or through the piriformis.) Entrapment results in sensory changes along the lateral and posterior portion of the leg and dorsal and plantar surface of the foot. Progressive weakness in the hamstring muscles, a portion of the adductor magnus muscle, and all the muscles of the leg and foot also develops.

b. *Obturator nerve*

Forms within the psoas muscle from nerve roots of L-2, L-3, and L-4 and enters the pelvis anterior to the sacroiliac joint. It then courses through the obturator canal along with the obturator vessels; there, it divides into the anterior and posterior branch. Injury or entrapment results in sensory changes along the medial aspect of the thigh and weakness primarily in the adductor muscles.

2. Referred pain

The hip is innervated primarily from the L-3 spinal level; hip joint irritation is usually felt along the L-3 dermatome reference from the groin, down the front of the thigh to the knee.[16]

F. Referred Pain Into the Hip and Buttock Region

If painful symptoms are referred to this region from other sources, primary treatment must be directed to the source of the irritation. Therapeutic stretching and strengthening exercise to the hip region may be used to develop a biomechanical balance of forces to minimize stresses to the regions above and below this joint. Common sources of referred pain into the hip and buttock region include:

1. Irritation of nerve roots or tissues derived from spinal segments L-1, L-2, L-3, S-1, and S-2
2. Lumbar intervertebral and sacroiliac joints

II. Joint Problems: Nonoperative Management

A. Related Diagnoses and Etiology of Symptoms

1. Osteoarthritis (degenerative joint disease [DJD]) is the most common arthritic disease of the hip joint. The etiology may be from aging, joint trauma, repetitive ab-

normal stresses, or disease. With the degenerative changes are articular cartilage degeneration, capsular fibrosis, and osteophyte formation at the joint margins. These effects usually occur in regions undergoing greatest loading forces, such as along the superior weight-bearing surface.

2. Other joint pathologies such as rheumatoid arthritis, aseptic necrosis, slipped epiphyses, dislocations, or congenital deformities can also lead to degenerative changes in the hip joint.

3. Tightness in the capsular tissues leading to joint hypomobilities as well as tightness in the surrounding periarticular tissues may occur any time the joint is immobilized following a fracture or surgery.

B. Common Impairments/Problems

1. Pain experienced in the groin and referred along the anterior thigh and knee in the L-3 dermatome.
2. Stiffness after rest.
3. Limited motion with a firm capsular end-feel. Initially limitation is only in internal rotation; in advanced stages the hip is fixed in adduction, has no internal rotation or extension past neutral, and is limited to 90 degrees of flexion.[16]
4. Antalgic gait usually with a compensated gluteus medius (abductor) limp.
5. Limited hip extension leading to increased extension forces on the lumbar spine and possible back pain.
6. Limited hip extension preventing full knee extension when standing or during gait leading to increased knee stresses.
7. Impaired balance and postural control.[23]

C. Common Functional Limitations/Disabilities[12,24]

1. Early stages. Progressive pain with continued weight bearing and gait or at the end of the day after many lower extremity activities. The pain may interfere with work (job specific) or routine household activities such as meal preparation, cleaning, and shopping.
2. Progressive degeneration. Increased difficulty rising up from a chair, climbing stairs, squatting, and other weight-bearing activities. Restricted routine ADL such as bathing, toileting, and dressing (putting on pants, hose, socks).

D. Management of Acute and Early Subacute Joint Lesions

Chapter 7 describes general principles and plan of care in the treatment of osteoarthritis and rheumatoid arthritis as well as general management of joints during acute, subacute, and chronic stages of tissue injury and repair. In conjunction with the medical management of the disease and inflammation, correction of faulty mechanics is an integral part of decreasing pain in the hip. In addition to pain and the degenerative changes that alter weight distribution through the joint, faulty hip mechanics may be caused by conditions such as obesity, leg-length differences, muscle imbalances, sacroiliac dysfunction,[12] joint capsule tightness, poor posture, or injury to other joints in the chain.[7]

1. To decrease pain at rest

a. Grade I or II oscillation techniques with the joint in the resting position

b. Rocking in a rocking chair (provides gentle oscillations to the lower extremity joints as well as stimulates the mechanoreceptors in the joints)[50]

2. To decrease pain by reducing mechanical stress

　　a. Use assistive devices for ambulation to help reduce stress on the hip joint. If the pain is unilateral, the patient can be taught to walk with a single cane or crutch on the side opposite the painful joint.

　　b. If a leg-length asymmetry is causing hip joint stress, gradually elevate the short leg with lifts in the shoe.

3. To decrease effects of stiffness and maintain available motion

　　a. Instruct the patient in the importance of moving the hips through their ROM every day. When the acute symptoms are medically controlled, the patient should perform active ROM if he or she can control the motion or with assistance if necessary.

　　b. Apply grade I or II joint-play techniques (sustained or oscillation) in pain-free positions.

E. Management of Late Subacute and Chronic Joint Lesions

1. To increase joint play

　　a. To distract the weight-bearing surface, use long-axis traction (see Fig. 6–46).

　　b. To increase flexion and internal rotation, apply a posterior glide to the femoral head (see Fig. 6–47).

　　c. To increase extension and external rotation, apply an anterior glide to the femoral head (see Fig. 6–48).

2. To increase range of motion

　　a. Use active inhibition techniques to any tight muscles (see Chapter 5).

　　b. Teach self-stretching procedures as described in Section VI.

3. To progress strength and functional usage in supporting muscles

　　a. Begin with isometric resistance; progress to isotonic resistance as the patient tolerates movement. If any exercises exacerbate the joint symptoms, reduce the intensity. Also reassess the patient's functional activities and adapt them to reduce the stress.

　　b. Progress to functional exercises as tolerated using closed-chain and weight-bearing activities. The patient may require assistive devices while weight bearing. Use of a pool or tank to reduce the effects of gravity may allow partial-weight-bearing exercises without stress.

　　c. Develop postural awareness and balance.

　　d. Progress to a low-impact aerobic exercise program such as swimming or cycling within the available ROM.

III. Joint Surgery and Postoperative Management

Many types of joint surgeries are available to treat chronic joint disease of the hip and some fractures of the hip that compromise the vascular supply to the head of the femur. The procedures include *osteotomy* (which is actually an extra-articular procedure), *arthrodesis*, and several variations of arthroplasty of the hip, such as *resurfacing, hemireplacement,* and *total joint replacement* procedures.[22,40,48] The goals of joint surgery and postoperative management are to provide a patient with (1) a pain-free hip, (2) a stable joint for lower extremity weight bearing and functional ambulation, and (3) adequate ROM and strength of the lower extremity for functional activities.

It is important for the therapist to have a basic understanding of the more common surgical procedures for management of joint disease and deformity and a thorough knowledge of appropriate therapeutic exercise procedures and their progression for an effective and safe postoperative rehabilitation program.

A. Total Hip Replacement

1. Indications for surgery[5,11,18,21,34,40]

a. Severe hip pain with motion and weight bearing as the result of joint deterioration and loss of articular cartilage associated with rheumatoid or traumatic arthritis, osteoarthritis, ankylosing spondylitis, or avascular necrosis

b. Marked limitation of hip motion

c. Instability or deformity of the hip

d. Failure of previous hip surgery (femoral stem hemiarthroplasty, total hip or resurfacing arthroplasty)

2. Procedures

a. *General background*

(1) Total hip replacements have been performed since the early 1960s. Charnley[11] and McKee,[34] surgeons from England, are credited with the early research. Earlier procedures, such as the Smith-Petersen cup arthroplasty,[22] required long postoperative periods of rehabilitation. Successful methods of prosthetic fixation such as the use of methyl methacrylate cement or cementless procedures using bioingrowth fixation have dramatically improved arthroplasty of the hip.

(2) A variety of designs of total hip replacement components have been developed since the early 1960s. Early designs included the Charnley,[11] the McKee-Ferrar,[34] and the Charnley-Mueller[37] replacements. Today all designs are made up of an inert metal (cobalt-chrome alloy, stainless steel) femoral stem and a high-density polyethylene acetabular replacement. In the 1960s and 1970s, the prosthetic components were cemented in place with an acrylic cement, methyl methacrylate. This revolutionized joint replacement surgery, because the use of cement allowed very early weight bearing and shortened the patient's period of rehabilitation.

The main postoperative complication after total hip arthroplasty has been loosening of the prosthetic components, which leads to recurrent hip pain and the need for surgical revision. The patients in which loosening most often occurs are those who are young and physically active. Loosening has not been a particular problem in elderly patients or in young patients with multiple joint involvement who tend to limit their physical activities.[19,20,33,36]

The long-term problem of loosening of the cemented prostheses at the bone-cement interface has given rise to the development of porous-coated total hip replacements. The porous-coated surfaces (beaded or wire mesh) of the femoral and acetabular components allow ingrowth of bone into the prostheses for fixation. Cementless fixation is sometimes called *biologic fixation.* Today, most total hip replacements involve cementless, precision-fit procedures.[19,20] Patients with osteoporosis and insufficient bone integrity require cemented fixation.[48] Weight bearing is more restricted over a longer period postoperatively with bioingrowth fixation than with cemented total hip arthroplasty, but it is anticipated that there will be a lower incidence of future loosening and less need for revision of the arthroplasty.[19,20,25,36,48]

b. *Overview of procedures*[5,11,26,35,40,48]

(1) A lateral, posterolateral, or anterolateral incision is made along the affected hip. The site of the incision affects the degree of exposure available to the surgeon during the surgery but also affects the postoperative stability of the hip replacement, particularly in the early postoperative period.[40] Anterior and anterolateral incisions were commonly used in the early years of total hip replacement surgery. These incisions provided the most stability post-operatively, but exposure of the surgical field was inadequate and often required a trochanteric osteotomy. The necessity for trochanteric osteotomy adds to potential postoperative complications such as nonunion of the osteotomized trochanter or pain and soft tissue irritation from a considerable amount of internal fixation. For these reasons the anterior and anterolateral incisions are rarely used today except when there is significant hip deformity. An alternative, the lateral incision, is used more frequently and provides good stability but requires a release of up to one-half of the proximal insertion of the gluteus medius muscle, which can lead to significant weakening of the hip abductors and a Trendelenburg gait postoperatively. Today, a posterolateral incision and approach are most frequently used. It provides excellent exposure and leaves the abductor muscles intact but results in the greatest amount of joint instability postoperatively and is associated with the highest incidence of dislocation of the prosthesis.

(2) The capsule is incised and removed (capsulectomy) and the hip is dislocated.

(3) The head of the femur is removed and replaced with an intramedullary femoral stem prosthesis.

(4) The acetabulum is remodeled and replaced with a high-density polyethylene cup. To increase stability and decrease the possibility of postoperative dislocation, the cup replacement can be built up posteriorly and superiorly.

3. Postoperative instruction[2,4,6,8,18,21]

If possible, preoperative contact should be made with the patient to:

a. Evaluate the patient.

b. Begin gait training with assistive devices to be used after surgery to prevent the adverse effects of bed rest, such as pulmonary and vascular complications.

c. Teach basic precautions for early bed mobility so the patient will avoid excessive flexion and adduction of the operated hip postoperatively.

d. Teach deep-breathing and coughing exercises to be started directly after surgery to prevent pulmonary complications.

e. Teach ankle pumping exercises to decrease the risk of deep vein thrombosis or pulmonary embolism.

4. Postoperative management[4,6,8,15,21,26,28,41,42,48]

a. *Immobilization*

After surgery when the patient is lying in bed in the supine position, the operated limb must remain in a position of slight abduction and neutral rotation. An abduction pillow or wedge is usually sufficient, but the operated limb may sometimes be placed in a balanced sling suspension with the thigh and calf supported.

b. *Exercise*

MAXIMUM-PROTECTION PHASE

The most important consideration in the very early stage of rehabilitation is protection of the healing structures of the hip joint to prevent dislocation or subluxation of the prosthesis.

(1) To prevent pulmonary and vascular complications postoperatively, begin deep-breathing, coughing, and ankle pumping exercises immediately.

(2) To maintain the strength and flexibility of the unoperated lower limb and upper extremities, initiate active ROM and resisted exercises as soon as possible, particularly if multiple joints are affected by arthritis.

(3) To prevent atrophy of musculature in the operated limb, begin low-intensity, pain-free isometric exercises against gentle resistance.

(4) To decrease postoperative edema of soft tissues and to decrease hypersensitivity and postoperative pain, begin gentle distal to proximal massage of the operated leg. Local edema and hypersensitivity often occur in the area of the IT band and respond well to gentle massage.[49]

(5) To maintain soft tissue and joint mobility, begin active or active-assisted ROM of the operated hip within a protected range while the patient is lying supine as early as the day after surgery. Some patients may also use continuous passive motion (CPM) while hospitalized despite indications that long-term ROM is only 3 to 5 percent better with the use of CPM than without.

(6) To ensure that bed mobility and transfers are performed safely, review or teach these techniques to the patient.

(7) When the patient is allowed out of bed, usually by 2 to 3 days postoperatively, begin the following activities:

(a) Short periods of sitting at the edge of the bed or in a chair with an elevated seat with the hips in no more than 45 degrees of flexion and with the hips slightly abducted

(b) Gait training in the parallel bars or with a walker or crutches with partial weight bearing on the operated side

(8) ***Precautions***

To prevent joint dislocation or subluxation when the hip joint is unstable in the early postoperative days and weeks, the patient must avoid full ROM of the operated hip.[25,35,44,48]

(a) If a posterolateral incision has been made, excessive hip flexion and adduction past neutral must be avoided. During the first few postoperative days, avoid hip flexion past 45 degrees and adduction past neutral during ROM and ADLs. By 2 to 3 weeks postoperatively the patient is usually allowed to flex the hip to 90 degrees. Adapt ADLs as follows[35,48]:

—Have the patient transfer to the sound side.

—Have the patient avoid sitting in low, soft chairs.

—Suggest that the patient use a raised toilet seat.

—Do not allow the patient to excessively bend the trunk over the operated hip when rising from a chair or to pick up an object from the floor.

—Do not allow the patient to cross the legs.

—Suggest to the patient that he or she sleep with an abduction pillow and to avoid sleeping on the side for at least 8 to 12 weeks postoperatively.

    (b) If the procedure involved an anterolateral incision, the patient should avoid hyperextension of the hip as well as adduction past neutral.

    (c) Excessive hip rotation must also be limited while tissues heal.

        —If a posterolateral incision was used, avoid internal rotation.

        —If an anterolateral incision was used, avoid external rotation.

MODERATE-PROTECTION PHASE

(1) The length of time a patient must protect the operated hip is dependent upon the type of surgical procedure, whether or not a trochanteric osteotomy was done, and the type of component fixation (cementless or cemented). Generally, all patients should expect moderate protection to be necessary for 6 weeks postoperatively.[25,26,48] This is approximately the amount of time it takes for soft tissues and bone to heal, for the joint to become encapsulated, and for adequate bioingrowth to provide fixation of the prosthetic components

    (a) If the prosthetic components have been cemented in place and no trochanteric osteotomy was necessary, exercises and weight bearing can progress quite rapidly. In some cases weight bearing to tolerance may be permissible immediately after surgery.

    NOTE: Remember, one of the criteria for using cement is when the patient is osteoporotic and has insufficient bone stock for a cementless procedure. This situation may necessitate more caution in the rehabilitation process.

    (b) If a trochanteric osteotomy was performed (although rarely used today), weight bearing and progression of exercises will be significantly restricted for at least 6 to 8 weeks to allow time for the trochanter to heal. Antigravity hip abduction should not be initiated for at least 6 to 8 weeks or as long as 12 weeks.

    (c) If the hip abductors were partially or totally reflected and resutured to the greater trochanter, restrictions on antigravity abduction also apply.

    (d) If a cementless arthroplasty was used, weight bearing will be restricted for a longer time than with a cemented procedure.

(2) With these considerations in mind, during the period of moderate protection:

    (a) Progress active ROM gradually and in a protected range; avoid hip flexion past 90 degrees and adduction past neutral.

    (b) Emphasize the development of neuromuscular control of hip musculature rather than strength by means of active and light resisted motions performed repetitively.

    (c) Perform movements in an open and closed kinematic chain. Have the patient maintain partial weight bearing on the operated leg by performing closed-chain exercises standing in the parallel bars or while using a walker.

(3) Avoid vigorous stretching during this stage of rehabilitation, but promote hip extension and prevent a hip flexion contracture by having the patient lie prone if tolerated.

(4) In general, when moderate protection is necessary, the patient should avoid too much activity too soon.

MINIMUM PROTECTION AND RETURN TO ACTIVITY PHASES

(1) Adequate strength in the hip extensors and abductors is most important for efficient ambulation. Emphasize closed- and open-chain strengthening and improving endurance in these muscles when safe.

(2) Use light weights and high repetitions in a PRE program. Use of heavy exercise loads are inappropriate and can cause micromotion of the femoral stem prosthesis and can contribute to potential loosening of the prosthesis.

(3) Have the patient make a transition from walker or crutches to a cane. This may occur as late as 12 weeks postoperatively.

(4) To improve muscular endurance and general conditioning, have the patient exercise on a stationary bicycle. Raise the height of the bicycle seat to prevent excessive hip flexion.

(5) Avoid high-impact recreational activities, such as jumping or resisted movements that impose heavy rotational forces on the limb. Both will contribute to loosening and failure of the hip replacement.

B. Hemireplacement of the Hip

1. Indications for surgery[1,10,40,48]

a. Subcapital fracture of the head of the femur

b. Degeneration of the head of the femur associated with disease, hip pain, and deformity but a relatively normal acetabulum

2. Procedure[1,40,48]

a. A lateral or posterolateral incision is made.

b. The head of the femur is removed and replaced with an inert metal femoral stem prosthesis.

c. Fixation is achieved with cement or, if bone integrity is adequate, cementless, press-fit fixation is used.

d. Since a young, active individual may occasionally be a candidate for a hemireplacement arthroplasty, a bipolar prosthesis with a polyethylene covering over the metal femoral head has been developed to minimize wear or tear on the patient's acetabulum.

3. Postoperative management

a. Considerations and precautions for positioning, as well as the components and progression of the exercise program and ambulation are similar to postoperative management of total hip arthroplasty.

b. Compressive forces on the unreplaced acetabulum during exercise are a greater concern with hemiarthroplasty than with total hip replacement. In the early postoperative period exercises that impose the greatest compressive or shearing forces and greatest potential for deterioration of the acetabular cartilage should be avoided. They include gluteal setting exercises and straight-leg raises. These exercises actually create greater compressive forces on the acetabulum than does lower extremity weight bearing during ambulation with crutches in the early postoperative period.[45]

IV. Fractures of the Proximal Femur and Postoperative Management

A. Background

One of the more common orthopedic problems in the elderly is fracture of the hip, or more correctly, fracture of the most proximal portion of the femur in the hip joint area. Osteoporosis, a condition associated with aging, weakens bone and commonly affects the neck of the femur. A sudden twisting motion can cause a pathologic fracture in osteoporotic bone. An elderly person may fall and break a hip, but in many patients the fall may occur as the result of a fracture. Occasionally a young, active individual may sustain a stress fracture of the proximal femur as the result of repetitive microtrauma or an avulsion fracture of the greater or lesser trochanters because of an exceptionally forceful contraction of either the hip abductor or flexor muscles. Common fractures of the hip are *extracapsular* around the areas of the greater and lesser trochanters and *intracapsular* at the neck of the femur.[10,13]

The acute signs of hip fracture are pain in the groin or hip region or pain with active or passive motion of the hip or with lower extremity weight bearing. The lower extremity appears to be shorter by several centimeters and assumes a position of external rotation.

In most cases *open reduction* of the fracture and internal fixation are indicated to stabilize the fracture site and minimize the risk of avascular necrosis of the head of the femur, nonunion, or delayed union. Occasionally a *closed reduction* may be appropriate for a nondisplaced fracture in a younger patient. After a closed reduction the fracture site may be immobilized with a hip spica cast, and weight bearing must be restricted for at least 6 to 8 weeks or longer.

B. Open Reduction and Internal Fixation of Hip Fracture

1. Indications for surgery[27,29,47]

   a. Intertrochanteric fracture (extracapsular)
   b. Subcapital femoral neck fracture (intracapsular)
   c. Subtrochanteric fracture
   d. Fracture of the proximal femur

2. Procedures

   a. A variety of internal fixation devices can be used to reduce and stabilize many different types of hip fractures. The type and severity of the fracture and the age and physical abilities of the patient are all considered by the surgeon.
   b. Internal fixation devices are chosen for their maximum stabilization of the fracture site. They include:
   (1) Multiple pins
   (2) Screws
   (3) Nail-plate fixation
   c. Prosthetic hemireplacement is indicated for subcapital fractures in which the vascular supply to the head of the femur is disturbed.

3. Postoperative management[3,26,27,29,41,47,49]

   a. The primary goal of postoperative care is to get the patient up and moving as quickly as possible. Internal fixation of the fracture site allows early movement and weight bearing on the involved extremity, which minimizes the complications of bed rest, edema, muscle atrophy, soft tissue contractures, and osteoporosis.
   b. With most forms of internal fixation, there is no need for external immobilization (i.e., a cast). If stabilization of the fracture site can be achieved only with external immobilization, a hip spica cast will have to be worn for 6 to 12 weeks, and the patient will have to avoid weight bearing on the involved leg. It is important for these patients that limited ambulation with a walker, inde-

pendence in transfers, and wheelchair mobility all be a part of their plan of care.

c. After internal fixation of a hip fracture, the following activities should be initiated:

(1) Active-assisted and active ROM of the involved hip to maintain mobility and prevent contractures. Continuous passive motion (CPM) may also be used in the early postoperative period.

(2) Muscle-setting exercises (gluteal and quadriceps setting) and neuromuscular electrical stimulation to minimize muscle atrophy.

(3) Active ankle exercises to maintain circulation and to decrease the possibility of thromboembolitic disease. Distal to proximal massage of the lower extremity will also improve fluid dynamics and minimize hypersensitivity of the operated extremity.[49]

(4) Resisted knee flexion and extension and *possibly* light manual resistance exercises to the involved hip to maintain strength postoperatively.

NOTE: There is lack of agreement whether or not light resistance exercise (2 to 3 lb of resistance) for the involved hip should be done before the fracture site has healed. (Bony healing may take 4 to 6 months.) Some therapists and surgeons believe that resistance to hip musculature may put undesirable stress on the internal fixation and jeopardize the stability of the fracture site. Others believe that light manual resistance will minimize postoperative weakness without undue stress at the fracture site. Close communication between the therapist and surgeon is necessary before resistance to the involved hip is added to a postoperative exercise program.

(5) Open- and closed-chain active-resistive exercises, emphasizing strengthening of the uninvolved lower extremity and the scapular depressors and triceps to enhance gait training and ADL.

(6) Early protected weight bearing and ambulation with a walker or crutches whenever the internal fixation device adequately stabilizes the fracture site to prevent complications associated with long-term bed rest.

(7) Progressive closed-chain exercises of the involved lower extremity when partial to full weight bearing is permissible to improve strength, endurance, stability, and balance.

V. Overuse Syndromes/Repetitive Trauma Syndromes: Nonoperative Management

A. Related Diagnoses and Etiology of Symptoms

1. Trochanteric bursitis

Pain is experienced over the lateral hip and possibly down the lateral thigh to the knee when the iliotibial band rubs over the trochanter. Discomfort may be experienced after standing asymmetrically for long periods with the affected hip elevated and adducted and pelvis dropped on the opposite side. Ambulation and climbing stairs aggravate the condition.

2. Psoas bursitis

Pain is experienced in the groin or anterior thigh and possibly into the patellar area. It is aggravated during activities requiring excessive hip flexion.

3. Ischiogluteal bursitis (tailor's or weaver's bottom)

Pain is experienced around the ischial tuberosities, especially when sitting. If the adjacent sciatic nerve is irritated from the swelling, symptoms of sciatica may occur.

4. Tendinitis or muscle pull

Overuse or trauma to any of the muscles in the hip region can occur from excessive strain while the muscle is contracting (often in a stretched position) or from repetitive use and not allowing the injured tissue to heal between activities. Common problems include hip flexor, adductor, and hamstring strains. Poor flexibility and fatigue may predispose an individual to strain and injury during an activity or sporting event or sudden falls such as slipping on ice may result in the strain.

B. Common Impairments/Problems

1. Pain when the involved muscle contracts, when it is stretched, or when the provoking activity is repeated.
2. Gait deviations; slightly shorter stance on painful side; may have a slight lurch when involved muscle contracts to protect the muscle.
3. Imbalance in muscle flexibility and strength. (Common imbalances and resulting faulty mechanics are discussed in Section I.C.4.)
4. Decreased muscular endurance.

C. Common Functional Limitations/Disabilities

1. Inability to do the provoking activity
2. Decreased ambulation

D. Management of Acute or Chronic Inflammation in Overuse Syndromes

1. To decrease acute pain

When there is chronic irritation, follow the guidelines as described in Chapter 7 with emphasis on rest to the involved tissue by not stressing or putting pressure on an inflamed bursa or by not doing the provoking activity. If necessary, decrease amount and time walking or use an assistive device.

2. To reduce mechanical irritation

Patient education and cooperation are necessary to reduce repetitive trauma.

E. Management in Subacute Phase

NOTE: When the acute symptoms have decreased, initiate a progressive exercise program within the tolerance of the involved tissues that emphasizes regaining a balance in length and strength and improving endurance in the muscles of the hip and rest of the lower extremity.

1. To develop a strong mobile scar and regain flexibility

Remodel the scar in muscle or tendon by applying cross-fiber massage to the site of the lesion followed by multiple-angle submaximal isometrics in pain-free positions.

2. To develop a balance in length and strength of the hip muscles

 a. Begin strengthening the injured muscle (or muscle related to the inflamed bursa) with low-intensity isotonic resistance through the range.

 b. Stretching the involved muscle is initiated with gentle, progressive inhibition techniques. When tolerated, the patient can be taught self-stretching techniques (Section VI).

 c. Muscles not directly injured should be stretched and strengthened if they are contributing to imbalanced forces. The patient may not have good trunk coordination or strength, which may be contributing to the overuse because of compensations in the hip. See Chapter 15 for suggestions in developing trunk control.

3. To develop stability and closed-chain function

 a. Initiate controlled weight-bearing exercises when tolerated (Section VI). Because the individual is probably standing and walking, he or she may not tolerate much more closed-chain activities as exercises early in the healing stage, so proceed with caution.

 b. Use total-chain exercises such as biking or partial weight bearing with shifting activities in the parallel bars. Observe coordination between trunk, hip, knee, and ankle motions and exercise only to the point of fatigue, substitute motions, or pain in the weakest segment in the chain.

4. To develop muscle endurance

Instruct the patient to safely perform each exercise from 1 to 3 minutes before progressing to the next level of difficulty.

F. Manage in Chronic Phase

1. To progress strength and functional control

 a. Progress closed-chain and functional training to include balance and muscular endurance for each activity.

 b. Use specificity principles; increase eccentric resistance and demand for controlled speed if necessary for return-to-work activity or sporting event.

 c. Progress to patterns of motion consistent with desired functional outcome. Use acceleration/deceleration drills; assess the total body functioning while doing the desired activity. Note timing and sequencing of events.

2. To return to function

Prior to returning to the desired function the patient practices the activity in a controlled environment and for a limited period. As tolerated, the environment becomes less controlled or more varied, and endurance activities are increased.

VI. Exercises for Muscle Strength or Flexibility Imbalance

NOTE: No matter what the cause, muscle strength or flexibility imbalance in the hip can lead to poor lumbopelvic mechanics as well as poor hip mechanics, which predisposes the patient to or perpetuates low-back, sacroiliac, or hip pain. See Chapters 14 and 15 for discussion and treatment of poor posture and low-back pain. Poor hip mechanics from muscle flexibility and strength imbalance can also affect the knee and ankle in weight-bearing activities, thus causing overuse syndromes or stress to these regions. The exercise techniques in this section are suggestions for correcting imbalances as well as for progressing the patient through the subacute healing and chronic rehabilitative phases of treatment. The choice of exercises and intensity of demand should be based on the goals of treatment and tissue response.

A. Techniques for Self-Stretching of Tight Muscles

Flexibility or self-stretching exercises, chosen according to the degree of limitation and ability of the patient to participate, can be valuable to reinforce therapeutic measures performed by the therapist. Active inhibition and passive stretching techniques are described in Chapter 5. Not all of the following exercises are appropriate for every patient; the therapist should choose the exercise and intensity appropriate for the level of patient function, and progress them when indicated. Whenever the patient is able to contract the muscle opposite the tight muscle, there are the added benefits of reciprocal inhibition of the tight muscles as well as training the agonist (the muscle opposite the tight muscle) to function for effective control in the gained range of motion.

1. To stretch tight hip flexor muscles and soft tissue anterior to the hip

    a. Position of patient: prone. The patient presses the thorax upward, allowing the pelvis to sag (see Fig. 14–1).

        Precaution: This exercise also stretches the lumbar spine into extension; if it causes pain to radiate down the patient's leg, rather than just a stretch sensation in the anterior trunk, hip, and thigh, it must not be performed.

    b. Position of patient: supine. He or she flexes the hip and knee on the side opposite the tight muscle, clasps the hands around the thigh, and holds it against the chest, thus stabilizing the pelvis. The extremity with the tight hip flexor muscles is placed in hip and knee flexion and is slowly lowered toward the table in a controlled manner. The thigh should not be allowed to rotate outward or abduct. The patient attempts to relax the tight muscles at the end of the available range and allow the weight of the leg to cause a pulling sensation in the anterior hip region.

    c. To progress the range as well as include stretching of the two-joint hip flexor muscles (rectus femoris and tensor fasciae latae), the patient is positioned with the hips at the end of the treatment table. The tight hip can then extend beyond neutral and the knee can flex. The hold-relax technique is added by applying resistance to the distal femur as the patient attempts to flex the hip. Following relaxation, the hip is moved into greater extension as allowed (see Fig. 5–14).

        The patient can attempt to further extend the hip by contracting the extensor muscles against the resistance of his or her own tissues, against manual resistance from the therapist, or against mechanical resistance from a pulley system.

    d. Position of patient: standing. The patient assumes a fencer's squatlike posture, with the back leg in the same plane as the front leg and the foot pointing forward. As the patient shifts the body weight on the anterior leg, he or she should feel a stretch sensation in the anterior hip region of the back leg (Fig. 11–1). If the heel of the back foot is kept on the floor, this exercise may also stretch the gastrocnemius muscle.

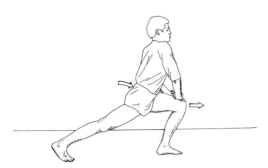

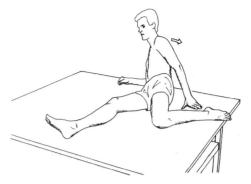

Figure 11–1. Self-stretching of hip flexor muscles and soft tissue anterior to the hip, using a modified fencer's squat posture.

Figure 11–2. Rectus femoris self-stretch. The leg to be stretched is abducted as far as possible with the knee flexed. The hip is then adducted and extended by leaning down onto the opposite elbow and rolling the trunk back. A pull should be felt in the anterior thigh, not medial to the knee.

2. **To isolate stretch to the rectus femoris muscle**

   a. Position of patient: prone, with the knee flexed on the side to be stretched. The patient grabs the ankle on that side and pulls the hip into extension as he or she flexes the knee until the stretch is felt in the anterior thigh. The patient may also place a strap around the ankle and pull on the strap to flex the knee. Do not let the hip abduct or laterally rotate or let the spine hyperextend.

   b. Position of patient: sitting on the floor, with one lower extremity forward and the one to be stretched abducted as far as possible with the knee flexed. The patient adducts and extends the hip on that side by leaning down onto the opposite elbow and rolling the trunk back until a pull is felt proximally in the anterior thigh (Fig. 11–2).

   Precaution: If done incorrectly, this exercise places significant stress on the medial supporting structures of the knee and therefore should be monitored carefully if a patient has instability or pain.

3. **To stretch tight gluteus maximus muscles and soft tissue posterior to the hip**

   a. Position of patient: supine. He or she brings both the knees toward the chest and grasps the thighs firmly. The patient flexes the hips until he or she feels the stretch sensation in the posterior hip, then holds the position. (If the patient flexes further, he or she would begin flexing the lumbar spine.) The therapist should monitor this exercise to influence where the stretch is applied.

   b. Position of patient: supine. The patient brings one knee to the chest and grasps the thigh firmly. This isolates the stretch force to the hip being flexed. To progress this stretch, pull the knee toward the opposite shoulder.

   c. Position of patient: on hands and knees (all-fours position). He or she rocks the pelvis into an anterior tilt, causing lumbar extension, then maintains lumbar extension, while shifting the buttocks back in an attempt to sit on the heels. The hands remain forward. It is important not to let the lumbar spine flex while holding the stretch position (Figs. 11–3A and B).

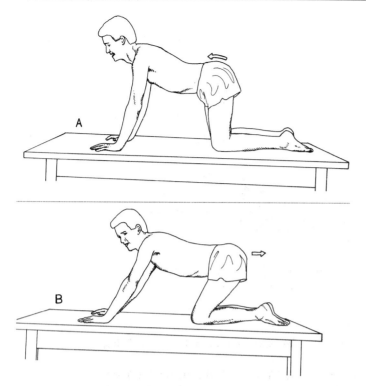

Figure 11–3. Gluteus maximus self-stretch with lumbar spine stabilization. (*A*) The patient on all fours rocks into an anterior pelvic tilt, causing lumbar extension. (*B*) While maintaining lumbar extension, the patient shifts the buttocks back, attempting to sit on the heels. When lordosis can no longer be maintained, the end-range of hip flexion is reached and held for the stretch.

d. The patient sits in a chair and arches (extends) the low back to stabilize the spine. He or she then grasps the front of the chair seat and pulls the trunk forward, keeping the back arched so the motion occurs only at the hips.

4. **To stretch the hamstring muscle group**

a. Position of patient: supine, with one leg in hip flexion and knee extension (straight-leg raising: SLR). If the patient can perform this actively, the therapist then adds a stretch force, using the hold-relax technique, or resists the SLR through the entire range of motion.

b. Position of patient: supine, on the floor, with one leg through a doorway and the other leg (the one to be stretched) propped up against the door frame. The knee should be kept extended. To increase the stretch, the patient should move the buttock closer to the door frame, keeping the knee extended (Fig. 11–4A). The patient can be taught to perform the hold-relax agonist contraction technique by forcing the heel of the leg being stretched against the door frame, causing an isometric contraction, relaxing it, then lifting the leg away from the frame (Fig. 11–4B). For an effective stretch, the pelvis and opposite leg must remain on the floor with the knee extended.

c. Position of patient: sitting, with the leg to be stretched extended across to another chair, or sitting at the edge of a treatment table, with the leg to be stretched extended along the treatment table and the opposite foot on the floor. The patient leans the trunk forward toward the thigh, keeping the back extended, so that there is motion only at the hip joint (Fig. 11–5).

d. Position of patient: supine, with both hips flexed 90 degrees, knees extended,

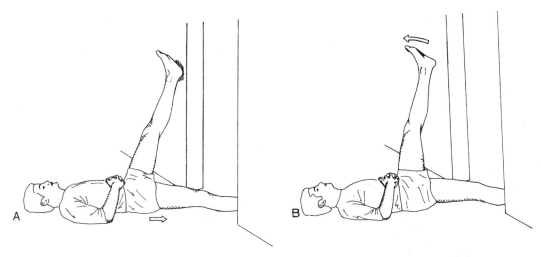

Figure 11–4. Self-stretching of the hamstring muscles. Additional stretch can occur if the person either (*A*) moves the buttock closer to the door frame or (*B*) lifts the leg away from the door frame.

and legs and buttocks against the wall. He or she alternately flexes each leg away from the wall.

e. Bilateral toe-touching exercises are often used to stretch the hamstring muscles. The therapist must recognize that having the patient reach for the toes does not selectively stretch the hamstrings but stretches the low and mid-back as well. Toe-touching is considered a general flexibility exercise and tends to mask tightness in one region and overstretch areas already flexible. Whether a person can touch the toes depends on many factors such as body type, arm,

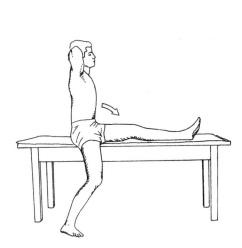

Figure 11–5. Self-stretching of the hamstring muscles by leaning the trunk toward the extended knee, flexing at the hips.

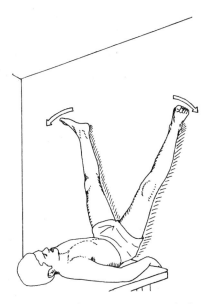

Figure 11–6. Self-stretching of the adductor muscles with the hips at 90 degrees of flexion.

trunk, and leg length, flexibility in thoracic and lumbar regions, as well as hamstring and gastrocnemius length.[30]

5. To stretch tight hip adductor and internal rotator muscles

   a. Position of patient: sitting, with soles of feet together and hands on the inner surface of the knees. He or she pushes the knees down toward the floor with a sustained stretch. The amount of stretch can be increased by pulling the feet closer to the trunk.

   b. Patient position: supine with soles of feet together. He or she lets the knees fall outward toward the floor, with the force of gravity applying the stretch force at the end of the available range.

   Precaution: The patient must be taught to stabilize the pelvis and lumbar spine by actively contracting the abdominal muscles and maintain a posterior pelvic tilt.

   c. Position of patient: supine, with both hips flexed 90 degrees, knees extended, and legs and buttocks against the wall. The hips are abducted bilaterally as far as possible (Fig. 11–6).

   d. Patient in a fencer's position, with the hind leg externally rotated. As the patient shifts the weight on the front leg, he or she should feel a stretch along the medial thigh in the hind leg.

6. To stretch tight tensor fasciae latae

   a. Position of patient: standing on the normal extremity, with the tight extremity crossed behind. Keeping both feet on the floor, the patient side bends away from the tight side, shifting the pelvis toward the tight side, allowing the normal knee to bend slightly. To place additional stretch on the tensor fasciae latae, position the extremity in external rotation as it is placed behind the normal extremity (Fig. 11–7).

   b. Position of patient: side-lying, with the leg to be stretched uppermost; the bottom leg is flexed for support. The top leg is abducted and aligned in the plane of the body in extension. While maintaining this position, the patient externally rotates the hip and then gradually lowers (adducts) the thigh to the point of stretch. If the extended and externally rotated position is not maintained, the iliotibial tract will slip in front of the greater trochanter and an effective stretch will not take place. Additional stretch can be obtained by having the knee flexed during this activity (Fig. 11–8).

B. Techniques to Isolate and Strengthen Weak Muscles

Begin at the functional level for each muscle group. A muscle that has not been properly used or that has been stretched because of antagonistic muscle tightness will require training by making the patient aware of its contracting in its new range as the antagonist is lengthened. On a manual muscle test, the patient may have good isometric strength, yet coordination and timing of muscle contractions may not be satisfactory as a result of faulty posture, poor gait habits, pain, improper lower extremity usage, or other problems. As a muscle is strengthened, it should be exercised as closely as possible in a manner similar to its intended functional use. For gait, the hip functions in both an open and closed kinematic chain and so should be exercised, if possible, with the extremity free as well as with the extremity fixed. Manual and mechanical resistance exercise techniques are described in Chapter 3.

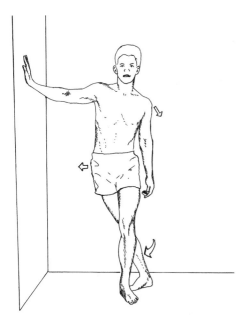

Figure 11–7. Self-stretching of the tensor fasciae latae occurs as the trunk bends away from and the pelvis shifts toward the tight side. Increased stretch occurs when the extremity is positioned in external rotation prior to the stretch.

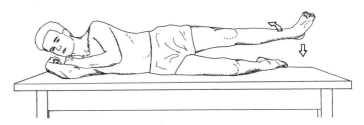

Figure 11–8. Tensor fasciae latae self-stretching: side-lying. The thigh is abducted in the plane of the body, then it is extended and externally rotated, then slowly lowered. Additional stretch can occur by flexing the knee.

1. **To train and strengthen the hip abductor (gluteus medius) and hip hiker (quadratus lumborum) muscles**

   a. Position of patient: standing, with one leg on a 2- to 4-inch block. Have the patient alternately lower and elevate the pelvis on the side of the unsupported leg (Fig. 11–9).

   b. Position of patient: standing. He or she abducts one leg, then the other. The

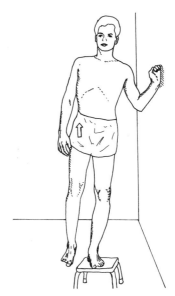

Figure 11–9. Training the hip abductor and hiker muscles.

motion should be only in the hips; there should be no side bending of the trunk. Adding ankle weights or securing an elastic resistance around the thighs provides mechanical resistance. This is a closed-chain, stabilizing exercise for the weight-bearing side. Be sure that the pelvis does not drop on the unsupported side (see Fig. 11–13B).

c. Position of patient: side-lying, with the bottom leg flexed for balance. Have the patient abduct the top leg, keeping the hip neutral to rotation and in slight extension. Do not allow the hip to flex or the trunk to roll backward. If this is too difficult, begin with the patient supine and have him or her concentrate on isolated hip abduction movements while keeping the trunk still. Adding ankle weights in the side-lying position provides resistance as the patient progresses in strength.

2. **To train and strengthen the hip extensor (gluteus maximus) muscle**

a. Position of patient: prone or supine. He or she is first taught gluteal setting exercises to increase awareness of the contracting muscle.

b. Patient stands at the edge of the treatment table, then flexes the trunk onto the table with the hips at the edge. He or she alternately extends one hip, then the other. This is done with the knee flexed to train the gluteus maximus while relaxing the hamstrings. If the hamstrings cramp from active insufficiency, the patient is attempting to use them and should practice relaxing them before progressing with this exercise. Progress by adding weights or elastic resistance to the distal thigh.

c. Position of patient: on hands and knees in an all-fours position. He or she then alternately extends the hips, keeping the knee flexed. Care is taken not to attempt extension beyond the available range in the hip, causing stress is in the sacroiliac joint or lumbar spine (Fig. 11–10).

d. Position of patient: hook-lying. *Bridging exercises* are carried out by having the patient press the upper back and feet into the mat and elevate the hips

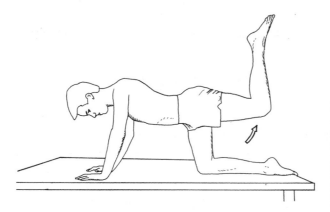

Figure 11–10. Isolated training and strengthening of the gluteus maximus. Starting in the all fours position, the knee is flexed to rule out substitution by the hamstring muscles. Care is taken not to hyperextend the back, thereby causing stress to the sacroiliac or lumbar spinal joints.

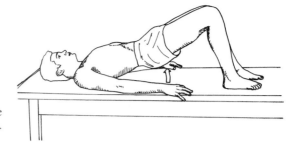

Figure 11–11. Training and strengthening the hip extensor muscles using bridging exercises. Resistance can be added against the pelvis.

(Fig. 11–11). Manual resistance can be applied against the pelvis or mechanical resistance can be applied by strapping a weighted belt around the pelvis.

3. To train and strengthen the external rotators of the hip

    a. Position of patient: prone, with knees bent and about 10 inches apart. The patient presses the heels together, causing an isometric contraction of the external rotators.

    b. Position of patient: standing, with feet parallel, about 4 inches apart. The patient flexes the knees slightly, then externally rotates the thighs (so that the knees are pointing laterally), keeping the feet stationary on the floor. He or she maintains the external rotation while extending the knees, then relaxes the rotation slightly until the patellae point forward. This activity is useful when the patient has functional medial rotation of the femur.[17]

    c. Position of patient: sitting, with knees flexed over the edge of the treatment table, with an elasticized material around the ankle and the table leg on the same side. The patient moves the foot toward the opposite side, pulling against the resistance, causing external rotation at the hip.

4. To train and strengthen the hip adductor muscles

    a. Position of patient: side-lying, with the bottom leg aligned in the plane of the trunk; the top leg is flexed forward with the foot on the floor or with the thigh resting on a pillow. The patient lifts the bottom leg upward in adduction. Weights can be added to the ankle to progress strengthening (Fig. 11–12A).

    b. Position of patient: side-lying, with both legs aligned in the plane of the trunk. The patient holds the top leg in abduction and adducts the bottom leg up to meet it (Fig. 11–12B).

C. Techniques to Increase Strength, Stability, and Control in Weight Bearing

Weight-bearing exercises in the lower extremity involve all of the joints in the closed chain and are therefore not limited to hip muscles. Most activities bring into play antagonistic two-joint muscles in which each muscle is being lengthened across one joint while it is shortening across another, thus maintaining an optimal length-tension relationship. In addition to causing motion, a prime function of the muscles in weight bearing is to control against the forces of gravity and momentum.

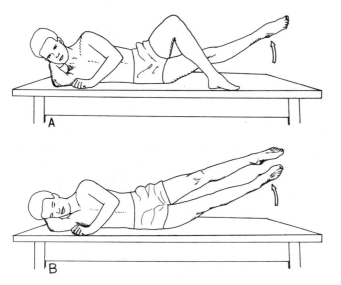

Figure 11–12. Training and strengthening the hip adductors. (*A*) The top leg is stabilized by flexing the hip and resting the foot on the mat while the bottom leg is adducted against gravity. (*B*) The top leg is isometrically held in abduction while the bottom leg is adducted against gravity.

1. **Weight-bearing control and stability**

   a. Develop ability to shift the body weight. If the patient cannot bear full weight, begin in the parallel bars with part of the weight borne on the hands. He or she shifts anteriorly to posteriorly, side to side, and obliquely. Manual resistance to the motion is added with pressure against the patient's pelvis.

   b. *Rhythmic stabilization* exercises develop postural adjustments to applied forces. Apply manual resistance against the pelvis and ask the patient to hold (isometric contractions); there should be little or no movement. Vary the force and direction of resistance. At first use verbal cuing; as the patient learns control, apply the varying forces without warning. Progress to unilateral standing.

   c. Marching in place requires shifting balance. Progress to resisted walking, either against the therapist's resistance at the pelvis or against an elastic or pulley resistance secured around the pelvis. With advanced training, use an obstacle course requiring changing directions, variable surfaces, changing speeds, and other adaptations based on return-to-function needs.

2. **Closed-chain resistance**

   The patient stands on the involved leg. An elastic resistance is looped around the thigh of the other extremity and secured to a stable upright structure. The patient extends, abducts, adducts, or flexes the thigh against the resistance (open-chain movement). Stabilization is required in the weight-bearing leg, and fatigue is determined when the patient can no longer hold the weight-bearing extremity or pelvis stable (Fig. 11–13).

3. **Balance training**

   The patient stands with bilateral support on a rocker board, wobble board, or BAPS board and begins with single-plane weight shifting forward/backward and side to side. He or she progresses by placing the extremities in a diagonal plane and shifts the weight. When able, the patient progresses to single-leg activities on the balance board (see Fig. 13–15).

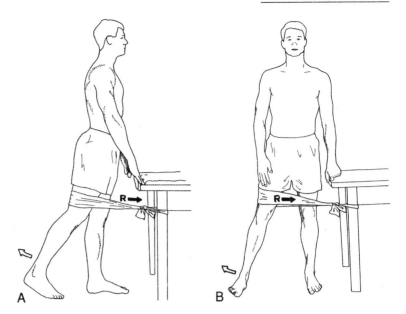

Figure 11–13. Closed-chain exercise with elastic resistance around the opposite leg. (*A*) Resisting extension on the right requires stabilization of anterior muscles of the left side. (*B*) Resisting abduction on the right requires stabilization of the left frontal plane muscles.

4. Step-ups

Begin with a low step, 2 to 3 inches in height, and progress height as the patient is able. The patient can step up sideways, forward, or backward. Be sure that the entire foot is planted on the step and that the body is lifted, then lowered with a smooth motion, not lurching of the trunk or pushing off with the trailing extremity. Resistance can be added with a weight belt, with weights in the hands, or around the ankle of the non–weight-bearing leg.

5. Lunges

The patient strides forward and flexes the hip and knee of the forward leg up to 90 degrees and returns upright. Repeat, or alternate legs. A cane or rod can be used for balance or the patient can learn control of the motion in the parallel bars or beside a treatment table. It is important to instruct the patient to keep the toes pointing forward, bend the knee in the same plane as the feet, and keep the back upright (Fig. 11–14). Progressions include using weights in the hands for resistance, taking a longer stride, or lunging forward onto a small step.

NOTE: A patient with an anterior cruciate ligament (ACL) deficiency or a surgically repaired knee should not flex the knee forward of the toes when performing lunges because this increases the sheer force and stress to the ACL. Individuals with patellofemoral compression syndrome will experience increased pain under these circumstances because the compressive force from the body weight is greater when it is kept posterior to the knee. Adapt the position of the knee based on the patient's symptoms and presenting pathology.

6. Wall slides

The patients rests the back against a wall with feet forward and shoulder-width apart. He or she slides the back down the wall by flexing the hips and knees and dorsiflexing the ankle, then slides up the wall by extending hips and knees and plantarflexing the ankles. If sliding is sticky, place a towel behind the patient's

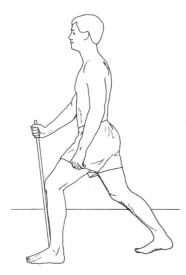

Figure 11–14. Lunge with cane assistance.

back. A large ball (Swiss ball) placed behind the back requires additional control because it is less stable. Arm motions and weights can be added to develop coordination or to add resistance (Fig. 11–15).

7. Partial squats

The patient lowers the trunk by flexing the hips and knees. To add resistance, the patient holds weights in the hands or uses elastic resistance secured under the feet (see Fig. 12–11). To protect the ACL, knee flexion range is limited from 0 to 60 degrees and the patient is instructed to lower the hips as if preparing to sit on a chair so that the knees stay behind the toes. To protect a patellofemoral compression problem, distribute the body weight by allowing the trunk to bend forward and the knees to move forward of the toes.

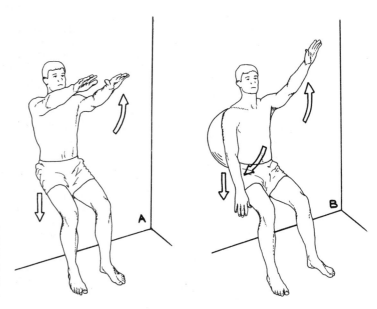

Figure 11–15. Wall slides/partial squats to develop eccentric control of body weight. (*A*) The back sliding down a wall, superimposing bilateral arm motion for added resistance. (*B*) The back rolling a gym ball down the wall, superimposing antagonistic arm motion to develop coordination.

8. Equipment

Use of mechanical equipment such as a leg press, treadmill, bicycle, and slide board is beneficial for strengthening, coordination, and endurance.

D. To Progress to Specificity of Training

General ideas include:
1. Progress exercises to the load and intensity needed to return to activity.
2. Plyometric drills such as jumping from a stool, flexing hips, knees, and ankles to absorb the impact of landing, and immediately jumping up.
3. Maximum eccentric loading using any of the exercises described.
4. Specific analysis of technique with biomechanical adaptations to avoid improper stresses.

VII. Summary

The anatomy and kinesiology of hip structure and function, as well as the functional relationships between hip motion and pelvic motion, have been reviewed. The action of the hip during gait, including hip motion and muscular control, and the role of the hip in relation to balance and coordination have also been discussed.

Guidelines for therapeutic exercise management of common musculoskeletal problems, such as joint and muscle lesions, and common surgical procedures, such as hip pinnings and hip replacements, have been outlined. Specific descriptions of self-stretching techniques and strengthening procedures for the hip, as well as suggestions for closed-chain exercises to progress the patient in functional weight-bearing activities, have been described and illustrated.

References

1. Apley, AG: System of Orthopedics and Fractures, ed 5. Butterworth, London, 1977.
2. Ball, PB, Wroe, MC, and MacLeod, L: Survey of physical therapy preoperative care in total hip replacement. Physical Therapy in Health Care 1:83, 1986.
3. Barnes, B: Ambulation outcomes after hip fractures. Phys Ther 64:317, 1984.
4. Beber, C, and Convery, R: Management of patients with total hip replacement. Phys Ther 52:823, 1972.
5. Benke, GJ: Joint replacement. In Downie, PA (ed): Cash's Textbook of Orthopedics and Rheumatology for Physiotherapists. JB Lippincott, Philadelphia, 1984.
6. Bentley, JA: Physiotherapy following joint replacement, etc. In Downie, PA (ed): Cash's Textbook of Orthopedics and Rheumatology for Physiotherapists. JB Lippincott, Philadelphia, 1984.
7. Bullock-Saxton, JE: Local sensation changes and altered hip muscle function following severe ankle sprain. Phys Ther 74:17, 1994.
8. Burton, D, and Imrie, S: Total hip arthroplasty and postoperative rehabilitation. Phys Ther 53:132, 1973.
9. Cailliet, R: Low Back Pain Syndrome, ed 4. FA Davis, Philadelphia, 1988.
10. Canale, ST: Intracapsular fractures. In Steinberg, ME (ed): The Hip and Its Disorders. WB Saunders, Philadelphia, 1991.
11. Charnley, J: Total hip replacement by low friction arthroplasty. Clin Orthop 72:721, 1974.
12. Cibulka, MT, and Delitto, A: A comparison of two different methods to treat hip pain in runners. Journal of Orthopaedic and Sports Physical Therapy 17:173, 1993.
13. Craik, RL: Disability following hip fracture. Phys Ther 74:388, 1994.
14. Crutchfield, CA, et al: Balance and coordination training. In Scully, RM, and Barnes, MR (eds): Physical Therapy. JB Lippincott. Philadelphia, 1989.
15. Cullen, S: Physical therapy program for patients with total hip replacement. Phys Ther 53:1293, 1973.
16. Cyriax, J: Textbook of Orthopaedic Medicine, Vol 1. Diagnosis of Soft Tissue Lesions, ed 8. Bailliere Tindall, London, 1982.
17. Daniels, L, and Worthingham, C: Therapeutic Exercise for Body Alignment and Function, ed 2. WB Saunders, Philadelphia, 1977.
18. Eftekhar, N: Preoperative management of total hip replacement. Orthop Rev 3:17, 1974.
19. Engh, CA: Bone ingrowth into porous coated canine acetabular replacements: The effect of pore size, apposition and dislocation. Hip 13:214, 1985.
20. Engh, CA, Bobyn, JD, and Matthews, JCH: Biological fixation of a modified Moore prosthesis. In Hip Society: The Hip. Proceedings of the Twelfth Open Scientific Meeting of the Hip Society. CV Mosby, St Louis, 1984.

21. Fortune, W: Lower limb joint replacement. In Nickel, VL (ed): Orthopedic Rehabilitation. Churchill-Livingstone, New York, 1982.

22. Friedebold, G: The Smith-Petersen cup arthroplasty: An analysis of fractures. In Chapchal, G (ed): Arthroplasty of the Hip. Georg Thieme, Stuttgart, 1973.

23. Goldstein, TS: Determining the cause of disability. In Functional Rehabilitation in Orthopedics. Aspen, Gaithersburg, MD, 1995.

24. Gucione, AA: Arthritis and the process of disablement. Phys Ther 74:408, 1994.

25. Harris, WH: The porous total hip replacement system. In Harris, WH (ed): Advanced Concepts in Total Hip Replacement. Slack, Thorofare, NJ, 1985.

26. Hielema, F, and Summerfore, R: Physical therapy for patients with hip fracture or joint replacement. Physical Therapy in Health Care 1:89, 1986.

27. Hielema, FJ: Epidemiology of hip fracture. Phys Ther 59:1221, 1979.

28. Hyde, SA: Physiotherapy in Rheumatology. Blackwell Scientific, Oxford, 1980.

29. Iversen, LD, and Clawson, DK: Manual of Acute Orthopedic Therapeutics, ed 2. Little, Brown, Boston, 1982.

30. Kendall, F: Criticism of current tests and exercises for physical fitness. Phys Ther 45:187, 1965.

31. Kopell, H, and Thompson, W: Peripheral Entrapment Neuropathies, ed 2. Robert E Krieger, Huntington, NY, 1976.

32. Lehmkuhl, LD, and Smith LM: Brunnstrom's Clinical Kinesiology, ed 5. FA Davis, Philadelphia, 1995.

33. Ling, RSM (ed): Current Problems in Orthopedics: Complications of Total Hip Replacement. Churchill-Livingstone, New York, 1984.

34. McKee, G: Development of total prosthetic replacement of the hip. Clin Orthop 72:85, 1970.

35. Melvin, J: Rheumatic Disease: Occupational Therapy and Rehabilitation, ed 2. FA Davis, Philadelphia, 1982.

36. Morrey, RF, and Kavanagh, BF: Cementless joint replacement: Current status and future. Bull Rheum Dis 37:1, 1987.

37. Muller, WE: Total hip prosthesis. Clin Orthop 72:460, 1970.

38. Norkin, C, and Levangie, P: Joint Structure and Function: A Comprehensive Analysis, ed 2. FA Davis, Philadelphia, 1992.

39. Normal and Pathological Gait Syllabus. Physical Therapy Department, Rancho Los Amigos Hospital, Downey, CA, 1977.

40. Nunley, JA, and Oser, ER: Surgical treatment of arthritis of the hip. Physical Therapy in Health Care 1:59, 1986.

41. Patton, F: Treatment of hip fractures in the geriatric patient. Phys Ther 42:314, 1962.

42. Richardson, R: Physical therapy management of patients undergoing total hip replacement. Phys Ther 55:984, 1975.

43. Sahrmann, SA: Diagnosis and treatment of muscle imbalances associated with musculoskeletal pain. Lecture outline. Ohio Chapter, APTA Conference, Columbus, OH, 1988.

44. Schamerloh, C, and Ritter, M: Prevention of dislocation or subluxation of total hip replacements. Phys Ther 57:1028, 1977.

45. Strickland, EM, et al: In vivo acetabular contact pressure during rehabilitation: Part I. Acute phase. Phys Ther 72:691, 1992.

46. Taylor, JR, and Twomey, LT: Age changes in lumbar zygapophyseal joint. Spine 11(7):739, 1986.

47. Trombly, CA: Occupational Therapy for Physical Dysfunction, ed 2. Williams & Wilkins, Baltimore, MD 1983.

48. Waugh, T: Arthroplasty rehabilitation. In Goodgold, J (ed): Rehabilitation Medicine. CV Mosby, St Louis, 1988.

49. Woolf, CH: Generation of acute pain: Central mechanisms. British Medical Bulletin 47:523, 1991.

50. Wyke, B: Neurological aspects of pain for the physical therapy clinician. Physical Therapy Forum, Ohio Chapter APTA Conference, Columbus, OH, 1982.

The Knee

The knee joint is designed for mobility and stability; it functionally lengthens and shortens the lower extremity to raise and lower the body or to move the foot in space. Along with the hip and ankle, it supports the body when standing, and it is a primary functional unit in walking, climbing, and sitting activities.

Highlights of the anatomy and function of the knee complex are reviewed in the first section of this chapter. For further study the reader is referred to several texts and references.[11,19,49,55,73] To design a therapeutic exercise program for a patient's knee, the reader should be familiar with the principles of management presented in Chapter 7.

OBJECTIVES

After studying this chapter, the reader will be able to:

1 Identify important aspects of the knee structure and function for review.
2 Establish a therapeutic exercise program to manage soft tissue and joint lesions in the knee region related to stages of recovery following an inflammatory insult to the tissues, recognizing unique circumstances in the knee and patella for their management.
3 Establish a therapeutic exercise program to manage patients following common surgical procedures for the knee.

I. Review of the Structure and Function of the Knee

A. Bony parts Include the Distal Femur, Proximal Tibia, and Patella (see Fig. 6–49).

B. Knee Joint Complex

The lax joint capsule encloses two articulations: the tibiofemoral and the patellofemoral joints. Recesses from the capsule form the suprapatellar, subpopliteal, and gastrocnemius bursae. Folds or thickenings in the synovium persist from embryologic tissue in up to 60 percent of individuals and may become symptomatic with microtraumas or macrotraumas.[6,52]

1. **The tibiofemoral joint**

   a. Characteristics

   The knee joint is a biaxial modified hinge joint with two interposed menisci supported by ligaments and muscles. Anterior-posterior stability is provided by the posterior and anterior cruciate ligaments, respectively; mediolateral stability is provided by the medial (tibial) and lateral (femoral) collateral ligaments, respectively.

   b. The convex bony partner is composed of two asymmetric condyles on the distal end of the femur. The medial condyle is longer than the lateral, which contributes to the locking mechanism at the knee.

   c. The concave bony partner is composed of two tibial plateaus on the proximal tibia with their respective fibrocartilaginous menisci. The medial plateau is larger than the lateral.

   d. The menisci improve the congruency of the articulating surfaces. They are attached to the joint capsule by the coronary ligaments. The medial meniscus is firmly attached to the joint capsule as well as to the medial collateral ligament, anterior cruciate ligament, and semimembranosus muscle; therefore, it is subject to injury when there is a lateral blow to the knee.

   e. With motions of the tibia (open kinematic chain), the concave plateaus slide in the same direction as the bone motion.

Physiologic Motions of the Tibia	*Direction of Slide of the Tibia*
Flexion	Posterior
Extension	Anterior

   f. With motions of the femur on a fixated tibia (closed kinematic chain), the convex condyles slide in the direction opposite to the bone motion.

   g. Rotation occurs between the femoral condyles and the tibia during the final degrees of extension. This is called the locking, or screw-home, mechanism.

   (1) When the tibia is free (open kinematic chain), terminal extension results in the tibia's rotating externally on the femur. To unlock the knee, the tibia rotates internally.

   (2) When the tibia is fixed with the foot on the ground (closed kinematic chain), terminal extension results in the femur's rotating internally (the medial condyle slides further posteriorly than the lateral). Concurrently, the hip goes into extension. If a person lacks hip extension, knee locking cannot occur when the foot is fixed. As the knee is unlocked, the femur rotates laterally. Unlocking of the knee occurs indirectly with hip flexion and directly from action of the popliteus muscle.

2. **The patellofemoral joint**

   a. Characteristics

   The patella is a sesamoid bone in the quadriceps tendon. It articulates with the intercondylar (trochlear) groove on the anterior aspect of the distal portion of the femur. Its articulating surface is covered with smooth hyaline cartilage. The patella is embedded in the anterior portion of the joint capsule and is connected to the tibia by the ligamentum patellae. Many bursae surround the patella.

   b. With flexion of the knee, the patella slides caudally along the intercondylar groove; with extension, it slides cranially. If patellar movement is restricted, it interferes with the range of knee flexion and may contribute to an extensor lag in active knee extension.[100]

C. Knee and Patellar Function

1. Patellar alignment

Normal alignment of the patella is defined as a 15-degree **Q angle.** The Q angle is the angle formed by two intersecting lines: one from the anterior superior iliac spine to the mid-patella, the other from the tibial tubercle through the mid-patella. The Q angle describes the lateral tracking or bowstring effect that the quadriceps muscles and patellar tendon have on the patella.

a. Forces maintaining alignment

Lateral fixation of the patella is provided by the iliotibial band and lateral retinaculum; these are opposed by the active medial pull of the vastus medialis obliquus (VMO) muscle. The patellar ligament fixates the patella inferiorly against the active pull of the quadriceps muscle superiorly.[76]

b. Patellar malalignment and tracking problems may be caused by:

(1) Increased Q angle. This can be from genu valgum, patella alta, pronated feet, wide pelvis, increased femoral anteversion, or external tibial torsion.

(2) Muscle and fascial tightness. Tight IT band and lateral retinaculum prevent medial gliding of the patella. Tight ankle plantarflexors result in pronation of the foot when the ankle dorsiflexes, causing medial torsion of the tibia and functional lateral displacement of the tibial tuberosity in relationship to the patella. Tight rectus femoris and hamstrings may affect the mechanics of the knee, leading to compensations.[63]

(3) Lax medial capsular retinaculum or an insufficient VMO muscle. The VMO may be weak from disuse or inhibited because of joint swelling or pain, leading to poor medial stability.[95] Poor timing of contraction, altering the ratio of firing between the VMO and vastus lateralis muscle, may lead to imbalanced forces.[85,103] Weakness or poor timing of VMO contraction will increase the lateral drifting of the patella.

2. Patellar compression

Compression of the posterior aspect of the patella against the femur rises sharply after 30 degrees knee flexion. Near 30 degrees, it approximates body weight; it rises to greater than three times body weight during stair climbing and eight times body weight during squatting and deep-knee-bending activities.[73,76] Contact area of the posterior surfaces of the patella also varies through the range of knee flexion. Normally this helps absorb the forces and maintain cartilage health.

3. Extensor muscles

a. The quadriceps femoris muscle group is the only muscle crossing anterior to the axis of the knee and is the prime mover for knee extension. Other muscles that can act to extend the knee require the foot to be fixated, creating a closed kinematic chain. In this situation, the hamstrings and also the soleus muscles can cause or control knee extension by pulling the tibia posteriorly.

b. During standing and the stance phase of gait, the knee is an intermediate joint in a closed kinematic chain. The quadriceps muscle controls the amount of flexion at the knee as well as causes knee extension through reverse muscle pull on the femur. In the erect posture, when the knee is locked, the quadriceps need not function when the gravity line falls anterior to the axis of motion (see Chapter 15). In this case, tension in the hamstring and gastrocnemius tendons supports the posterior capsule.

c. The patella improves the leverage of the extensor force by increasing the distance of the quadriceps tendon from the knee joint axis. Its greatest effect on the leverage of the quadriceps is during extension of the knee from 60 to 30 degrees and rapidly diminishes from 15 to 0 degrees of full extension.[36,73]

d. The peak torque of the quadriceps muscle occurs between 70 and 50 degrees.[10] The physiologic advantage of the quadriceps rapidly decreases during the last 15 degrees of knee extension because of its shortened length. This, combined with its decreased mechanical advantage in the last 15 degrees, requires the muscle to significantly increase its contractile force when large demands are placed on the joint during terminal extension.[36] During standing, assistance for extension comes from the hamstrings and soleus muscles as well as from the mechanical locking mechanism of the knee. In addition, the anterior cruciate ligament and the pull of the hamstring muscle group counter the anterior translation force of the quadriceps muscle.[36,77] During open-chain knee extension exercises in the sitting or supine position, when the resistive force is maximum in terminal extension because of the moment arm of the resistance, a relatively strong contraction of the quadriceps muscle is required to overcome both the physiologic and mechanical disadvantages of the muscle to complete the final 15 degrees of motion.[36]

4. **Flexor muscles**

a. The hamstring muscles are the primary knee flexors and also influence rotation of the tibia on the femur. Because they are two-joint muscles, they contract more efficiently when they are simultaneously lengthened over the hip (during hip flexion) as they flex the knee. In closed-chain activities, the hamstring muscles can act to extend the knee by pulling on the tibia.

b. The gastrocnemius muscle can also function as a knee flexor, but its prime function at the knee on weight bearing is to support the posterior capsule against hyperextension forces.

c. The popliteus muscle supports the posterior capsule and acts to unlock the knee.

d. The pes anserinus muscle group (sartorius, gracilis, semitendinosus) provides medial stability to the knee and affects rotation of the tibia in a closed chain.

5. **The knee and gait[73,74]**

a. Range of motion of the knee during gait
During the normal gait cycle, the knee goes through a range of 60 degrees (0 degrees extension at initial contact or heel strike to 60 degrees at the end of initial swing). There is some medial rotation of the femur as the knee extends at initial contact and just prior to heel-off.

b. Muscle control of the knee during gait
(1) The quadriceps muscle controls the amount of knee flexion during initial contact (loading response), then extends the knee toward mid-stance. It again controls the amount of flexion during preswing (heel-off to toe-off) and prevents excessive heel rise during initial swing. With loss of quadriceps function, the patient lurches the trunk anteriorly during initial con-

tact to move the center of gravity anterior to the knee so it is stable or rotates the extremity outward to lock the knee.[97] With fast walking, there may be excessive heel rise during initial swing.

(2) The hamstring muscles primarily control the forward swinging leg during terminal swing. Loss of function may result in the knee's snapping into extension during this period. The hamstrings also provide posterior support to the knee capsule when the knee is extended during stance. Loss of function results in progressive genu recurvatum.[97]

(3) The unijoint ankle plantarflexor muscles (primarily the soleus) help control the amount of knee flexion during preswing by controlling the forward movement of the tibia. Loss of function results in hyperextension of the knee during preswing (also loss of heel rise at the ankle and thus a lag or slight dropping of the pelvis on that side during the preswing phase).

(4) The gastrocnemius muscle provides tension posterior to the knee when it is in extension (end of loading response or foot flat, and just prior to preswing or heel-off). Loss of function results in hyperextension of the knee during these periods as well as loss of plantarflexion during preswing or push-off.

c. Because the knee is the intermediate joint between the hip and foot, problems in these two areas will interfere with knee function during gait. Examples:

(1) Inability to extend the hip will prevent the knee from extending just before terminal stance (heel-off).

(2) Most of the muscles functioning to control the hip are two-joint muscles and also cross the knee. With asymmetries in length and strength, imbalanced forces may stress various structures in the knee, giving rise to pain when walking or running (see Chapter 11).

(3) The position and function of the foot and ankle affect the stresses transmitted to the knee. For example, with pes planus or pes valgus there is medial rotation of the tibia and an increased bowstring effect on the patella, increasing the lateral tracking forces.

D. Referred Pain

1. Common sources for referred pain to the knee include[18]:
   a. Nerve roots and tissues derived from spinal segments L-3, referring to the anterior aspect, and from S-1 and S-2, referring to the posterior aspect of the knee
   b. The hip joint (which is primarily L-3)
2. Treatment of the source of irritation is necessary to relieve the pain. Therapeutic exercise to the knee is beneficial only in preventing disuse of the part; primary treatment must be directed to the source of the irritation.

II. Joint Problems and Capsular Restrictions: Nonoperative Management

A. Related Diagnoses and Etiology of Symptoms

Rheumatoid arthritis and osteoarthritis as well as acute joint trauma can affect the knee articulations at the tibiofemoral joint. Tightness and adhesions from immobilization develop in the joints and surrounding tissues any time the joint is splinted or casted. Chapter 7 describes the etiology of these arthritic and joint symptoms.

B. Common Impairments/Problems

With tibiofemoral joint involvement, the pattern of restriction at the knee is usually more loss of flexion than extension. When there is effusion (swelling within the joint), the joint assumes a position near 25 degrees of flexion, at which there is greatest capsular distensibility. Little motion is possible because of the swelling. Symptoms of joint involvement, such as distention, stiffness, pain, and reflex quadriceps inhibition may cause **extensor (or quadriceps) lag** (the active range of knee extension is less than the passive range).[96]

1. Rheumatoid arthritis (RA)

Early in the disease, the hands and feet are usually involved first; with progression of RA, the knees may also become involved. The joints become warm and swollen, with limitation as described. In addition, a genu valgum deformity commonly develops in the advanced stages of this disease.

2. Osteoarthritis (degenerative joint disease, DJD)

Pain, muscle weakness, and joint limitations progressively worsen. Genu varum commonly develops.

3. Joint trauma

Following trauma, immediate swelling indicates bleeding into the joint. Slowly progressive swelling (4 or more hours) indicates serous effusion, which may occur with ligament and meniscal tears. When acute there will be muscle guarding, weakness, and limited motion from the swelling. When swelling recedes, evaluate for ligamentous and meniscal tears (see Sections V and VI).

4. Joint restrictions after a period of immobilization

When the knee has been immobilized for several weeks or longer, such as following healing of a fracture or post surgery, the capsule, muscles, and soft tissue become restricted. Adhesions may restrict patellar mobility. Usually, this will limit knee flexion and may cause pain as the patella is compressed against the femur. With lack of superior gliding of the patella, there may be an extensor lag with active knee extension even with full passive knee extension.[100] This usually occurs after operative repairs of some knee ligaments, when the knee has been immobilized in flexion for a prolonged period. The best therapy is prevention. To keep the patella mobile whenever the knee is to be immobilized, the patient should be taught quadriceps-setting exercises to be performed frequently every day.

C. Common Functional Limitations/Disabilities[29]

1. With acute symptoms there is pain on motion, with weight bearing, and during gait, which may interfere with work or routine household activities.
2. Limitation or difficulty controlling weight-bearing activities with the knee flexed such as rising from a chair or a commode, descending or ascending stairs, stooping, or squatting.

D. Management of Acute Joint Lesions

See Chapter 7 for general guidelines as well as specific guidelines for RA and DJD.

1. To control the pain

In addition to using modalities and providing rest with an elastic wrap or splint, *gentle joint-play oscillation techniques* (grade I) may inhibit the pain. If these techniques increase the pain or swelling, they should not be attempted for several days.

2. To minimize stiffness

a. *Passive or active-assistive ROM* within the limits of pain and available motion are performed. The patient may be able to perform active ROM in the gravity-eliminated, side-lying position.

b. *Grade I or II tractions or glides*, if tolerated, with the joint in resting position (25 degrees flexion), are performed; stretching is contraindicated at this stage.

3. To minimize muscle atrophy and prevent patellar adhesions (see description of exercise techniques in Section VIII)

a. *Multiple-angle gentle muscle-setting techniques* including quadriceps femoris (quad sets) and hamstring contractions in pain-free positions.

b. *Gentle closed-chain quad sets.* Begin with the patient sitting and the knee extended as far as possible without provoking pain and have the patient press the heel on the floor while pressing the thigh into the chair.

c. *Quad sets with straight-leg raising (SLR).* Vary the angle of knee flexion/extension during the SLR, including full knee extension; the patient should be able to maintain each knee position without pain.

NOTE: SLR primarily affects the hip flexors and is done in conjunction with quad sets to vary the effect of gravity on the quadriceps while maintaining the knee in extension.

4. To prevent deformity and to protect the joint in RA or DJD

a. Minimize full weight-bearing activities during an acute flair of arthritis. If necessary, use crutches, canes, or a walker to distribute forces through the upper extremities while walking.

b. Instruct the patient and family members in good bed positioning to avoid flexion contractures.

c. Make functional adaptations to reduce the amount of knee flexion and patellar compression when the person moves from flexion to extension in activities such as standing up from sitting or stair climbing. Instruct the patient to minimize stair climbing, to use elevated seats on commodes, and to avoid deep-seated or low chairs.

E. Management of Subacute and Chronic Joint Problems[29]

1. To decrease the effects of stiffness from inactivity

Instruct the patient to perform active ROM and muscle-setting techniques.

2. To decrease pain from mechanical stress

Continue use of assistive devices for ambulation, if necessary. The patient may progress to using less assistance or may continue for periods without assistance.

Continue use of elevated seats on commodes and chairs, if needed, to reduce the mechanical stresses imposed when attempting to stand up.

3. To increase range of motion (ROM)

a. When there is loss of joint play and decreased mobility, joint mobilization techniques should be used.

   Precaution: Do not increase ROM unless the patient has strength to control the motion already available. A mobile joint with poor muscle control causes knee instability and makes lower extremity function difficult.

   (1) To increase flexion of the joint
      (a) Long-axis traction to the tibia (see Fig. 6–50A, B, and C)
      (b) Posterior glide to the tibia (see Figs. 6–51 and 6–52A and B)
      (c) Caudal glide of the patella if restricted (see Fig. 6–54)
      (d) Medial-lateral glide of the patella (see Fig. 6–55)

   (2) As the available range of flexion plateaus, progress by flexing the knee to the limit of its motion, then apply a posterior glide to the tibia; or position the tibia in medial rotation; then apply a posterior glide.

   (3) To increase extension of the joint
      (a) Long-axis traction (see Fig. 6–50A, B, and C).
      (b) Anterior glide of the tibia (see Fig. 6–53).
      (c) Progress by positioning the tibia in lateral rotation; then apply an anterior glide.
      (d) Superior-glide the patella if restricted in a caudal position.

b. When there is decreased flexibility in the muscles affecting knee motion, muscle elongation (inhibition) techniques should be used. Muscles typically involved include hamstrings, quadriceps, and gastrocsoleus.

   Precaution: Strong muscle contractions may exacerbate joint symptoms; adapt the dosage according to the patient's tolerance level.

c. When there is decreased flexibility in the noncontractile soft tissue preventing knee motion, passive stretching techniques should be used.

   (1) Apply low-intensity, long-duration stretch within the patient's tolerance.

   Precaution: Passive stretching using the tibia as a lever tends to exacerbate joint symptoms; use these techniques only when joint play is available.

   (2) Apply soft tissue massage or friction massage to loosen adhesions or contractures. Include deep massage around the border of the patella.

4. To develop strength and endurance in supporting muscles (see Section VIII for description of exercises)

a. Strengthen the quadriceps femoris and hamstring muscles within the patient's pain-free tolerance with multiple-angle isometrics, short-arc terminal extension exercises in open- and closed-chain positions, and a moderate progression of repetitions and resistance in wider arcs of motion as long as the motion is pain free. When doing open-chain exercises, patients experience less pain with faster speeds and lighter resistance than when doing the exercises slowly with heavy resistance. Resistance through the mid-range (45 to 90 degrees) tends to exacerbate joint pain because of the compressive forces of the patella. Apply resistance in arcs of motion that are pain free on either side of the symptomatic range. This could be done using manual resistance in the pain-free ranges, limiting the range with mechanical resistance exercises as well as using a range-limiting device on an isokinetic unit.

b. Because the patellofemoral joint is frequently symptomatic in arthritis of the knee, develop patellar balance with patellar mobilization and vastus medialis training (Section IV).

c. Strengthen hip- and ankle-stabilizing muscles in open- and closed-chain activities. (See respective chapters for exercises.)

d. To improve endurance, increase repetitions at each resistance level before progressing.

5. To improve knee function

a. Begin functional training. With improved strength and muscular endurance, the patient may increase the level of functional activities, beginning with swimming and bicycling and progressing to unassisted walking when the muscle is functioning at a "good" strength grade (⅘ or 80 percent) on a manual muscle test.

(1) When bicycling, adjust the seat so that the knee goes into complete extension when the pedal is down. Resistance from pedaling should be minimal.

(2) For some patients, progression to running or jumping rope and other high impact, faster paced or more intense activities can be undertaken as long as the joint remains asymptomatic. If joint deformity is present and proper biomechanics cannot be restored, the patient probably cannot progress to these activities.

b. With degenerative and rheumatoid arthritis, the patient should be cautioned to alternate activity with rest.

III. Joint Surgery and Postoperative Management

Surgical management of arthritis of the knee is indicated when joint pain and effusion cannot be controlled with conservative therapy and appropriate medical management or when destruction of articular surfaces, deformity, or restriction of motion have progressed to the point that functional abilities are significantly impaired.

The goals of surgery and postoperative management include: (1) relief of pain, (2) correction of deformity or instability, and (3) restoration of function in the involved knee.

The choice of surgical procedure will depend on the patient's age, type of arthritis, severity of joint destruction, and involvement of other joints. *Synovectomy* may be the procedure of choice in a young patient with unremitting joint effusion, synovial proliferation, and pain as the result of RA but with minimal deterioration of joint surfaces. *Osteotomy* of the tibia, an extra-articular procedure, will correct joint deformity, redistribute weight-bearing forces on the tibia and femur, and subsequently reduce joint pain during ambulation and delay the need for arthroplasty of the knee. When erosion of articular surfaces becomes severe, *total joint replacement* is the surgical procedure of choice to relieve pain, correct deformity, and restore functional movement. Only in very selective situations is *arthrodesis* of the knee chosen to provide the patient with a stable and pain-free knee. *Arthroscopic chondroplasty* and *abrasion arthroplasty* for deterioration of the articular cartilage of the posterior aspect of the patella (chondromalacia patellae) will be discussed in Section V of this chapter.

Regardless of the type of surgery chosen to relieve joint symptoms, a thorough preoperative evaluation followed by postoperative exercises and progressive ambulation are necessary components of an effective postoperative treatment plan.

A. Synovectomy

1. Indications for surgery[3,31,46,67,72,110]

a. Chronic synovitis and pain of the knee lasting 6 months or longer secondary to unremitting rheumatoid arthritis or osteoarthritis that cannot be controlled by medical management

b. Synovial hypertrophy and joint pain secondary to recurrent hemarthrosis associated with hemophilia

c. Intact or minimally eroded articular surfaces

d. Decreased ROM secondary to chronic synovitis and joint pain

e. A means of deferring total joint arthroplasty in the young patient with chronic synovitis usually associated with RA

2. Procedures[3,46,67,72,110]

a. Open procedure. Longitudinal medial and/or lateral longitudinal parapatellar incisions are made to allow access to the anterior and posterior compartments of the joint; the capsule and deep fascia are incised.

b. Arthroscopic procedure. Multiple portals are necessary for access to all portions of the joints.

c. As much synovium as possible (usually 80 to 90 percent) is excised.

d. If the menisci show signs of significant deterioration, a meniscectomy is also performed.

3. Postoperative management[45,46,67,72,112]

a. *Immobilization*

The knee is immobilized for 24 to 48 hours in a bulky compressive dressing and a posterior splint. During that time the leg is elevated to decrease postoperative edema.

b. *Exercise*

MAXIMUM-PROTECTION PHASE

(1) To prevent peripheral edema and decrease the risk of deep vein thrombosis, initiate ankle pumping exercises.

(2) To regain or maintain neuromuscular control of hip and knee musculature on the operated side, begin:

(a) Quadriceps-setting exercises

(b) Straight-leg raises in the supine, prone, and side-lying positions

(3) To minimize postoperative pain and swelling, after the compressive dressing can be removed, begin gentle distal-to-proximal massage.

(4) To prevent postoperative contractures and regain full ROM of the knee, patients are routinely placed on a continuous passive motion (CPM) machine shortly after surgery. In addition, during therapy have the patient perform:

(a) Active-assisted knee flexion and extension exercises within the pain-free ROM

(b) Gentle active inhibition and muscle elongation techniques to the quadriceps and hamstrings

(5) Ambulation with crutches is begun the day after surgery, with weight bearing as tolerated. The patient should wear the posterior splint until full active knee extension has been achieved.

MODERATE- TO MINIMUM-PROTECTION PHASES

(1) To regain or improve control and strength of the knee musculature, continue quadriceps setting and straight-leg raising (SLR) exercises and begin submaximal multiple-angle isometrics against manual resistance. Progress to low-intensity isotonic resistance exercises in an open kinetic chain. Add progressive closed-chain strengthening activities as weight bearing allows. Emphasize control of the quadriceps in full knee extension for safe and efficient ambulation.

(2) If limitation of motion persists, begin joint mobilization and soft tissue stretching when swelling has subsided.

(3) Exercises and weight bearing are progressed rapidly after arthroscopic synovectomy but more slowly after an open synovectomy. A patient often regains normal ROM and will be able to ambulate without assistive devices as early as 7 to 10 days after an arthroscopic procedure. Full ROM, unassisted ambulation, and return to full functional activities should be attained more gradually over a 6-week postoperative period after an open synovectomy.

(4) The patient should be encouraged to become involved in or resume low-impact, low-intensity but progressive conditioning activities such as swimming or bicycling.

4. Expected results[46,72,110]

Synovectomy has been shown to alleviate chronic synovitis and joint pain and in most cases improve ROM and postpone joint destruction. There is little evidence to support the claim that synovectomy can reverse the disease process. Full active and passive knee extension, at least 100 degrees of knee flexion, and adequate strength and stability of the knee are necessary for most functional activities.

B. Total Knee Replacement

1. Indications for surgery[14,30,31,46,82,94,112]

a. Severe joint pain with weight bearing or motion that compromises functional abilities

b. Extensive destruction of articular cartilage of the knee secondary to arthritis

c. Gross instability or limitation of motion

d. Marked deformity of the knee such as genu varum or valgum

e. Failure of a previous surgical procedure

2. Procedures

a. *Background and development of total knee arthroplasty*
Prosthetic replacement of one or both surfaces of the knee joint began to develop in the late 1950s and early 1960s.

(1) MacIntosh[58,59] and then McKeevor[66] replaced the tibial plateau (hemi-arthroplasty) with an acrylic and, later, an inert metal implant as a treatment for severe degenerative arthritis and varus or valgus deformities of the knee.

(2) In 1951, Walldius[51,68,104] designed the first constrained total knee arthroplasty, which consisted of a stemmed and hinged (articulated) metal prosthetic replacement for the distal femur and proximal tibia. All ligaments and soft tissue stabilizers of the knee were removed, but the articulated prosthesis provided stability to the knee joint. The prosthetic components allowed 90 degrees of knee flexion and full extension but did not take into account the rotary motion between the femur and the tibia. Consequently this early design had a high failure rate because of eventual loosening of the prosthesis in the intramedullary canals. In addition, this procedure required a very long period of total immobilization of the knee after surgery, which made it very difficult for patients to regain a functional degree of knee flexion. Today the constrained design is used only in cases of severe joint instability and after a previous unconstrained total knee replacement has failed.

(3) A nonarticulated unconstrained multicondylar replacement was developed by Gunston[38,39] in the late 1960s and was designed to resurface the articular surfaces of the tibia and femur. The prosthesis allowed all normal motions of the knee and consisted of two high-density polyethylene troughlike tibial components and two metal disklike femoral components, all of which were held in place with acrylic cement. The replacement provided no internal stability of the knee; therefore, intact, balanced collateral ligaments were a necessary prerequisite. This resurfacing system allowed approximately 120 degrees of knee flexion and full extension. From this design a unicondylar (unicompartmental) replacement was also developed to separately resurface either the medial or lateral joint surfaces when only one side of the joint was involved.[46]

(4) Other variations of nonarticulated knee replacements consisted of two components, a polyethylene tibial and a metal femoral replacement held in place with cement.* The patellofemoral joint was not resurfaced.

(5) Today there are two basic classifications of knee replacement prostheses: resurfacing (unconstrained) and constrained.[46,90,110,112]

(a) *Resurfacing (unconstrained) prostheses* can be unicondylar, unicompartmental, bicondylar, or total condylar. Replacements that resurface the entire knee joint can be *cruciate excising* or *cruciate retaining*. If the design is cruciate retaining, the posterior collateral ligament (PCL) is spared and must provide posterior stability to the knee. If the PCL is not intact, a cruciate-excising prosthesis, which has posterior stability built into the design, is most appropriate. In all cases, a patient must have intact collateral ligaments to be considered for a resurfacing replacement. Resurfacing replacements are composed of an inert metal femoral component and a polyethylene tibial component. In a total condylar replacement, the posterior aspect of the patella is also resurfaced with a polyethylene dome-shaped component.

(b) *Constrained prostheses,* which are hinged and allow no significant accessory motions of the knee, or partially articulated, *semiconstrained*

---

*Refs. 17, 30, 31, 46, 78, 82, 91, 94.

replacements that allow a small degree of varus, valgus, or rotation are rarely used today. Constrained designs sacrifice the collateral and cruciate ligaments and are indicated only for patients with severe instability and deformity of the knee.

b. *Fixation**

Total knee replacements are either held in place with acrylic cement or utilize biologic fixation (bony ingrowth). Initially almost all total knee replacements involved cement fixation. The most common long-term problem, which can cause pain and contribute to failure of a total knee procedure, is loosening of the tibial component at the bone-cement interface. To counteract this problem, biologic, cementless fixation that relies on rapid growth of bone into the surfaces of a porous-coated prosthesis was developed. It has been suggested that biologic fixation may be the most appropriate choice for young, active patients in which long-term loosening may be most likely to occur. To date, the long-term effectiveness of cemented versus cementless fixation has not been determined.

c. *Overview of procedures*[30,46,82,110,112]

(1) A longitudinal incision is made along the anteromedial aspect of the knee.

(2) A synovectomy, if necessary, and a meniscectomy are performed. Other soft tissue procedures may include a retinacular release or extensor mechanism realignment.

(3) The tibial and femoral articulating surfaces are prepared and the components implanted and held in place with biologic or cement fixation. The posterior aspect of the patella may also be prepared and resurfaced.

3. Postoperative management[†]

a. *Immobilization*

The knee is immobilized in a bulky compression dressing for a day or two postoperatively. After the bulky dressing is removed, a posterior knee splint is often worn but is removed for daily exercise. Cementless arthroplasty may require a longer period of immobilization than a cemented procedure to allow ingrowth of bone into the prosthesis. A posterior knee splint may be indicated for use at night for as long as 12 weeks postoperatively.

b. *Exercise*

MAXIMUM-PROTECTION PHASE

(1) To regain neuromuscular control of hip and knee musculature while the knee is immobilized, have the patient perform the following exercises numerous times each day:

(a) Quadriceps- and hamstring-setting exercises, possibly coupled with neuromuscular electrical stimulation[16]

(b) Straight-leg raises in supine, prone, and side-lying positions[47]

(2) To promote circulation and decrease postoperative edema and pain, initiate:

(a) Ankle pumping exercises immediately after surgery.

---

*Refs. 43, 44, 70, 71, 81, 82, 110, 112.
†Refs. 14, 16, 34, 35, 45, 61, 67, 105–107.

(b) Gentle distal-to-proximal massage of the operated lower extremity.[112]

(c) Continuous passive motion (CPM). CPM is routinely used in the early postoperative days after total knee replacement surgery. It has been suggested that CPM decreases postoperative pain, promotes wound healing, decreases the incidence of deep vein thrombosis, and decreases hospital stay, but these benefits have not been consistently supported in the research literature.[4,25,32,34,48,57,65] Therefore, CPM is recommended as an adjunct to, not a replacement for, a supervised postoperative exercise program.

(3) Early protected motion

To prevent postoperative contractures, initiate and progress active-assisted and active knee flexion and extension to patient tolerance. Soft tissue pain, swelling, and muscle spasm make it difficult to flex the knee. Reciprocal inhibition of the quadriceps by means of the agonist-contraction technique of muscle elongation (described in Section VI.A.3 of Chapter 5) is an effective method of relaxing the quadriceps and increasing knee flexion.

Precaution: Vigorous passive stretching to increase knee flexion or extension is not appropriate during the very early postoperative period when soft tissues are just beginning to heal.

(4) Weight bearing

The extent to which weight bearing is allowable is dependent upon the type of prosthesis implanted and the type of fixation used.

(a) If biologic fixation has been used, weight bearing is usually restricted up to 6 weeks postoperatively and gradually progressed over the duration of rehabilitation. Full weight bearing and ambulation without assistive devices may not be permissible for up to 12 weeks postoperatively.

(b) With cement fixation, weight bearing as tolerated is permissible immediately after surgery and increased to full weight bearing over 6 weeks. The patient should continue to use crutches or a cane through the moderate- and minimum-protection phases of rehabilitation until adequate strength and stability have returned to the operated lower extremity.

MODERATE-PROTECTION PHASE

(1) Exercises to increase strength

(a) As healing progresses, multiple-angle isometrics and light isotonic resistance exercises of the quadriceps and hamstrings can be added. Adequate strength of the knee extensors is most important for stability of the knee during weight-bearing activities.

(b) Resisted straight-leg raises in various positions should be included to increase the strength of hip musculature with emphasis on the hip extensors and abductors.

(c) As weight bearing permits, closed-chain mini-squats and short-arc lunges can be added to improve stability and functional control of the knee.

(2) Exercises to increase ROM

(a) Gentle self-stretching (low-intensity, prolonged stretch) or contract-relax exercises are also added to continue to increase knee ROM if limited motion persists.

NOTE: The use of joint mobilization techniques to increase ROM may or may not be appropriate, depending on the design of the prosthetic components of the total knee arthroplasty. It is advisable to discuss the use of joint mobilization with the surgeon before initiating these techniques.

(b) When using a stationary bicycle, the patient may first have the seat positioned as high as possible. To increase knee flexion, the seat can be gradually lowered.

(c) If a patient has not achieved 75 to 90 degrees of knee flexion by the time of discharge from the hospital, some surgeons manipulate the knee while the patient is under general anesthesia.

MINIMUM-PROTECTION AND RETURN-TO-ACTIVITY PHASES

(1) By the 12th week after surgery the emphasis in rehabilitation is on muscle conditioning so that the patient will have the strength and endurance to return to a full level of functional activities.

(2) Ambulation activities, stair climbing, and so on are gradually increased.

(3) Stationary bicycling and aquatic exercises are excellent nonimpact conditioning activities.

4. **Expected results**[46,61,90,92,106,107]

a. Almost all patients who undergo total knee arthroplasty report a significant relief of pain with knee motion and weight bearing.

b. Although patients are encouraged to achieve full functional ROM of the knee (full active extension and at least 95 to 100 degrees of flexion) by the time of discharge after surgery, improvement in ROM may continue up to 12 to 24 months postoperatively. Long-term postoperative follow-up of patients after knee replacement suggests that only minimal changes occur in ROM. Patients with restricted ROM preoperatively usually continue to have restrictions in knee flexion or extension postoperatively, despite an aggressive postoperative exercise program.

c. It may take at least 3 months postoperatively for a patient to regain strength in the quadriceps and hamstrings to a preoperative level. Quadriceps weakness tends to persist longer after knee arthroplasty than does knee flexor weakness. As the patient's level of functional activity continues to increase, he or she may see further gains in strength and endurance for more than a year postoperatively.[92,107]

IV. Patellofemoral Dysfunction: Nonoperative Management

A. Related Diagnoses[89]

1. **Chondromalacia patellae** refers to softening and fissuring of the cartilaginous surface of the patella and is diagnosed with arthroscopy or arthrogram.[33,63] It may eventually predispose the joint to degenerative arthritis or basal degeneration of the middle and deep zones of the cartilage.[33] Causes of the degeneration may include trauma, surgery, prolonged or repeated stress, or lack of normal stress, such as during periods of immobilization.[76] The patella femoral grinding test is positive,[42] and palpation elicits tenderness along the medial aspect of the articular surface of the patella.[33] It is common in young people, and girls have a greater tendency to develop symptoms than do boys.[33] In older people, it is associated with osteoarthritis. An increased Q angle is often seen.

2. **Plica syndrome, plica synovalis, medial shelf syndrome, suprapatellar plica synovitis, and medial plica synovitis**[6] describe conditions related to irritation of remnants of embryologic synovial tissue around the patella, which may occur as a result of microtrauma or macrotrauma. With chronic irritation, the tissue becomes an inelastic fibrotic band. When acute, the tissue is painful on palpation; when chronic, the plical band is tender. The band is usually palpable medial to the patella, although there are variations in its location.[6,52]

3. **Patellofemoral pain, patellar malalignment, extensor mechanism malalignment or dysfunction, lateral patellar compression syndrome, runner's knee, and tendinitis** describe a condition of insidious onset characterized by pain and aching in the patellar region brought on by stair climbing; prolonged sitting or squatting with flexed knees; or occupational, sports, and recreational activities.

4. **Patellar subluxation, or patellar dislocation,** describes excessive lateral movement of the patella. With dislocation, the patella displaces laterally out of the trochlear groove from direct trauma to the patella or from a forceful quadriceps contraction while the foot is planted and the femur is externally rotating while the knee is flexed. A shallow trochlear groove or flat lateral femoral condyle, weak or overstretched medial structures, and patella alta predispose the patella to dislocation.

B. Etiology of Symptoms[23,63,85,89,103,111]

Other than direct trauma or anatomic variations in bony structure of the patella or trochlear groove, anterior knee pain is related to an imbalance of soft tissues aligning the patella in the trochlear groove and influencing patellar tracking. As described in Section I.C, malalignment or tracking problems may be caused by factors that increase the Q angle, muscle or fascial tightness along the lateral aspect of the patella, or an insufficient VMO muscle.

C. Common Impairments/Problems[23,63,85,89,103,111]

1. Weakness, inhibition, or poor recruitment or timing of firing of the VMO
2. Overstretched medial retinaculum
3. Tight lateral retinaculum, IT band, or fascial structures around the patella
4. Decreased medial glide or medial tipping of the patella
5. Pronated foot
6. Pain on palpation
7. Tight gastrocsoleus, hamstring, or rectus femoris muscles
8. Irritated patellar tendon or subpatellar fat pads

D. Common Functional Limitations/Disabilities

1. Pain or poor knee control when descending or ascending stairs
2. Pain with jumping or running interfering with sport and recreational activities
3. Pain with prolonged sitting or squatting with the knee in flexion

E. Nonoperative Management of Acute Patellofemoral Symptoms

When symptoms are acute, treat as any acute joint with modalities, rest, gentle motion, and muscle-setting exercises in pain-free positions. Pain and joint effusion inhibit the quadriceps, so it is imperative to reduce irritating forces. Splinting the patella with a brace or tape may unload the joint and relieve the irritating stress.[63]

F. Nonoperative Management of Subacute Patellofemoral Symptoms

1. **To increase flexibility of the lateral fascia and insertion of the IT band[64]**

   a. *Mobilize the patella* with a medial glide (Fig. 12–1; see also Fig. 6–55). Position the patient side-lying. Stabilize the femoral condyles with one hand under the femur and glide the patella medially with the base of the hand. There is usually greater mobility with the knee near extension. To progress stretching, position the knee in greater flexion.

   b. *Friction massage* around the lateral aspect of the patella.

   c. *Medial tipping* of the patella (Fig. 12–2). The thenar eminence at the base of the hand is placed over the medial aspect of the patella. A direct posterior force tips the patella medially. While the patella is held in this position, friction massage can be applied with the other hand along the lateral border. The patient can be taught to self-stretch in this manner.

   d. *Patellar taping* can be used to realign the patella and apply a prolonged stretch as well as maintain alignment of the patella for nonstressful training.[63,64]

   e. *Self-stretch insertion of IT band* (Fig. 12–3). The patient is side-lying with a belt or sheet strapped around the ankle and the other end placed over the shoulder and held in the hand. The hip is positioned in extension, adduction, and slight lateral rotation and the knee in flexion. First flex the knee and abduct the hip, then extend the hip (this ensures that the IT band is over the greater trochanter). The femur is then adducted with slight lateral rotation until tension is felt in the IT band along the lateral knee. The patient stabilizes self in this position by holding onto the strap. If tolerated, a 2- to 5-lb weight is placed distally over the lateral thigh for added stretch and the position is maintained for 20 to 30 minutes.

2. **To stretch other tight structures**

   Identify any tight muscles and selectively stretch. Techniques to stretch the hamstrings and rectus femoris at the knee are described in Section VIII; to stretch the hamstrings, tensor fasciae latae, and rectus femoris at the hip, see Chapter 11; to stretch the gastrocnemius and soleus, see Chapter 13.

3. **To train and strengthen the VMO in non–weight bearing**

   NOTE: The exercises are described in greater detail in the exercise section of this chapter (Section VIII).

   a. Use tactile cues over the muscle belly, electrical stimulation, or biofeedback to reinforce VMO contraction

   b. *Quadriceps setting (quad sets) in pain-free positions.* The patient sets the quads with the knee in various positions while focusing on tension development in the VMO. Opinions vary as to the best knee angles for training. Because the site of irritation will vary between patients, identifying pain-free positions for each patient should ensure nondestructive loading.[89,111]

   c. *Quad sets with straight-leg raising (SLR).* Because many fibers of the VMO

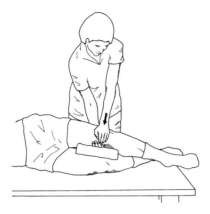

Figure 12–1. Medial glide of the patella.

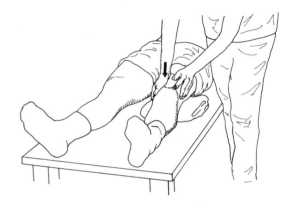

Figure 12–2. Medial tipping of the patella with friction massage along the lateral border.

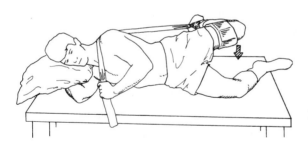

Figure 12–3. Self-stretch to the insertion of IT band.

originate on the adductor muscle, some popular exercise programs suggest that by laterally rotating the femur while performing SLR exercises the adductors will contract and provide a firm base for the VMO,[2,23,63] but EMG studies do not support this claim.[50]

  d. *Short-arc terminal extension* (see Fig. 12–8). Begin with the knee flexed around 20 degrees. If tolerated and the motion is not painful, light resistance is added at the ankle. Strengthening in terminal extension trains the muscle to function where it is least efficient because of its shortened position and where there is minimal patellar compression because it is superior to the femoral groove.

4. **To train and strengthen functional control of VMO in weight bearing**

   NOTE: See Section VIII for detailed descriptions of the exercises. The patient should perform the repetitions of the appropriate exercise until symptoms or loss of control just begin in order to develop endurance but not push beyond that point.

   a. If weight bearing is painful, initiate closed-chain quad sets in *partial weight bearing*. Begin with the patient seated with the knee in near extension and the heel on the floor and instruct the patient to push the thigh into the chair and the heel into the floor to cause a hamstring contraction while simultaneously performing quad sets, concentrating on VMO contractions.
   b. When weight bearing is tolerated, initiate unilateral terminal knee extension against elastic resistance (see Fig. 12–10). Begin with the patient bearing most weight on the sound lower extremity. Gradually, increase body weight on the involved leg.
   c. Progress to standing in a forward-stride position and have the patient rock forward onto the extremity, controlling the amount of knee flexion and amount of weight while focusing on contraction of the VMO. During training, do not use strong resistance or the patient may focus on the sensation of heavy exertion rather than on control.
   d. Add activities such as low step-ups, partial lunges, mini-squats, and stationary bicycling at low resistance (see Fig. 12–11) within only pain-free ranges.

5. **To modify biomechanical stresses**

   a. If the patient has foot pronation, a foot orthosis may relieve the stresses at the knee.[27]
   b. Assess any lower chain faulty mechanics and modify if possible.

6. **To educate the patient**

   a. Until the knee is symptom free, the patient should avoid positions and activities that provoke the symptoms. Avoid stair climbing and descending until the muscles are strengthened to a level at which they can function without symptoms. The patient should not sit with the knees flexed excessively for prolonged periods.
   b. Use a home exercise program to reinforce the training.

G. Nonoperative Management of Chronic Patellofemoral Symptoms

1. Progress resistance in pain-free arcs of motion using light weights and more repetitions. If the motion is painful in the mid-range, resist on either side of the painful arc.
2. Progress functional control by increasing step height, lunges, partial squats, single-knee dips, resistive walking, elastic resistance while standing, balance board activities, and leg presses as described in Chapter 11 and Sections V and VIII of this chapter.
3. Progress to activity-specific drills.

V. Patellofemoral and Extensor Mechanism Surgery and Postoperative Management

When conservative (nonoperative) management of patellofemoral dysfunction fails, surgery may be indicated. Surgical intervention can be used to alter the alignment of the patellofemoral joint, correct soft tissue imbalances, decrease an abnormal Q angle, improve tracking of the patella, and débride the articular surface of the patella. All of these factors can contribute to chronic patellofemoral pain and crepitation and recurrent dislocation or subluxation of the patella. Before any surgery is chosen, the etiology of symptoms and identification of contributing factors must be determined by a thorough physical examination and arthroscopic and radiographic evaluation. Surgical options include *release of the lateral retinaculum, chondroplasty* or *abrasion arthroplasty* of the patella, *proximal or distal realignment of the extensor mechanism,* and *patellectomy.* A combination of procedures may also be indicated.

The goals of postoperative rehabilitation are to[5,40]: (1) reduce or control postoperative pain and swelling, (2) prevent or reduce the adverse effects of immobilization, (3) restore postoperative knee ROM quickly and safely, (4) maximize the function of the knee extensor mechanism, especially the VMO, to restore full active knee extension and prevent a postoperative quadriceps lag, and (5) educate the patient and possibly alter lifestyle to prevent recurrence of patellofemoral pain and dysfunction.

A. Lateral Retinacular Release

1. Indications for surgery[5,41,46,80]

a. Chronic lateral subluxation (displacement) and excessive tilting of the patella
b. Abnormal patellar tracking as the result of extensor mechanism malalignment associated with long-standing patellofemoral pain and swelling
c. Tight lateral structures and lax, overstretched, and weak medial structures of the knee
d. Nonimprovement in symptoms after 3 to 6 months of conservative (nonoperative) management, including exercise, bracing, taping, anti-inflammatory medication, or modification in daily activities

2. Procedures[46,69,83]

a. Either an open or an arthroscopic release may be performed.
b. If an open procedure is used, a vertical incision is made along the lateral aspect of the patella. This allows the surgeon to visualize the lateral patellar retinaculum and lower fibers of the vastus lateralis muscle.
   (1) A longitudinal incision is made in the deep and superficial fibers of the retinaculum and possibly the distal vastus lateralis fibers. This allows the patella to move more medially for more normal patellar tracking.
   (2) A medial capsular reefing or plication may also be performed to tighten or reinforce medial structures of the knee.
c. If an arthroscopic approach is used, the same procedures are performed through multiple portals around the patella.
d. This procedure may be performed separately or in conjunction with realignment of the extensor mechanism or arthroscopic chondroplasty (débridement and smoothing) for chondromalacia patellae.

3. Postoperative management[5,40,46,80]

a. *Immobilization*
   The knee is immobilized in full extension with a compression dressing and patella-stabilizing orthosis or posterior splint for 0 to 3 days. A CryoCuff,

which combines cold and compression, may be applied to minimize postoperative swelling and pain and prevent hemarthrosis.

b. *Exercise*

MAXIMUM-PROTECTION PHASE

(1) To decrease pain and swelling and minimize muscle atrophy, initiate pain-free submaximal muscle-setting exercises of the quadriceps and hamstrings and active SLR exercises for the hip and knee musculature in the supine, side-lying, and prone positions.[47] These exercises are performed while wearing the knee immobilizer. To further facilitate recruitment of the quadriceps, particularly the VMO, use electrical muscle stimulation or biofeedback in conjunction with quadriceps-setting exercises.

(2) To prevent deep vein thrombosis and promote circulation in the operated lower extremity, perform ankle pumping exercises immediately after surgery.

(3) To maintain passive mobility of the patella, perform superior, inferior, and medial glides of the patella. (See Figs. 6–54, 6–55, and 12–1.)

(4) To restore full knee ROM, especially flexion, which can be limited postoperatively, remove the knee immobilizer and begin gentle active or active-assisted knee flexion using heel slides in supine or sitting positions or initiate active inhibition techniques to elongate the quadriceps.

(5) Partial weight bearing on the operated lower extremity and ambulation with crutches while wearing the knee immobilizer is permissible the day of or the day after surgery. Weight bearing is progressed based on pain and patient tolerance.

    Precaution: If arthroscopic articular surgery of the patellofemoral joint was also performed, the patient may need to be non–weight bearing (NWB) on the operated lower extremity for up to 4 to 6 weeks postoperatively. (See Section V.B of this chapter.)

(6) NOTE: If an arthroscopic lateral release was performed, there will be minimal trauma and compromise of soft tissues. Approximately 7 to 10 days is necessary for healing of the incision. Exercises and weight bearing can be progressed rapidly, similar to nonoperative management of patellofemoral dysfunction.[5,40,69]

MODERATE-PROTECTION PHASE

By 2 to 4 weeks postoperatively the rehabilitation program can be progressed as follows:

(1) To restore full flexion and extension, progress active knee motion. If knee motion continues to be restricted, initiate gentle joint mobilizations and soft tissue stretching when indicated.

(2) To recondition, strengthen, and improve endurance of knee musculature, particularly the VMO, add the following exercises at the end of the first week or during the second week postoperatively:

  (a) Multiple-angle isometrics against resistance

  (b) Stationary bicycling against light resistance

  (c) Open-chain short-arc submaximal resisted knee extension and resisted hamstring curls against light manual or mechanical resistance

(3) To restore stability and functional control at the knee, begin closed-chain exercises in partial and later full weight bearing on the operated leg. Include partial squats, partial lunges, and step-ups. Have the patient slightly externally rotate the legs to place the VMO in the optimum line of pull during contraction.

(4) **Precaution:** Avoid open- and closed-chain exercises in portions of the ROM that cause patellofemoral pain, crepitation, or joint effusion. Avoid exercises against heavy loads or in positions that increase compressive forces on the patellofemoral joint.

(5) By 3 weeks postoperatively, full weight bearing out of the immobilizer during ambulation and functional activities is permissible.

(6) To facilitate balance, emphasize proprioceptive input through progressive weight-bearing activities. Start with static bilateral standing activities and progress to dynamic bilateral and then unilateral standing activities on a balance board.

(7) NOTE: After use of the knee immobilizer is discontinued, it may be useful to fit the patient with a lateral patellar tracking orthosis that should be worn during exercises and functional activities.

MINIMUM-PROTECTION AND RETURN-TO-FULL-ACTIVITY PHASES

(1) Progress open-chain lower extremity resistance exercises by increasing repetitions and add isokinetic strengthening exercises at intermediate and fast velocities.

(2) Increase the speed and intensity of closed-chain resistance exercises with progressive plyometric training.

(3) Add closed-chain functional exercises on a slide board, NordicTrack, or stair-stepping exercise unit.

(4) Add agility training and simulated recreational, occupational, and functional activities, always avoiding activities that produce pain and crepitation.

(5) Discontinue use of patellar tracking orthosis if activities can be carried out without recurrence of patellofemoral symptoms.

(6) NOTE: Patients can usually return to full activities by 6 to 8 weeks after a lateral retinacular release.

B. Chondroplasty and Abrasion Arthroplasty

1. Indications for surgery[5,46]

a. Pain and crepitation in the patellofemoral joint often associated with restriction of knee motion and functional activities

b. Deterioration of the articular surface of the patellofemoral joint resulting in osteophytic formation, loose bodies, and synovitis

2. Procedures[9,46,83]

a. Chondroplasty or abrasion arthroplasty, two common débridement procedures, may be performed independently or in conjunction with other patellofemoral surgery such as lateral retinacular release or proximal or distal realignment of the extensor mechanism.

b. The procedures are usually done arthroscopically and involve a smoothing (shaving) and débridement of the posterior articular surfaces of the patella.

c. Osteophytes, if present, are removed. Necrotic bone is removed and vascular bone is exposed to stimulate growth of fibrocartilage and facilitate cartilage repair.

d. A partial synovectomy may also be performed if significant synovitis is present.

3. **Postoperative management**[5,40,54]

   a. *Immobilization*

   A brief period of immobilization in a compressive dressing is necessary. Cold packs or a CryoCuff is used to minimize postoperative pain and swelling.

   b. *Exercise*

   (1) Weight bearing must be totally or significantly restricted for 4 to 6 weeks postoperatively. Weight bearing in the early weeks postoperatively can increase compressive forces at the patellofemoral joint and inhibit cartilage regeneration. Full weight bearing may not be permissible for 8 to 12 weeks.

   (2) Exercises for postoperative rehabilitation include those carried out in a nonoperative management program or after arthroscopic lateral retinacular release. Early low-intensity open-chain motion is stressed to restore and maximize nutrition to articular surfaces. Closed-chain exercises are restricted for a longer period of time than after lateral retinacular release. Full weight-bearing closed-chain activities may not be permissible for 6 to 12 weeks postoperatively.

   (3) All exercises or activities that cause compressive forces on the patella, increased joint crepitation, pain, or joint effusion must be avoided.

   c. NOTE: Long-term results of arthroscopic articular surgeries alone are, at best, only slightly better than nonoperative management. Because the causes of joint deterioration are not corrected by articular surgery, the joint surfaces may continue to deteriorate.

C. Realignment of the Extensor Mechanism

1. **Indications for surgery**[9,41,46,80,83]

   a. Recurrent dislocation or subluxation of the patella occurring with sudden contraction of the quadriceps

   b. Increased patellar Q angle

   c. Lateral tracking of the patella and insufficiency of the VMO

   d. Painful, compressive forces at the patellofemoral joint

2. **Procedures**[9,46,80,83]

   a. Either a distal or a proximal realignment procedure may be chosen. Variations include the Elmslie-Trillat, Hauser, or Maquet procedures.

   b. In a *distal realignment* procedure, the distal insertion of the patellar tendon with a portion of the tibial tubercle is incised and osteotomized and repositioned more distally and medially on the tibia and fixed in place with a screw. The procedure may be combined with bony elevation (anteriorization) of the tibial tubercle with a local bone graft to decrease compressive forces on the patella for patients with chondromalacia patellae.

   c. In a *proximal realignment* procedure, which involves the proximal aspect of the patellar tendon, the VMO muscle is transferred distally to increase the resting length-tension relationship of the muscle and to provide a dynamic restraint to decrease the lateral tracking of the patella. This procedure is also known as an *advancement of the quadriceps*.

   d. In both procedures, a long parapatellar incision is made to expose soft tissues and the tibial tubercle.

3. Postoperative management*

a. *Immobilization*

The knee is immobilized in a hinged knee brace or a posterior splint in full extension up to 10 days to 2 or 3 weeks. Some surgeons allow removal of the immobilizer for passive ROM, while other surgeons advocate continuous immobilization for a period after surgery.

b. *Exercise*

MAXIMUM-PROTECTION PHASE

(1) In the early postoperative days, the knee immobilizer is removed for CPM or manual passive motion in a limited and protected range to minimize the adverse effects of immobilization. Knee flexion is often limited to 40 to 60 degrees when knee motion is first initiated. NOTE: Knee motion is progressed more slowly after proximal realignment surgery than after distal realignment surgery.

(2) Weight bearing is restricted to touch-down or non–weight bearing while wearing the knee immobilizer in the maximum-protection phase.

(3) Exercises similar to those indicated after lateral retinacular release may be initiated. Emphasis is placed on repeated pain-free exercises and activation of the VMO, which may be augmented with electrical muscle stimulation and biofeedback. Every effort is made to prevent an **extensor (quadriceps) lag**.

MODERATE-PROTECTION PHASE

(1) Weight bearing, ROM, and reconditioning and strengthening of the quadriceps mechanism must be progressed more slowly after bony procedures than after soft tissue procedures. All must be carefully limited for 6 to 8 weeks postoperatively. Otherwise, exercises are similar to those incorporated into an exercise plan after lateral retinacular release.

(2) By 6 weeks postoperatively the patient should have 100 to 120 degrees of knee flexion and full active knee extension after a distal realignment procedure. Knee flexion is progressed more slowly after a proximal realignment procedure.

NOTE: A quadriceps lag of 5 to 10 degrees may persist because of knee effusion, quadriceps atrophy, or poor mechanical advantage of the quadriceps mechanism for several months after surgery.

MINIMUM-PROTECTION AND RETURN-TO-ACTIVITY PHASES

(1) By 6 to 8 weeks the knee orthosis and crutches may be discontinued. Strength, endurance, stabilization, ROM, and balance exercises can all be progressed if the patient is pain free. Efforts should be made to modify the patient's lifestyle, and any activities that cause patellofemoral pain and compression or compromise the stability of the patella should be avoided.

(2) Return to full, functional activities can occur by 20 to 24 weeks after distal realignment and 24 weeks after a proximal realignment procedure.

*Refs. 2, 5, 12, 23, 40, 50, 56, 80, 96, 100, 101.

VI. Sprains and Minor Ligamentous Tears

A. Related Diagnoses and Mechanisms of Injury

Ligamentous injuries occur most often in individuals between 20 and 40 years of age as the result of sport injuries (e.g., skiing, soccer, and football). The anterior cruciate ligament (ACL) is the most commonly injured ligament. The injury occurs when the knee is forcefully hyperextended. The medial collateral ligament, as well as the ACL, can be injured with a valgus strain and external rotation of the tibia when the foot is planted. The posterior cruciate ligament (PCL) can be injured with a forceful blow to the anterior portion of the tibia while the knee is flexed. Often more than one ligament is damaged as the result of a single injury.[46]

B. Common Impairments/Problems

Following trauma, the joint usually does not swell for several hours. Once swollen, motion is restricted. The joint assumes a position of minimum stress, usually around 25 degrees of flexion. If tested when the joint is not swollen, the patient feels pain when the injured ligament is stressed. If there is a complete tear, instability is detected when the torn ligament is tested.

C. Common Functional Limitations/Disabilities

1. When acute, cannot bear weight or ambulate without assistance.
2. With complete tear, knee may give way when stressed.

D. Nonoperative Management

Acute sprains and partial ligamentous tears of the knee can be treated conservatively with rest, joint protection, and exercise. After the acute stage of healing, exercises should be geared toward regaining normal ROM and strength of the muscles supporting and stabilizing the joint during functional activities. The degree of instability with ligamentous tears will affect the demands the patient can place on the knee when returning to full activity.

1. If possible, evaluate and treat the problem with cold, compression, and quadriceps-setting exercises before effusion sets in.
2. When the joint is swollen, treat it like an acute joint lesion as described in Section II. The knee may not fully extend for muscle-setting exercises, so begin the exercises in the range most comfortable for the patient.
3. As the swelling decreases, initiate active range of motion and strengthening exercises to the flexors and extensors of the knee in both open- and closed-chain positions.

    Precaution: Open-chain terminal knee extension exercises (from 60 degrees to zero) with resistance applied to the distal leg, and closed-chain squatting between 60 and 90 degrees cause increased anterior translation of the tibia and stress to the ACL. Exercises using either of these activities in the designated ranges should not be attempted with ACL injuries.[36,108,109] Instruct the patient in closed-chain strengthening activities from 60 to 0 degrees and open-chain strengthening from 90 to 60 degrees.[108]

    Isolated open-chain knee flexion exercises increase posterior translation of the tibia and should not be done with PCL injuries.

4. If the collateral or coronary ligaments are involved, cross-fiber massage to the structure helps align the healing fibers and maintain mobility in them.

5. Protective bracing may be necessary in weight-bearing activities to decrease stress to the healing ligament or to provide stability where ligament integrity has been compromised. The patient must be instructed to decrease vigorous activities until appropriate stability is obtained.

6. Progress to functional training with closed-chain resistive exercises, steps, agility drills, and plyometrics.

E. Reconstruction of Ligamentous Lesions and Postoperative Management

The ligaments that surround the anatomically unstable knee joint are extremely vulnerable to acute or chronic injury. Acute tears or chronic insufficiencies of the cruciate, collateral, capsular, or oblique ligaments can significantly compromise an individual's functional capabilities at work or during recreational activities.[12,41,46,53,84] Severe tears or ruptures of ligaments can cause gross joint instability, articular erosion, pain, and limitation of motion. As noted earlier, the most commonly injured ligament of the knee is the ACL.

Surgical intervention is indicated when joint instability causes disability and functional limitations or could eventually lead to deterioration of joint surfaces.[40,46,79] Acute ligamentous lesions as the result of macrotrauma to the knee joint are repaired after the joint is less acute and an accurate diagnosis can be made. Chronic deficits are treated surgically if conservative (nonoperative) intervention fails.

Ligamentous surgery, using an arthroscopically assisted or open approach, involves a *direct repair* of the torn ligament, an *intra-articular or extra-articular reconstruction* of joint structures, or a combination of procedures to restore stability to the knee.[1,46,53,75] In most instances, direct repair by means of suturing the torn ligament affords the least acceptable outcome. Direct repairs are often unsuccessful because ligaments have a very poor vascular supply, necessitating long periods of immobilization and restricted weight bearing so that the ligament is not disrupted as it heals.

Extra-articular reconstruction procedures, which involve the transposition of dynamic musculotendinous stabilizers or inert restraints around the knee such as the semitendinosus muscle, capsular ligament, or iliotibial band are designed to provide external stability to the knee joint.[40,46] They were commonly used in the past but are used infrequently today because they do not restore normal arthrokinematics to the knee. Over time, transferred structures often stretch out, resulting in a recurrence of joint instability. Today extra-articular procedures are primarily used as an adjunct to an intra-articular reconstruction in difficult cases or in adolescents who have not reached bony maturity and still have open epiphyses.

The most successful surgical intervention for ligamentous injury is the intra-articular reconstruction, which has been used most often for anterior or posterior cruciate lesions. The procedure involves use of an autograft (the patient's own tissue), an allograft (donor tissue), or a synthetic graft such as Gore-Tex. The patellar tendon has been shown to have tensile strength equal to the ACL and is the most commonly chosen graft material for intra-articular reconstruction. Other substitutes that are not as strong as the patellar tendon are a portion of the iliotibial band or semitendinosus or gracilis tendons. An allograft or synthetic graft is used when an autogenous graft in a previous reconstruction has failed. Recent advances in graft placement and fixation and improvement and refinement of arthroscopic techniques have lessened the need for long periods of immobilization of the operated knee and protected weight bearing during ambulation as the graft heals.

The goals of surgery and postoperative rehabilitation are (1) restoration of joint stability and motion, (2) pain-free and stable weight bearing, (3) appropriate postoperative strength and endurance, and (4) the ability to return to preinjury functional activities.

A successful postoperative outcome starts with a preoperative program including edema control, exercise to minimize atrophy and maintain as much ROM as possible, protected ambulation, and patient education. Exercises are similar to those used for nonoperative management of ligament injuries already discussed in Section VI.D of this chapter. Preoperative exercises should not further irritate the injured tissues or cause additional swelling or pain.[22,40,46,59,87]

The *rate* and *progression* of postoperative rehabilitation programs vary; no one program has been shown to be most effective or most efficient. Emphasis is placed on preventing postoperative complications while always protecting the healing graft. Early controlled motion and weight bearing have been shown to decrease the incidence of postoperative complications, such as contracture, patellofemoral pain, and muscle atrophy, and to allow patients to return to activity more quickly without compromising the integrity of the reconstructed ligament.[88]

There is a move away from strict time-based protocols to programs that are progressed based on the attainment of specific criteria and measurable goals or performance on functional tests.[22,26,60] For example, an exercise program will be progressed to a higher level only after full active knee extension has been achieved or joint arthrometer testing indicates a particular level of joint stability. It is the responsibility of the therapist to be familiar with testing procedures and to have a thorough understanding of the operative procedure and the impact of exercise on healing structures. Open communication with the surgeon enables the therapist to discuss any precautions or concerns specific to individual patients and procedures.

F. Intra-articular Anterior Cruciate Ligament (ACL) Reconstruction

1. Indications for surgery[41,46,53]

   a. Severe acute tear or chronic insufficiency of the ACL leading to abnormal anterior transition of the tibia on the femur and instability or buckling of the knee. The pivot-shift test is also abnormal. An ACL deficit is often associated with a lesion of other structures of the knee, such as the medial collateral ligament (MCL), resulting in rotatory instability of the joint.

   b. Partial tear that results in limitation of functional activities in active individuals.

   c. Failed conservative (nonoperative) management of an ACL tear.

2. Procedures[1,8,46,53,79]

   a. *Background*

   A variety of surgical procedures for the ACL-deficient knee are available, specifically intra-articular or extra-articular reconstruction or direct repair of the torn ligament. The type of procedure chosen depends upon the severity and location of the tear as well as the age of the patient and the level of activity to which the patient would like to return.

   As mentioned previously, the most successful and most commonly used procedure today is an intra-articular reconstruction with a patellar tendon autogenous graft that replaces the torn ACL.

b. The intra-articular reconstruction either involves an arthrotomy or is performed as an arthroscopically assisted procedure.[113] If an arthrotomy is used, a medial or lateral parapatellar incision is made. This method allows visualization of the knee joint and injured tissues but involves a capsular incision and dislocation or subluxation of the patella that compromises the extensor mechanism and increases quadriceps pain postoperatively. The arthroscopically assisted ACL reconstruction requires three small incisions for portals as well as an incision at a donor site if an autograft is used. The endoscopic procedure is less disruptive to structures of the knee and allows more vigorous postoperative rehabilitation than an open procedure.

c. In an intra-articular ACL reconstruction with a patellar tendon graft, the torn ACL is removed and bone tunnels are drilled in the tibia and femur. The intracondylar notch may be widened (a notchplasty) if it is abnormally narrow. The central one-third of the patellar tendon with bone plugs on both ends is then harvested and placed in prepared drill holes in the tibia and femur. Graft fixation is achieved with sutures and reinforced with headless screws or staples. The bony donor sites are filled with cancellous bone from the drill holes into the tibia and femur.

d. The graft is placed in the same position as was the torn ACL. *Isometric placement* of the graft is sought that allows relatively equal stresses (tension) to be placed on the graft as the knee joint is moved through the ROM. This makes it possible to initiate ROM early after surgery.

e. The knee is drained (if an arthroscopic procedure is used) and the incision site is closed. A small compression dressing and motion-controlling orthosis is immediately placed on the knee.

3. **Postoperative management***

NOTE: Just one or two decades ago rehabilitation after ACL reconstruction involved long periods of complete immobilization in a position of knee flexion and an extended period (often 6 to 8 weeks) of restricted weight bearing. Return to full activity often took a full year.[8,21,60] In recent years, with advances in surgical techniques and a better understanding of tissue healing, early postoperative motion and early weight bearing are possible.[22,26,87,88,102,108]

a. *Immobilization*[22,26,60,87,88]

(1) Position of immobilization

(a) After an intra-articular ACL reconstruction the knee is placed in a controlled-motion brace that is locked in extension or slight flexion. Even though the greatest stress on the graft occurs between 20 degrees of flexion and full extension of the knee, isometric placement of the graft allows the patient to safely extend the knee without disrupting the autograft.

(b) If an intra-articular ACL procedure has been combined with an extra-articular procedure, a collateral ligament reconstruction, or a repair of the medial meniscus, the knee must be immobilized in approximately 20 to 30 degrees of knee flexion.

*Refs. 8, 15, 21, 22, 26, 53, 79, 87, 88, 101, 102, 108, 112.

(2) Duration of immobilization
   (a) Complete immobilization in a hinged but locked orthosis is usually not necessary after reconstruction with an autogenous patellar graft. Continuous passive motion (CPM) is often initiated within a safe ROM immediately after surgery.[24,26,62,75]
   (b) The knee is kept immobilized when the patient is ambulating or sleeping. The immobilizer is removed or unlocked for CPM use or supervised exercises. This may be necessary for 4 to 6 weeks after surgery.
   (c) CPM is not initiated for several weeks after extra-articular ACL reconstruction or MCL repair.[75]

b. *Exercise**

NOTE: The rate and progression of exercise after ACL reconstruction will depend upon the type of surgical procedure and type of graft. Exercise and weight bearing can progress most rapidly after an arthroscopic, autogenous patellar tendon graft reconstruction.[88,108] Procedures that use an open procedure or less strong autografts, such as a portion of the semitendinosus tendon or iliotibial band or prosthetic graft materials, require a more cautious progression of exercises and weight bearing. A delicate balance exists in the early postoperative period between adequate protection of healing tissues with immobilization or restricted motion and early controlled knee motion and weight bearing to prevent or minimize contractures, articular degeneration, and muscle atrophy. Even though early movement will create a stronger, better oriented scar in the healing ligament, too-vigorous exercises or too-rapid progression of weight bearing can stretch and damage the repaired structures. A period of protected movement is necessary so that proper vascularization and organization of collagen fibers can occur during healing and so that the tensile strength of the collagen fibers of the ligament can increase.[53,108]

MAXIMUM-PROTECTION PHASE (0 TO 6 WEEKS)

(1) To control postoperative pain and edema, use ice, compression, and massage.[26,40,87,112]
(2) To prevent muscle atrophy, initiate electrical stimulation, quadriceps- and hamstring-setting exercises, and straight-leg raises in supine, prone, and side-lying positions with the brace locked in full knee extension. Little to no anterior translation of the tibia on the femur occurs with a quadriceps muscle contraction when the knee is fully extended because this is the closed-pack position of the knee.
(3) To prevent contractures and maintain ROM, use:
   (a) CPM or therapist-assisted passive ROM from full knee extension to 90 degrees of flexion for the first week or two after surgery. CPM has also been found to decrease pain after ACL reconstruction.[63,79] To prevent anterior translation of the tibia and excessive stress to the graft site while using a CPM device, it has been suggested that the unit should be used without a calf band.[24]
   (b) Gravity-assisted supine wall slides (see Fig. 12–5) to increase knee flexion. The lower leg must be passively extended to the starting position by the therapist or with the uninvolved leg.

*Refs. 15, 22, 26, 40, 60, 87, 88, 102, 108.

(c) Patellar glides to prevent contracture of the extensor mechanism. Full, passive knee extension may not be achieved for a week or two until tissue swelling subsides.

(4) Ambulation with crutches with weight bearing as tolerated is initiated the day after surgery with the motion-controlled brace locked in extension. Full–weight bearing (FWB) in the knee immobilizer may be achieved and crutch use discontinued as early as 2 to 3 weeks after surgery if the patient has full active knee extension. In a more conservative rehabilitation program the patient may be required to delay any weight bearing on the operated leg for up to 1 week postoperatively. Then weight bearing is gradually progressed over 6 weeks.

(5) To improve neuromuscular control of the operated lower extremity in the later portion of the maximum-protection phase (from 2 to 6 weeks postoperatively), bilateral closed-chain exercises such as toe raises with the knee brace locked in extension, closed- and open-chain pool exercises, *assisted* open-chain knee extension, multiple-angle isometric quadriceps and hamstring exercises and, later, stationary bicycling can be added and progressed.

(6) ***Precaution:*** Despite the fact that by 4 weeks the bone plugs of a patellar tendon graft are well healed within the drill hole and vascularization of the graft is beginning, the graft itself is weakest and slightly necrotic at 4 to 6 weeks postoperatively. Therefore, to protect the healing graft, *avoid* activities such as open-chain unassisted terminal knee extension that can cause shear forces and forceful anterior tibial translation.

MODERATE-PROTECTION PHASE (6 TO 12 WEEKS)

(1) At the beginning of this phase, if full knee extension is possible, FWB is established and crutches may be discontinued, but the patient must continue to wear the knee orthosis and in most cases must keep it locked when ambulating or performing weight-bearing activities. NOTE: In carefully selected patients the knee orthosis is unlocked at 6 weeks postoperatively.[108]

(2) Before proceeding to more vigorous and demanding exercises, the integrity of the ACL graft, as reflected by stability of the knee joint, is measured with an arthrometer.

(3) The moderate-protection phase is characterized by exercises that are designed to increase strength of the lower extremity and re-establish full ROM of the knee. By 9 weeks, revascularization of the graft is becoming well established and, therefore, exercises can be more vigorous.

(4) Progressive stretching to increase ROM and closed- and open-chain eccentric and concentric resistance exercises to increase strength, stability, and endurance of the quadriceps, hamstrings, and hip musculature are emphasized in this phase of rehabilitation.

(a) The patient should acquire 120 degrees of knee flexion and full extension during this phase.

(b) Emphasis is placed on strengthening both the knee extensors and knee flexors. The quadriceps deteriorate quickly in the early postoperative period when joint effusion persists despite early muscle re-education. Hamstring strengthening is also emphasized to maximize dynamic stability of the posterior aspect of the knee. Resistance training is carried out in functional weight-bearing positions whenever possible. **_Precaution:_** Avoid closed-chain squatting exercises between 60 and 90 degrees of flexion and open-chain terminal knee extension with resistance placed at the distal tibia. Both cause anterior tibial translation and can disrupt the graft.[108,109]

(5) The hinged brace is removed several times a day for graded, straight-line ambulation.

MINIMAL-PROTECTION AND RETURN-TO-ACTIVITY PHASES

(1) From 12 to 20 weeks postoperatively emphasis is placed on incorporating light functional activities such as walking, jogging, and agility drills into the rehabilitation program if the patient has regained approximately 75 to 80 percent of knee muscle strength. The unlocked knee brace is worn during most functional activities, particularly the more vigorous activities that involve turning, twisting, or light jumping motions.

(2) Plyometrics and velocity spectrum isokinetic rehabilitation can also be added to the rehabilitation program.

(3) By 20 to 24 weeks most individuals return to a preinjury activity level. Functional bracing may still be required during high-demand recreational activities.

G. Posterior Cruciate Ligament (PCL) Reconstruction

1. Indications for surgery[13,28,40]

a. Complete tear or avulsion of the PCL with posterolateral and rotary instability of the knee.

b. Chronic PCL insufficiency associated with posterolateral instability, limitations in functional activities, and deterioration of articular surfaces of the knee.

c. NOTE: Many patients with complete PCL tears return to a preinjury level of activity without surgical intervention. There is far less consensus on indications for surgery after PCL injury than after ACL injury. Reconstructive surgery is a much more common method of treatment of ACL lesions than of PCL lesions.

2. Procedures[13,28,40]

a. The arthroscopically assisted intra-articular reconstruction of the PCL using the central one-third of the patellar tendon or a synthetic graft is the most common procedure. The procedure is similar to ACL reconstruction except that the graft is secured to the anterior aspect of the medial femoral condyle and then advanced through drill holes and attached to the posterior aspect of the tibial plateau to mimic the function of the PCL.

b. The extra-articular reconstruction with transposition of the gracilis or semitendinosus tendon to simulate the action of the PCL is less common.

c. Direct repair may also be undertaken but is not as successful as reconstruction because of the poor vascularity of the PCL.

3. Postoperative management[28,40]

a. _Immobilization_

The knee is usually immobilized in full extension in a locked brace or cast brace. In some instances the knee may be immobilized in 15 degrees of flexion. The immobilizer is worn at all times except for CPM or supervised and home exercise.

b. *Exercise*

NOTE: Many of the postoperative exercises in the maximum-, moderate- and minimum-protection phases after PCL reconstruction are similar to those in a postoperative ACL reconstruction rehabilitation program. Only the differences, not the similarities, are pointed out here.

MAXIMUM-PROTECTION PHASE (0 TO 6 WEEKS)

(1) After intra-articular reconstruction CPM is initiated immediately after surgery but only within a protected range of full knee extension or slight flexion to a maximum of 60 degrees of flexion. Knee flexion past 60 degrees places excessive stress on the graft and could contribute to failure of the reconstruction.

(2) Weight bearing is more restricted after PCL surgery than after ACL reconstruction. Partial weight bearing and ambulation with crutches are required for at least 4 to 6 weeks or longer after PCL surgery.

(3) To increase neuromuscular control of the knee, begin quadriceps-setting exercises in full extension and multiple-angle isometric exercise to the quadriceps between full extension and 60 degrees of knee flexion. Add active knee extension from 60 degrees of flexion to full extension.

> *Precaution:* Avoid strong muscle contractions of the hamstrings, as this will cause a posterior translation of the tibia on the femur and could disturb the healing graft.

MODERATE- AND MINIMUM-PROTECTION PHASES

(1) Exercises and functional training activities are progressed more slowly after PCL surgery than in postoperative ACL rehabilitation.

(2) Emphasis continues to be placed on quadriceps strengthening in functional positions.

(3) Open-chain resisted knee flexion causes a posterior translation of the tibia on the femur and, therefore, is delayed for 6 to 12 weeks postoperatively to protect the graft or transposed structures. Hamstring control and strengthening is achieved with closed-chain exercises and resisted hip extension rather than with resisted knee flexion.

(4) Closed-chain functional activities are added to the program later after PCL reconstruction than after ACL surgery because weight bearing is delayed or restricted longer after a PCL procedure.

(5) Overall it takes approximately 3 months longer to return to full occupational or recreational activities after PCL surgery than after ACL surgery.

VII. Meniscal Tears

A. Related Diagnoses and Mechanisms of Injury

Most frequently injured is the medial meniscus. Insult may occur when the foot is fixed on the ground and the femur is rotated internally, as when pivoting, getting out of a car, or receiving a clipping injury. An anterior cruciate ligament injury often accompanies a medial meniscus tear. Lateral rotation of the femur on a fixed tibia may tear the lateral meniscus. Simple squatting or trauma may also cause a tear.

B. Common Impairments/Problems

Meniscal tears can cause an acute locking of the knee as well as chronic symptoms with intermittent locking, pain along the joint line from stress to the coronary ligament, joint swelling, and some degree of quadriceps atrophy. When there is joint locking, the knee does not fully extend and there is a springy end-feel when passive extension is attempted. If the joint is swollen, there is usually slight limitation of flexion or extension. The McMurray or Apley grinding tests may be positive.[42]

C. Common Functional Limitations/Disabilities

1. When the meniscus tear is acute, the patient may be unable to bear weight on the involved side.
2. Unexpected locking or giving way during ambulation often occurs, causing safety problems.

D. Nonoperative Management

1. Often the patient can actively move the leg to "unlock" the knee, or the unlocking happens spontaneously.
2. Passive manipulative reduction of the medial meniscus (Fig. 12–4)
   Position of patient: supine. Passively flex the involved knee and hip as you simultaneously internally and externally rotate the tibia. When the knee is fully flexed, laterally rotate the tibia and apply a valgus stress at the knee. Hold the tibia in this position as you extend the knee. The meniscus may click into place.[42] Once reduced, the knee will respond as an acute joint lesion; treat as described in Section II in this chapter.
3. Exercises should be performed in open- and closed-chain positions to improve strength and endurance in isolated muscle groups and to prepare the patient for functional activities.

E. Surgical Repair of Meniscal Tears

When a significant tear or rupture of the medial or lateral meniscus occurs or if nonoperative management of a partial tear has been unsuccessful, surgical intervention is often necessary. Every effort is made to retain as much of the meniscus

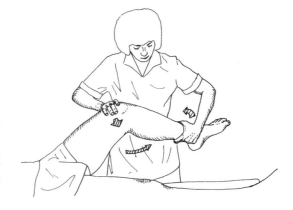

Figure 12–4. Manipulative reduction of a medial meniscus. Internally and externally rotate the tibia as you flex the hip and knee (not shown), then laterally rotate the tibia and apply a valgus stress at the knee as you extend it. The meniscus may click into place.

as possible to minimize long-term degeneration of the articular surfaces of the knee. To preserve the load transmission and shock absorbing functions of the menisci and reduce stresses on articular surfaces of the knee, surgical *repair of a meniscus* or *partial meniscectomy* is preferable to total meniscectomy.[20,98] A central tear that involves the avascular portion of the meniscus is usually treated with partial meniscectomy. A peripheral tear that involves the vascular portion of the meniscus can often be repaired surgically. If there is extensive damage to the peripheral and central portions of the meniscus, a total meniscectomy must be performed. In many instances arthroscopic repair or removal of the torn meniscus is possible, but in some instances an open procedure with arthrotomy is necessary.

Many patients with chronic meniscal lesions have a more successful outcome from surgery and can return to full activity sooner if they participate in a preoperative exercise program. The progression of postoperative rehabilitation and the time required to return to full activity will depend upon the extent and location of the tear and the type of surgical approach and procedure chosen. Rehabilitation will proceed more conservatively after repair of a meniscus or total meniscectomy than after partial meniscectomy. Damage and repair of other soft tissues of the knee will also affect the course and progression of rehabilitation after surgery.

F. Arthroscopic Repair of the Meniscus and Postoperative Management

1. Indications for surgery[7,20]

a. If a lesion occurs in the vascular portion (outer one-third) of the medial or lateral meniscus, surgical repair of the cartilage is possible.

b. Repairs are more successful with acute injuries of a meniscus than with chronic meniscal lesions.

2. Procedure[7,20,54,98]

a. Small incisions are made at the knee for portals, and saline is arthroscopically introduced into the knee joint to distend the knee.

b. The torn portion of the peripheral meniscus is sutured in place. Any loose bodies or debris are endoscopically removed.

c. The knee is irrigated and drained and skin incisions at portal sites are closed. A compression dressing is applied.

d. A meniscal repair may be accompanied by repair or reconstruction of other soft tissues of the knee such as the ligaments.

e. NOTE: An open procedure requiring an arthrotomy is also a surgical option.

3. Postoperative Management[7,15,40,47,86,101]

a. *Immobilization*

(1) Complete immobilization is not necessary postoperatively. CPM within a limited ROM is appropriate.

(2) To protect the sutured cartilage and restrict motion to a safe portion of the range, a controlled-motion orthosis is worn at all times in the early phases of rehabilitation. Depending on the site of the lesion and repair, motion is controlled to allow 0 to 90 or 20 to 90 degrees of flexion.

(3) Cryotherapy and elevation of the operated limb are used to control postoperative edema. An intermittent compression cryogenic pump such as CryoCuff effectively combines cold and compression to control edema.

b. *Exercise*

MAXIMUM-PROTECTION PHASE (0 TO 2 OR 3 WEEKS)

(1) To minimize atrophy and re-establish neuromuscular control of knee musculature, begin comfortable submaximal quadriceps- and hamstring-setting exercises as soon as possible after surgery. Complement isometric exercises with electrical muscle stimulation or biofeedback.

(2) To maintain strength in hip musculature on the operated side, begin SLR exercises in supine, prone, and side-lying positions, with most emphasis on the prone position to prevent weakness in the hip extensors as well as other hip musculature.

(3) To prevent contractures, begin active-assisted and active ROM within a comfortable and protected range and cautiously progress the exercises while the patient wears the controlled-motion brace. Exercises may include:

(a) Heel slides in supine

(b) Gravity-assisted knee flexion in sitting

(c) Therapist or self-assisted knee extension in sitting

(4) Weight bearing is limited to non–weight bearing to protect the healing meniscus. The extent of articular damage associated with the acute lesion may also dictate the degree to which weight bearing must be restricted. Instruct the patient in independent ambulation with crutches.

MODERATE-PROTECTION PHASE (3 OR 4 TO 6 OR 8 WEEKS)

(1) To progress ROM in flexion and extension, the range allowed by the controlled-motion orthosis is increased by approximately 10 degrees per week until full, pain-free active range is attained. The patients should achieve 120 degrees of knee flexion and full knee extension by 8 weeks postoperatively.

(2) Weight bearing

During the moderate-protection phase the patient is slowly weaned from crutches, and weight bearing is *gradually* increased for ambulation and functional closed-chain exercises to avoid compromising the repair site. The location and vascularity of the repair site and whether or not full extension of the knee (closed-packed position) is permissible in the brace will dictate how quickly weight bearing can be safely progressed. Full weight bearing is usually achieved by 6 weeks after a peripheral repair and 8 weeks after a central repair.

(3) To increase strength and dynamic control of knee musculature in functional positions, begin closed-chain exercises such as bilateral mini-squats (without and then against elastic resistance) (see Fig. 12–11) and unilateral terminal knee extension against elastic resistance (see Fig. 12–10).

(4) Gradually progress open-chain knee flexion and extension exercises to increase strength with PRE such as submaximal resisted knee extension in sitting and hamstring curls in prone or standing (see Fig. 12–9); add submaximal, medium- to high-speed isokinetic exercises in a safe, protected range.

NOTE: Avoid resistance exercises against maximum resistance for approximately 6 to 8 weeks until soft tissues are well healed.

(5) To increase muscular endurance and improve general lower extremity conditioning, begin stationary bicycling or swimming.

(6) To re-establish balance, initiate proprioceptive training using weight-bearing activities.

MINIMUM-PROTECTION AND RETURN-TO-ACTIVITY PHASES

NOTE: The minimum-protection phase of rehabilitation begins at approximately the 8th postoperative week. Return to full activity usually does not begin until the 20th to 24th week. Progression is dependent upon ROM, knee muscle strength and endurance, and absence of joint effusion and pain.

(1) Progress strengthening, stabilization, and balance activities in functional positions with marching, lunges, step-up and step-down exercises, and plyometric training or slide board and balance board exercises.

(2) Progress strengthening with isokinetic exercises for the lower extremity with velocity spectrum rehabilitation.

(3) Continue to improve general endurance and conditioning with aerobic activities such as bicycling, swimming, and walking.

(4) If mild restrictions in ROM persist, stretch tight structures with joint mobilization or soft tissue stretching techniques.

(5) When meniscal integrity tests are normal, restore functional abilities with simulated activities that mimic functional skills. Add light jogging activities, sprinting, or jumping, if appropriate.

G. Partial Arthroscopic Meniscectomy and Postoperative Management

1. Indications for surgery[7,20,46,54,113]

a. Tears or ruptures of the inner two-thirds (the avascular portion) of the medial or lateral menisci of the knee

b. Displacement of the meniscus associated with locking of the knee

2. Procedure[7,46,113]

a. Small incisions are made at the knee for portals (usually 3), and the knee is injected and distended with saline solution through one of the portals.

b. The torn portion of the meniscus is identified, grasped, and divided endoscopically by knife or by scissors and removed by vacuum. Intra-articular debris or loose bodies are also removed.

c. A soft compression dressing is applied after the knee is irrigated and drained, and skin incisions at portal sites are closed.

d. If the meniscus tear occurs in conjunction with tears or ruptures of other soft tissues of the knee, such as the cruciate or collateral ligaments, surgical management for repair of these structures must also be considered.

e. If a total meniscectomy is performed, as in the case of a complete tear, an open procedure with arthrotomy may be necessary.

3. Postoperative Management[7,40,54,86]

a. *Immobilization*

(1) A compression dressing is placed on the knee, but it is not necessary to immobilize the knee postoperatively with a splint or motion-controlled orthosis.

(2) For the first few postoperative days cryotherapy, massage, and elevation of the operated leg are used to minimize edema and pain.

b. *Exercise*

NOTE: Although the ideal situation is to begin exercise instruction on the day after surgery, most patients undergo a partial meniscectomy on an outpatient basis and do not see a therapist for at least a week postoperatively. Under these circumstances it is helpful to teach the patient initial exercises to reduce atrophy and prevent contracture *preoperatively* so that he or she may initiate the exercises at home immediately after surgery.

MODERATE-PROTECTION PHASE

(1) There is no need for a maximum-protection phase postoperatively as there is little soft tissue trauma during surgery. Moderate protection is needed for approximately 3 to 4 weeks. All exercises and weight-bearing activities should be pain free and progressed gradually during the first few postoperative weeks.

(a) The patient may immediately begin setting exercises, straight-leg raises, active knee ROM, and weight bearing as tolerated.

(b) Full weight bearing is usually achieved by 4 to 7 days and 90 degrees of knee flexion and full extension by 10 days.

(c) Closed-chain exercises and stationary bicycling may be initiated a few days after surgery to regain dynamic control and endurance of the knee.

(2) *Precautions:* Patients who have undergone partial arthroscopic meniscectomy must be cautioned not to push themselves too quickly. Too rapid progression of exercise will cause recurrent joint effusion and possible damage to articular cartilage of the knee.

MINIMUM-PROTECTION AND RETURN-TO-ACTIVITY PHASES

(1) By the third to fourth postoperative week minimal protection of the knee is necessary, but full active knee ROM should be achieved before progressing to high-demand exercises. Resistance training, endurance activities, functional closed-chain exercises in full weight bearing, and balance training can all be progressed rapidly.

(2) Advanced activities such as plyometrics, maximum-effort isokinetic training, and simulated high-demand functional activities can be initiated as soon as 4 to 6 or 6 to 8 weeks postoperatively.

(3) *Precaution:* High-impact weight-bearing activities such as jogging or jumping, if included in the program, should be added and progressed cautiously to prevent future or additional articular damage to the knee.

VIII. Exercises for Muscle Strength and Flexibility Imbalances

NOTE: Strength and flexibility imbalances between muscle groups can occur from a variety of causes, some of which are disuse, faulty joint mechanics, surgery, immobilization (from fracture, surgery, trauma), and nerve injury. Besides the hamstrings and rectus femoris, most of the two-joint muscles crossing the knee primarily function either at the hip or at the ankle, yet they have an effect on knee function. If there is an imbalance in length or strength in the hip or ankle muscles, there are usually altered mechanics throughout the lower extremity. See also the chapters on the hip and the ankle and foot for a complete picture. When attempting to increase ROM and strength, the mechanics of the tibiofemoral and patellofemoral joints and their importance in lower extremity function must be respected (see Section I of this chapter). When the patient has patellofemoral pain or when predisposing factors associated with immobilization could lead to articular cartilage degeneration, heavy resistance against the quadriceps in open-chain exercises or with the knee in greater than 30 degrees of flexion should be avoided to prevent destructive compressive forces to the patellar cartilage until healing has occurred. In addition, special adaptations to exercises must be made with specific surgical procedures. These have been highlighted in the surgical sections of this chapter. Because the knee is a weight-bearing joint, the need for stability takes precedence over the need for mobility, although mobility coupled with adequate strength is also necessary for normal function.

A. Techniques to Stretch Tight Muscles

1. To stretch tight hamstring muscles

Flexibility in the hamstring muscle group is necessary for knee extension as well as many functional activities in which the muscle group is elongated over the hip and knee simultaneously.

a. *Active inhibition techniques (hold-relax or contract-relax)*

(1) If the knee extends to 0 degrees but the hamstrings limit straight-leg raising (the knee begins to flex as the hip is flexed), active inhibition techniques for the hamstrings, emphasizing hip flexion while the knee is held in extension as described in Chapters 5 and 11 (The Hip), should be used.

(2) If the knee cannot extend even when the hip is extended because of extreme tightness in the hamstrings, active inhibition techniques are used, but emphasis is placed on increasing knee extension rather than straight-leg raising.

(a) Position of patient: supine, with the hip and knee extended as much as possible. Isometrically resist knee flexion with your hand proximal to the ankle; have the patient relax and then passively extend the knee.

(b) Position of patient: prone with the hip and knee extended as much as possible. Place the small pad or folded hand towel under the femur proximal to the patella to protect the patella from compressive forces. Stabilize the pelvis to prevent hip flexion and then apply the hold-relax technique to increase knee extension.

b. *Passive stretching techniques*

(1) Always use a low-intensity long-duration stretch to ensure that the patient will stay as relaxed as possible.

(2) Position of patient: prone, hips extended with the patient's foot off the edge of the treatment table. Place a rolled towel under the patient's femur just proximal to the patella and a cuff weight around the ankle. As the muscle relaxes, the weight will place a sustained passive stretch on the hamstrings, which will increase knee extension.

2. To stretch tight quadriceps femoris muscles

Before stretching the muscle group, be sure the patella is mobile (see Section II.B) so it can glide in the trochlear groove as the knee flexes.

a. *Active inhibition techniques*

Position of patient: sitting, with the knee at the edge of the treatment table and flexed as far as possible. Apply hold-relax, contract-relax, or agonist contraction techniques to increase knee flexion.

b. *Self-stretching: gravity-assisted supine wall slides* (Fig. 12–5)
Position of patient: supine with buttocks against the wall and lower extremities vertically resting against the wall (hips flexed, knees extended). Slowly flex the involved knee by sliding the foot down the wall, hold in a comfortable position, then slide the foot back up the wall.

c. *Self-stretching: rocking forward on a step* (Fig. 12–6)
Position of patient: standing with the foot of the involved knee on a step. The patient rocks forward over the stabilized foot, flexing the knee to the limit of its range. He or she can rock back and forth in a slow, rhythmic manner or hold the stretched position. Begin with a low step or stool; progress the height as more range is obtained.

d. *Self-stretching while sitting* (Fig. 12–7)
Position of patient: Sitting in a chair with the involved knee flexed to the end of its available range and the foot firmly planted on the floor. Have the patient move forward in the chair, not allowing the foot to slide. Have the patient hold the stretch position for a comfortable, sustained stretch to the knee extensors.

e. *Rectus femoris stretch*
(1) To stretch the rectus femoris, the patient lies supine with the opposite hip flexed to stabilize the spine and pelvis (Thomas test position). With the

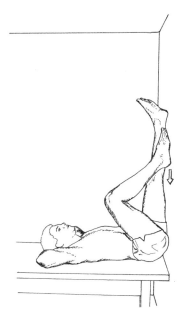

Figure 12–5. Gravity-assisted supine wall slide. The patient flexes the knee to the limit of its range and holds it there for a sustained stretch to the quadriceps femoris muscle.

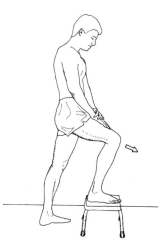

Figure 12–6. Self-stretching rock on step. The patient places the foot of the involved side on a step, then rocks forward over the stabilized foot to the limit of knee flexion to stretch the quadriceps femoris muscle. Use a higher step for greater flexion.

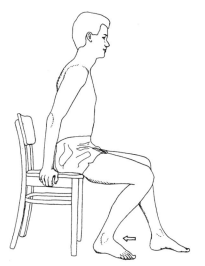

Figure 12–7. Self-stretching in a chair. The patient fixates the foot of the involved leg on the floor, then moves forward in the chair over the stabilized foot to place a sustained stretch on the quadriceps femoris muscle and increase knee flexion.

hip in extension the knee is progressively flexed using inhibition techniques.

(2) Self stretching: prone-lying

Position of patient: prone with hips extended and involved knee flexed as far as possible. The patient grasps the foot or a belt secured around the distal tibia and pulls the heel toward the buttocks.

(3) Self-stretching; standing

Position of patient: standing on the uninvolved lower extremity and holding onto a table with one hand for balance. The patient extends the hip and flexes the knee of the leg to be stretched as far as possible. He or she then grasps the distal tibia and brings the foot toward the buttocks to further flex the knee.

> **Precaution:** Have the patient keep the low back flat so the stretch does not increase the lumbar lordosis. This can be accomplished by having the patient first perform a posterior pelvic tilt, then hold the tilt by contracting the abdominals while stretching the rectus femoris.

(4) Self stretch: hurdler's position (see Fig. 11–2).

B. Techniques to Isolate, Train, and Strengthen Weak Muscles

When strengthening exercises for knee musculature are selected, implemented, and progressed in a rehabilitation program, stability of the knee, which involves co-contraction of the quadriceps and hamstrings muscles and safe patellofemoral and extensor mechanism biomechanics, which allow appropriate patellar tracking, are primary concerns. Once stability and patellar mechanics are well established, coordination and timing of muscle contractions as well as endurance are emphasized. *Closed-chain exercises* with an emphasis on low-intensity (low-resistance) high-repetition activities are more effective than open-chain exercises for improving stability and muscular endurance of the knee for dynamic control during weight-bearing activities. Closed-chain exercises are also less likely to cause joint and soft tissue irritation than open-chain exercises against heavy resistance. Closed-chain exercises are described and illustrated in Section VIII.C.

Although closed-chain control of the knee is essential, remember that the knee functions in both an open and a closed kinematic chain during most activities of daily living. The quadriceps and hamstrings must contract simultaneously (co-contraction), as well as contract concentrically and eccentrically during functional activities. Therefore, exercises in all of these varying conditions should be incorporated into a comprehensive knee rehabilitation program. It is also important to change the position of the hip during quadriceps- and hamstring-strengthening exercises to affect the length-tension relationship of the rectus femoris and hamstrings.[29] Only after a thorough evaluation and understanding of the patient's impairments and functional limitations can a therapist select and design an exercise plan to meet an individual patient's needs.

In the exercises that follow, open-chain exercises are described before closed-chain exercises simply because weight bearing after knee injury or surgery is often restricted for a time. Isolated activation of knee musculature is also necessary for ADL that involve open-chain movement such as lifting the leg to get in and out of bed or in and out of a car or flexing and extending the knee for dressing. Closed-chain exercises in partial and later full weight bearing should be initiated as soon as healing allows to progress to related functional weight-bearing activities.

1. **To isolate, train, and strengthen the extensor muscles (quadriceps femoris and rectus femoris)**

   A wide variety of static and dynamic exercises can be used to improve the function of the quadriceps femoris muscles in an open kinematic chain. Because of variations in muscle fiber orientation and attachments of the knee extensor muscles, individual components of the quadriceps femoris muscle group place different biomechanical stresses on the patella. Emphasis is often placed on isolation and activation of the vastus medialis obliquus (VMO) and vastus medialis (VM) muscles because of their ability to stabilize the patella and to maintain appropriate patellar tracking. Tactile cues, biofeedback, and electrical muscle stimulation over the VMO can reinforce selective strengthening of this portion of the quadriceps for patellar control. In this section the effectiveness of various quadriceps exercises with regard to training and strengthening the VMO will be discussed.

   a. *Quadriceps setting (quad sets)*

      NOTE: Of the many variations of static and dynamic exercises that have been proposed to selectively train the VMO, quadriceps setting coupled with biofeedback has been shown to be most effective.[93]

      (1) Position of the patient: supine, or sitting in a chair (with the heel on the floor) and long-sitting with the knee extended (or flexed a few degrees) but not hyperextended.

      (2) Have the patient contract the quadriceps isometrically, causing the patella to glide proximally; then hold for a count of 10.

         (a) Use verbal cues such as "Try to push your knee back and tighten your thigh muscle" or "Try to tighten your thigh muscle and pull your kneecap up." When the patient sets the muscle properly, offer verbal reinforcement immediately and then have the patient repeat the activity.

         (b) Have the patient dorsiflex the ankle and then hold an isometric contraction of the quadriceps against resistance.[2]

   b. *Straight-leg raising (SLR)*

      Position of the patient: supine with the knee extended. This exercise combines dynamic hip flexion and static knee extension. To stabilize the pelvis and low back, the opposite hip and knee are flexed and the foot is placed flat on the exercise table.

      NOTE: Straight-leg raising in supine generates an isometric contraction of the quadriceps with the added resistance of gravity. The effective resistance decreases as the lower extremity elevates because of the decreasing moment arm of gravity. The rectus femoris is the primary muscle in the quadriceps group that is active during SLR exercise.[93]

      (1) Instruct the patient to first set the quadriceps muscle; then lift the leg to about 45 degrees of hip flexion while keeping the knee extended; hold the leg in that position for a count of 10; then lower it.

      (2) As the patient progresses, have the patient lift to only 30 degrees of hip flexion and hold the position. Later, have the patient flex the hip to only 15 degrees. The most significant resistance to the quadriceps is during the first few degrees of SLR.

      (3) To increase resistance to the rectus femoris, place a cuff weight around the patient's ankle.

      (4) It has been proposed that if SLR in the supine position is coupled with lateral rotation or isometric adduction of the hip, the VMO or VM muscles

can be preferentially activated and strengthened.[2,5,10,23,63] The rationale for advocating these exercises is that many fibers of the VMO muscle originate from the adductor magnus tendon.[2,50] Although a number of authors[2,5] have advocated these adaptations to SLR to increase the medially directed forces on the patella, there is lack of scientific evidence to back up these suggestions. In two quantitative studies comparing quadriceps muscle activity during quad sets and variations of SLR, quad sets were found to be associated with significantly greater VMO or VM activity than several variations of SLR.[50,93] Therefore, as noted earlier, a combination of quad sets and biofeedback appears to be the best way to selectively activate the VMO.

c. *Straight-leg lowering*

Position of the patient: supine. If the patient cannot perform SLR because of a quadriceps lag or weakness, begin by passively placing the leg in 90 degrees of SLR (or as far as the flexibility of the hamstrings allows) and have the patient gradually lower the extremity while keeping the knee fully extended. Be prepared to control the descent of the leg with your hand under the heel as the torque created by gravity increases. If the knee begins to flex as the extremity is lowered, have the patient stop at that point, then raise the extremity upward to 90 degrees. Repeat the motion, attempting to lower the extremity a little further each time while keeping the knee extended. Once the patient can keep the knee extended while lowering the leg through the full ROM, SLR can be initiated.

d. *Multiple-angle isometric exercises*

(1) Position of the patient: supine or long-sitting. Bent leg raises with the knee in multiple angles of flexion strengthen the knee extensors isometrically.

(2) Position of the patient: seated at the edge of a treatment table. When tolerated, resistance is applied at the ankle either manually or mechanically, to isometrically strengthen the quadriceps in varying degrees of knee flexion. An effective co-contraction with the hamstrings can be activated (except in the last 10 to 15 degrees of knee extension) by having the patient push the thigh downward into the table while attempting knee extension against maximum resistance.[37]

e. *Short-arc terminal extension* (Fig. 12–8)

NOTE: Although in the past it was thought that the VMO was responsible for the terminal phase of knee extension, it is now well documented that all components of the quadriceps femoris muscle group are active throughout active knee extension.[93]

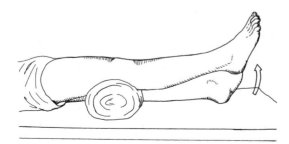

Figure 12–8. Short-arc terminal extension exercise to strengthen the quadriceps femoris muscle. When tolerated, resistance is added proximal to the ankle.

Position of patient: supine or long-sitting. Place a rolled towel or bolster under the knee to support it in flexion. The patient can also assume a short-sitting position at the edge of a table with the seat of a chair or a stool placed under the heel to stop knee flexion at the desired angle.

(1) Begin with the knee in a few degrees of flexion. Progress the degrees of flexion as tolerated by the patient or dictated by the condition.

(2) Initially the patient extends the knee only against the resistance of gravity. Later cuff weights around the ankle can be added to increase the resistance if the patient does not experience pain or crepitation.

> **Precaution:** When adding resistance to the distal leg, the amount of torque generated by the quadriceps muscle increases significantly in the terminal ranges of knee extension. In this portion of the range the quadriceps has a poor mechanical advantage and poor physiologic length while having to contract against an external resistance force that has a long lever arm. The amount of muscle force generated causes an anterior gliding force on the tibia, which is restrained by the ACL. This exercise is not appropriate for a person with an unstable knee after an ACL injury or during postoperative rehabilitation before the ligament has healed.

(3) Short-arc terminal extension can be combined with an isometric hold and/or SLR when the knee is in full extension.

(4) To prevent lateral shear forces at the knee, the patient can invert the foot as he or she extends the knee.[2,36]

f. *Full-arc extension*

Position of patient: sitting or supine.

(1) Resistance can be applied through the arc of 90 degrees of flexion to full extension. Resistance from 90 to 60 degrees causes less anterior tibial translation than closed-chain squatting in this range. But resistance applied in open-chain extension from 30 to 0 degrees increases anterior translation more than does performing mini-squats in the same range.[108] Resistance should be applied only in the ranges tolerated by the patient during the subacute and moderate-protection phases of treatment resistance through the full arc of motion and should be done only in the later stages of rehabilitation (chronic stage of healing) if the knee is pain free and asymptomatic. If there is pain, resistance should be applied only through those parts of the range with no symptoms.

(2) Various forms of mechanical resistance equipment discussed in Chapter 3 can be used to strengthen the knee extensors in an open kinematic chain.

(a) Emphasize high-repetition low-resistance training with isotonic equipment and medium- to high-speed training with isokinetic equipment to minimize compressive and shear forces to knee joint structures during exercise. The tibial pad against which the patient pushes when extending the knee against resistance can also be placed more proximally than distally on the lower leg to minimize excessive stresses to supporting structures of the knee.

(b) If a cuff weight is applied to the tibia to provide resistance, it will also cause a distraction to the joint and stress on the ligaments when the patient sits or lies supine with the knee flexed to 90 degrees and the tibia over the edge of the treatment table. To avoid this stress to ligaments, place a stool under the foot so it can be supported when the leg is in the dependent position.[11]

2. **To isolate, train, and strengthen the knee flexor muscles (primarily the hamstrings)**

   a. *Hamstring-setting exercises (hamstring sets)*
   Position of patient: supine or long-sitting with the knee in extension or slight flexion over a towel roll. Have the patient isometrically contract the knee flexors just enough to feel tension developing in the muscle group by gently pushing the heel into the treatment table and holding the contraction. Have the patient relax and then repeat the setting exercise.

   b. *Multiple-angle isometric exercises*
   Position of patient: supine or long-sitting.
   (1) Either manual or mechanical resistance is applied to a static hamstring muscle contraction with the knee flexed to several positions in the ROM.
   (2) Placing the tibia in internal or external rotation prior to resisting knee flexion will emphasize the medial or lateral hamstring muscles, respectively.
   (3) The patient can be taught to give self-resistance at multiple points in the ROM by placing the opposite foot behind the ankle of the leg to be resisted.

   c. *Hamstring curls (open-chain knee flexion)*
   (1) Position of patient: standing, holding onto a solid object for balance. The patient picks up the foot and flexes the knee (Fig. 12–9). Maximum resistance from gravity occurs when the knee is at 90 degrees flexion. Add resistance with ankle weights or a weighted boot. If the patient flexes the hip, stabilize it by having the patient place the anterior thigh against a wall or solid object.
   (2) Position of patient: prone. Place a small towel roll or foam rubber under the femur just proximal to the patella to avoid compression of the patella between the treatment table and femur. With a cuff weight around the

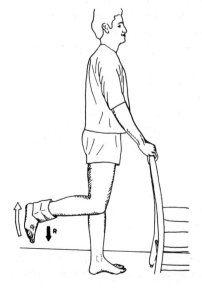

Figure 12–9. Hamstring curls: resistance exercises to the knee flexors with the patient standing. Maximum resistance occurs when the knee is at 90 degrees.

ankle, the patient flexes the knee to only 90 degrees; maximum resistance from gravity occurs when the knee first starts to flex at 0 degrees. To strengthen hamstrings eccentrically, the patient then lowers the weight and fully extends the knee. If hamstring curls are performed in prone using manual resistance, a weight-pulley system or isokinetic equipment resistance to the knee flexors can be applied throughout the range of knee flexion.

(3) *Precaution*: Open-chain hamstring curls performed against resistance placed on the distal tibia causes posterior tibial translation. A patient with a PCL injury or reconstruction should avoid this exercise in the early stages of rehabilitation.

C. Techniques to Develop Strength, Stability, and Control in Weight Bearing

Closed-chain progressive exercises are beneficial for activating and training the musculature of the lower extremity to respond in specific functional patterns. As the quadriceps contract eccentrically to control knee flexion or contract concentrically to extend the knee, the hamstrings and soleus function to stabilize the tibia against the forward translating force of the quadriceps at the knee joint as well as assist in controlling the knee flexion moment from gravity. This synergy provides support to the cruciate ligaments.[77] In addition, because the hip extends and the ankle plantarflexes as the knee extends (and vice versa) during closed-chain activities, the two-joint hamstrings and gastrocnemius and the one-joint soleus are maintaining favorable length-tension relationships through action at the hip and ankle, respectively.

In a rehabilitation program, closed-chain exercises can be incorporated in an exercise regimen as soon as partial or full weight bearing is safe. Closed-chain strengthening exercises generate fewer shear forces on knee ligaments, particularly anterior tibial translation, than open-chain quadriceps-strengthening activities.[26] Therefore, resistance can be added to closed-chain activities more quickly after injury or surgery than to open-chain exercises while still protecting healing structures such as the ACL. Clinically, closed-chain exercises enable a patient to develop strength, endurance, and stability of the lower extremity in functional patterns sooner after knee injury or surgery than do open-chain exercises. The progression of closed-chain exercises described in Chapter 11 (The Hip) are also appropriately used in knee rehabilitation programs.

If the patient does not tolerate full weight bearing, begin exercises in the parallel bars or in a pool to partially unload the body weight. During the healing phase following surgical procedures or with anterior knee pain problems, the knee should be splinted, taped, or braced while exercising. Exercises are begun at the level tolerated by the patient at which there is complete control and no exacerbation of symptoms.

1. Closed-chain isometric exercises

a. *Setting exercises* (to facilitate co-contraction of the quads and hamstrings)
Position of patient: sitting on a chair with the knee extended or slightly flexed and the heel on the floor.

(1) Have the patient press the heel against the floor and the thigh against the seat of the chair and concentrate on contracting the quadriceps and ham-

strings simultaneously to facilitate co-contraction around the knee joint. Hold the muscle contraction, relax, and repeat.

(2) Co-contraction can be learned more easily or enhanced with biofeedback.

b. *Rhythmic stabilization*

(1) Position of the patient: standing with bilateral weight bearing. Apply manual resistance to the pelvis in several directions as the patient holds the position. This will facilitate isometric contraction of muscles in the ankles, knees, hips, and trunk.

(2) Progress rhythmic stabilization activity by having the patient bear weight only on the involved lower extremity while resistance is applied.

c. *Closed-chain isometrics against elastic resistance*

Position of patient: standing on the involved extremity with elastic resistance looped around the thigh of the opposite extremity and secured to a stable object. See Figs. 11–13A and B.

(1) The patient flexes and extends the hip of the non–weight-bearing lower extremity to facilitate co-contraction of muscles and stability of the weight-bearing leg.

(2) This closed-chain exercise also facilitates proprioceptive input and balance on the weight-bearing (involved) lower extremity.

2. Closed-chain dynamic exercises

a. *Unilateral closed-chain terminal knee extension*

Position of patient: standing with elastic resistance looped around the distal thigh and secured to a stationary structure (Fig. 12–10). The patient actively performs terminal knee extension while bearing partial to full weight on the involved extremity.

b. *Mini-squats; short-arc training*

(1) Begin by having the patient stand and bend both knees up to 30 to 45 degrees, then extend them. Progress by using elastic resistance placed under both feet (Fig. 12–11) or by holding weights in the hands. The patient should maintain the trunk upright and concentrate on the sensation of the quadriceps muscle contracting, not pulling back of the femur with the hip extensors.

(2) Progress squats to greater ranges of knee flexion in the rehabilitative phase of treatment if necessary for the patient's function.

NOTE: Squatting can be accomplished in one of two ways, each with positive and negative effects. Having the knees move anterior to the toes as the hips descend increases the shear forces on the tibia and strains the ACL. This can be dangerous if the patient squats while carrying considerable weight or following ACL surgery. Yet this is a more normal method for squatting and maintaining balance over the base of support. Squatting, as if sitting on a chair, in which the tibia remains relatively vertical requires greater trunk flexion to maintain balance and stronger quadriceps contraction to support the load of the pelvis posterior to the knee axis at an angle where patellar compressive loads are great. Yet this method reduces stress on the ACL. The choice of method should be based on the patient's symptoms and pathologic condition.

(3) Increase the difficulty of the exercise by performing unilateral resisted mini-squats.

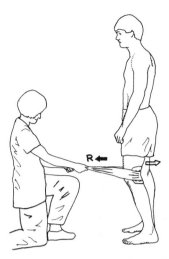

Figure 12–10. Unilateral closed-chain extension.

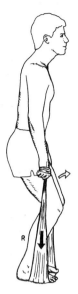

Figure 12–11. Resisted mini-squats; closed-chain short-arc training. Elastic resistance to knee extension is provided for short-arc motion. It is important to use the quadriceps femoris muscles rather than substitute with the hamstring muscles for proper strengthening.

    (4) NOTE: It has been suggested but not documented in research that, if partial squats are performed with the legs slightly externally rotated, the VMO muscle is in an optimum line of pull and may be more readily activated.[5]

  c. *Forward, backward, and lateral step-ups and step-downs*

    (1) Begin with a low step, 2 to 3 inches in height, and increase the height as the patient is able. Make sure the patient keeps the trunk upright.

    (2) Emphasize control of body weight during concentric (step-up) and eccentric (step-down) quadriceps activity. To emphasize the quadriceps and minimize pushing off with the plantarflexors of the trailing extremity, instruct the patient that the heel is to be the last to leave the floor and first to return or to "keep the toes up."

    (3) Resistance is added with a weight belt, with hand-held weights or ankle weights around the non–weight-bearing leg if there is good ligamentous integrity.

  d. *Standing wall slides*

    (1) Position of patient: standing with back against the wall (see Fig. 11–15A). The patient flexes the hips and knees and slides the back down and then up the wall, lifting and lowering the body weight.

    (2) As control improves, the patient moves into greater knee flexion, up to a maximum of 60 degrees. Knee flexion beyond 60 degrees is not advocated in order to avoid excessive shear forces on ligamentous structures of the knee and compressive forces on the patellofemoral joint.

(3) Isometric training can be added by having the patient stay in the lowered (partial squat) position. If the patient is able, he or she maintains the partial squat and alternately extends one leg and then the other.

(4) Wall slides performed with a gym ball behind the back decrease stability and require more control (see Fig. 11–15B).

e. *Partial and full lunges*

(1) Position of patient: a step-forward stance position with weight acceptance on the forward foot. Have the patient rock body weight forward, allowing the knee to flex slightly, and then rock backward and control knee extension.

(2) Progress the activity with full lunges (see Fig. 11–14). The patient begins with the feet together, then lunges forward with the involved extremity, beginning with a small stride and small amount of knee flexion, and returns upright by extending the knee and then bringing the foot back beside the other foot. Instruct the patient to keep the flexing knee in alignment with the toes and not to flex beyond a vertical line coming up from the toes. As the patient gains control, the stride length is increased and knee flexion is increased accordingly. Weights can be added to the trunk or in the patient's hands for progressive strengthening. The speed of the activity is also increased as control improves.

D. Techniques to Stimulate Functional Activities, Develop Endurance, and Progress to Specificity of Training

Activities previously described are progressed for endurance by increasing the number of repetitions or time element at each resistance level. Once control has developed, emphasis is placed on coordination, timing, and skill acquisition specific to the desired activity of the patient.

1. Strength and endurance training

Mechanical equipment such as a leg press, treadmill, stationary bicycle, and stair-stepping units is useful for strengthening and endurance training and provides motivational feedback to the patient.

2. Low-impact conditioning activities

Activities such as swimming and progressive walking are designed for general conditioning and are graded to the patient's tolerance.

3. Balance activities

Training on a balance board or slide board is used to stimulate proprioception, balance, coordination, and agility.

4. Plyometric training (Fig. 12–12)

High-speed, stretch-shortening exercises, which are designed to improve power, are appropriate for selected patients intending to return to high-demand functional or recreational activities. Jumping on and off varying height surfaces and incorporating directional changes in the movements are also appropriate in the later stages of knee rehabilitation.

5. Drills

Running, sprinting, jumping rope or on a small trampoline, agility drills, and sport-specific simulation drills are initiated and carefully monitored for appropriate progression and correct mechanics.

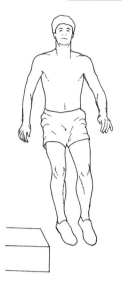

Figure 12–12. Plyometric training using lateral jumps from a step. When the patient lands on the ground, the hips and knees flex, then quickly extend to jump up on the step. This applies a quick lengthening prior to shortening of the quadriceps muscle.

6. Work-Hardening activities

For a patient returning to a repetitive lifting job, strength in the hip extensors as well as knee extensors is necessary for good body mechanics. Progression in lifting tasks with squats should also include good body mechanics. This is described in greater detail in Chapter 15.

IX. Summary

The anatomy and kinesiology of knee structure and function have been briefly reviewed, including the tibiofemoral and patellofemoral relationships, muscle function, and muscle control of the knee during gait.

Guidelines for therapeutic exercise management of common musculoskeletal problems such as joint, muscle, meniscus, and ligamentous lesions, as well as common surgical procedures for the knee and techniques for preoperative and postoperative management, have been outlined. Similarities and differences in the management of various surgical procedures and precautions during exercise have been delineated.

Descriptions of stretching techniques and static and dynamic closed- and open-chain muscle conditioning and strengthening procedures for the knee region have been described and illustrated in this chapter.

References

1. Amiel, D, Kleiner, JB, and Akeson, WH: The natural history of the anterior cruciate ligament autograft of patellar tendon origin. Am J Sports Med 14: 449–462, 1986.
2. Antich, TJ, and Brewster, CE: Modification of quadriceps femoris muscle exercises during knee rehabilitation. Phys Ther 66:1246, 1986.
3. Arthritis & Rheumatism Council, British Orthopaedic Association: Controlled trial of synovectomy of the knee and MCP joints in rheumatoid arthritis. Ann Rheum Dis 35:437, 1976.
4. Basso, DM, and Knapp, L: Comparison of two continuous passive motion protocols for patients with total knee implants. Phys Ther 67:360, 1987.
5. Bennett, JG: Rehabilitation of patellofemoral joint dysfunction. In Greenfield, BH (ed): Rehabilitation of the Knee: A Problem-Solving Approach. FA Davis, Philadelphia, 1993.
6. Blackburn, TA, Eiland, WG, and Bandy, WG: An introduction to the plica. Journal of Orthopaedic and Sports Physical Therapy 3:171, 1982.
7. Boyce, DA, and Hanley, ST: Functional based reha-

bilitation of the knee after partial meniscectomy or meniscal repair. Orthopedic Physical Therapy Clinics of North America 3:555–574, 1994.

8. Brewster, CE, Moynes, DR, and Jobe, FW: Rehabilitation for anterior cruciate reconstruction. Journal of Orthopaedic and Sports Physical Therapy 5:121, 1983.

9. Brown, DE, Alexander, AH, and Lichtman, DM: The Elmslie-Trillat procedure: Evaluation in patellar dislocation and subluxation. Am J Sports Med 12:104–109, 1984.

10. Brownstein, BA, Lamb, RL, and Mangine, RE: Quadriceps, torque, and integrated electromyography. Journal of Orthopaedic and Sports Physical Therapy 6:309, 1985.

11. Cailliet, R: Knee Pain and Disability, ed 3. FA Davis, Philadelphia, 1992.

12. Campbell, D, and Glenn, W: Rehabilitation of knee flexor and knee extensor muscle strength in patients with meniscectomies, ligamentous repairs and chondromalacia. Phys Ther 62:10, 1982.

13. Clancy, WG, Shelbourne, KD, and Zoellner, GB: Treatment of knee joint stability secondary to rupture of the posterior cruciate ligament. Report of a new procedure. J Bone Joint Surg Am 65:310, 1983.

14. Convery, RF: Total knee arthroplasty; Indications, evaluation and post-operative management. Clin Orthop 94:42, 1973.

15. Costill, DL, Fink, WJ, and Habansky, AJ: Muscle rehabilitation after knee surgery. The Physician and Sportsmedicine 5:71, 1977.

16. Coutts, RD, et al: The effect of muscle stimulation in the rehabilitation of patients following total knee replacement. In Rand, JA, and Dorr, LD (eds): Total Arthroplasty of the Knee: Proceedings of the Knee Society, 1985–1986. Aspen Publishers, Rockville, MD, 1987.

17. Coventry, MB, et al: A new geometric knee for total knee arthroplasty. Clin Orthop 83:157, 1972.

18. Cyriax, J: Textbook of Orthopaedic Medicine, Vol 1. Diagnosis of Soft Tissue Lesions, ed 8. Bailliere Tindall, London, 1982.

19. Davies, G, Malone, T, and Bassett, F: Knee examination. Phys Ther 60:1565, 1980.

20. DeHaven, KE: Rationale for meniscus repair or excision. Clin Sports Med 4:267–273, 1985.

21. DePalma, BF, and Zelko, RR: Rehabilitation following anterior cruciate ligament surgery. Athletic Train 21:200, 1986.

22. Dietrichson, J, and Souryal, TO: Preoperative and postoperative rehabilitation of anterior cruciate ligament tears. Orthopedic Physical Therapy Clinics of North America 3:539–554, 1994.

23. Doucette, SA, and Goble, EM: The effect of exercise on patellar tracking in lateral patellar compression syndrome. American Journal of Sports Medicine 20:434, 1992.

24. Drez, D, et al: In vivo measurement of anterior tibial translation using continuous passive motion devices. American Journal of Sports Medicine 19:381, 1991.

25. Ecker, ML, and Lotke, PA: Postoperative care of the total knee patient. Orthopedic Physical Therapy Clinics of North America 20:55, 1989.

26. Einhorn, AR, Sawyer, M, and Tovin B: Rehabilitation of intra-articular reconstructions. In Greenfield, BH (ed): Rehabilitation of the Knee: A Problem-Solving Approach. FA Davis, Philadelphia, 1993.

27. Eng, JJ, and Peirrynowsk, MR: Evaluation of soft foot orthotics in the treatment of patellofemoral pain syndrome. Phys Ther 73:840, 1993.

28. Engle, RP, Meade, TD, and Canner, GC: Rehabilitation of posterior cruciate ligament injuries. In Greenfield, BH (ed): Rehabilitation of the Knee; A Problem-Solving Approach, FA Davis, Philadelphia, 1993.

29. Fisher, NM, et al: Quantitative effects of physical therapy on muscular and functional performance in subjects with osteoarthritis of the knees. Arch Phys Med Rehabil 74:840, 1993.

30. Fortune, WP: Lower limb joint replacement. In Nickel, VL (ed): Orthopedic Rehabilitation. Churchill-Livingstone, New York, 1982.

31. Freeman, MAR: Arthritis of the Knee: Clinical Features and Surgical Managment. Springer-Verlag, New York, 1980.

32. Goll, SR, Lotke, PA, and Ecker, ML: Failure of CPM as prophylaxis against deep venous thrombosis after total knee arthroplasty. In Rand, JA, and Dorr, LD (eds): Total Arthroplasty of the Knee. Aspen Publishers, Rockville, MD, 1987.

33. Goodfellow, J, Hungerford, D, and Woods, C: Patellofemoral joint mechanics and pathology of chondromalacia patellae. J Bone Joint Surg Br 58:291, 1976.

34. Gose, JC: CPM in the postoperative treatment of patients with total knee replacements. Phys Ther 67:39, 1987.

35. Greene, B: Rehabilitation after total knee replacement. In Greenfield, BH (ed): Rehabilitation of the Knee: A Problem-Solving Approach. FA Davis, Philadelphia, 1993.

36. Grood, ES, et al: Biomechanics of the knee: Extension exercise. J Bone Joint Surg Am 66:725, 1984.

37. Gryzlo, SM, et al: Electromyographic analysis of knee rehabilitation exercises. Journal of Orthopaedic and Sports Physical Therapy 20:36, 1994.

38. Gunston, FH: Complications of polycentric knee arthroplasty. Clin Orthop 120:11, 1976.

39. Gunston, FH: Polycentric knee arthroplasty: Prosthetic stimulation of normal knee movement. J Bone Joint Surg Br 53:272, 1971.

40. Harrelson, GL: Knee rehabilitation. In Andrews, JR, and Harrelson, GL (eds): Physical Rehabilitation of the Injured Athlete. WB Saunders, Philadelphia, 1991.

41. Helfet, AJ: Disorders of the Knee. JB Lippincott, Philadelphia, 1982.

42. Hoppenfeld, S: Physical Examination of the Spine and Extremities. Appleton-Century-Crofts, New York, 1976.

43. Hungerford, DS, Krackhow, KA, and Kenna, RV: Two to five years experience with cementless, porous-coated total knee prosthesis. In Rand, JA, and Dorr, LD (eds): Total Arthroplasty of the Knee. Aspen Publishers, Rockville, MD, 1987.

44. Hungerford, DS, Kenna, RV, and Krackhow, KA: The porous-coated anatomic total knee. Orthopedic Physical Therapy Clinics of North America 13:103, 1982.

45. Hyde, SA: Physiotherapy in Rheumatology. Blackwell Scientific, Oxford, 1980.

46. Insall, JN: Surgery of the Knee. Churchill-Livingstone, New York, 1984.

47. Jaramillo, J, Worrell, TW, and Ingersoll, CD: Hip isometric strength following knee surgery. Journal of Orthopaedic and Sports Physical Therapy 20:160–165, 1993.

48. Johnson, DP: The effect of continuous passive motion on wound healing and joint mobility after knee arthroplasty. J Bone Joint Surg Am 72:421, 1990.

49. Kapandji, IA: The Physiology of the Joints, Vol II. Churchill-Livingstone, Edinborgh, 1970.

50. Karst, GM, and Jewett, PD: Electromyographic analysis of exercises proposed for differential activation of medial and lateral quadriceps femoris muscle components. Phys Ther 73:286–295, 1993.

51. Kluge, L: The Walldius prosthesis: A total treatment program. Phys Ther 52:26, 1972.

52. Kegerreis, S, Malone, T, and Ohnson, F: The diagonal medical plica: An underestimated clinical entity. Journal of Orthopaedic and Sports Physical Therapy 9:305, 1988.

53. King, S, and Butterwick, D: The anterior cruciate ligament: A review of recent concepts. Journal of Orthopaedic and Sports Physical Therapy 8:110, 1986.

54. Kuland, DN: The Injured Athlete, ed 2. JB Lippincott, Philadelphia, 1988.

55. Lemkuhl, LD, and Smith, LK: Brunnstrom's Clinical Kinesiology, ed 4. FA Davis, Philadelphia, 1983.

56. Lennington, KR, and Yanchuleff, TT: The use of isokinetics in the treatment of chondromalacia patellae: A case report. Journal of Orthopaedic and Sports Physical Therapy 4:176, 1983.

57. Lynch, PA, et al: Deep venous thrombosis and continued passive motion after total knee arthroplasty. J Bone Joint Surg Am 70:11, 1988.

58. MacIntosh, DL, and Hunter, GA: The use of the hemiarthroplasty prosthesis for advanced osteoarthritis and rheumatoid arthritis of the knee. J Bone Joint Surg Br 54:244, 1972.

59. MacIntosh, DL: Hemiarthroplasty of the knee using a space-occupying prosthesis for painful varus and valgus deformities. J Bone Joint Surg Am 40:1431, 1958.

60. Malone, TR, and Garrett, WE: Commentary and historical perspective of anterior cruciate ligament rehabilitation. Journal of Orthopaedic and Sports Physical Therapy 15:265–269, 1992.

61. Manske, PR, and Gleason, P: Rehabilitation program following polycentric total knee arthroplasty. Phys Ther 57:915, 1977.

62. McCarthy, MR, et al: The effects of immediate continuous passive motion on pain during the inflammatory phase of soft tissue healing following anterior cruciate ligament reconstruction. Journal of Orthopaedic and Sports Physical Therapy 17:96–101, 1993.

63. McConnell, J: The management of chondromalacia patellae: A long term solution. Australian Journal of Physiotherapy 32:215, 1986.

64. McConnell, J: McConnell Institute Workshop on Management of Patella femoral pain. Columbus, OH, 1994.

65. McInnes, J, and Larson, M: A controlled evaluation of continuous passive motion in patients undergoing total knee arthroplasty. JAMA 268:1423–1428, 1992.

66. McKeaver, DC: Tibial plateau prosthesis. Clin Orthop 18:86, 1960.

67. Melvin, J: Rheumatic Disease: Occupational Therapy and Rehabilitation, ed 2. FA Davis, Philadelphia, 1982.

68. Merriweather, R: Total knee replacement: The Walldius arthroplasty. Orthopedic and Physical Therapy Clinics of North America 4:585, 1973.

69. Metcalf, RW: An arthroscopic method for lateral release of the subluxating or dislocating patella. Clin Orthop 167:9, 1982.

70. Miller, J: Fixation in total knee arthroplasty. In Insall, JN (ed): Surgery of the Knee. Churchill-Livingstone, New York, 1984.

71. Morrey, RD, and Kavanagh, BF: Cementless joint replacement: Current status and future. Bull Rheum Dis 37:1, 1987.

72. Newman, AP: Synovectomy. In Sledge, CB, et al (eds): Arthritis Surgery. WB Saunders, Philadelphia, 1994.

73. Norkin, C, and Levangie, P: Joint Structure and Function: A Comprehensive Analysis. FA Davis, Philadelphia, 1983.

74. Normal and Pathological Gait Syllabus. Physical Therapy Department, Rancho Los Amigos Hospital, Downey, CA, 1977.

75. Noyes, FR, and Mangine, RE: Early knee motion after open and arthroscopic anterior cruciate ligament reconstruction. Am J Sports Med 15:149, 1987.

76. Outerbridge, RE, and Dunlop, J: The problem of chondromalacia patellae. Clin Orthop Rel Res 110:177, 1975.

77. Palmitier, RA, et al: Kinetic chain exercises in knee rehabilitation. Sports Med 11:402, 1991.

78. Paradis, D, and Hamlin, C: Geometric and polycentric knee prosthesis. Phys Ther 53:762, 1973.

79. Paulos, L, et al: Knee rehabilitation after anterior cruciate ligament reconstruction and repair. American Journal of Sports Medicine 9:140, 1981.

80. Paulos, L, et al: Patellar malalignment: A treatment rationale. Phys Ther 60:1624, 1980.

81. Rand, JA, Bryan, RS, and Chao, EYS: A comparison of cemented versus cementless porous-coated anatomic total knee arthroplasty. In Rand, JA, and Dorr, LD (eds): Total Arthroplasty of the Knee. Aspen, Rockville, MD, 1987.

82. Rand, JA, and Dorr, LD (eds): Total Arthroplasty of the Knee: Proceedings of the Knee Society, 1985–1986. Aspen, Rockville, MD, 1987.

83. Riegler, HF: Recurrent dislocations and subluxations of the patella. Clin Orthop 227:201–209, 1988.

84. Sandor, SM, Hart, JAL, and Oakes, BW: Case study: Rehabilitation of a surgically repaired medial collateral knee ligament using a limited motion cast and isokinetic exercise. Journal of Orthopaedic and Sports Physical Therapy 7:154, 1986.

85. Scaepanski, TL, et al: Effect of contraction type, angular velocity, and arc of motion on VMO:VL EMG ratio. Journal of Orthopaedic and Sports Physical Therapy 14:256, 1991.

86. Seto, JL, and Brewster CE: Rehabilitation of meniscal injuries. In Greenfield, BH: Rehabilitation of the Knee: A Problem-Solving Approach. FA Davis, Philadelphia, 1993.

87. Seto, JL, Brewster, CE, Lomardo, SJ, and Tibone, JE: Rehabilitation of the knee after anterior cruciate lig-

ament reconstruction. Journal of Orthopaedic and Sports Physical Therapy 11:8–18, 1989.

88. Shelbourne, KD, and Nitz, P: Accelerated rehabilitation after anterior cruciate ligament reconstruction. Journal of Orthopaedic and Sports Physical Therapy 15:256–264, 1992.

89. Shelton, GL, and Thigpen, LK: Rehabilitation of patellofemoral dysfunction: A review of literature. Journal of Orthopaedic and Sports Physical Therapy 14:143, 1991.

90. Shoji, H, and Solomonov, M: Factors affecting postoperative flexion in total knee arthroplasty. Clin Orthop 13:643–649, 1990.

91. Skolnick, MD, Coventry, MB, and Ilstrop, OM: Geometric total knee arthroplasty. J Bone Joint Surg Am 58:749, 1976.

92. Smidt, GL, Albright, JP, and Deusinger, RH: Pre- and postoperative functional changes in total knee patients. Journal of Orthopaedic and Sports Physical Therapy 6:25, 1984.

93. Sodeberg, GL, and Cook, TM: An electromyographic analysis of quadriceps femoris muscle setting and straight leg raising. Phys Ther 63:1434–1438, 1983.

94. Sonstegard, D, et al: The surgical replacement of the human knee joint. Scientific American 238:1, 1978.

95. Spencer, JD, Hayes, KC, and Alexander, IJ: Knee joint effusion and quadriceps reflex inhibition in man. Arch Phys Med Rehabil 65:171, 1984.

96. Sprague, R: Factors related to extension lag at the knee joint. Journal of Orthopaedic and Sports Physical Therapy 3:178, 1982.

97. Steindler, A: Kinesiology of the Human Body Under Normal and Pathological Conditions. Charles C Thomas, Springfield, IL, 1955.

98. Stone, RC, Frewin, PR, and Gonzales, S: Long term assessment of arthroscopic meniscus repair. A two to six year follow-up study. Arthroscopy 6:73, 1990.

99. Stratford, P: Electromyography of the quadriceps femoris muscles in subjects with normal and acutely effused knees. Phys Ther 62:279, 1982.

100. Tamburello, et al: Patella hypomobility as a cause of extensor lag. Research presentation, Overland Park, KS, May 1985.

101. Timm, KE, and Patch, DG: Case study: Use of Cybex II velocity spectrum in the rehabilitation of postsurgical knees. Journal of Orthopaedic and Sports Physical Therapy 6:347, 1985.

102. Tovin, BJ, et al: Comparison of the effects of exercise in water and on land on the rehabilitation of patients with intraarticular anterior cruciate ligament reconstructions. Phys Ther 74:710–719, 1994.

103. Voight, ML, and Wieder, DL: Comparative reflex response times of vastus medialis obliques and vastus lateralis in normal subjects and subjects with extensor mechanism dysfunction. American Journal of Sports Medicine 19:131, 1991.

104. Walldius, B: Arthroplasty of the knee using an endoprosthesis. Acta Orthop Scand 30:137, 1960.

105. Waters, EA: Physical therapy management of patients with total knee replacement. Phys Ther 54:936, 1974.

106. Waugh, T: Arthroplasty rehabilitation. In Goodgold J (ed): Rehabilitation Medicine. CV Mosby, St Louis, 1988.

107. Wigren, A, et al: Isokinetic muscle strength and endurance after knee arthroplasty with the modular knee in patients with osteoarthritis and rheumatoid arthritis. Scand J Rheumatol 12:145, 1983.

108. Wilk, KE, and Andrews, JR: Current concepts in the treatment of anterior cruciate ligament disruption. Journal of Orthopaedic and Sports Physical Therapy 15:279, 1992.

109. Wilk, KE, and Andrews, JR: The effects of pad placement and angular velocity on tibial displacement during isokinetic exercise. Journal of Orthopaedic and Sports Physical Therapy 17:24, 1993.

110. Windsor, RE, and Insall, JN: Surgery of the knee. In Sledge, CB, et al (eds): Arthritis Surgery. WB Saunders, Philadelphia, 1994.

111. Woodall, W, and Welsh, J: A biomechanical basis for rehabilitation programs involving the patellofemoral joint. Journal of Orthopaedic and Sports Physical Therapy 11:535, 1990.

112. Woolf, CJ: Generation of pain: Central mechanisms, Br Med Bull 47(3):523–533, 1991.

113. Zarins, B: Arthroscopy and arthroscopic surgery. Bull Rheum Dis 34:1, 1984.

The Ankle and Foot

The joints and muscles of the ankle and foot are designed to provide stability as well as mobility in the terminal structures of the lower extremity. The foot must bear the body weight when standing, with a minimum of muscle energy expenditure. The foot also must be able to adapt to absorb forces and to accommodate uneven surfaces, and then it must be able to become a rigid structural lever to propel the body forward when walking or running.

The anatomy and kinesiology of the ankle and foot are complex, but it is important to understand them to effectively treat problems in that area. The first section of this chapter reviews highlights of these areas that the reader should know and understand. For greater depth and explanation, the reader is referred to several texts and articles for study of the material.[2,17,19,21,28,34,36] Chapter 7 presents information on principles of management; the reader should be familiar with that material before proceeding with establishing a therapeutic exercise program for the ankle and foot.

OBJECTIVES

After studying this chapter, the reader will be able to:

1   Identify important aspects of the structure and function of the ankle and foot for review.
2   Establish a therapeutic exercise program to manage soft tissue and joint lesions in the ankle and foot related to stages of recovery following an inflammatory insult to the tissues, recognizing unique circumstances in the ankle and foot for their management.
3   Establish a therapeutic exercise program to manage common surgical procedures in the ankle and foot.

I. Review of the Structure and Function of the Ankle and Foot

A. Bony Parts (see Figs. 6-49 and 6-58)

1. Leg

Tibia and fibula

2. Hindfoot (posterior segment)

Talus and calcaneus

3. Midfoot (middle segment)

Navicular, cuboid, and three cuneiforms

4. Forefoot (anterior segment)

Five metatarsals and 14 phalanges, which make up the 5 toes (3 phalanges for each toe except the large toe, which has 2 phalanges)

B. Motions of the Foot and Ankle

1. Primary plane motions defined

a. Sagittal plane motion is *dorsiflexion* (in a dorsal direction) and *plantarflexion* (in a plantar direction).

b. Frontal plane motion is *inversion* (turning inward) and *eversion* (turning outward).

c. Transverse plane motion is *abduction* (away from midline) and *adduction* (toward the midline).

2. Triplanar motions occurring about oblique axes defined

a. *Pronation* is a combination of dorsiflexion, eversion, and abduction.

b. *Supination* is a combination of plantarflexion, inversion, and adduction.

NOTE: The terms inversion and supination, as well as eversion and pronation, are often interchanged.[36] This text will use the terms as defined above.

C. Joints and Their Characteristics[34]

1. The tibiofibular joints

Anatomically, the superior and inferior tibiofibular joints are separate from the ankle but provide accessory motions that allow greater movement at the ankle; fusion or immobility in these joints may impair ankle function.

a. *Superior tibiofibular joint*

A plane synovial joint made up of the fibular head and a facet on the posterolateral aspect of the rim of the tibial condyle; the facet faces posteriorly, inferiorly, and laterally.

b. *Inferior tibiofibular joint*

A syndesmosis with fibroadipose tissue between the two bony surfaces; it is supported by the crural tibiofibular interosseous ligament and the anterior and posterior tibiofibular ligaments.

c. With dorsiflexion and plantarflexion of the ankle, there are slight accessory movements of the fibula.[17]

(1) As the ankle plantarflexes, the lateral malleolus (fibula) rotates medially and is pulled inferiorly, and the two malleoli approximate. At the superior joint, the fibular slides inferiorly. The opposite occurs with dorsiflexion.

(2) As the foot supinates, the head of the fibula slides distally and posteriorly (external rotation); with pronation, the head of the fibula slides proximally and anteriorly (internal rotation).

2. The ankle (talocrural) joint

This is a synovial hinge joint supported by a structurally strong mortise and medial (deltoid) and lateral collateral ligaments (anterior and posterior talofibular and calcaneofibular ligaments).

a. The concave articulating surface is the mortise, which is made up of the distal tibia and the tibial and fibular malleoli. The fibular malleolus extends farther distally than the tibial malleolus. The combined surfaces are congruent with the body of the talus. Integrity of the mortise is provided by the tibiofibular joints and their associated ligaments.

b. The convex articulating surface is the body of the talus. The surface is wedge shaped, being wider anteriorly, and is also cone shaped, with the apex pointing medially. As a result, when the foot dorsiflexes, the talus also abducts and slightly everts; and when the foot plantarflexes, the talus also adducts and slightly inverts around an oblique axis.

c. With physiologic motions of the foot, the body of the talus slides in the opposite direction.

	Direction of Slide
Physiologic Motion	*of the Talus*
Dorsiflexion	Posterior
Plantarflexion	Anterior

See also accessory motions of the fibula listed in Section 1.c.

3. Subtalar (talocalcaneal) joint

This is a uniaxial joint with an oblique axis of motion lying approximately 42 degrees from the transverse plane and 16 degrees from the sagittal plane, which allows the calcaneus to pronate and supinate in a triplanar motion on the talus. Frontal plane inversion (turning heel inward) and eversion (turning heel outward) can be isolated only with passive motion. The subtalar joint is supported by the medial and lateral collateral ligaments, which support the talocrural joint; by the interosseous talocalcaneal ligament in the tarsal canal; and by the posterior and lateral talocalcaneal ligaments. In closed-chain activities, the joint attenuates the rotatory forces between the leg and foot so that, normally, excessive inward or outward turning of the foot does not occur.

a. There are three articulations between the talus and calcaneus; the posterior is separated from the anterior and middle by the tarsal canal. The canal divides the subtalar joint into two joint cavities.

b. The posterior articulation has its own capsule; the facet on the bottom of the talus is concave, whereas the opposing facet on the calcaneus is convex.

c. The anterior articulations are enclosed in the same capsule as the talonavicular articulation, forming the *talocalcaneonavicular* joint. Functionally, these articulations work together. The facets of the anterior and middle articulations on the talus are convex, whereas the opposing facets on the calcaneus are concave.

d. With physiologic motions of the subtalar joint, the convex posterior portion of the calcaneus slides opposite to the motion; the concave anterior and middle facets on the calcaneus slide in the same direction.

Physiologic Motion	*Direction of Slide of Posterior Articulation*
Supination with inversion	Lateral
Pronation with eversion	Medial

4. Talonavicular joint

Anatomically and functionally part of the talocalcaneonavicular joint, this joint is supported by the spring, the deltoid, the bifurcate, and the dorsal talonavicular ligaments. The triplanar motions of the navicular on the talus function with the subtalar joint, resulting in pronation and supination. With pronation, the accessory motions of the navicular are dorsal sliding with abduction and eversion. In the weight-bearing foot this occurs as the head of the talus drops plantarward and medially, resulting in a pliable foot and a decreased medial longitudinal arch. The opposite accessory motions occur with supination, resulting in a rigid foot and an increased medial longitudinal arch.

a. The head of the talus is convex; the proximal articulating surface of the navicular is concave.

b. With physiologic motions of the foot, the navicular slides in the same direction as the motion of the forefoot.

c. In the weight-bearing foot (closed chain), the motions of the talus and navicular are in the opposite directions, so that if the head of the talus drops plantarward and rotates medially, the navicular slides dorsally and rotates laterally.

Physiologic Motion of the Foot	*Direction of Slide of the Navicular on the Head of the Talus*
Supination	Plantar (and medial)
Pronation	Dorsal (and lateral)

5. Transverse tarsal joint

A functionally compound joint including the anatomically separate talonavicular and calcaneocuboid joints.

a. *Talonavicular joint* (see Section 4 above).

b. The *calcaneocuboid joint* is saddle shaped. The articulating surface of the calcaneus is convex in a dorsal-to-plantar direction and concave in a medial-to-lateral direction; the articulating surface of the cuboid is reciprocally concave and convex.

c. The transverse tarsal joint participates in the triplanar pronation-supination activities of the foot and makes compensatory movements to accommodate variations in the ground. Passive accessory motions include abduction-adduction, inversion-eversion, and dorsal-plantar gliding.

6. The remaining intertarsal and tarsometatarsal joints

These are plane joints whose functions reinforce those of the hind foot (see Section D).

7. The metatarsophalangeal (MTP) and interphalangeal (IP) joints of the toes

These joints are the same as the metacarpophalangeal and interphalangeal joints of the hand except that, in the toes, extension range of motion is more important than is flexion (the opposite is true in the hand). Extension of the MTP joints is necessary for normal walking. Also, the large toe does not function separately as does the thumb.

D. Functional Relationships of the Ankle and Foot[34]

1. Normally, an external torsion exists in the tibia, so that the ankle mortise faces approximately 15 degrees outward.[13] With dorsiflexion, the foot moves up and slightly laterally; with plantarflexion, the foot moves down and medially. Dorsiflexion is the closed-packed, stable position of the talocrural joint. Plantarflexion is the loose-packed position. This joint is more vulnerable to injury when walking in high heels because of the less stable plantarflexed position.

2. In a closed-chain, weight-bearing foot, supination of the subtalar and transverse tarsal joints with a pronation twist of the forefoot (plantarflexion of the first and dorsiflexion of the fifth metatarsals) increases the arch of the foot and is the closed-packed or stable position of the joints of the foot. This is the position the foot assumes when a rigid lever is needed for propelling the body forward during the push-off phase of ambulation.

3. During weight bearing, pronation of the subtalar and transverse tarsal joints causes the arch of the foot to lower, and there is a relative supination of the forefoot with dorsiflexion of the first and plantarflexion of the fifth metatarsals. This is the loose-packed or mobile position of the foot and is assumed when the foot absorbs the impact of weight bearing and rotational forces of the rest of the lower extremity and when the foot conforms to the ground.

4. In the weight-bearing foot, subtalar motion and tibial rotation are interdependent. Supination of the subtalar joint results in or is caused by lateral rotation of the tibia and, conversely, pronation of the subtalar joint results in or is caused by medial rotation of the tibia.

5. The arches of the foot are visualized as a twisted osteoligamentous plate, with the metatarsal heads being the horizontally placed anterior edge of the plate, and the calcaneus being the vertically placed posterior edge. The twist causes the longitudinal and transverse arches. When bearing weight, the plate tends to untwist and flatten the arches slightly.

   a. Primary support of the arches comes from the spring ligament, with additional support from the long plantar ligament, the plantar aponeurosis, and short plantar ligament. During push-off in gait, as the foot plantarflexes and supinates and the metatarsal phalangeal joints go into extension, increased tension is placed on the plantar aponeurosis, which helps increase the arch (windlass effect).

   b. In the normal static foot, muscles do little to support the arches. They contribute to support during ambulation.

6. A person with a varus deformity of the calcaneus (observed non–weight bearing) may compensate by standing with a pronated (or everted) calcaneus posture. *Pes planus, pronated foot,* and *flat foot* are terms often interchanged to mean a pronated posture of the hindfoot and decreased medial longitudinal arch. *Pes cavus* and *supinated foot* describe a high-arched foot.[36]

E. Muscle Function in the Ankle and Foot

1. Plantarflexion is primarily caused by the two-joint gastrocnemius muscle and the one-joint soleus muscle; they attach to the calcaneus via the Achilles tendon.

2. Other muscles passing posteriorly to the axis of motion for plantarflexion contribute little to that motion, but they do have other functions.
    a. Tibialis posterior is a strong supinator and invertor that helps to control and reverse pronation during gait.
    b. Flexor hallucis longus and flexor digitorum longus flex the toes and help support the medial longitudinal arch. To prevent clawing of the toes (MTP extension with IP flexion), intrinsic muscles must also function at the MTP joints.
    c. Peroneus longus and brevis primarily evert the foot, and the longus gives support to the transverse and lateral longitudinal arches.
3. Dorsiflexion of the ankle is caused by the tibialis anterior muscle (which also inverts the ankle), the extensor hallucis longus and extensor digitorum longus muscles (which also extend the toes), and the peroneus tertius.
4. Intrinsic muscles of the foot are similar to the hand in the functioning of the toes (except there is no thumblike function in the foot), and they also provide support of the arches during gait.
5. In normal standing, the gravitational line falls anteriorly to the axis of the ankle joint, creating a dorsiflexion moment. The soleus muscle contracts to counter the gravitational moment through its pull on the tibia. Other extrinsic foot muscles help stabilize the foot during postural sway.
6. The ankle and foot during gait[34,35]
    a. During the normal gait cycle, the ankle goes through a range of motion of 35 degrees; 15 degrees of dorsiflexion occurs at the end of mid-stance and 20 degrees of plantarflexion occurs at the end of stance.
    b. Shock-absorbing, terrain-conforming, and propulsion functions of the ankle and foot
        (1) From heel strike to foot flat (loading response), the anterior tibialis muscle contracts to control the foot as it lowers to the ground and also to untwist the forefoot to its loose-packed position.[21] The entire lower extremity rotates inward, which reinforces the loose-packed position of the foot. With the joints in a lax position, they can conform to variations in the ground contour as the foot is lowered and absorb some of the impact forces.
        (2) Once the foot is fixed on the ground, dorsiflexion begins as the tibia comes up over the foot; the tibia continues to rotate internally, which reinforces pronation of the subtalar joint and loose-packed position of the foot.
        (3) During mid-stance, the tibia begins to rotate externally, which initiates supination of the hindfoot and locking of the transverse tarsal joint. This brings the foot into its closed-packed position, which is reinforced as the plantar aponeurosis tightens through the windlass effect with toe extension. This stable position converts the foot into a rigid lever, ready to propel the body forward as the ankle plantarflexes from the pull of the gastrocsoleus muscle group.
    c. Muscle control of the ankle during gait
        (1) The ankle dorsiflexors function during the initial foot contact and loading response (heel strike to foot flat) to counter the plantarflexion torque and to control the lowering of the foot to the ground. They also function during the swing phase to keep the foot from plantarflexing and dragging on the ground. With loss of the dorsiflexors, foot slap occurs at initial foot contact, and the hip and knee flex excessively during swing (or else the toe drags on the ground).

(2) The ankle plantarflexors begin functioning near the end of mid-stance and during terminal stance and preswing (heel-off to toe-off) to control the rate of forward movement of the tibia and also to plantarflex the ankle for push-off. Loss of function results in slight lag of the lower extremity during terminal stance with no push-off.

F. Major Nerves Subject to Pressure and Trauma[23]

The foot is where several major nerves terminate. Injury or entrapment of the nerves may be anywhere along their course, from the lumbosacral spine to near their termination. For treatment to be effective, it must be directed to the source of the problem. Therefore, a thorough history is obtained and a selective tension examination is performed when referred pain patterns or sensory changes are reported by the patient.[3,13,21]

1. Common peroneal nerve

After it bifurcates from the sciatic nerve, it passes between the biceps femoris tendon and lateral head of the gastrocnemius muscle and then comes laterally around the fibular neck and passes through an opening in the peroneus longus muscle. Pressure or force against the nerve in this region can cause a neuropathy. Sensory changes occur in the distal lateral surface of the leg and dorsum of the foot (except the little toe); muscles affected may include the dorsiflexors of the ankle and evertors of the foot (peroneus longus and brevis, tibialis anterior, extensor digitorum longus and brevis, extensor hallucis longus, and peroneus tertius).

2. Posterior tibial nerve

This nerve occupies a groove behind the medial malleolus along with the tendons of the tibialis posterior, flexor hallucis longus, and flexor digitorum longus muscles; the groove is covered by a ligament, forming a tunnel. Entrapment usually from a space-occupying lesion is known as a tarsal tunnel syndrome. Sensory innervation includes the plantar surface of the foot and toes and the dorsum of the distal phalanges. Muscles affected include intrinsic muscles of the foot (abductor hallucis, flexor hallucis brevis, lumbricals, interossei, and quadratus plantae); weakness and postural changes in the foot (pes cavus and clawing of the toes) may occur.

3. Plantar and calcaneal nerves

These branches of the posterior tibial nerve may become entrapped as they turn under the medial aspect of the foot and pass through openings in the abductor hallucis muscle. Overpronation presses the nerves against these openings. Irritation of the nerves may elicit symptoms similar to acute foot strain (tenderness at the posteromedial plantar aspect of the foot), painful heel (inflamed calcaneal nerve), and pain in a pes cavus foot. The degree of muscle weakness will depend on which of the branches is involved.

4. Common sources of segmental sensory reference in the foot

  a. Lumbosacral spine
    (1) Vertebral joints between L-4 and L-5 or between L-5 and S-1 vertebrae
    (2) Nerve roots L-4, L-5, and S-1
  b. Dermatomal reference from tissue derived from the same spinal segments as L-4, L-5, and S-1

II. Joint Problems: Nonoperative Management

A. Related Diagnoses

Chapter 7 provides a general discussion of arthritic conditions and etiology of symptoms. The following is specific to joint conditions in the ankle and foot:

1. **Rheumatoid arthritis (RA).** This pathology commonly affects the talocrural, subtalar and MTP joints of the foot leading to instabilities and painful deformities that increase with the stress of weight bearing.

2. **Degenerative joint disease (DJD) and joint trauma.** Degenerative symptoms occur in joints that are repetitively traumatized, and acute joint symptoms are often seen in conjunction with ankle sprains.

3. **Postimmobilization stiffness.** Tightness in the capsular tissues leading to joint hypomobilities as well as tightness in the surrounding periarticular tissues may occur any time the joint is immobilized following a fracture or surgery.

4. **Gout.** Symptoms commonly affect the metatarsophalangeal joint of the great toe, causing pain during terminal stance so that there is a shorter stance and no smooth push-off.

B. Common Impairments/Problems[3,6]

1. **Restricted motion.** When symptoms are acute, there is swelling and restricted, painful motion; when chronic, there is restricted motion, decreased joint play, and a firm capsular end-feel in the affected joint.

   a. *Talocrural joint.* Passive plantarflexion is more limited than is dorsiflexion (unless the gastrocsoleus muscle group is also tight, in which case dorsiflexion will be limited accordingly).

   b. *Subtalar and transverse tarsal joints.* Progressive limitation of supination develops until eventually the joint fixes in pronation with flattening of the medial longitudinal arch. The closed-packed position of the tarsals (supination) becomes more and more difficult to assume during the terminal stance (push-off) phase of gait.

   c. *Metatarsophalangeal (MTP) joint of the large toe.* Gross limitation of extension and some limitation of flexion develop; the rest of the MTP joints are variable. Lack of extension restricts the terminal stance phase of gait with inability to rock up onto the metatarsal heads.

2. **Hallux valgus.** This deformity develops as the proximal phalanx shifts laterally toward the second toe. Eventually the flexor and extensor muscles of the great toe shift laterally and further accentuate the deformity. The bursa over the medial aspect of the metatarsal head may become inflamed, causing a painful bunion.

3. **Dorsal dislocation of the proximal phalanges on the metatarsal heads.** If this occurs, the fat pad, which is normally under the metatarsal heads, migrates dorsally with the phalanges and the protective cushion on weight bearing is lost, leading to pain, callus formation, and potential ulceration.

4. **Claw toe (MTP hyperextension and IP flexion) and hammer toe (MTP hyperextension, PIP flexion, and DIP hyperextension).** These result from muscle imbalances between the intrinsic and extrinsic muscles of the toes. Friction from shoes may cause calluses to form where the toes rub.

5. **Decreased mobility in the proximal and distal tibiofibular joints.** Restricted accessory motion in these joints usually occurs with periods of immobility and will limit ankle and subtalar joint motion.[24]

6. **Muscle weakness and poor muscular endurance.**

7. **Poor balance and postural control.**

8. Gait deviations. Antalgic gait occurs usually with a short stance phase from pain and inability to plantarflex the ankle and supinate the foot for an effective push-off during terminal stance.

C. Common Functional Limitations/Disabilities

1. When symptoms are acute, any weight-bearing activities will be painful, preventing independent ambulation and causing difficulty rising from a chair and ascending and descending stairs.
2. When symptoms are subacute or chronic with joint restrictions and weakness, ambulation will be decreased. At best there will be limitations on distance and the person may require use of assistive devices for ambulation; at worst the person will be unable to ambulate and therefore be bound to a wheelchair for mobility.

D. Management of Acute and Early Subacute Joint Problems and Restrictions

Management will depend on the signs and symptoms present. Follow the general outline as presented in Chapter 7 for acute, subacute, and chronic joint problems. Protection from deforming weight-bearing forces and additional trauma imposed by improperly fitting footwear is an integral part of managing arthritis in the ankles and feet. Use of orthotics and well-constructed shoes may be necessary to help protect the joints by realigning forces or providing support from faulty foot postures.[29,30]

1. To treat pain and maintain mobility

a. Grade I or II joint distraction and oscillation techniques.
b. Gentle cross-fiber massage to associated ligaments.
c. Active-assistive (or active, if the acute symptoms are managed with medical intervention) ROM; no stretch force or resistance is used when acute.

2. To maintain muscle integrity and circulation

Muscle-setting techniques to associated muscles.

3. To decrease mechanical stress

Use assistive devices for ambulation.

E. Management of Late Subacute and Chronic Joint Lesions

Evaluate for signs of muscle tightness, joint restrictions, or muscle weakness, and initiate exercises and mobilization procedures at a level appropriate for the condition of the patient.

1. To increase mobility of the talocrural joint

a. General mobility: joint traction (see Fig. 6–59).
b. To increase plantarflexion: anteriorly glide the talus (see Fig. 6–61).
c. To increase dorsiflexion: posteriorly glide the talus (see Fig. 6–60).
d. To increase accessory motions of the fibula: anteriorly glide the fibular head (see Fig. 6–56) and glide the fibular malleolus (see Fig. 6–57).

2. To increase mobility of the subtalar joint

a. General mobility: joint traction (see Fig. 6–62).
b. To increase inversion: laterally glide the calcaneus (see Fig. 6–63B).
c. To increase eversion: medially glide the calcaneus (see Fig. 6–63A).

3. To increase mobility of intertarsal and tarsometatarsal joints

a. For the accessory motion of plantarflexion, necessary for supination and increasing the longitudinal arches: Plantarglide the distal articulating bone on the stabilized proximal bone at the restricted joint (see Fig. 6–64).

b. For the accessory motion of dorsiflexion, necessary for pronation and decreasing the longitudinal arches: dorsalglide the distal articulating bone on the stabilized proximal bone at the restricted joint (see Fig. 6–65).

NOTE: Since weight-bearing forces and joint changes with arthritis reinforce pronation, usually mobilizing to increase pronation should not be undertaken in the arthritic foot. Perform these techniques only in the stiff foot following immobilization when the foot does not effectively pronate during weight acceptance in gait.

4. To increase mobility of the MTP and IP joints of the toes

Glide the distal articulating bone on the stabilized proximal bone in the direction of restriction, as is performed with the joints of the fingers (see Fig. 6–42, 6–43, and 6–44).

5. To increase mobility in the soft tissue and muscles

Passive stretching and active inhibition techniques are performed as described in Chapter 5. Self-stretching techniques are described later in this chapter.

6. To regain a balance in muscle strength

Begin resistive exercises at a level appropriate for the weakened muscles. Begin with isometric resistance in pain-free positions and progress to isotonics through pain-free ranges using open- and closed-chain exercises. Additional resistive exercises are described later in this chapter. Low-load weight-bearing exercises may be performed in a pool or tank.

7. To protect the joint from deforming forces

In degenerative or systemic arthritic conditions, proper orthotic devices should be fabricated to support the patient's foot, and proper shoe fit should be emphasized.[1] Continued use of assistive devices for ambulation may be necessary.

8. To stimulate balance and proprioception

Initiate protected closed-chain balance exercises as described in Section VI.

9. Patient education

Teach patients to be aware of signs of systemic fatigue (especially in RA), local muscle fatigue, and joint stress so that they can exercise and remain active within safe levels. Emphasize the importance of daily range of motion and endurance activities and joint protection, including avoidance of faulty foot and ankle postures.

III. Joint Surgery and Postoperative Management

Chronic arthritis of the ankle and foot can lead to severe pain, limitation of motion, gross instability or deformity, and significant loss of functional use of the lower extremities. Surgical management includes *synovectomy, arthrodesis, total joint replacement,* or *excision arthroplasty.* The choice of surgery depends upon the degree of articular damage, the severity of joint deformity or instability and the postoperative functional goals of the patient. Arthrodesis of the ankle, such as a *triple arthrodesis* or a *subtalar arthrodesis*, provides pain-free weight bearing and stability of the ankle for the person with high functional demands but sacrifices mobility of one or more joints of the ankle. Pain-free compensatory movements must be available in other ankle or foot joints to absorb weight-bearing forces during ambulation. Arthroplasty of the ankle, which is used less frequently than arthrodesis, is an alternative for patients with severe bilateral disease but low functional demands in which bilateral ankle fusions would be impractical and would dramatically restrict functional mobility such as ascending or descending stairs or rising from a chair.

The goals of joint surgery and a postoperative rehabilitation program include (1) relief of pain with weight bearing and joint motion, (2) stability of the ankle and foot joints for ambulation and functional activities, (3) improvement of joint motion and strength, and (4) correction of deformity. The rehabilitation program includes postoperative exercise, gait training with assistive devices, patient education including information on shoe fit and selection, as well the appropriate choices of recreational and daily living activities.

A. Total Ankle Joint Replacement

1. Indications for surgery[8,41,44,48,52,54]

a. Severe tibiotalar joint deterioration and pain secondary to rheumatoid arthritis or degenerative joint disease.
b. Marked limitation of motion of the ankle joint bilaterally.
c. Avascular necrosis of the ankle joint, secondary to repeated ankle injury.
d. An alternative to arthrodesis for the patient with low-intensity functional demands but good ligamentous stability at the ankle. (The components of a total ankle arthroplasty do not improve stability of the ankle.)

NOTE: Patients with a very unstable ankle, vascular deficiency, inadequate bone density, or muscle imbalances at the ankle are not good candidates for this procedure.

2. Procedure[41,42,44,55]

a. An anterior mid-line incision or sometimes a posterior incision is made.
b. Minimal bone is excised from the tibiotalar joint.
c. An all-plastic tibial replacement (the Mayo single-axis prosthesis) or a metal-stemmed tibial prosthesis with a polyethylene articulating surface (the Waugh-Smith multiaxis prosthesis) is implanted and held in place with biologic fixation (bone ingrowth) or cement.
d. A talar component made of metal is affixed to the talus with cement or cementless fixation.
e. Biologic fixation, although requiring a longer period of restricted weight bearing and rehabilitation, is now preferred as it decreases the incidence of loosening of the components over time.

3. Postoperative management[41,46,52]

a. *Immobilization*
   (1) If biologic fixation is used, the ankle is immobilized in a cast or splint in a neutral position for up to 6 weeks.
   (2) If cement fixation is used, the ankle is immobilized in a bulky dressing or splint in a neutral position for 3 to 5 days.

(3) The foot is elevated at all times in the early postoperative period when the patient is in bed. Elevation prevents or minimizes edema, which can cause poor wound healing.

(4) During the early postoperative period the patient must be non–weight bearing during transfers, and ambulation with crutches is necessary while the bulky dressing or short leg cast is in place.

b. *Exercise*

MAXIMUM-PROTECTION PHASE

(1) While the ankle is immobilized, begin isometric (muscle-setting) exercises of the ankle musculature, gluteal, and quadriceps muscles. Gentle active-resisted hip and knee exercises can also be performed in preparation for walking.

(2) To strengthen the nonoperated lower extremity and upper extremities, begin resisted exercises in preparation for ambulation.

(3) To regain ROM when the immobilization is removed and if wound healing is sufficient, initiate active open-chain dorsiflexion and plantarflexion. The patient will need about 10 degrees of dorsiflexion and 25 degrees of plantarflexion for normal walking and about 50 to 60 degrees of ankle motion for ascending and descending stairs.[41] If the design of the prosthetic components allows, active open-chain inversion, eversion, and circumduction can also be initiated.

MODERATE- AND MINIMUM-PROTECTION PHASES

(1) To strengthen ankle musculature in an open chain, add isotonic resistance exercises against elastic tubing.

(2) To strengthen ankle musculature in a closed chain, begin active and resisted ankle exercises on a BAPS (balance or rocker) board in a *seated* position while weight bearing must be restricted (see Fig. 13–2). Closed-chain dorsiflexion, plantarflexion inversion, and eversion exercises can be progressed by applying rhythmic stabilization to the pelvis or lower extremities while the patient is standing or by having the patient stand on a balance board when partial or full weight bearing is permissible.

(3) To stretch the plantarflexors, if dorsiflexion is restricted, add towel stretches in a long-sitting position or have the patient stand on a wedge for an extended period (see Fig. 13–1).

4. Long-term results[41,52,54]

The long-term success of total ankle arthroplasty is still limited. The most common postoperative complication is loosening of the prosthetic components. There is also a high degree of wound-healing problems. Although patients are relieved of pain, return of motion is often poor and limited to 5 to 10 degrees of ankle motion.

B. Arthrodesis at the Ankle and Foot

1. Indications for surgery[16,37,41,50]

a. Severe articular damage and pain with weight bearing at any number of joints of the ankle or foot secondary to rheumatoid, degenerative, or traumatic arthritis

b. Instability of a weight-bearing joint

c. Deformity of the toes, foot, or ankle

d. Appropriate for patients with high functional demands and pain-free compensatory movements in adjacent joints

2. Procedures[16,37,41,50]

a. The procedures, all of which provide bony ankylosis, will vary depending on the joints involved.

b. Some common procedures include:

(1) Triple arthrodesis of the ankle

    (a) Fusion of the talocalcaneal, calcaneocuboid, and talonavicular joints.

    (b) Provides permanent medial-lateral stability and relief of pain in the subtalar joint.

    (c) Eversion and inversion of the ankle are lost.

(2) Arthrodesis of the tibiotalar joint

    (a) Fusion of the tibia and talus in approximately 5 degrees of plantarflexion provides relief of pain and stability at the tibiotalar joint

    (b) Dorsiflexion and plantarflexion are lost, significantly affecting the biomechanics of gait.

    (c) The forefoot must be stable and pain free to compensate for the loss of motion at the ankle.

    (d) NOTE: Bilateral tibiotalar arthrodesis is usually not appropriate as it makes it difficult to get up from a chair or to ascend or descend stairs.

(3) Arthrodesis of the first toe

    (a) Fusion of the first metatarsophalangeal (MTP) joint for hallux rigidus and hallux valgus

    (b) Provides relief of pain during ambulation in the MTP joint of the first toe

(4) Arthrodesis of the interphalangeal (IP) joints of the toes

    (a) Fusion of the IP joints of the toes for hammer toes, usually occurring in the second and third toes

    (b) Provides relief of pain for ambulation and correction of deformities of the toes

3. Postoperative management[1,16,41]

a. The fused joints are immobilized in plaster or with skeletal pins for approximately 6 to 12 weeks.

b. During this time the patient must be non–weight bearing or partially weight bearing. Gait training with assistive devices is necessary.

c. Active range of motion exercises must be performed to maintain mobility in any other joints affected by arthritis.

d. The patient should be advised of proper shoe selection and fit when the immobilization device is removed.

C. Excision Arthroplasty for Metatarsalgia

1. Indications for surgery[16,32,37,40,50]

a. Metatarsalgia involves severe pain in the metatarsophalangeal (MTP) region of the foot with weight bearing and ambulation.

(1) Chronic synovitis of the MTP joints secondary to rheumatoid arthritis causes erosion and deterioration of the joint surfaces.

(2) Metatarsalgia is associated with volar subluxation of the heads of the metatarsals because of destruction of the joint capsule and stretching of the plantar intertarsal ligaments.

b. Hammer toes develop because of shortening of the long extensor muscles of the toes and pull on the long toe flexor muscles.[32]

c. Hallux valgus of the first toe is also an associated deformity of the foot seen with metatarsalgia.

d. Surgery is indicated when conservative management such as shoe modifications and foot orthoses[1,32] no longer relieve MTP pain during ambulation.

2. Procedures[16,32,37,40,41,50]

a. The involved metatarsal heads and the proximal portion of the proximal phalanges are resected (Fowler procedure).

b. If the first toe is primarily involved, the exostosis is removed from the medial aspect of the first metatarsal, and the proximal third to half of the first proximal phalanx is resected (Keller procedure).

3. Postoperative management

a. Weight bearing is partially restricted for several weeks. Gait training with assistive devices is necessary.

b. Active exercise to the intrinsic muscles of the foot is begun at approximately 1 month.[16,41]

c. The patient may be fitted with a metatarsal pad of polyethylene foam to be worn on the inside of the shoe. Use of the pad will equalize the pressure forces on the plantar aspect of the foot and will transfer the weight proximal to the metatarsal heads during weight bearing.[1,12,43]

IV. Overuse Syndromes/Repetitive Trauma Syndromes[11]

A. Related Diagnoses and Etiology of Symptoms

An overuse syndrome is a local inflammatory response to stresses from repetitive microtrauma, which may be from faulty alignment problems in the lower extremity, muscle imbalances or fatigue, changes in exercise or functional routines, training errors, improper footwear for the ground or functional demands placed on the feet, or a combination of several of these factors. The syndrome occurs because continued demand is placed on the tissue before it is adequately healed, so the pain and inflammation continue. A common cause predisposing the foot to overuse syndromes is abnormal pronation of the subtalar joint. The abnormal pronation could be related to a variety of causes including excessive joint mobility, leg-length discrepancy, femoral anteversion, external tibial torsion, genu valgum, or muscle flexibility and strength imbalances.

1. Tendinitis or tenosynovitis

Any of the tendons of the extrinsic muscles to the foot may become irritated as they approach and cross over the ankle or where they attach in the foot. Pain occurs during or following repetitive activity. When the foot and ankle are tested, pain is experienced at the site of the lesion as resistance is applied to the muscle action and also when the involved tendon is placed on a stretch or palpated.[3] A common site for symptoms is proximal to the calcaneus in the Achilles tendon or its sheath (Achilles tendinitis or peritendinitis). Symptoms may develop when the person switches from high-heeled shoes to low-heeled shoes and then does a lot of walking.[25] Symptoms are also associated with athletic activities such as running, tennis, and basketball.[27,39] Usually there is a tight gastrocsoleus complex and abnormal foot pronation.

2. Plantar fascitis

Pain is usually experienced along the plantar aspect of the heel where the plantar fascia inserts on the medial tubercle of the calcaneus. The site of the injury is very tender to palpation. Excessive pronation of the subtalar joint, which may be reinforced by tight gastrocsoleus muscles, predisposes the foot to abnormal forces and irritation of the plantar fascia. Conversely, stress forces on the fascia can also occur with an excessively high arch (cavus foot). Pressure to the irritated site with weight bearing or stretch forces to the fascia as when extending the toes during push-off causes pain.

3. Shin splints

This term is used to describe activity-induced leg pain along the posterior medial or anterior lateral aspects of the proximal two-thirds of the tibia. It may include different pathologic conditions such as musculotendinitis, stress fractures of the tibia, periosteitis, increased pressure in a muscular compartment, or irritation of the interosseous membrane.

  a. Anterior shin splints. Most common is overuse of the anterior tibialis muscle. A tight gastrocsoleus complex and a weak anterior tibialis muscle, as well as foot pronation, are associated with anterior shin splints. Pain increases with active dorsiflexion and when the muscle is stretched into plantarflexion.

  b. Posterior shin splints. A tight gastrocsoleus complex and a weak posterior tibialis muscle, along with foot pronation, are associated with posterior medial shin splints. Pain is experienced when the foot is passively dorsiflexed with eversion and with active supination. Muscle fatigue with vigorous exercise, such as running or aerobic dancing, may precipitate the problem.

B. Common Impairments/Problems

1. Pain with repetitive activity, on palpation to the involved site, when the involved musculotendinous unit is stretched, and with resistance to the involved muscle
2. Pain with gait
3. Muscle length-strength imbalances, especially tight gastrocsoleus muscle group
4. Abnormal foot posture (may be from faulty footwear)

C. Common Functional Limitations/Disabilities

1. Decreased distance or speed of ambulation
2. Restriction of sport or recreational activities
3. May limit wearing of nonsupportive footwear

D. Management of Acute Symptoms in Overuse/Repetitive Trauma Syndromes

While inflamed, the leg or foot problem should be treated as an acute condition with rest and appropriate modalities[5] (see Chapter 7). Immobilization in a cast or splint with the foot slightly plantarflexed or use of a heel lift inside the shoe may be used to relieve stress.[27,31,39]

1. Apply cross-friction massage to the site of the lesion.
2. Initiate gentle muscle-setting contractions or electrical stimulation to the involved muscle in pain-free positions.
3. Teach active ROM within the pain-free ranges.
4. Instruct the patient to avoid the activity that provokes the pain.

E. Management in Subacute and Chronic Phases of Treatment

When symptoms become subacute, the entire lower extremity as well as the foot should be evaluated for abnormal alignment or muscle flexibility and strength imbalances. Eliminating or modifying the cause is important to prevent recurrences.

1. Correct abnormal foot alignment with appropriate foot orthoses if necessary.[7,27,29,39]
2. Stretch tight structures such as the gastrocsoleus complex. (See Section VI for suggestions.)
3. Strengthen the involved muscles, beginning with resistive isometric and progressing to resistive isotonic and isokinetic exercises in open- and closed-chain activities. This usually involves strengthening the dorsiflexors but should also include the invertors (especially the posterior tibialis) and evertors for proper medial and lateral support.
4. As the patient gains a balance between flexibility and strength, emphasis needs to be placed on endurance and on training the involved muscles to respond to eccentric loading.
5. When returning to the previously stressful activity, the patient should be taught prevention, which includes stretching, gentle repetitive warm-ups, and use of proper foot support. The importance of allowing time for recovery from fatigue and microtrauma after high-intensity workouts also must be emphasized.

V. Traumatic Soft Tissue Injuries

A. Sprains and Minor Tears of Ligaments

1. Mechanisms and sites of injuries

Following trauma, the ligaments of the ankle may be stressed or torn. The most common type of ankle sprain is caused by an inversion stress and can result in a partial or complete tear of the anterior talofibular ligament[14,20]; the posterior talofibular ligament is torn only with massive inversion stresses. If the inferior tibiofibular ligaments are torn following stress to the ankle, the mortise becomes unstable. Rarely do the components of the deltoid ligament become stressed; there is greater likelihood of an avulsion from or fracture of the medial malleolus with an eversion stress. Depending on the severity, the joint capsule may also be involved, resulting in symptoms of acute (traumatic) arthritis.

2. Common impairments/problems

a. Pain when the injured tissue is stressed in mild to moderate injuries
b. Excessive motion or instability of the related joint with complete tears
c. Proprioceptive deficit manifested as decreased ability to perceive passive motion and development of balance problems[9]
d. Related joint symptoms and reflex muscle inhibition

3. Common functional limitations/disabilities

a. When symptoms are acute, may not be able to bear weight, thus requiring assisted ambulation
b. Recurrences of injuries with instabilities; may have increased incidence of falling and safety problems

4. **Nonoperative management: acute phase of treatment**

   See Chapter 7 for principles of treatment during stages of inflammation and repair.

   a. If possible, evaluate and treat the problem before swelling or joint effusion begins. To minimize the swelling, use compression, elevation, and cold.

   b. Grades I and II (mild and moderate) sprains do not cause gross instability of the ankle and are treated conservatively. The ankle is usually immobilized in neutral or in slight dorsiflexion and eversion.

   c. While symptoms are acute, decrease the stress of weight bearing with crutches for ambulation.[38,53]

   d. Muscle-setting techniques are used to help maintain muscle integrity and assist circulation.

5. **Subacute phase of treatment**

   a. As the acute symptoms decrease, continue to provide protection for the involved ligament with a splint when weight bearing. Fabricating a stirrup out of thermoplastic material and holding it in place with an elastic wrap or Velcro straps provide stability to the joint structures while allowing for the stimulus of weight bearing for proprioceptive feedback and proper healing.[38] Commercial splints such as an air splint are also available to provide medial-lateral stability while allowing dorsiflexion and plantarflexion.[22]

   b. Begin cross-fiber massage to the ligaments as tolerated.

   c. Use grade II joint mobilization techniques to maintain mobility of the joint.

   d. During the subacute phase the splint is removed and ROM is performed several times a day within the tolerance of the tissue. Also begin mild passive stretching to the healing ligament by having the patient actively move the ankle opposite the line of pull of the ligament within the pain-free range. For the anterior talofibular ligament, the motion is plantarflexion and inversion. Stretch to the gastrocsoleus muscle group is important so that adequate dorsiflexion can be obtained. Progress the stretching to weight-bearing stretches as indicated by the patient's recovery.

6. **Chronic phase of treatment**

   a. Increase strength in the supporting muscles. Resistance exercises to the peroneal muscles are important for lateral ankle support.[19] Any other muscles that test weak on evaluation should also be strengthened.

   b. Training to improve proprioceptive feedback for ankle stability, coordination, and reflex response begins with use of a rocker or balance board and progresses to other balance activities.[10] Depending on the final goals for rehabilitation, train the ankle with weight-bearing activities such as walking, jogging, and running and with agility activities such as controlled twisting, turning, and lateral weight shifting. (Exercises are described in Section VI.)

   c. When the patient is involved in sports activities, the ankle should be splinted, taped, or wrapped, and proper shoes should be worn to protect the ligament from reinjury.[19]

B. Complete Ligament Tears: Surgical Repair of and Postoperative Management

A third-degree (grade 3) sprain of the lateral ankle, which usually occurs as the result of a severe inversion injury, often causes complete tears of the anterior talofibular (ATF) and calcaneofibular (CF) ligaments. A transverse fracture of the lateral malleolus or an avulsion fracture of the base of the fifth metatarsal may also occur with severe inversion injuries.[33] A complete tear of one or more ligaments of the ankle causes marked instability of the ankle and significantly impairs an individual's functional activities.[18,22,25]

Lateral ankle reconstruction is often indicated for patients with acute third-degree ligament injuries or for patients with chronic lateral ankle instability that has not been corrected with conservative management who wish to return to vigorous sports or recreational activities.[45,47] The goal of surgery and postoperative management is to restore joint stability but retain functional ROM.[20,25,47]

1. Indications for surgery[18,20,25,45,47]

a. Third-degree lateral ankle sprain
b. Complete tear of the ATF and/or CF ligaments
c. Gross instability of the ankle

2. Procedure[18,25,45,47]

a. A lateral incision is made posterior and inferior to the lateral malleolus.
b. A direct repair involves reopposing and suturing the torn ligament.
c. The torn lateral ligament(s) may be replaced with a portion of the peroneus brevis tendon (peroneal graft).

3. Postoperative management[14,15,25,30,31,33]

a. *Immobilization*

(1) The ankle is immobilized in a short-leg cast-brace in 0 degrees of dorsiflexion and slight eversion for 6 to 8 weeks. While the immobilization is in place, the patient must be non–weight bearing on the operated lower extremity for the first 2 to 3 weeks after surgery. From 2 to 6 weeks postoperatively partial weight bearing in a walking cast is permissible.

(2) In the early postoperative days the foot should be elevated when the patient is seated or supine to minimize peripheral edema.

b. *Exercise*

MAXIMUM-PROTECTION PHASE

(1) While the ankle is immobilized, perform active or gentle resisted exercises of the hip and knee on the involved side to maintain strength in the lower extremity.

(2) Gentle, pain-free muscle setting to the ankle musculature is also appropriate when the ankle is immobilized.

MODERATE- AND MINIMUM-PROTECTION PHASES

(1) When the immobilization is removed at 6 to 8 weeks, perform exercises to:

(a) Restore ROM of the ankle with grade III joint mobilizations but avoid stretch mobilization of the subtalar joint in a lateral direction. Add contract-relax procedures and gentle manual or self-stretching activities to restore muscle flexibility. Initially open-chain stretching or closed-chain stretching in a seated position is advisable in the early stages of rehabilitation when weight bearing is restricted. Closed-chain stretching with the patient standing imposes significant ground reaction forces on the repaired ligaments. Emphasize restoration of dorsiflexion and plantarflexion before inversion and eversion.

(b) Increase strength in open- and closed-chain positions. After surgical repair of the lateral ligaments, strength of the evertors is particularly important for increased support of the ankle. Isometric strengthening of the evertors can be achieved by having the patient cross the ankles and press the lateral borders of the feet together. Dynamic strengthening of the evertors against elastic resistance is also appropriate (see Fig. 13–4).

    (c) Retrain balance and postural control with proprioceptive exercises on a balance board. Begin with bilateral and progress to unilateral standing activities on a balance board.

  (2) Progression of exercises is similar to exercises associated with conservative (nonoperative) management of ankle sprains. Include isotonic and isokinetic resistance exercises as well as progressive closed-chain functional activities.

  (3) Most patients can return to full activity by 4 to 6 months postoperatively and when strength of ankle musculature reaches 80 to 90 percent as compared with the normal ankle.

4. Long-term results[47]

A good postoperative result will provide lateral ankle joint stability, but a slight (10 degrees) loss of inversion may occur.

C. Complete Rupture of the Achilles Tendon: Surgical Repair and Postoperative Management

Rupture of the Achilles tendon occurs as the result of a forceful eccentric contraction of the gastrocnemius and soleus muscles (triceps surae), most frequently in older adults with compromised blood supply to the tendon. In young, active individuals a rupture can occur during high-intensity weight-bearing activities such as jumping or movements that require rapid deceleration. A complete rupture leads to pain, swelling, and significant weakness of the plantarflexors and is associated with a positive Thompson test[51] (absence of reflexive plantarflexion when the patient is prone-lying and the calf is squeezed). Although rupture of the Achilles tendon can be managed conservatively, surgery is indicated when the torn fragments cannot be reapposed with positioning and immobilization.[25,45,49]

1. Indications for surgery[25,31,49]

Complete rupture of the Achilles tendon in which end-to-end apposition cannot be achieved by conservative means.

2. Procedure[24,45,49]

a. A medial longitudinal incision of the ankle is made.
b. The tendon fragments are reapposed and sutured together.
c. A plantaris tendon graft may be used to reconstruct the tendon.

3. Postoperative management[15,25,31,33,49]

a. *Immobilization*

The ankle is immobilized in a short leg cast for 3 to 4 weeks with the ankle positioned in plantarflexion but with some tension on the newly sutured tendon. Then a new cast or splint is applied with the ankle in more dorsiflexion with slightly more tension on the tendon for 2 to 4 weeks. In the early postoperative period the patient must remain non–weight bearing on the operated side and ambulate with crutches. The foot and lower leg are elevated when the patient is seated or lying down.

b. *Exercise*

MAXIMUM-PROTECTION PHASE

(1) While the immobilization is in place, begin submaximal muscle-setting exercises of the ankle musculature as soon as it is comfortable for the patient. As healing progresses, increase the intensity of the isometric exercises.

(2) Maintain hip and knee strength on the operated side.

MODERATE- AND MINIMUM-PROTECTION PHASES

(1) When the immobilization can be removed for exercise but weight bearing is still restricted, begin exercises to:

(a) Increase ROM of the ankle. This may include joint mobilization of any restricted ankle or foot joints and low-intensity open-chain muscle stretching, particularly of the gastrocnemius and soleus muscles.

(b) Increase strength of ankle musculature in an open-chain with multiple-angle isometrics, isotonic resistance exercises against elastic tubing (see Figs. 13–3, 13–4, and 13–5) or cuff weights around the forefoot, or isokinetic exercises. Start with short-arc exercises in a protected range and progress to full-arc exercises.

(c) Increase musculature endurance with bicycling or walking activities in a pool.

(2) When weight bearing is permissible, add exercises to:

(a) Improve balance, stability, and closed-chain lower extremity control by applying rhythmic stabilization exercises in standing (see Fig. 13–6) or by having the patient stand on a balance or BAPS board (see Fig. 13–7).

(b) Improve closed-chain eccentric strength of the plantarflexors with partial squatting activities, heel drops, and so on.

(c) Increase muscle flexibility, especially in the gastrocnemius and soleus muscles, by self-stretching on a wedge or against a wall.

(3) In the early stages of weight bearing after cast removal, the patient should wear a ½- to 1-inch heel lift to decrease stress on the Achilles tendon and decrease ground reaction forces during ambulation.

(4) As the patient prepares to return to full activity, add functional exercises such as toe walking, jogging, hopping, plyometric drills, and sport-specific training. Most patients can usually return to full activity by 6 to 9 months postoperatively.

VI. Exercises for Muscle Strength and Flexibility Imbalances

NOTE: Causes of strength and flexibility imbalances in the ankle and foot include disuse, immobilization, nerve injury, and progressive joint degeneration. In addition, imbalances occur from the weight-bearing stresses that are imposed on the feet. Imbalances can be the cause or the effect of faulty lower extremity mechanics. Because the lower extremities bear weight, realignment by strengthening exercises alone is of limited value. Strengthening exercises undertaken in conjunction with conscious correction, appropriate stretching, balance training, and other necessary measures (such as using orthotic inserts or adaptations for shoes, bracing, splinting, or surgery) improve alignment so that structurally safe weight bearing is possible. In addition, observation of the types of shoes and surfaces that the person uses for walking or sports activities may lead to the source of faulty mechanics, which can then be adjusted. (Techniques of orthopedic adaptations for shoes, bracing, and splinting are beyond the scope of this text.) When attempting to gain a balance of strength and flexibility of the muscles, use of progressive weight bearing is important to simulate functional activities.[9,26] For all exercises appropriate precautions should be followed as outlined in Chapters 3 through 7. These chapters also describe manual stretching and resistive techniques that may be appropriately used early in a rehabilitation program.

NOTE: Faulty foot postures such as *toeing in* or *pigeon-toed feet* may be due to internal rotation at the hips (anteversion), internal torsion of the tibia, or excessive adduction of the forefoot (metatarsus varus). *Toeing out* may be associated with external rotation of the hips (retroversion), external torsion of the tibia, or flat feet. The problems may be congenital or acquired and may or may not be correctable with stretching and training exercises.

A. Techniques for Self-Stretching of Tight Muscles

1. Self-stretching tight ankle plantarflexors

Precaution: When the patient uses weight-bearing exercises to stretch the plantarflexor muscles, shoes with arch supports should be worn or a folded washcloth can be placed under the medial border of the foot[31] to minimize the stress to the arches of the foot. To isolate the stretch force to the soleus, the knee is flexed. The two-joint gastrocnemius is stretched by maintaining the knee in extension while dorsiflexing the ankle.

a. Position of patient: long-sitting (knees extended). The patient strongly dorsiflexes the feet, attempting to keep the toes relaxed.

b. Position of patient: long-sitting. The patient places a towel or belt under the forefoot and pulls it dorsally.

c. Position of patient: sitting with the foot flat on the floor. The patient slides the foot backward, keeping the heel on the floor (see Fig. 12–7).

d. Position of patient: standing. The patient strides forward with one foot, keeping the heel of the back foot flat on the floor. To provide stability to the foot, the patient partially rotates the hind leg inward so the foot assumes a supinated position and locks the joints. He or she then shifts body weight forward onto the front foot (similar to Fig. 11–1). To stretch the gastrocnemius muscle, the patient keeps the knee of the back leg extended; to stretch the soleus, he or she flexes the knee of the back leg.

e. Position of patient: standing, facing a wall, with the hands placed against the wall at shoulder level. The patient leans into the wall, keeping heels on the floor. To increase the stretch force, increase the distance the feet are placed from the wall. Stretch either the gastrocnemius or the soleus muscle by keeping the knees extended or flexed, respectively.

f. Position of patient: standing on an inclined board with feet pointing upward and heels downward (Fig. 13–1). Greater stretch will occur if the patient leans forward. Because the body weight is on the heels there is little stretch on the long arches of the feet. Little effort is required to maintain this position for extended periods.

g. Position of patient: standing, with forefoot on the edge of a step or stool and heel over the edge. The patient slowly lowers the heel over the edge (heel drop).

Precaution: This stretch may create muscle soreness because it requires that the patient control an eccentric contraction of the plantarflexors.

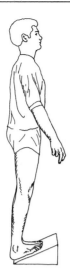

Figure 13–1. Self-stretching the ankle plantarflexor muscles.

2. Self-stretching the evertor muscles of the ankle and foot

a. Position of patient: sitting, with the foot to be stretched placed across the opposite knee. The patient uses the opposite hand and lifts the foot into inversion. Emphasize to the patient that the heel must be turned inward and to not twist only the forefoot (similar to the position in Fig. 2–34).

b. Position of patient: sitting or standing, with feet pointing forward. The patient rolls the weight to the lateral border of the feet. If possible, he or she walks a short distance on the lateral borders.

c. Position of patient: standing or walking, with the involved foot on a slanted board, placing the lateral aspect of the foot to be stretched on the lower side and the medial side of the foot on the top side of the board. Bilateral stretching can be accomplished if hinged planks are placed in an inverted-**V** position and the patient stands or walks on them.

3. Self-stretching the extrinsic muscles of the toes

a. Position of patient: sitting, with the foot crossed onto the opposite knee. The patient stabilizes the foot under the metatarsophalangeal (MTP) joints with the thumbs and passively flexes the MTP joints by applying pressure against the proximal phalages. Or he or she attempts active flexion of the MTP joints, assisting the motion if necessary.

b. Position of patient: standing,, with the toes over the edge of a stool or book. The MTP joints are at the edge. The patient attempts to flex the MTP joints, keeping the IP joints of the toes extended.

B. Techniques to Train and Strengthen Muscles Necessary for Postural Control of the Ankle and Foot

Most functional demands on the ankle and foot occur in weight-bearing postures. Kinesthetic input from skin, joint, and muscle receptors and the resulting joint and muscle responses are different in open and closed kinematic chain activities; therefore, whenever possible, lower extremity exercises should be progressed to closed-chain positions. In addition to the closed-chain exercises described in this section, refer to Chapter 11 for total lower extremity functional exercises.

1. **Training activities for muscle control**

    a. Position of patient: long-sitting. First the patient dorsiflexes and inverts the feet to emphasize the anterior tibialis muscles, then plantarflexes and inverts to emphasize the posterior tibialis muscles.

    b. Position of patient: sitting, with feet on the floor. The patient curls the toes against the resistance of the floor. A towel is placed under the feet, and he or she attempts to wrinkle it up by keeping the heel on the floor and flexing the toes. This may also be done with the patient standing.

    c. Position of patient: sitting, with feet on the floor. The patient attempts to raise the medial longitudinal arches while keeping the forefoot and hindfoot on the floor (lateral rotation of the tibia should occur but not abduction of the hips). The activity is repeated until the patient has good control, then progresses to performing the motion while standing.

    d. Position of patient: sitting, with both feet or just the involved foot on a rocker or balance board. The patient performs controlled ankle and foot motions (with or without the assistance of the normal foot) into dorsiflexion and plantarflexion and inversion and eversion (Fig. 13–2). If a disk is used, the patient can also perform circumduction in each direction. This activity is progressed to the standing position to further develop control and to develop balance.

    e. Patient practices walking, concentrating on the placement of the feet and the shifting of the body weight with each step. The patient begins by accepting the body weight on the heel, then shifts the weight along the lateral border of the foot to the fifth metatarsal head and across to the first metatarsal head and great toe for the push-off.

2. **Open-chain strengthening activities**

    a. Position of patient: sitting, with a tennis ball placed between the soles of the feet. The patient rolls the tennis ball back and forth from heel to forefoot.

    b. Position of patient: sitting. A number of small objects, such as marbles or dice, are placed to one side of the patient's foot. He or she picks up one object at a

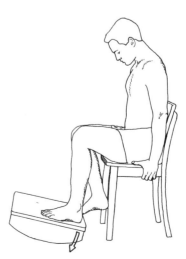

Figure 13–2. Using a rocker board to develop control of ankle motions with the patient sitting. When both feet are on the board, the normal foot can assist the involved side. With only the involved foot on the board, the activity is more difficult.

time by curling the toes around it and then places it in a container on the other side of the foot. This emphasizes the plantar muscles as well as inversion and eversion.

c. Position of patient: sitting, progressing to standing. Sand, foam, or other distensible material in a box can be used to offer resistance to the various foot motions as the patient rocks forward, backward, and side to side or curls the toes.

d. Position of patient: long-sitting, holding onto an elasticized material that is also placed under the forefoot. The patient plantarflexes the foot against the resistance (Fig. 13–3).

e. Position of patient: long- or short-sitting with ankles crossed. The patient presses the lateral borders of both feet together against each other and isometrically contracts the evertor muscles.

f. Position of patient: long-sitting or supine, with a loop of elasticized material placed around both feet. The patient everts one or both feet against the resistance (Fig. 13–4).

g. Position of patient: long-sitting or supine. An elasticized material is tied to the foot end of the bed (or other object) and is placed over the dorsum of the patient's foot. He or she then dorsiflexes against the resistance (Fig. 13–5).

3. Closed-chain strengthening and stabilization activities

Position of patient: standing. If the patient does not initially tolerate full weight bearing without reproduction of symptoms, begin with standing in the parallel bars or in a pool to reduce weight-bearing forces.

a. Begin developing isometric strength and control for stability. As the patient stands, apply resistance to the patient's pelvis while he or she attempts to maintain control (rhythmic stabilization). The resistance is applied in various directions, first with verbal cues, then without warning.

b. The patient and the therapist each hold onto a wooden dowel or cane with both hands. The therapist applies resistance through the rod in various directions as the patient attempts to remain stable (Fig. 13–6). Progress the patient to standing only on the involved foot.

c. For dynamic strength training the patient performs bilateral toe raises, heel raises, and rocking outward to the lateral borders of the feet; he or she then progresses to unilateral toe raises, heel raises, and lateral border standing. When tolerated, resistance is added with a weight belt or hand-held weights.

d. Training advances to walking on heels, toes, then lateral borders of the feet,

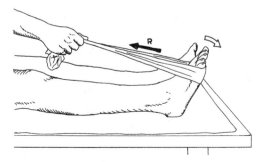

Figure 13–3. Resisting the ankle plantarflexor muscles with an elasticized material.

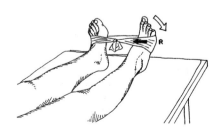

Figure 13–4. Resisting the evertor muscles of the foot with an elasticized material.

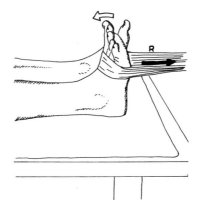

Figure 13–5. Resisting the ankle dorsiflexor muscles with an elasticized material.

progressively increasing the distance. For strengthening, the therapist applies resistance to the patient's pelvis.

4. Balance activities

Use a rocker board or balance board and have the patient shift the weight from side to side and front to back while attempting to control the ankle and maintain balance. A variety of commercial exercise boards are available with gradations in size of the rocker or half-sphere as well as adaptations for resistance. Gradations in difficulty can be adapted according to the patient's ability.

a. Position of patient: sitting. The patient begins sitting to learn to control the direction of motion of the board. (See Fig. 13–2.)

b. Position of patient: standing. If necessary, the patient is supported with both hands in the parallel bars or on a solid object. He or she begins with both feet on the board, then progresses to one-legged activities (Fig. 13–7). Additional

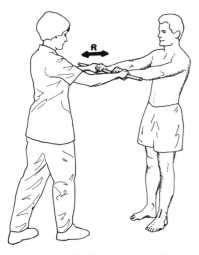

Figure 13–6. Rhythmic stabilization exercises with the patient standing and maintaining balance against the alternating resistance forces from the therapist. The therapist applies force through the rod in backward/forward, side-to-side, and rotation directions.

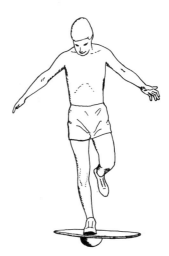

Figure 13–7. Advanced training for balance and coordination on a balance board requires that the patient not hold on while balancing with one leg.

progression would be to change the amount of motion allowed by the board by using a larger sphere or rocker, then balancing without hand support.

5. Stimulation and practice of functional activities

   a. Progress weight-bearing activities to walking on uneven surfaces, side-to-side weight shifting, walking on a balance beam, obstacle maneuvering, and agility drills.

   b. Develop endurance by increasing the amount of time spent performing the various drills.

   c. Develop power with plyometric drills such as jumping and hopping off boxes by increasing the velocity of movement.

   d. Using the principle of specificity of training, replicate whatever functional activity the individual requires, first in controlled patterns, then with increased speed and decreased control.

VII. Summary

The anatomy, joint characteristics, and functional relationships of joints and muscles of the ankle and foot have been briefly reviewed for background information in the first section of this chapter. Therapeutic exercise management of common musculoskeletal problems has been presented, including joint problems, sprains, minor tears, imbalances of muscle strength and flexibility, and muscle overuse syndromes. Exercise techniques for the ankle and foot not previously described in other chapters have been included. A discussion of total ankle joint replacement surgery, arthrodesis of several joints of the ankle and foot, excision arthroplasty for metatarsalgia, and repair of soft tissues have also been included in this chapter.

References

1. Bistevins, R: Footwear and footwear modifications. In Kottke, FJ, Stillwell, GK, and Lehmann, JF (eds): Krusen's Handbook of Physical Medicine and Rehabilitation, ed 3. WB Saunders, Philadelphia, 1982.
2. Cailliet, R: Foot and Ankle Pain, ed 2. FA Davis, Philadelphia, 1983.
3. Cyriax, J: Textbook of Orthopaedic Medicine, Vol 1. Diagnosis of Soft Tissue Lesions, ed 8. Bailliere Tindall, London, 1982.
4. DeLacerda, F: A study of anatomical factors involved in shinsplints. Journal of Orthopaedic and Sports Physical Therapy 2:55, 1980.
5. DeLacerda, F: Iontophoresis for treatment of shinsplints. Journal of Orthopaedic and Sports Physical Therapy 3:183, 1982.
6. Dimonte, P, and Light, H: Pathomechanics, gait deviations and treatment of the rheumatoid foot. Phys Ther 62:1148, 1982.
7. Donatelli, R, et al: Biomechanical foot orthotics: A retrospective study. Journal of Orthopaedic and Sports Physical Therapy 10:205, 1988.
8. Fortune, WP: Lower limb joint replacement. In Nickel, VL (ed): Orthopedic Rehabilitation. Churchill-Livingstone, New York, 1982.
9. Garn, SN, and Newton, RA: Kinesthetic awareness in subjects with multiple ankle sprains. Phys Ther 68:1669, 1988.
10. Gauffin, H, Trupp, H, and Odenieck, P: Effect of ankle disk training on postural control in patients with functional instability of the ankle joint. International Journal of Sports Medicine 9:141, 1988.
11. Greenfield, B: Evaluation of overuse syndromes in the lower extremities. In Donatelli, R (ed): Mechanics of the Foot and Ankle. FA Davis, Philadelphia, 1990.
12. Haslock, DI, and Wright, V: Footwear for arthritic patients. Arch Phys Med 10:236, 1970.
13. Hoppenfeld, S: Physical Examination of the Spine and Extremities: Appleton-Century-Crofts, New York, 1976.
14. Howell, DW: Therapeutic exercise and mobilization. In Hunt, GC (ed): Physical Therapy of the Foot and Ankle. Churchill-Livingstone, New York, 1988.
15. Hunter, SL: Rehabilitation of ankle injuries. In Prentice, WE (ed): Rehabilitation Techniques in Sports Medicine. Times Mirror/Mosby, St Louis, 1990.
16. Hyde, SA: Physiotherapy in Rheumatology. Blackwell Scientific Publications, Oxford, 1980.
17. Kapandji, IA: The Physiology of the Joints, Vol 11, ed 5. Churchill-Livingstone, Edinburgh, 1987.
18. Kaplan, EG, et al: A triligamentous reconstruction for lateral ankle instability. J Foot Surg 23:24, 1984.
19. Kaumeyer, G, and Malone, T: Ankle injuries: Anatomical and biomechanical considerations neces-

sary for the development of an injury prevention program. Journal of Orthopaedic and Sports Physical Therapy 1:171, 1980.

20. Kay, DB: The sprained ankle: Current therapy. Foot Ankle 6:22, 1985.

21. Kessler, R, and Hertling, D: Management of Common Musculoskeletal Disorders. Harper & Row, Philadelphia, 1983.

22. Kimura, IF, et al: Effect of the air stirrup in controlling ankle inversion stress. Journal of Orthopaedic and Sports Physical Therapy 9:190, 1987.

23. Kopell, H, and Thompson, W: Peripheral Entrapment Neuropathies, ed 2. Robert E Krieger, Huntington, NY, 1976.

24. Kramer, P: Restoration of dorsiflexion after injuries to the distal leg and ankle. Journal of Orthopaedic and Sports Physical Therapy 1:159, 1980.

25. Kuland, DN: The Injured Athlete. JB Lippincott, Philadelphia, 1988.

26. Lattanza, L, Gray, GW, and Kantner, R: Closed vs open kinematic chain measurements of subtalar joint eversion: Implications for clinical practice. Journal of Orthopaedic and Sports Physical Therapy 9:310, 1988.

27. Leach, RE, James, S, and Wasliewski, S: Achilles tendinitis. Am J Sports Med 9:93, 1981.

28. Lehmkuhl, LD, and Smith, LK: Brunnstrom's Clinical Kinesiology, ed 4. FA Davis, Philadelphia, 1983.

29. Lockard, MA: Foot orthoses. Phys Ther 68:1866, 1988.

30. McPoil, TG: Footwear. Phys Ther 68:1857, 1988.

31. McPoil, TG, and McGarvey, TC: The foot in athletics. In Hunt, GC (ed): Physical Therapy of the Foot and Ankle. Churchill-Livingstone, New York, 1988.

32. Moncur, C, and Shields, M: Clinical management of metatarsalgia in patients with arthritis. Clinical Management 3:7, 1983.

33. Mulligan, E: Lower leg, ankle and foot rehabilitation. In Andres, JR, and Harrelson, FL (eds): Physical Rehabilitation of the Injured Athlete. WB Saunders, Philadelphia, 1991.

34. Norkin, C, and Levangie, P: Joint Structure and Function: A Comprehensive Analysis, ed 2. FA Davis, Philadelphia, 1992.

35. Normal and Pathological Gait Syllabus. Physical Therapy Department, Rancho Los Amigos Hospital, Downey, CA, 1977.

36. Oatis, CA: Biomechanics of the foot and ankle under static conditions. Phys Ther 68:1815, 1988.

37. Opitz, JL: Reconstructive surgery of the extremities. In Kottke, FJ, Stillwell, GK, and Lehmann, JF (eds): Krusen's Handbook of Physical Medicine and Rehabilitation, ed 3. WB Saunders, Philadelphia, 1982.

38. Quillen, W: An alternative management protocol for lateral ankle sprains. Journal of Orthopaedic and Sports Physical Therapy 2:187, 1981.

39. Reynolds, NL, and Worrell, TN: Chronic Achilles peritendinitis: etiology, pathophysiology, and treatment. Journal of Orthopaedic and Sports Physical Therapy 13:717, 1991.

40. Salter, RB: Textbook of Disorders and Injuries of the Musculoskeletal System, ed 2. Williams & Wilkins, Baltimore, 1983.

41. Saltzman, CL, and Johnson, KA: Surgery of the foot and ankle. In Sledge, CB, et al (eds): Arthritis Surgery. WB Saunders, Philadelphia, 1994.

42. Samuelson, K, Tuke, M, and Freeman, MAR: A replacement arthroplasty for the three articular surfaces of the ankle, utilizing a posterior approach. J Bone Joint Surg Br 59:376, 1977.

43. Schnell, MD, Bowker, JH, and Bunch, WH: The orthotist. In Nickel, VL (ed): Orthopedic Rehabilitation. Churchill-Livingstone, New York, 1982.

44. Scholz, KC: Total ankle arthroplasty using biological fixation components compared to ankle arthrodesis. Orthopedics 10:125, 1987.

45. Schon, LC, and Ouzounian, TJ: The ankle. In James, MH (ed): Disorders of the Foot and Ankle. Medical and Surgical Management, ed 2. WB Saunders, Philadelphia, 1991.

46. Smith, CL: Physical therapy management of patients with total ankle replacement. Phys Ther 60:303, 1980.

47. Snook, GA: Lateral ankle reconstruction for chronic instability. In Torg, JS, Welsh, RP, and Shephard, RJ (eds): Current Therapy in Sports Medicine, ed 2. BC Decker, Toronto, 1990.

48. Stauffer, RN: Total ankle joint replacement. Arch Surg 112:105, 1977.

49. Sullivan, JM: Rupture of the Achilles tendon. In Torg, JS, Welsh, RP, and Shephard, RJ (eds): Current Therapy in Sports Medicine, ed 2. BC Decker, Toronto, 1990.

50. Thomas, WH: Surgery of the foot in rheumatoid arthritis. Orthop Clin North Am 6:831, 1975.

51. Thompson, TC, and Doherty, JH: Spontaneous rupture of tendon of Achilles: A new clinical diagnostic test. J Trauma 2:126–129, 1962.

52. Unger, AS, Inglis, AE, and Mow, CS: Total ankle arthroplasty in rheumatoid arthritis: A long-term follow-up study. Foot Ankle 8:173, 1988.

53. Wallace, L, Knortz, K, and Esterson, P: Immediate care of ankle injuries. Journal of Orthopaedic and Sports Physical Therapy 1:46, 1979.

54. Waugh, T: Arthroplasty rehabilitation. In Goodgold, J (ed): Rehabilitation Medicine. CV Mosby, St Louis, 1988.

55. Waugh, TR, and Evanski, PM: Irvine ankle arthroplasty: Prosthetic design and surgical technique. Clin Orthop 114:180, 1976.

The Spine: Acute Problems

In theory, treating musculoskeletal conditions of the spinal column and trunk is the same as treating musculoskeletal conditions of the extremities. The complex functional relationships of the facet joints, the intervertebral joints, the muscles, and the nervous system in the axial skeleton provide a challenge for the therapist in evaluation, assessment of the problems, and development of a therapeutic exercise program that deals with the problems. Often symptoms and testing procedures cannot point to one anatomic structure at fault or the symptoms are inconsistent with the apparent physical findings, leading to the dilemma of choosing the best treatment. Currently there is discussion in the literature regarding classification systems for spinal problems, whether to categorize patients based on pathology of anatomic structures[5,68] or based on categories such as symptoms[14] or occupational disability.[33,71] Because of the difficulty in establishing criteria for consistent classifications of patients, there have been few well-controlled research studies to substantiate valid and reliable treatment approaches.[56]

However, research has substantiated the healing process in tissues following injury. These basic principles are described in Chapter 7 and are used in designing programs for treating any musculoskeletal injury. The only complicating factor in the spine is the close proximity of key structures to the spinal cord and nerve roots. It is recognized that following a traumatic injury or repetitive microtrauma the tissues will react with inflammation and swelling. The constant pain from the chemical irritants and tissue distention and the limited motion from swollen tissue and muscle guarding are the same as in the extremities. Therefore, when signs of inflammation are present, the initial treatment approach is to decrease the effects of inflammation, relieve the stress on the inflamed tissues, and provide a healthy environment for the tissues to begin the healing process. Current thought is challenging the historical practice of complete bed rest for extended periods because of ensuing weakness and loss of tissue integrity.[49,57,59,67,71] Early, nondestructive motion results in earlier return to function and reduction in pain intensity.

Functional limitations and disabilities are not known at the time of injury. Usually 80 to 90 percent of acute injuries resolve within 1 month.[33] Disabilities will be dependent on the extent of the injury. If it involves the spinal cord, levels of complete paralysis may occur. If it involves the nerve roots (also the cauda equina), various amounts of muscle weakness in specific myotomes may occur, which may or may not interfere with the individual's daily personal and work-related activities. Upper quarter nerve roots will affect function of the arms and hands; lower quarter nerve roots will affect function of the lower extremities, especially in weight-bearing activities. Studies on chronic-pain syndromes as a result of back injuries seem to conclude that the degree of disability is related to psychologic, economic, and sociologic factors and prior incidence of injury more than the actual tissues involved.[21,33] A recent study in Norway documented that nerve root involvement and pain provocation with active movements in several directions were more common in patents who developed chronic pain.[21] Discussion of treatment for spinal cord injuries and chronic-pain syndromes is beyond the scope of this book.

Highlights of the anatomy and function of the spine are reviewed in the first section of this chapter. Defining basic skills of exercise intervention that the therapist should have to treat patients with acute spinal problems (other than spinal cord injuries) is the overall purpose of the remainder of this chapter. Every therapist should have basic skills in evaluating and identifying problems associated with the back; this chapter is based on the assumption that those skills have already been learned. Chapter 15 describes principles and techniques for treating postural faults and dysfunctions, including scoliosis, and for treating spinal conditions during the subacute healing and chronic rehabilitation phases of recovery. Principles and techniques of applying spinal traction are in Chapter 16.

OBJECTIVES

After studying this chapter, the reader will be able to:

1. Identify major components of spinal structure and function for review.
2. Describe functional spinal positions and how they relate to symptom control.
3. Describe intervertebral disk function and mechanical factors that influence it.
4. Establish a treatment program for managing disk lesions based on the patient's response to testing procedures.
5. Identify contraindications to movement during an acute disk lesion.
6. Describe the biomechanical relationship between the intervertebral disk and facet joints.
7. Establish treatment programs for managing acute joint, muscle, and soft tissue problems in the spinal region based on the problems identified.
8. Establish treatment programs for managing torticollis, tension headaches, and temporomandibular joint dysfunction.
9. Identify safe techniques to use to meet the goals of treatment during the acute stage.

I. Review of the Structure and Function of the Spine

A. Functional Units of the Spinal Column[12,25]

1. The anterior pillar, made up of the vertebral bodies and intervertebral disks, is the hydraulic, weight-bearing, shock-absorbing portion.
2. The posterior pillars, made up of the articular processes and facet joints, are the gliding mechanism for movement. Also part of the posterior unit are the two vertebral arches, two transverse processes, and a central posterior spinous process. Muscles attach to the processes from which they cause and control motion.

B. Structure and Function of the Intervertebral Disks[7,12,24,40,41]

1. The intervertebral disk, consisting of the annulus fibrosus and nucleus pulposus, is one component of a three-joint complex between two adjacent vertebrae.

2. The *annulus fibrosus* is made up of dense layers of collagen fibers and fibrocartilage. The collagen fibers in any one layer are parallel and angled around 60 to 65 degrees to the axis of the spine, with the tilt alternating in successive layers.[22,29] Because of the orientation of the fibers, tensile strength is provided by the annulus when the spine is compressed, twisted, or bent, which helps restrain the various spinal motions. The annulus is firmly attached to adjacent vertebrae, and the layers are firmly bound to one another. Fibers of the innermost layers blend with the matrix of the nucleus pulposus. The annulus fibrosus is supported by the anterior and posterior longitudinal ligaments.

3. The *nucleus pulposus* is a gelatinous mass that normally is contained within but whose loosely aligned fibers merge with the inner layer of the annulus fibrosus. It is located centrally in the disk, but in the lumbar spine, it is situated closer to the posterior border than the anterior border of the annulus. Aggregating proteoglycans, normally in high concentration in a healthy nucleus, have a great affinity for water. The resulting fluid mechanics of the confined nucleus functions to evenly distribute pressure throughout the disk and from one vertebral body to the next under loaded conditions. Because of the affinity for water, the nucleus imbibes water when pressure is reduced on the disk and water is squeezed out under compressive loads. These fluid dynamics provide transport for nutrients and help maintain tissue health in the disk.

4. The *cartilaginous end-plates* cover the nucleus pulposus superiorly and inferiorly and lie between the nucleus and vertebral bodies. Each one is encircled by the apophyseal ring of the respective vertebral body. The collagen fibers of the inner annulus fibrosus insert into the end-plate and angle centrally, thus encapsulating the nucleus pulposus. Nutrition diffuses from the marrow of the vertebral bodies to the disk via the end-plates.[50]

5. With flexion (forward bending) of a vertebral segment, the anterior portion of the disk is compressed and the posterior is distracted. The nucleus pulposus generally does not move in a healthy disk but may have a slight distortion with flexion, potentially to redistribute the load through the disk.[32] Asymmetric loading in flexion results in distortions of the nucleus toward the contralateral posterolateral corner, where the fibers of the annulus are more stretched.[2]

C. Physiologic Curves: Description and Function

1. Anterior curves are in the cervical and lumbar regions. **Lordosis** is a term also used to denote anterior curve, although some sources reserve the term lordosis to denote abnormal conditions such as those that occur with sway back.[15]

2. Posterior curves are in the thoracic and sacral regions. **Kyphosis** is a term used to denote a posterior curve. Kyphotic posture refers to an excessive posterior curving of the thoracic spine.[15]

3. The line of gravity transects the spinal curves, which are balanced anteriorly and posteriorly. Deviation of one portion of the spinal column results in shifting of another portion to compensate and maintain balance.

4. The flexibility of the curves gives the vertebral column 10 times the resistance to axial compression forces as that of a straight column.[25,72] Flexibility and balance in the spinal column are necessary to withstand the effects of gravity and other external forces.

D. Inert Structures Influencing Movement and Stability in the Spinal Column[12,25]

When a structure limits movement in a specific direction, it provides stability in that direction.

1. **The slant and direction of the articulating facets**

   a. In the cervical region, the facets are generally in the frontal plane, with some oblique angulation toward the transverse plane, allowing relatively free forward bending (flexion) and backward bending (extension). From the second cervical vertebra to the third thoracic vertebra, side bending and rotation of the vertebrae always occur together and are toward the same side whether in the upright position or in the forward-bent position.

   b. In the upper thoracic region, the facets are in the frontal plane with slight angulation toward the sagittal plane. In the lower thoracic region, they lie more in the sagittal plane. Rotation, side bending, and forward bending are allowed to various degrees by the facets but are restricted by the ribs. The facets markedly restrict backward bending along with the spinous processes. The upper three or four thoracic vertebrae function with the cervical spine on side bending and rotation. The remainder of the thoracic vertebrae function similar to the lumbar vertebrae so that when upright, side bending of the vertebrae results in vertebral rotation in the opposite direction for the vertebrae below the third thoracic level.

   c. In the lumbar region, the facets are typically in the sagittal plane with some curvature in the frontal plane, although variations in shape and orientation occur,[8,65] allowing some forward, backward, and side bending, but limiting rotation except in the lower lumbar segments. At the end of the range of forward bending, the facet surfaces in the frontal plane approximate and provides stability against further movement.[69] When upright, side bending occurs with rotation in opposite directions. When forward bent, side bending and rotation of the vertebrae occur together in the same direction.

2. **The ligaments[51]**

   a. The ligaments posterior to the axis of motion limit forward bending (flexion) of the spinal segments. Ligaments subjected to highest strains on forward bending are the interspinous and supraspinous ligaments. The capsular ligaments, ligamentum flavum, and posterior longitudinal ligament also become taut and stabilize the spine at the end of the flexion range.

   b. The anterior longitudinal ligament limits backward bending.

   c. The contralateral intertransverse ligaments, as well as ligamentum flavum and capsular ligaments, limit side bending.

   d. The capsular ligaments limit rotation.

3. **The thoracolumbar (lumbodorsal) fascia**

   a. The thoracolumbar fascia reinforces the posterior ligamentous system through the orientation of its fibers and attachments in the lumbar spine and pelvic region.

   b. Passive tension in the posterior layer of the fascia occurs with forward bending of the lumbar spine on the pelvis or posterior tilt of the pelvis. The increased tension supports the lower lumbar vertebrae by stabilizing against flexion moments.[8]

c. The thoracolumbar fascia also provides dynamic trunk stability in conjunction with its muscular attachments as described in Section E to follow.

4. The shape and slant of the spinous processes limit extension

5. The relative size of the intervertebral disk and bodies

The greater the ratio of disk thickness to vertebral body height, the greater the mobility. The cervical spine ratio is 2:5 and is most mobile; the thoracic ratio is 1:5 and is least mobile; the lumbar ratio is 1:3.[25]

6. The annulus fibrosus of the intervertebral disk

The organized concentric rings of the annulus provide tensile strength to the disk. Movement is allowed, yet some fibers will be taut, whichever direction the spinal column bends, twists, or shears, and therefore behave similar to ligaments.[8]

7. The ribs in the thoracic region

a. The ribs limit all motions of the thorax.
b. During side bending, the thorax is elevated and enlarged on the contralateral side (side of the convexity) and is compressed on the ipsilateral side.
c. During rotation, the ribs protrude posteriorly on the side on which the vertebral body rotates and are flattened on the contralateral side.

8. Muscles

Muscles with normal elasticity do not cause limitations to spinal movement. When tight, they restrict movement opposite to their direction of contraction. Muscles provide dynamic stability and control of the spine as described in the following section.

E. Muscle Function: Dynamic Stabilization in the Spinal Column

1. Eccentric control

Muscles of the neck and trunk primarily act as stabilizers (guy wires) of the spinal column in upright posture. They are the dynamic control against the force of gravity as the weight of various segments shifts away from the base of support.[36]

a. When the line of gravity shifts forward, control is provided by the extensor muscles. They are the erector spinae group and the posterior cervical muscles, including the upper trapezius.
b. When the line of gravity shifts backward, control is provided by the flexor muscles, which are the abdominal and intercostal muscles, as well as psoas major, longus colli, longus capitis, rectus capitis, anterior scalenes, and sternocleidomastoid.
c. When the line of gravity shifts laterally, the contralateral muscles provide control. They include the psoas major, quadratus lumborum, scalenes, sternocleidomastoid, erector spinae, internal and external obliques, and intercostal muscles.

2. Effect of poor postural support from trunk muscles

Little muscle activity is required to maintain upright posture, but with total relaxation of muscles the spinal curves become exaggerated and passive structural support is called on to maintain the posture.

a. When there is continued end-of-range loading, strain occurs with creep and fluid redistribution in the supporting tissues, making them vulnerable to injury.[67]

b. Continual exaggeration of the curves leads to faulty posture and muscle strength and flexibility imbalances as well as other soft tissue tightness or hypermobility.

c. Muscles that are habitually kept in a stretched position beyond the physiologic resting position tend to weaken; this is known as **stretch weakness.**[27]

d. Muscles kept in a habitually shortened position tend to lose their elasticity. These muscles test strong only in the shortened position but become weak as they are lengthened.[17] This is known as **tight weakness**.[23]

3. Effect of limb muscles on spinal stability

a. Without adequate stabilization of the spine, contraction of the limb-girdle musculature will transmit forces proximally and cause motions of the spine that will place excessive stresses on spinal structures and the supporting soft tissue. For example, stabilization of the pelvis and lumbar spine by the abdominal muscles against the pull of the iliopsoas muscle is necessary when flexing the hip to avoid increased lumbar lordosis and anterior shearing of the vertebrae. Stabilization of the ribs by the intercostal and abdominal muscles is necessary for an effective pushing force from the pectoralis major and serratus anterior muscles.

b. Localized fatigue in the stabilizing spinal musculature may occur in unconditioned individuals when a lot of repetitive activity or heavy exertion is done with the extremities. There is greater chance of injury in the supporting structures of the spine when the stabilizing muscles fatigue.

c. Imbalances in the flexibility and strength of hip, shoulder, and neck musculature will cause asymmetric forces on the spine.

4. Dynamic support for the lumbar spine and intervertebral disks[7,8,18–20,54,64,65,69]

a. The thoracolumbar (lumbodorsal) fascia consists of three layers of fascia and the aponeuroses of several muscles—the latissimus dorsi, serratus posterior inferior, internal obliques, and transverse abdominis (Fig. 14–1).

(1) The posterior layer of the fascia attaches to the spinous processes in a triangular pattern and covers the back muscles (Figs. 14–2A and B). It blends with the other layers of fascia at the *lateral raphe,* along the lateral border of the iliocostalis lumborum.

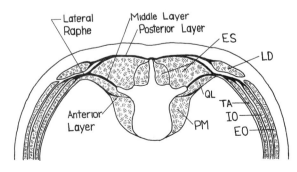

Figure 14–1. Transverse section in the lumbar region showing the relationships of the three layers of the thoracolumbar fascia to the muscles in the region and their attachments to the spine. ES = erector spinae; TA = transversus abdominus; IO = internal obliques; EO = external obliques; LD = latissimus dorsi; PM = psoas major; QL = quadratus lumborum muscles.

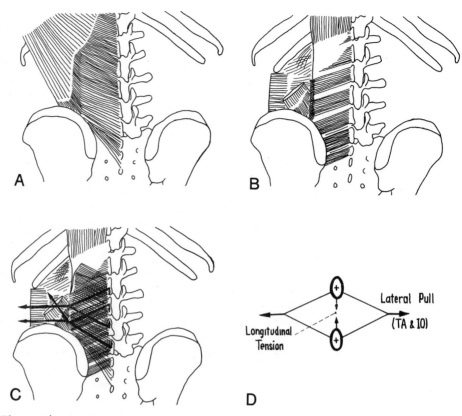

Figure 14–2. Orientation and attachments of the posterior layer of the thoracolumbar fascia. From the lateral raphe, (*A*) the fibers of the superficial lamina are angled inferiorly and medially and (*B*) the fibers of the deep lamina are angled superiorly and medially. (*C*) Tension in the angled fibers of the posterior layer of the fascia is transmitted to the spinous processes in opposing directions, resisting separation of the spinous processes. (*D*) Diagrammatic representation of a lateral pull at the lateral raphe, resulting in a tension between the lumbar spinous processes that oppose separation, thus creating an antiflexion moment. (*A, B,* and *C* adapted from Bogduck and MacIntosh,[7] pp 166–167, 169; *D* adapted from Gracovetsky, Farfan, and Helleur,[18] p 319.)

    (2) The middle layer is posterior to the quadratus lumborum and attaches to the tips of the transverse processes and intertransverse ligaments. Laterally, it blends with the lateral raphe and is continuous with the transversus abdominis. It, with the posterior layer, envelops the erector spinae muscles.

    (3) The anterior layer is a thin sheet anterior to the quadratus lumborum and attaches to the anterior aspect of the transverse processes and intertransverse ligaments.

  b. The muscle attachments are designed to converge forces via the fascia into the ligamentous system to provide stability and support as they function in the dynamics of the lumbar spine. Increased tension in or participation of any of the muscles attached to or surrounded by the fascia increases the support and equalizes forces at the lumbar spine.

    (1) Tension in the posterior layer of the fascia is transmitted upward and downward through the angled fibers, resulting in opposing vectors that re-

sist separation of the lumbar spinous processes, thus opposing any flexion moment (Figs. 14–2C and D).

(2) Because the posterior and middle layers of the thoracolumbar fascia envelop the erector spinae muscles of the lumbar spine, when these muscles contract, they expand against the fascial envelope, thereby increasing tension in the fascia. This creates a hydraulic amplifier mechanism (which is similar to filling a flexible tube with fluid, resulting in greater stability of the tube).[18] This increased fascial tension reinforces the back extensor muscles in countering the flexion moment on the spine during forward bending and extending against gravity.

(3) Contraction of the transversus abdominis and internal oblique muscles increases the intra-abdominal pressure. The increased intra-abdominal pressure pushes out against these muscles, increasing their tension and pull on the lateral raphe, which is transmitted to the angled fibers of the lumbodorsal fascia (Fig. 14–3).[20] This pressure mechanism, coupled with the pull of the muscles and increased tension in the lumbodorsal fascia, helps counter the flexion moment in the lumbar spine with lifting activities (see also Fig. 14–2C and D).

(4) Contraction of the latissimus dorsi with lifting activities results in the force being transmitted through the thoracolumbar fascia to reinforce the antiflexion moment of the fascia, thus providing additional support for the lumbar spine when bending and lifting.

(5) With flexion of the spine, the deep lamina of the posterior layer of the fascia becomes taut and thus supports the L-4 and L-5 vertebral segments via the attachments of the fascia from the spinous processes to the ilium. This is in addition to the ligamentous system supporting the entire lumbar spine.

5. Dynamic support for the head and cervical spine[55] (Fig. 14–4)

a. The fulcrum of the head on the spine is through the occipital/atlas joints. The center of gravity of the head is anterior to the joint axis and therefore has a flexion moment. The weight of the head is counterbalanced by the cervical extensor muscles.

b. The mandible is maintained in its resting position with the jaw partially closed through action of the mandible elevators (masseter, temporalis, and internal pterygoid muscles).

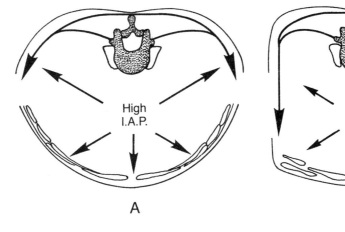

Figure 14–3. (A) Increased intra-abdominal pressure (IAP) pushes outward against the transversus abdominus and internal obliques, creating increased tension on the thoracolumbar fascia, resulting in an antiflexion moment. (B) Reduced pressure allows flexion of the spine. (Adapted from Gracovetsky,[20] p 114.)

High I.A.P.   Low I.A.P.

A   B

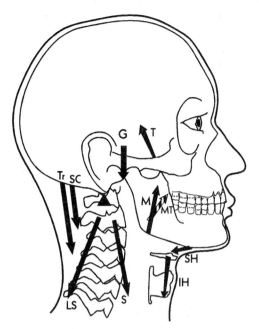

Figure 14–4. Head balance on the cervical spine. The posterior cervical muscles (trapezius and semispinalis capitis) counter the weight of the head. The mandibular elevating muscles (masseter, temporalis, and medial pterygoid) maintain jaw elevation opposing the mandibular depression force of gravity and tension in the anterior throat muscles (suprahyoid and infrahyoid groups). The scalene and levator muscles stabilize against the posterior and anterior translatory forces on the cervical vertebrae. (Tr = trapezius; SC = semispinalis capitis; M = masseter; T = temporalis; MT = medial pterygoid; SH = suprahyoid; IF = infrahyoid; S = scalene; LS = levator scapulae; G = center of gravity; ▲ = axis of motion.)

    c. The anterior throat muscles (suprahyoid and infrahyoid muscle groups) assist with swallowing and balancing the jaw against the muscles of mastication. These muscles also function to flex the neck when rising from the supine position. With a forward head posture, they tend to be stretched and weak so that the person lifts the head with the sternocleidomastoid muscles.

    d. The scalene and levator scapulae muscles act as guy wires to counterstabilize against the posterior and anterior translatory forces on the neck.

II. General Guidelines for Treating Acute Symptoms

When dealing with acute pain in the spine following trauma, fractures and instability must be ruled out before allowing movement. If these critical conditions are not present but there are symptoms of pressure against the spinal cord or a nerve root, the cause must be identified and treated. Causes of neurologic signs frequently seen by physical therapists include intervertebral disk protrusions, stenosis of the spinal canal or intervertebral foramina from bony impingement as a result of degenerative changes or from tissue inflammation, and nerve root entrapment. Whether the patient has symptoms of pain or has positive neurologic signs, if positioning or movement reduces the pressure against the involved tissue, mechanical techniques are attempted to treat the problem. If a disk lesion is the cause of the acute episode of back pain, treatment techniques are directed toward managing this structure first.

A. Establish a Position of Symptom Relief or Comfort

If a patient is experiencing acute inflammation from a traumatic injury, there will be constant pain, yet often an optimal position of comfort or symptom reduction can be determined in which there is the least amount of stress on the inflamed, irritated, or swollen region. The term **functional position** or **functional range** is used to describe this position.[47] The functional range may change for the individual as the tissues heal and the person gains mobility and strength in the region. Some of the pathologic conditions typically tend to cause symptoms in one portion of the range and are relieved in another range.[47] The following terms have been popularized based on the work of Morgan[47] and Saal and Saal.[60]

1. **Extension bias**[9]

The patient's symptoms are lessened in positions of extension (lordosis). Sustained flexed postures or repetitive flexion motions load the anterior disk region and facet joints, causing fluid redistribution from the compressed areas and swelling and creep in the distended areas. This is frequently the mechanism of symptom production in posterior or posterolateral intervertebral disk lesions or injury to the posterior longitudinal ligament. Whether the pathology is an injured disk or stressed and swollen tissues, repeated extension motions and positions relieve the symptoms by massaging the swollen tissues and moving the fluid to reverse the stasis (these techniques are described in Section III under disk lesions).

2. **Flexion bias**[9]

The patient's symptoms are lessened in positions of spinal flexion and provoked in extension. This is often the case when there is compromise of the intervertebral foramen or spinal canal, as in bony spinal stenosis, spondylosis, and spondylolisthesis.

3. **Non–weight-bearing bias**

The patient's symptoms are lessened when in non–weight-bearing positions such as when lying down or in traction or when reducing spinal pressure by leaning on the upper extremities (using arm rests to unweight the trunk), when leaning the trunk against a support, or when in a pool. The condition is considered *gravity sensitive*[9] because the symptoms are worsened when standing, walking, running, coughing, or similar activities that increase spinal pressure.

B. Initial Treatment

A trial treatment is given using either an extension approach, flexion approach, or non–weight-bearing approach. Usually the trial treatment begins with repeated extension motions (described in Section III).[59] Use of modalities and massage to decrease pain and swelling from the acute symptoms is appropriate during the acute stage. Nondestructive movement in the pain-free range may be appropriate if it does not exacerbate the symptoms. Specific techniques for various tissues or biases are described in the following sections.

C. Patient Education and Involvement With Acute Care

1. The patient is taught to identify and assume the spinal position that is most comfortable and reduces the symptoms by using pelvic tilts for lumbar spine positioning and head nods and chin tucks for cervical spine positioning. Corsets or cervical collars are used to provide support during the acute stage if necessary. The patient is taught how to use *passive positioning* to help maintain the functional position during the acute stage.
   a. When supine, hook lying flexes the spine; legs extended extends the spine. A pillow under the head flexes the neck; a small roll under the neck stabilizes a mild lordosis with the head neutral.

b. When prone, use of a pillow under the abdomen flexes the spine; no pillow extends the spine. To maintain the cervical spine in neutral alignment, a small towel roll is placed under the forehead so the patient does not turn the head.

c. Sitting usually causes spinal flexion, especially if the hips and knees are flexed. To emphasize flexion, prop the feet up on a small footstool to increase hip flexion; to emphasize extension, use a lumbar pillow or support in the low-back region. To unweight the spine, rest the arms on an arm rest or use a reclining chair.

d. Standing usually causes spinal extension; to emphasize flexion, stand with a small stool under one of the feet.

2. If tolerated, the patient is taught to perform simple movements while protecting the spine in the functional position.

a. Gentle pelvic tilting or chin tucks are taught in every position tolerated by the patient, including supine, prone, side-lying, sitting, and standing. The patient learns how much motion he or she can do without causing increased symptoms.

b. The patient is made aware of the effect of arm and leg motions on the position of the spine. Every time the arms reach overhead or the lower extremities extend, the back extends; every time the extremities are brought closer to the front of the body, the back flexes. These gentle extremity motions are practiced so that the patient can feel what is happening to the spine and can learn to avoid motions (during the acute stage) that exacerbate the symptoms. In the subacute stage, the patient is taught to control the spinal position while doing the extremity motions.

c. The patient is taught to use the "logroll" technique to turn from supine to side-lying to prone and return. The patient practices maintaining spinal alignment by keeping the shoulders aligned with the pelvis while rolling the trunk over as a unit (a log) and not twisting the spine.

d. The patient is taught to sit from the lying position by logrolling on to the side, pushing the body up with the hands while bringing the legs forward over the side of the bed. While moving through the sitting-up pattern, emphasis is placed on keeping the back in lordosis if there is an extension bias or in flexion if there is a flexion bias.

e. The patient is taught to go from standing to sitting and the reverse with spinal control. He or she first finds the functional position, then flexes or extends at the hips while maintaining the spinal position. The trunk moves as a whole.

3. Any special precautions for the condition are reviewed with the patient. Condition-specific precautions are described in the following sections.

III. Intervertebral Disk and Flexion Load Lesions

A. Injury and Degeneration of the Disk[1,2,10,16,22,24,37]

1. Fatigue loading and traumatic rupture

Breakdown in the annulus fibrosus may occur with fatigue loading over time or with traumatic rupture.[1,2]

a. Fatigue breakdown usually occurs with repeated overloading of the spine in flexion with asymmetric forward bending and torsional stresses.[1,2,16,29]

b. With torsional stresses, the annulus becomes distorted, most obviously at the posterolateral corner opposite the direction of rotation. The layers of the outer annulus fibrosus lose their cohesion and begin to separate from each other.

Each layer then acts as a separate barrier to the nuclear material. Eventually, radial tears occur and there is communication of the nuclear material between the layers.[16]

c. With repeated forward bending and lifting stresses, the layers of the annulus are strained; they become tightly packed together in the posterolateral corners, radial fissures develop, and the nuclear material migrates down the fissures.[1,2] Outer layers of annular fibers can contain the nuclear material as long as they remain a continuous layer.[1] Following injury, there is a tendency for the nucleus to swell and distort the annulus. Distortion is more severe in the region where the annular fibers are stretched.[2,37] If the outer layers rupture, the nuclear material may extrude through the fissures.

d. Healing is attempted, but there is poor circulation in the disk. There may be self-sealing of a defect with the nuclear gel[41] or proliferation of cells of the annulus to seal the defect.[37] Any fibrous repair is weaker than normal and takes a long time because of the relative avascular status of the disk.

e. Traumatic rupture of the annulus can occur as a one-time event or can be superimposed on a disk where there has been gradual breakdown of the annular rings. This is seen most commonly in traumatic hyperflexion injuries.[2]

2. Axial overload

Axial overload of the disk usually results in end-plate damage or vertebral body fracture before there is any damage to the annulus fibrosus.[40]

3. Age

Individuals are most susceptible to symptomatic disk injuries between the ages of 30 and 45 years. During this time, the nucleus is still capable of imbibing water, but the annulus weakens from fatigue loading over time and, therefore, is less able to withstand increased pressures when there are disproportionately high stresses. The nuclear material may protrude into the tears of fissures, which most commonly are posterolateral and, with increased pressures, may bulge against the outer annular fibers, causing an annular distortion; or the nuclear material may extrude from the disk through complete fissures in the annulus.[1,16]

4. Degenerative changes

Any loss of integrity of the disk from infection, disease, herniation, or an end-plate defect becomes a stimulus for degenerative changes in the disk.[37]

a. Degeneration is characterized by progressive fibrous changes in the nucleus, loss of the organization of the rings of the annulus fibrosus, and loss of the cartilaginous end-plates.[37]

b. As the nucleus becomes more fibrotic, it loses its capacity to imbibe fluid. Water content decreases and there is an associated decrease in the size of the nucleus.[38] Acute disk protrusions caused by a bulging nucleus pulposus against the annulus or extrusions of the nucleus through a torn annulus are rare in older people.

c. It is possible to have protrusions of the annulus fibrosus without nuclear pressure. Myxomatous degeneration with annular protrusion has been demonstrated in disk lesions in older people.[73]

5. Effect on spinal mechanics

Injury or degeneration of the disk affects spinal mechanics in general.[52] Initially there is increased mobility of the segment with greater than normal flexion-extension and forward and backward sliding of the vertebral body.[40] Force distribution through the entire segment is altered, causing abnormal forces in the facets and supporting structures[11,16,32] (see Section IV.B).

B. Related Diagnoses

Disk protrusions (derangements), tissue fluid stasis, diskogenic pain, and swelling from inflammation are conditions that may occur from prolonged flexion postures, repetitive flexion microtrauma, or traumatic flexion injuries. Initially symptoms may be exacerbated when attempting extension but then may be decreased when using carefully controlled extension motions. Several studies have documented that patients with herniated nucleus pulposus who have symptom reduction with an extension approach to treatment respond favorably to the conservative nonsurgical treatment.[3,30]

1. Diskogenic pain[61]

Symptoms may be from early stages of disk degeneration or possibly from a compression fracture of the end-plate of the vertebral body. Pain occurs without nerve root involvement, although there may be referred pain into the extremities.

2. Disk protrusions (derangements)[40]

a. Disk protrusion

Any change in the shape of the annulus that causes it to bulge beyond its normal perimeter.

b. Disk herniation

(1) Prolapse

A protrusion of the nucleus that is still contained by the outer layers of the annulus and supporting ligamentous structures.

(2) Extrusion

A protrusion in which the nuclear material ruptures through the outer annulus and lies under the posterior longitudinal ligament.

(3) Free sequestration

The extruded nucleus has moved away from the prolapsed area.

NOTE: Various authors use these terms differently. The above descriptions are from MacNab.[40] Bogduk[8] defines **prolapse** as a frank rupture of nuclear material into the vertebral canal and **herniation** as the nuclear material being partially expelled into the canal with the majority remaining in a defect in the annulus.

3. Tissue fluid stasis

With sustained flexed postures in the spine, the disks, facet joints, and ligaments are placed under sustained load. The intradiskal pressure increases, and there is compression loading on the cartilage of the facets and a distractive tension on the posterior longitudinal ligament and posterior fibers of the annulus fibrosus. Creep and fluid transfer occur. Sudden movement into extension does not allow for redistribution of the fluids and increases the vulnerability of the distended tissue to injury and inflammation.[67] Symptoms may be similar to those described as disk lesions because they lessen with repeated extension motions and respond to treatment described in the following sections.

C. Signs and Symptoms of Disk Lesions

1. Etiology of Symptoms

a. The disk is largely aneural; not all disk protrusions are symptomatic.

b. Symptoms of pain arise from pressure of the protrusion against pain-sensitive structures (ligaments, dura mater, and blood vessels around nerve roots).

c. Neurologic signs arise from pressure against the spinal cord or nerve roots. The only true neurologic signs are specific motor weaknesses and specific dermatome sensory changes. (Radiating pain in a dermatomal pattern, increased myoelectrical activity in the hamstrings, decreased straight-leg raising, and depressed deep tendon reflexes can also be associated with referred pain stimuli from spinal muscles, interspinous ligaments, the disk, and facet joints and, therefore, are not true signs of nerve root pressure.[13,26,44]

d. Symptoms are variable depending on the degree and direction of the protrusion as well as the spinal level of the lesion.

   (1) Posterior or posterolateral protrusions are most common.

   (2) With a small posterior or posterolateral lesion, there may be pressure against the posterior longitudinal ligament or against the dura mater or its extensions around the nerve roots. The patient may describe a severe mid-line backache or pain spreading across the back into the buttock and thigh.

   (3) A large posterior protrusion may cause spinal cord signs such as loss of bladder control and saddle anesthesia.

   (4) A large posterolateral protrusion may cause partial cord or nerve root signs.

   (5) An anterior protrusion may cause pressure against the anterior longitudinal ligament, resulting in back pain. There may be no neurologic signs.

e. Symptoms may shift if there is integrity of the annular wall, because the hydrostatic mechanism is still intact.[42]

f. Contents of the nucleus pulposus in the neural canal may cause an inflammatory reaction and irritate the dural sac, its nerve root sleeves, or the nerve roots. The symptoms may persist for extended periods and are not responsive to purely mechanical changes. The back pain may be worse than leg pain on the straight-leg-raising test. Poor resolution of this inflammatory stimulus may lead to fibrotic reactions and chronic pain.[39,58,60] Early medical intervention with anti-inflammatory agents is usually necessary.[60]

2. Onset and behavior of symptoms[28,40,42]

a. Onset is usually between 20 and 55 years of age but most frequently from mid 30s through 40s.

b. Except in cases of trauma, symptomatic onset is usually associated simply with bending, bending and lifting, or attempting to stand up after having been in a prolonged sitting or forward-bent posture. The person may or may not have the sensation of something tearing.

c. Many patients have a predisposing history of a faulty flexion posture (flat-back or forward-head postures; see Chapter 15).

d. Pain may increase gradually when the person is inactive, such as when sitting or after a night's rest. The patient often describes the onset of pain as when attempting to get out of bed in the morning.

e. With a posterior or posterolateral protrusion, symptoms are usually aggravated with activities that increase the intradiskal pressure, such as sitting, forward bending, coughing, or straining or when attempting to stand after being in a flexed position. Usually, symptoms are lessened when walking.

f. During the acute phase, the pain is almost always present but varies in intensity, depending on the person's position or activity.

g. The most common levels of protrusion are the segments between the fourth and fifth lumbar vertebrae and between the fifth lumbar vertebra and sacrum.

h. Initially, discomfort is noticed in the lumbosacral or buttock region. Some patients experience aching that extends into the thigh. Numbness or muscle weakness (neurologic signs) are not noted unless the protrusion has progressed to a degree in which there is nerve root, spinal cord, or cauda equina compression.

3. **Objective clinical findings**[28,42]

NOTE: The following information relates to a contained posterior or posterolateral nuclear protrusion in the lumbar spine. For the less frequently seen anterior protrusion, see the brief description in Section H.4.

a. The patient usually prefers standing and walking to sitting.

b. The patient may have a decrease in or loss of lumbar lordosis and may have some lateral shifting of the spinal column.

c. Forward bending is limited. When repeating the forward-bending test, the symptoms increase or peripheralize. *Peripheralization* means the symptoms are experienced farther down the leg.

d. Backward bending is limited; when repeating the backward-bending test, the pain lessens or centralizes. *Centralization* means the symptoms recede up the leg or become localized to the back. Important exceptions are[42]:

   (1) If there is a lateral shift of the spinal column, backward bending increases the pain. If the lateral shift is first corrected (see Section H.2.b), then repeated backward bending lessens or centralizes the pain.

   (2) If the protrusion cannot be mechanically reduced, backward bending peripheralizes or increases the symptoms.

   (3) If there is an anterior protrusion, backward bending increases the pain and forward bending relieves the pain.

e. Testing passive lumbar flexion when in the supine position and passive extension when in the prone position usually produces signs similar to those of the standing tests, but results may not be as dramatic because gravity is eliminated.

f. Pain between 30 and 60 degrees of straight-leg raising is considered positive for interference of dural mobility but not pathognomonic for a disk protrusion.[28,70]

g. A contained nuclear protrusion can be influenced by movement because the hydrostatic mechanism is still intact. An extruded or sequestrated nucleus with a complete annular tear disrupts the hydrostatic mechanism and cannot be influenced by movement.[42]

D. Principles of Treatment[24,28,48]

1. Effects of postural changes and activities

Relative changes in posture and activities affect intradiskal pressure. When compared with standing, intradiskal pressure is least when lying supine, increases by almost 50 percent when sitting with hips and knees flexed, and almost doubles if leaning forward while sitting.[24,48] Sitting with a back rest inclination of 120 degrees and lumbar support 5 cm in depth provides the lowest load to the disk while sitting.[4,28] Therefore, sitting with the hips and knees flexed or leaning forward should be avoided in acute disk lesions. If sitting is necessary, there should be support for the lumbar spine with the trunk reclined 120 degrees.

2. Effects of fluid stasis and inhibition

When a person is lying down, compression forces to the disk are reduced, and with time, the nucleus potentially can absorb more water to equalize pressures. Then, upon rising, body weight compresses the disk with the increased fluid, and intradiskal pressure greatly increases. The pain or symptoms from a protrusion are accentuated. To avoid exacerbating symptoms, absolute bed rest during the acute phase should be avoided. Bed rest during the first 2 days when symptoms are highly irritable is needed to promote early healing, but it should be interspersed with short intervals of standing, walking, and appropriately controlled movement.[71]

3. Effects of prolonged traction

The phenomenon of imbibition during reduced pressures also occurs during periods of prolonged traction or with postures of prolonged flexion. Therefore, static traction of longer than 10 minutes should not be used during the acute stage (see Chapter 16). Similarly, sustained bed positioning with lumbar flexion should be avoided unless it is the only position that decreases symptoms.

4. Effects of flexion and extension

Rest in a slightly forward-bent position often lessens pain because of the space potential for the nucleus. The patient may also deviate laterally to minimize pressure against a nerve root. Movement into extension initially causes increased symptoms. In acute disk lesions in which there is protective lateral shifting and lumbar flexion, techniques that cause lateral shifting of the spine opposite to the deviation followed by passive spinal extension to mechanically compress the protrusion and shift it anteriorly have been found to relieve the clinical signs and symptoms.[30,42,43]

5. Effects of isometric activities

Isometric activities (resisted pelvic tilt exercises, straining, Valsalva maneuver) as well as active back flexion or extension exercises increase intradiskal pressures above normal and, therefore, *must be avoided* during the acute stage.

6. Effects of muscle splinting

Reflex muscle splinting often accompanies an acute disk lesion and adds to the compressive forces. Modalities and gentle oscillatory traction to the spine may help decrease the splinting (see Chapter 16).

E. Acute Impairments/Problems Summarized

1. Pain from protrusion against a pain-sensitive structure and accompanying protective muscle spasm
2. Neurologic signs only if protrusion is against nerve root or spinal cord
3. Abnormal spinal posture and intradiskal pressure
4. Peripheralization of symptoms with repeated forward bending or sustained flexion
5. May have limited straight-leg raising (SLR)

F. Functional Limitations/Disabilities

With proper healing and safe progression through rehabilitation, there should be no long-term disabilities. Short-term functional limitations may include:
1. Inability to sustain flexed postures or sit for extended periods

2. Inability to stoop, squat, or lift objects over 10 lb
3. With neurologic involvement, may affect lower extremity strength and ambulation

G. General Treatment Goals and Plan of Care During Acute Phase

Goals

1. Relieve pain and promote muscle relaxation.

2. Relieve swelling and pressure against pain-sensitive or neurologic structures.

3. Educate the patient.

Plan of Care

1. Rest interspersed with periods of controlled movement.
   Modalities, massage, traction.

2. Motions that decrease the size and effect of the swollen disk or ligaments (trial of repeated extension).
   Avoid positions, exercises, and activities that increase intradiskal pressure (flexion).

3. Teach self-management.
   Posture control.
   Safe positions and movement patterns.

Precautions and Contraindications

a. A patient with acute pain in the spinal region that is not influenced by changing the patient's position or by movement must be screened by a physician for signs of serious pathology.

b. Any movement that peripheralizes the symptoms signals a movement that is contraindicated during the acute and early subacute period of treatment. Peripheralization with extension motions may indicate stenosis, large lateral disk protrusion, or pathology in a posterior element.[59]

c. Extension of the spine is contraindicated[42]:
   (1) When no position or movement decreases or centralizes the described pain
   (2) When saddle anesthesia and/or bladder weakness is present
   (3) When a patient is in such extreme pain that he or she rigidly holds the body immobile with any attempted correction

d. Flexion of the spine should be avoided:
   (1) When extension relieves the symptoms
   (2) When flexion movements increase the pain or peripheralize the symptoms

e. Any form of exercise or activity that increases intradiskal pressure, such as the Valsalva maneuver, active pelvic tilt, or trunk-raising exercises, should be avoided during this stage.

H. Techniques to Mechanically Reduce a Nuclear Disk Protrusion or Swollen Tissues in the Lumbar Spine

NOTE: These techniques are used only if the test movements have shown that the postures and movements used improve the symptoms.[28,42] If no test movements decrease the symptoms, this mechanical approach to treatment should not be used.

1. Severe symptoms

If symptoms are severe, bed rest is indicated with short periods of walking at regular intervals. Walking usually promotes lumbar extension and stimulates fluid mechanics to help reduce swelling in the disk or connective tissues. The patient should use crutches, if he or she cannot stand upright, to help relieve the increased pressure of the forward-bent posture.[28]

2. Posterior or posterolateral protrusion

If repeated flexion test movements increase the symptoms and if repeated extension test movements decrease or centralize the symptoms, all flexion activities should be avoided during this phase of treatment. Treatment begins with:

a. *Passive extension*

(1) Position of patient: prone. If the flexion posture is severe, place pillows under the abdomen for support. Gradually increase the amount of extension by removing the pillows, and then progress by having the patient prop himself or herself up on the elbows, allowing the pelvis to sag (Fig. 14–5). When propping, pillows placed under the thorax help take strain off the shoulders. Wait 5 to 10 minutes between each increment of extension to allow for reduction of water content and size of the bulge. There should be an accompanying centralization of or decrease in symptoms. Progress to having the patient prop himself or herself up on the hands, allowing the pelvis to sag (see Fig. 15–8A).

(2) If the sustained postures are not well tolerated, have the patient perform passive lumbar extension intermittently by repeating the *prone press-ups* (same end position as Fig. 15–8A) rather than just propping up.

Precaution: Carefully monitor the patient's experience of symptoms. Symptoms should lessen in the thigh and buttock, but they may increase in the low back (centralize). If the symptoms progress down the leg (peripheralize), immediately stop the exercises and reassess.[42]

b. *Lateral shift correction*

If the patient has lateral shifting of the spine (Fig. 14–6), extension alone will not reduce the nuclear protrusion until the shift is corrected. Once the shift is corrected, the patient must extend as in (a) above to maintain the correction. Methods to correct the shift include the following:

(1) The therapist stands on the side to which the thorax is shifted and places his or her shoulder against the patient's elbow (which is flexed against the rib cage). The therapist then wraps his or her arms around the patient's pelvis on the opposite side and simultaneously pulls the pelvis toward him or her while pushing the patient's thorax away (Fig. 14–7). This is a gradual maneuver. Continue with the lateral shifting if centralization of the pain occurs.[43] If there is overcorrection, the pain and lateral shift may move to the contralateral side. It is corrected by shifting the thorax back. The purpose is to centralize the pain and correct the lateral shift. Once the shift is corrected, immediately have the patient backward bend (see Fig. 15–8B). Again, allow time. Progress to passive extension with prone propping and prone press-ups as previously described.

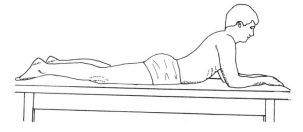

Figure 14–5. Passive lumbar extension accomplished by having the patient prop up the elbows.

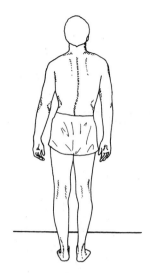

Figure 14–6. Patient with lateral shift of the thoracic cage toward the right. The pelvis is shifted toward the left.

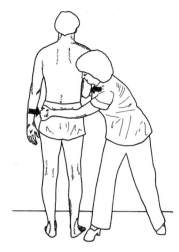

Figure 14–7. A lateral gliding technique used to correct a lateral shift of the thorax is applied against the patient's elbow and thoracic cage as the pelvis is pulled in the opposite direction.

(2) Alternate method

Place the patient in a side-lying position, with the side to which the thorax is shifted placed downward. A small pillow or towel roll is placed under the thorax. The patients remains in this position until the pain centralizes, then rolls prone and begins passive extension with prone propping and prone press-ups.

(3) Alternate method

With the patient prone, the therapist attempts to manually side-glide the thorax and pelvis toward the mid-line. The forces are in equal and opposite directions. Once the symptoms centralize, begin passive extension with prone propping and prone press-ups.

3. Patient education

a. Help the patient recognize what positions and motions increase or decrease the pain or symptoms by practicing them under supervision.

b. Instruct the patient to frequently repeat the extension activities, with lateral shift correction, if necessary, during the first couple of days.

(1) To teach *self-correction of the lateral shift*, the patient places the hand on the side of the shifted rib cage on the lateral aspect of the rib cage and places the other hand over the crest of the opposite ilium. He or she then gradually pushes these regions toward the mid-line and holds (Fig. 14–8). Eventually, he or she can voluntarily correct the shift.

(2) If appropriate, the patient could also be instructed to correct the shift by side-lying or prone-lying as previously described.

c. Caution the patient that if pain worsens or peripheralizes when exercising, he or she must immediately stop the activity.

d. Instruct the patient to maintain an extended posture with passive support while the lesion is healing.

(1) The patient should sit with lumbar support. This could be a towel roll or

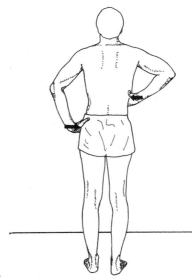

Figure 14–8. Self-correction of a lateral shift.

lumbar pillow. This is especially important when riding in a car or sitting in a soft chair.

(2) When going to bed, he or she should pin a towel, folded lengthwise four times, around the waist.

e. Instruct the patient to avoid flexion activities, lifting, or any other functions that increase intradiskal pressure while symptoms are acute.

f. Teach safe movement patterns to protect the back as described in Section II.

4. Anterior protrusion

If repeated flexion tests decrease the symptoms and repeated extension tests increase the symptoms and if the patient demonstrates an accentuated lordosis that came on suddenly, treatment begins with[42]:

a. *Correction of a lateral shift if present*

Position of patient: standing and placing the leg opposite the shift on a chair so the hip is in about 90 degrees of flexion. The leg on the side of the lateral shift is kept extended. The patient then flexes the trunk onto the raised thigh and applies pressure by pulling on the ankle (Fig. 14–9). Repeat several times but not to the point that the symptoms shift to the opposite side.

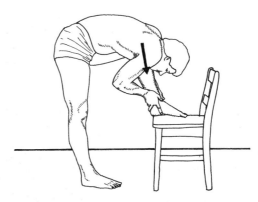

Figure 14–9. Self-correction of a lateral shift when there is deviation of the trunk as it flexes.

b. *Passive flexion*

Position of patient: supine. When no lateral shift is present, the patient brings both knees to the chest and holds this position with the arms around the thighs for several minutes (see Fig. 15–5). He or she can lower the legs partway down and pull them back up to the chest in an intermittent rhythm to create a slow, oscillating motion in the spine. Progress after several days to flexion of the spine when sitting and standing.

NOTE: Patients with symptoms of nerve root compression from causes other than nuclear protrusion, such as spinal stenosis or spondylosis, may also benefit from passive flexion exercises to relieve the symptoms because flexion of the spine widens the foramina.

5. Traction

Traction may be tolerated by the patient during the acute stage and has the benefit of widening the disk space and possibly reducing the nuclear protrusion by decreasing the pressure on the disk or by placing tension on the posterior longitudinal ligament[63] (see Chapter 16).

a. Time of the traction should be short; osmotic forces soon equalize. Then upon release of the traction force, there could be an increase in the disk pressure, leading to increased pain.
   (1) Less than 15 minutes of intermittent traction
   (2) Less than 10 minutes of sustained traction
b. High poundage; greater than half the patient's body weight is necessary for separation of the lumbar vertebrae.
c. If there is complete relief initially, often there will be an exacerbation of symptoms later.

I. Subacute Healing Phase of a Disk Lesion

Usually the acute symptoms decrease in 4 to 6 days and the patient learns to control the symptoms.

1. Teach simple spinal movements in pain-free ranges using gentle pelvic tilts. The patient is taught to be aware of how far forward and backward he or she can rock the pelvis and move the spine without increasing symptoms. The pelvic rocking is done supine, sitting, in the hand-knee all-fours position, prone-lying, side-lying, and standing. It is important to stay within the patient's ability to control the symptoms. Finish all exercise routines with the pelvis tilted anteriorly and the spine in extension.
2. Teach the patient how to set the abdominal and back extensor muscles to maintain control of the extended spinal position while performing simple extremity motions. It is important to caution against holding the breath and causing the Valsalva maneuver in order to not excessively increase the intradiskal pressure.
3. Encourage activities within the tolerance of the individual, such as walking or swimming.
4. Initiate passive straight-leg raising to maintain mobility in the nerve roots of the lumbar spine.

J. Management When Disk Symptoms Have Stabilized

1. Signs of improvement

Improvement is noted with loss of spinal deformity, increased motion in the back, and negative dural mobility signs.[28] Loss of back pain with increased true neurologic signs is an indication of worsening. The patient is tested to determine whether the symptoms have stabilized by performing repeated flexion and extension tests with the patient standing, then lying supine and prone as done initially. The tests may be positive for dysfunction (tightness, tension) but should not cause peripheralization of the symptoms as when the condition was acute.[42]

2. Impairments/problems found in the late subacute and chronic phases

a. Pain when adaptively shortened structures are stretched
b. Decreased range of motion
c. Muscle strength imbalances
d. Faulty kinesthetic awareness and control of normal spinal alignment
e. Patient unaware of how to prevent recurrences

3. Treatment emphasis

The emphases during this stage are *recovery of function, development of a healthy back care plan*, and *teaching the patient how to prevent recurrences*. Goals, plan of care, and suggested exercises to correct the identified impairments are described in Chapter 15. The pain from adaptive shortening will decrease as normal flexibility, strength, and endurance are restored. Following any flexion exercises, the patient should conclude with extension exercises such as prone press-ups or standing back extension (see Figs. 15–8A and B).[42]

4. Patient education/prevention

a. Teach the patient posture awareness, stabilization principles, trunk-strengthening and endurance exercises, and safe body mechanics as described in Chapter 15. Include lower extremity strengthening to support the body and to use for body mechanics. Strengthen the upper extremities to carry objects without undue shifting and stress to the trunk.
b. Assess the patient's daily activities at work, home, and recreational settings and recommend ergonomically effective adaptations.
c. Emphasize to the patient that if he or she must be in a flexed posture, the flexion should be interrupted with backward bending at least once every hour.
d. Emphasize that if the patient feels the symptoms of a protrusion developing, he or she should immediately perform press-ups in the prone position or backward bending while standing to prevent progression of the symptoms (see Figs. 15–8A and B).

IV. Facet Joint Lesions in the Spine

A. Pathology of the Zygapophyseal[1] (Facet) Joints

1. Facet joints are synovial articulations that are enclosed in a capsule and supported by ligaments; they respond to trauma and arthritic changes similar to any peripheral joint.
2. Various types of meniscoid-like structures or invaginations of the facet capsules are present in the zygapophyseal joints of the spine. They are synovial reflections containing fat and blood vessels. In some cases, dense fibrous tissue develops as a result of mechanical stresses.[6,7] Some people describe an entrapment of these structures between the articulating surfaces with sudden or unusual movement as a source of pain and limited motion via tension on the well-innervated capsule.[31,66] Bogduk describes the *locked-back mechanism* as being an extrapment of the meniscoids in the supracapsular or infracapsular folds, which then blocks the return to ex-

tension from the flexed position.[6,7] (It is called an **extrapment** because the meniscoid fails to re-enter the joint cavity; it becomes a space-occupying lesion in the capsular folds, causing pain as it impacts and stretches the capsules.)

B. Pathomechanical Relationships of the Intervertebral Disk and Facet Joints

1. The disk and facets make up a three-joint complex between two adjoining vertebrae and are biomechanically interrelated. Asymmetric disk injury affects the kinematics of the entire unit plus the joints above and below, resulting in asymmetric movements of the facets, abnormal stresses, and eventual cartilage degeneration.[52]

2. Abnormal movement caused by disk degeneration puts a stress on the supporting ligaments and paraspinal muscles, causing abnormal proprioceptive input, further affecting fine control of movement.

3. As the disk degenerates, there is a decrease in both water content and disk height. The vertebral bodies approximate and the intervertebral foramina and spinal canal narrow.[11,12]

   a. Initially, there is increased slack with increased mobility in the spinal segment.[40] Opposition of the facet surfaces changes and the capsules are strained, resulting in irritation, swelling, and muscle spasm.

   b. Eventually, with the repeated irritation from the faulty mechanics, there are progressive degenerative changes in the facets and vertebral bodies. Osteophyte formation along the facets and spondylitic lipping and spurring along the vertebral bodies occur and hypomobility develops.[32,45] These lead to additional narrowing of the associated foramina and spinal canal.

   c. In the cervical spine, the uncovertebral joints thicken, roughen, and distort.

4. Stenosis is a narrowing of a passage or opening. In the spine, stenosis is any compromise of the space in the spinal canal (central stenosis), nerve root canal, or foramen (lateral stenosis) and may be congenital or acquired. The narrowing may be from soft tissue structures such as a disk protrusion, fibrotic scars, or joint swelling or from bony narrowing as with spondylitic osteophyte formation or spondylolisthesis.

5. Spinal nerve roots or the spinal cord becomes involved:

   a. When a protrusion of the disk compresses against the cord or nerve roots

   b. When there is decreased disk height from degenerative changes resulting in a decreased foraminal space[53] or excessive gliding of the vertebra from shear forces[40]

   c. When there is an inflammatory response from trauma, degeneration, or disease with accompanying edema and stenosis

   d. When a facet joint subluxes and the nerve root becomes impinged between the tip of the superior articulating facet and the pedicle

   e. When spondylosis results in osteophytic growth on the articular facets or along the diskal borders of the vertebral bodies that decrease spinal canal or intervertebral foraminal size

   f. When there is spondylolisthesis, or when there is scarring or adhesion formation following injury or spinal surgery

6. In all cases, the cycle of dysfunction from injury, pain, and muscle splinting leads to further restriction of movement, pain, and muscle splinting unless appropriate therapy is introduced.

C. Common Diagnoses and Impairments/Problems

1. Facet sprain/joint capsule injury

There is usually a history of trauma such as falling or a motor vehicle accident. The joints react with effusion (swelling), with limited range of motion, and with accompanying muscle splinting. The swelling may cause foraminal stenosis and neurologic signs.

2. Osteoarthritis, degenerative joint disease, spondylosis[12,62]

a. Usually there is a history of faulty posture, prolonged immobilization following injury, severe trauma, repetitive trauma, or degenerative changes in the disk.

b. In early stages of degenerative changes, there is greater play, or hypermobility, in the three-joint complex. Over time, stress from the altered mechanics leads to osteophyte formation with spurring and lipping along the joint margins and vertebral bodies. Progressive hypomobility with bony stenosis results.

c. Usually, where there is hypomobility, compensatory hypermobility occurs in neighboring spinal segments.

d. Pain may occur from the stresses of excessive mobility or from stretch to hypomobile structures. Pain may also occur from encroachment of developing osteophytes against pain-sensitive tissue or from swelling and irritation because of excessive or abnormal mobility of the segments.

e. The encroachment of osteophytes on the spinal canal and intervertebral foramina may cause neurologic signs.

f. The degenerating joint is vulnerable to facet impingement, sprains, and inflammation, as is any arthritic joint.

g. In some patients, movement relieves the symptoms; in others, movement irritates the joints and painful symptoms increase.

3. Rheumatoid arthritis (RA)[46]

a. Symptoms of RA can affect any of the synovial joints of the spine and ribs. There will be pain and swelling.

b. RA in the cervical spine presents special problems. There are neurologic symptoms wherever degenerative change or swelling impinges against neurologic tissue. There is increased fragility of tissues affected by RA, such as osteoporosis with cyst formation and erosion of bone, and instabilities from ligamentous necrosis. Most common of the serious lesions are atlantoaxial subluxation and C-4/5 and C-5/6 vertebral dislocations.

c. Pain or neurologic signs originating in the spine may or may not be related to subluxation. Therefore, these signs should be used as a precaution whenever dealing with this disease because of the potential damage to the spinal cord.

d. X-ray examinations are important in ruling out instabilities; signs and symptoms alone are not conclusive.

Precaution: Inappropriate movements of the spine could be life threatening or extremely debilitating because of the potential of subluxations and dislocations to cause damage to the cervical cord or vertebral artery.

4. Facet joint impingement (blocking, fixation, extrapment)[6,31,61,62,67]

a. With a sudden or unusual movement, the meniscoid of a facet capsule may be extrapped, impinged, or stressed, which causes pain and muscle guarding. The onset is sudden and usually involves forward bending and rotation.

    b. There is loss of specific motions, and attempted movement induces pain. At rest the individual has no pain.

    c. There are no true neurologic signs, but there may be referred pain in the related dermatome.

    d. Over time, stress is placed on the contralateral joint and on the disk, leading to problems in these structures.

D. Functional Limitations/Disabilities

1. Decreased trunk flexibility and susceptibility to pain reduces any activity requiring flexibility or prolonged repetition of trunk motions such as repetitive lifting and carrying of heavy objects.
2. When stenosis is associated with joint problems, the individual will be unable to perform repetitive or sustained activities requiring extension, as with reaching overhead or prolonged walking.

E. Management of Acute Joint Symptoms

1. To provide rest and support

    a. A cervical collar or lumbar corset may be helpful during the acute stage to provide rest to the inflamed joints. The support is also beneficial in RA or other disorders with hypermobilities or instabilities.

    b. Assist the patient in finding the functional position for comfort. Often the position is in the flexion range of the motion (flexion bias), especially if there are neurologic signs. The joint swelling or irritation from osteophytic spurs or lips decreases the foraminal space for the nerve roots, and this is exaggerated with extension positions.

2. To relieve pain and relax the muscles

    a. The use of modalities and massage is appropriate. Gentle intermittent joint distraction and gliding techniques may inhibit painful muscle responses and provide synovial fluid movement within the joint for healing. Dosages must be only grade I or II in order to not stretch the capsules and are best applied with manual techniques during the acute stage. (See Chapter 16.)

    b. If a patient has rheumatoid arthritis, traction or joint mobilizations in the spine are potentially dangerous because of ligamentous necrosis and vertebral instability and, therefore, are ***contraindicated***.[46]

    c. With spondylosis, if a patient does not have signs of acute joint inflammation but does have signs of nerve root irritation, stronger traction forces to cause opening of the intervertebral foramina may be beneficial to help temporarily relieve the pressure.

3. To decrease fluid stasis

Gentle range of motion within the limits of pain and muscle-setting techniques are initiated. The muscle contractions are gentle because strong contractions will cause joint compression and increase pain or cause a guarding response. Use techniques as described in the muscle section (Section V).

4. To teach self-management

Teach the patient how to control his or her functional spinal position while performing simple activities of rolling, side-lying to sit, sit to stand, and reverse as described in Section II.

Precaution: Because of the narrowed foramina and spinal canal, backward bending and backward bending with rotation should be avoided, because these motions narrow the foramina further.[6,12]

5. To manage meniscoid impingements

Release of the trapped meniscoid will relieve the pain and accompanying muscle guarding. The joint surfaces need to be separated and the joint capsules made taut.[31] General techniques include:

a. *Traction*

This may be applied manually or mechanically (see Chapter 16). Enough force is needed to cause separation of the vertebrae; thus a gliding traction of the facets occurs.

b. *Self-traction*

(1) To treat the lumbar spine, self-traction may be applied by pulling both thighs to the chest (see Fig. 15–5). Contralateral rotation will cause a distraction force on the facets (see Fig. 16–4B).

(2) To treat the cervical spine, the person axially extends the neck and places the hand under the occiput to lift the weight of the head.

c. *Spinal mobilization and manipulation*

These techniques require advanced training and are beyond the scope of this text.

F. Management of Subacute and Chronic Joint Problems

1. Chapter 15 describes techniques to relieve tension and improve patient's function through appropriately graded stretching and strengthening exercises, postural awareness, stabilization training, body mechanics, and environmental adaptations.

2. *Precautions*

a. Hypomobile joints require stretching but not if the techniques stress a hypermobile region. Traction techniques may be effective if the hypermobile region is stabilized while stretching (see Chapter 16). For those trained in joint manipulation techniques, they are effective for selective facet joint stretching.

b. If there are bony changes and osteophytic spurs, the patient should avoid postures and activities of hyperextension such as reaching overhead for prolonged periods of time. Adaptations in the environment might include using a step stool so that reaching is at shoulder level. Postures and motions emphasizing flexion of the spine that increase the size of the intervertebral foramina are usually preferred.

c. For patients with RA, emphasis is on stabilization and control. Because of the potential instabilities from necrotic tissue and bone erosion, subluxations and dislocations may cause damage to the spinal cord or vascular supply and be extremely debilitating or life threatening.

V. Muscle and Soft Tissue Lesions: Strains, Tears, and Contusions From Trauma or Overuse

A. Etiology of Symptoms and Impairments/Problems

1. General symptoms from trauma

Often more than one tissue is injured as a result of trauma. The extent of the tissue involvement may not be detectable during the acute phase.

a. There is pain, localized swelling, and tenderness on palpation.

b. There is protective muscle guarding regardless of whether the injured tissue is inert or contractile. Muscle guarding serves the immediate purpose of immobilizing the region. If the muscle contraction is prolonged, it results in the buildup of metabolic waste products and sluggish circulation. This altered local environment results in irritation of the free nerve endings so that the muscle continues to contract and becomes the source of additional pain (see Fig. 7–1).

c. Ligamentous strains will cause pain; then the ligament is stressed. If torn, there will be hypermobility of the segment.

d. As healing of the involved structures occurs, there may be adaptive shortening or scar tissue adhering to surrounding tissue and restricting tissue mobility and postural alignment.

2. Sites of lumbar strain

A common site for injury in the lumbar region is along the iliac crest. This is where many forces converge around the attachment of the lateral raphe of the lumbodorsal fascia, quadratus lumborum, erector spinae, and iliolumbar ligament. Injury to this region frequently occurs with falls and with repeated loading of the region during lifting or twisting motions.

3. Sites of cervical injury

Common injuries in the neck and upper thoracic region occur with flexion-extension trauma.

a. When the head rapidly accelerates into extension, if nothing stops it (such as a headrest in a car), the occiput is stopped by the thorax. The posterior structures, especially the joints, are compressed. The anterior structures (suprahyoid and infrahyoid muscles) are stretched. The mandible is pulled open and the condylar head of the temporomandibular joint translates forward, stressing the joint structures, and the muscles controlling jaw elevation are stretched (masseter, temporalis, and internal pterygoid).

b. When the head rapidly accelerates into flexion, if nothing stops it (such as the steering wheel or air bag in a car), the chin is stopped by the sternum. The mandible is forced posteriorly so the condylar head is forced into the retrodiskal pad within the joint. The posterior cervical muscles, ligaments, and fasciae are stretched.

4. Postural strain

Strain to the posterior cervical, scapular, and upper thoracic muscles and fasciae is common with postural stresses such as prolonged sitting at a computer terminal, drafting board, or desk.

5. Emotional stress

Emotional stresses are often expressed as increased tension in the posterior cervical or lumbar region.

B. Management During the Acute Phase

If the symptoms present with an acute inflammation, even if it is superimposed on an old injury or is the result of repetitive microtrauma, the condition is treated as an acute lesion until the inflammation is under control. It is important to eliminate the symptom-provoking stress to allow healing.

1. **To relieve pain and control edema and inflammation**

   Use appropriate modalities and massage. Passive support may be necessary to relieve the muscles from the job of supporting or controlling the injured part.

   a. *Cervical region*

   Cervical collars provide passive support. The length of time a collar is worn during the day relates to the severity of the injury and the amount of protection required. Collars often place the neck in a forward-head posture. This will cause healing in a faulty position, which will lead to future postural problems or painful syndromes. Usually, turning the collar around or cutting down the portion under the mandible will allow the neck to assume a correct alignment.

   b. *Lumbar region*

   Corsets provide passive support. As with the cervical region, the length of time that a corset is worn should be related to the amount of protection required. Some patients tend to become dependent on the corset and continue to wear it even after healing, when it no longer serves its intended purpose. After healing, it is better to strengthen the body's natural corset (abdominal muscles and others attached to the lumbodorsal fascia) and develop good spinal mechanics (see Chapter 15).

2. **To maintain muscle integrity**

   Identify the functional position in which the patient has reduced symptoms. With a muscle injury, this is often with the muscle in its shortened position. In this position, begin gentle muscle-setting techniques. Dosage is critical; resistance is minimal; use only enough to generate a setting contraction.

   a. *Cervical region*

   Position of patient: supine, with the therapist at the head of the treatment table, supporting the patient's head with the hands. Start with the guarding muscle in its shortened position. Ask the patient to hold as a gentle resistance (light enough to barely move a feather) is applied. Both the contraction and the relaxation should be gradual. There should be no neck movement or jerky resistance.

   (1) If there has been muscle injury, the technique is repeated with the muscle kept in the shortened range for several days before lengthening it.

   (2) If there is no muscle injury, progress the treatment by gradually lengthening the guarded muscle after each contraction and relaxation. Movement is performed only within the patient's pain-free range; no stretching is performed when there is muscle guarding.

   b. *Lumbar region*

   Position of patient: prone, with arms resting at the side. Have the patient lift the head. This will initiate a setting (stabilizing) contraction of the lumbar erector spinae muscles. A stronger contraction of the lumbar extensor muscles will occur if the head and thorax are extended. Alternate hip extension will also cause a setting contraction of the lumbar extensor muscles.

   (1) When there is muscle injury, the muscle is kept in this shortened range for several days.

   (2) For progression, if there is no muscle injury or as the muscle heals, gradually allow the muscle to elongate after each contraction by putting a pillow under the abdomen and then extending the thorax on the lumbar spine through a greater range. Elongation is performed only within tolerance during the early healing phase. There should be no increase in symptoms.

(3) Alternate position: supine. The patient presses the head and neck into the bed, causing a setting contraction of the spinal extensors.

3. To prevent fluid stasis and reduce stress to the region

The patient learns to find the functional position of comfort and then moves the part through its pain-free range, even if the range is very slight.

a. *Cervical region*

The patient lies supine and practices axial extension with chin tucks, using gentle motions. When tolerated, this motion is practiced sitting and standing.

b. *Lumbar region*

The patient lies supine, prone, or side-lying and practices gentle pelvic tilts. When tolerated, this is practiced sitting and standing.

4. To teach control of the functional position[9]

Begin early stabilization exercises. The exercises are initiated only when they do not increase the acute symptoms. The patient first explores the range of comfort as described in 3 above, then maintains that position while performing gentle arm and leg motions. The patient's attention is directed to the feel of the stabilizing contraction and is instructed to stay within the tolerance of the injured tissue.

a. Begin supine. First the patient alternately picks up one arm, then the other, noting the muscle response. The farther overhead the arm is lifted, the greater the stabilizing contraction. If there is increased pain, a smaller range of arm motion is used. A stronger contraction occurs if the legs are alternately slid up and down the table.

b. Positions of prone, sitting, and standing are used and the same sequence is followed.

5. To maintain integrity and promote relaxation of the muscles when there is no direct trauma to them

Use *reverse muscle action techniques*. These are valuable when neck motions cause pain and muscle guarding. The neck is not moved, but the muscles are called on to contract and relax through a functional range. The motions include active scapular elevation, depression, adduction, and rotation and active shoulder flexion, extension, abduction, adduction, and rotation. The shoulder motions may be carried out as circumduction or patterned activities as long as they do not stress the neck.

6. Use of traction

Gentle oscillating traction may reflexively inhibit the pain and help maintain synovial fluid and joint-play motion during the acute stage when the muscles do not allow full range of motion. Gentle techniques are most effectively applied using manual traction. Position the part with the injured tissue in a shortened position, and use a dosage less than that which causes vertebral separation. Traction techniques may aggravate a muscle or soft tissue injury if the tissue is placed in a lengthened position during the setup or with a high dosage of pull during treatment.

7. Adapt the environment

If there are activities or postures that caused the trauma or are continuing to provoke symptoms, identify the mechanism and modify the activity or environment to eliminate the potential for repeating the problem.

C. Management in the Subacute and Chronic Stages of Healing and Rehabilitation

Exercise techniques to progress the patient through the healing and rehabilitative stages are described in Chapter 15.

1. When the acute symptoms begin to diminish, the intensity of the exercise program can progress. Identify any muscle weaknesses or areas of reduced flexibility and progress stretching and strengthening within the tolerance of the tissues.

2. Identify any postural problems and retrain the patient's kinesthetic senses and proprioceptive awareness for correct posture. Include postural endurance training.

3. Teach the patient relaxation exercises to reduce muscle tension.

4. Often with low-back problems, muscle imbalances in the hip region perpetuate stresses in the low back. Refer to the muscle section in Chapter 11 for exercises to correct flexibility and strength imbalance problems in the hip.

5. Often with cervical and upper back problems, imbalances in the shoulder girdle perpetuate faulty posture and stresses. Refer to the muscle section in Chapter 8 for exercises to realign the shoulder girdle.

6. Functional activities can be resumed at a safe level as soon as the patient is able. Progressively increase the level of function as strength and stabilization improve. Patient education should include suggestions for adaptation of the environment as well as exercise techniques to prevent recurrences of problems.

VI. Selected Conditions

A. Torticollis (Wryneck, Cervical Scoliosis)

This involves asymmetry in strength or functioning of the sternocleidomastoid muscle (SCM). There is cervical rotation opposite to and side bending toward the side of the contracting or shortened muscle.

1. Congenital torticollis

  a. Causes

   Injury in utero or at birth to the SCM, which then becomes fibrotic and shortens. The injury may be from a faulty position of the fetus, nerve injury, or direct trauma to the muscle.

  b. Management

   Gentle passive range of motion and stretching are initiated as soon as the diagnosis is made. The head is rotated toward and side-bent away from the side of tightness, using the same technique as for scalene stretches (see Fig. 15–3).

2. Asymmetric weakness (muscle imbalance)

  a. Causes

   A common cause is hemiplegia, in which the stronger muscle turns the head toward the side of weakness. The functional problem may develop into a static limitation if the neck is not periodically taken through full range of motion.

  b. Management

   If there is innervation and control of the weaker muscle, initiate strengthening exercises. Active or passive range of motion is performed several times a day.

3. Hysterical torticollis

a. Causes

There may be many causes; sometimes it is described as the person's turning away from an unpleasant situation.

b. Management

Physical therapy consists of resistive exercises to the opposite muscle and range of motion to maintain flexibility. Relaxation exercises may be helpful if the person tends to be tense. Close communication is maintained with the psychiatrist or psychologist working with the cause of the disorder.

B. Tension Headache

This usually involves tension in the posterior cervical muscles, pain at the attachment of the cervical extensors, and/or pain radiating across the top and side of the scalp.

1. Causes

Tension headaches may follow soft tissue injury or may be caused by faulty or sustained postures, nerve irritation or impingement (the greater occipital nerve emerges through the neck extensor muscles where they attach at the base of the skull), or sustained muscle contraction (from faulty posture or emotional tension) leading to ischemia. Medical causes include migraine, allergy, or sinusitis. Whatever the cause, there usually is a cycle of pain, muscle contraction, decreased circulation, and more pain, which leads to decreased function and potential soft tissue dysfunction.

2. Management

a. Break into the cycle of pain and muscle tension using modalities, massage, and muscle-setting exercises to increase circulation to the part and carry off waste products.

b. Evaluate the flexibility and strength of the muscles in the cervical, upper thoracic, and shoulder girdle, and design an exercise program to regain a balance in length and strength in preparation for posture correction and training. Chapter 15 describes these procedures. Be sure there is adequate flexibility in the suboccipital muscles to relieve tension in that region.

c. Educate the patient in proper techniques to relieve the source or manage the irritation.

   (1) If there is poor posture, teach posture correction and ways to manage posture.

   (2) If the person is in tension-producing situations, teach relaxation techniques, range of motion and muscle-setting techniques, and proper spinal mechanics.

C. Temporomandibular Joint Dysfunction (Syndrome)[34,35,55]

1. Clinical picture

Pain from a variety of sources is often cited as part of the temporomandibular joint (TMJ) syndrome.

a. Pain may occur locally in the TMJ, in the retrodiskal pad located in the posterior region of the joint, or in the ear.

b. Pain from muscle spasm or myofascial pain in the masseter, temporalis, or pterygoid internis or externis muscles may be described as a headache.

c. Tension in the muscles of the cervical spine may itself be painful or cause referenced pain from irritation of the greater occipital nerve that may be described as a tension headache.

2. Causes

Imbalance occurs between the head, jaw, neck, and shoulder girdle. Causes may be:

a. Malocclusion, decreased vertical dimension of the bite, or other dental problems.

b. Faulty joint mechanics from inflammation, subluxation of the meniscus (disk), dislocation of the condylar head, joint contractures, or asymmetric forces from jaw and bite imbalances. Restricted motion results from periods of immobilization after reconstructive surgery or fracture of the jaw.

c. Muscle spasm in the muscles of mastication, causing abnormal or asymmetric joint forces. Muscle spasm can be the result of emotional tension, faulty joint mechanics, direct or indirect injury, or a postural dysfunction.

d. Sinus problems, resulting in the individual's being a mouth breather, which indirectly affects posture and jaw position.

e. Postural dysfunctions (see Chapter 15 for related material). With a forward-head posture, there is retraction of the mandible and resulting stretch on the anterior throat muscles. Consequently there is increased activity in the muscles that close the jaw to counter the changed forces. The muscles and soft tissue in the suboccipital region become tight, and the nerves and joints become compressed or irritated.

f. Trauma such as a flexion/extension accident in which the jaw forcefully opens when the head whips back into hyperextension. A direct blow from an auto accident, boxing, a fall or similar trauma, or sustained trauma as occurs in prolonged dental surgery in which the mouth is held open for lengthy periods of time may initiate symptoms in the TMJ or supporting tissue. Excessive stresses such as biting or chewing on large pieces of hard food may also traumatize the joints.

3. Management

a. The approach to management will depend on the cause. In simple cases in which posture, joint dysfunction, or muscle imbalances are the source of the problem, physical therapy treatment with therapeutic exercise can directly address the problems. In many cases, a dental referral, ear, nose, and throat referral, or psychologic support may be necessary to deal with primary causes. A complete evaluation is necessary prior to the initiation of any treatment.

b. *To decrease the pain and muscle guarding,* use modalities, massage, and relaxation techniques. In addition, the person should eat soft foods and avoid items requiring excessive jaw opening or firm biting and chewing motions.

c. *To correct muscle imbalances,* relax and stretch tight postural muscles, then retrain for proper muscle control. Cervical and shoulder postural stretching and retraining exercises are described in Chapters 15 and 8, respectively.

d. *To teach control of the jaw muscles*

(1) First teach recognition of the resting position of the jaw. The lips are closed, teeth slightly apart, and tongue resting lightly on the hard pallet behind the front teeth. The patient should breathe in and out slowly through the nose, using diaphragmatic breathing.

(2) Teach control while opening and closing the jaw through the first half of

the ROM. With the tongue on the roof of the mouth, the patient opens the mouth, trying to keep the chin in mid-line. Use a mirror for visual reinforcement. The patient is also taught to lightly palpate the lateral poles of the condyle of the mandible bilaterally and to attempt to maintain symmetry between movement on the two sides when opening and closing the mouth.

(3) If the jaw deviates while opening or closing, have the patient practice lateral deviation to the opposite side. The lateral motion should not be excessive or cause pain.

(4) Progress to applying gentle resistance with the thumb against the chin. Do not overpower the muscles.

e. *To increase range of motion if necessary*

(1) Begin by placing layered tongue depressors between the central incisors. The patient can gradually work to increase the amount of tongue depressors used until he or she can open approximately far enough to insert the knuckles of the index and middle fingers.

(2) Self-stretching is carried out by placing each thumb under the upper teeth and the index or middle fingers over the lower teeth and stretching the mouth open.

(3) Placing cotton dental rolls between the back teeth while the patient bites will distract the condyle from the fossa in the joint.

(4) Joint mobilization techniques are performed by using a gloved hand or hands. Determination of dosages and precautions for administration of mobilization techniques are described in Chapter 6.

(a) Unilateral distraction (Fig. 14–10A). The patient may be supine or sitting with the head supported. Use the hand opposite the side on which you are working. Place your thumb in the patient's mouth on the back molars; the fingers are outside and wrapped around the jaw. The force is in a downward (caudal) direction.

(b) Unilateral distraction with glide (Fig. 14–10B). After distracting the jaw as described in (a), pull it in a forward (anterior) direction. The other hand can be placed over the TMJ to palpate the amount of movement.

(c) Bilateral distraction (Fig. 14–11). If the patient is supine, stand at the head of the treatment table. If the patient is sitting, stand in front of the patient. Use both thumbs, placing them on the molars on each side of the mandible. The fingers are wrapped around the jaw. The force from the thumbs is equal, in a caudal direction.

VII. Summary

The initial section of this chapter has presented information to assist the reader in reviewing basic spinal mechanics and muscle function in preparation for designing exercise programs for patients with painful back and neck problems. The remainder of chapter has presented information to help the reader to be able to design a therapeutic exercise program for common acute neck and back problems based on typical clinical pictures and necessary precautions. Included have been intervertebral disk lesions, facet joint problems, muscle and soft tissue lesions, and several specific problems including torticollis, tension headaches, and TMJ syndrome. Within the section on soft tissue lesions, management techniques for muscle guarding and spasm have been described. Progression of treatment has been related to information presented in Chapter 15.

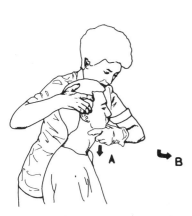

Figure 14–10. Unilateral mobilization of the temporomandibular joint. (*A*) Distraction is in a caudal direction. (*B*) Arrow indicating distraction with glide in a caudal, then anterior direction.

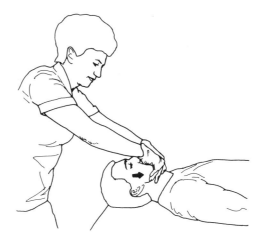

Figure 14–11. Bilateral distraction of the temporomandibular joint with the patient supine.

References

1. Adams, MA, and Hutton, WC: Gradual disc prolapse. Spine 10(6):524, 1985.
2. Adams, MA, and Hutton, WC: The effect of fatigue on the lumbar intervertebral disc. J Bone Joint Surg Br 65(2):199, 1983.
3. Alexander, AH, Jones, AM, and Rosenbaum, DH: Nonoperative management of herniated nucleus pulposus: Patient selection by the extension sign. Orthop Rev 21:181, 1992.
4. Anderson, B, et al: The influence of backrest inclination and lumbar support on lumbar lordosis. Spine 4:52, 1979.
5. Binkley, J, et al: Diagnostic classification of patients with low back pain: Report on a survey of physical therapy experts. Phys Ther 73:139, 1993.
6. Bogduk, N, and Engle, R: The menisci of the lumbar zygapophyseal joints: A review of their anatomy and clinical significance. Spine 9(5):454, 1984.
7. Bogduk, N, and MacIntosh, JE: The applied anatomy of the thoracolumbar fascia. Spine 9:164, 1984.
8. Bogduk, N, and Twomey, LT: Clinical Anatomy of the Lumbar Spine. Churchill-Livingstone, New York, 1987.
9. Bondi, BA, and Drinkwater-Kolk, M: Functional stabilization training. Workshop notes, Northeast Seminars, October 1992.
10. Burkart, S, and Beresfore, W: The aging intervertebral disk. Phys Ther 59:969, 1979.
11. Butler, D, et al: Discs degenerate before facets. Spine 15:111, 1990.
12. Cailliet, R: Low Back Pain Syndrome, ed 4. FA Davis, Philadelphia, 1988.
13. Cloward, R: The clinical significance of the sino-vertebral nerve of the cervical spine in relation to the cervical disc syndrome. J Neurol Surg Psychiatry 23:321, 1960.
14. DeRosa, CP, and Porterfield, JA. A physical therapy model for the treatment of low back pain. Phys Ther 72:261, 1992.
15. Daniels, L, and Worthingham, C: Therapeutic Exercise for Body Alignment and Function, ed. 2. WB Saunders, Philadelphia, 1977.
16. Farfan, HF, et al: The effects of torsion on the lumbar intervertebral joints: The role of torsion in the production of disc degeneration. J Bone Joint Surg Am 52(3):468, 1970.
17. Gossman, M, Sahrmann, S, and Rose, S: Review of length-associated changes in muscle. Phys Ther 62: 1977, 1982.
18. Gracovetsky, S, Farfan, H, and Helleur, C: The abdominal mechanism. Spine 10:317, 1985.
19. Gracovetsky, S, and Farfan, H: The optimum spine. Spine 11:543, 1986.
20. Gracovetsky, S: The Spinal Engine. Springer-Verlag Wein, New York, 1988.
21. Hellsing, AL, Linton, SL, and Kaluemark, M: A prospective study of patients with acute back and neck pain in Sweden. Phys Ther 74:116, 1994.
22. Hickey, DS, and Hukins, DEL: Aging changes in the macromolecular organization of the intervertebral disc: An x-ray diffraction and electron microscopic study. Spine 7(3):234, 1982.
23. Hughes, P: Advanced Upper Extremity Course. Workshop Notes, St Louis, 1979.
24. Jensen, G: Biomechanics of the lumbar intervertebral disc: A review. Phys Ther 60:765, 1980.
25. Kapandji, IA: The Physiology of the Joints, Vol 3. Churchill-Livingstone, New York, 1974.
26. Kellegren J: Observations on referred pain arising from muscle. Clin Sci 3:175, 1983.
27. Kendall, FP, McCreary, EK, and Provance, PG: Mus-

cles Testing and Function, ed 4. Williams & Wilkins, Baltimore, 1993.

28. Kessler, R: Acute symptomatic disk prolapse. Phys Ther 59:978, 1979.

29. Klein, JA, and Hukins, DWL: Collagen fiber orientation in the annulus fibrosus of intervertebral disc during bending and torsion measured by x-ray defraction. Biochem Biophys Acta 719:98, 1982.

30. Kopp, JR, et al: The use of lumbar extension in the evaluation and treatment of patients with acute herniated nucleus pulposus. Clin Orthop 202:211, 1986.

31. Kos, J, and Wolf, J: Intervertebral menisci and their possible role in intervertebral blockage (translated by Burkart, S). Bulletin of the Orthopaedic and Sports Medicine Sections, American Physical Therapy Association 1(3):8, 1976.

32. Krag, MH, et al: Internal displacement distribution from in vitro loading of human thoracic and lumbar spinal motion segments: Experimental results and theoretical predictions. Spine 12:1001, 1987.

33. Krause, N, and Ragland, DR: Occupational disability due to low back pain: A new interdisciplinary classification based on a phase model of disability. Spine 19:1011, 1994.

34. Kraus, SL: TMJ Craniomandibular Cervical Complex: Physical Therapy and Dental Management. Clinical Education Associates, Atlanta, 1986.

35. Kraus, SL: Temporomandibular joint and dentistry. Workshop notes, Detroit, 1987.

36. Lehmkuhl, LD, and Smith, LK: Brunnstrom's Clinical Kinesiology, ed 4. FA Davis, Philadelphia, 1983.

37. Lipson, SJ, and Muir, H: Proteoglycans in experimental intervertebral disc degeneration. Spine 6(3):194, 1981.

38. Lyons, G, Eisenstein, SM, and Sweet, MBI: Biochemical changes in intervertebral disc degeneration. Biochem Biophys Acta 673:443, 1981.

39. McCarron, RF, et al: The inflammatory effect of nucleus pulposus: A possible element in the pathogenesis of low-back pain. Spine 12:760, 1987.

40. MacNab, I: Backache. Williams & Wilkins, Baltimore, 1977.

41. Markolf, LK, and Morris, JM: The structural components of the intervertebral disc. J Bone Joint Surg Am 56(4):675, 1974.

42. McKenzie, R: The Lumbar Spine: Mechanical Diagnosis and Therapy. Spinal Publications, New Zealand, 1981.

43. McKenzie, R: Manual correction of sciatic scoliosis. N Z Med J 89:22, 1979.

44. Mooney, V, and Robertson, J: The facet syndrome. Clin Orthop 115:149, 1976.

45. Mooney, V: The syndromes of low back disease. Orthop Clin North Am 14(3):505, 1983.

46. Moneur, C, and Williams, HJ: Cervical spine management in patients with rheumatoid arthritis. Phys Ther 68:509, 1988.

47. Morgan, D: Concepts in functional training and postural stabilization for the low-back injured. Topics in Acute Care and Trauma Rehabilitation 2:8, 1988.

48. Nachemson, A: The lumbar spine: An orthopaedic challenge. Spine 1:59, 1976.

49. Nachemson, A: Recent advances in the treatment of low back pain. Int Orthop 9:1, 1985.

50. Ogata, K, and Whiteside, LA: Nutritional pathways of the intervertebral disc. Spine 6(3):211, 1981.

51. Panjabi, MM, Geol, VK, and Takata, K: Physiologic strains in the lumbar spinal ligaments. Spine 7:192, 1982.

52. Penjabi, MM, Krag, MH, and Chung, TQ: Effects of disc injury on mechanical behavior of the human spine. Spine 9:707, 1984.

53. Porter, RW, Hibbert, C, and Evans, C: The natural history of root entrapment syndrome. Spine 9:418, 1984.

54. Porterfield, JA: Dynamic stabilization of the trunk. Journal of Orthopaedic and Sports Physical Therapy 6:271, 1985.

55. Rocobado, M: Temporomandibular joint dysfunctions. Workshop notes, Cincinnati, 1979.

56. Rothstein, JM: Patient classification. Editor's note. Phys Ther 73:214, 1993.

57. Saal, JA: Dynamic muscular stabilization in the nonoperative treatment of lumbar pain syndromes. Orthop Rev 19:691, 1990.

58. Saal, JS, et al: High levels of inflammatory phospholipase A_2 activity in lumbar disc herniations. Spine 15:674, 1990.

59. Saal, JA, and Saal, JS: Nonoperative treatment of herniated lumbar intervertebral disc with radiculopathy; an outcome study. Spine 14:431, 1989.

60. Saal, JA, Saal, JS, and Herzog, RJ: The natural history of lumbar intervertebral disc extrusions treated nonoperatively. Spine 15:683, 1990.

61. Saunders, JD: Evaluation and Treatment of Musculoskeletal Disorders. Educational Opportunities, Minneapolis, 1985.

62. Saunders, JD: Classification of musculoskeletal spinal conditions. Journal of Orthopaedic and Sports Physical Therapy 1:89, 1979.

63. Saunders JD: Lumbar traction. JOSPT 1:36, 1978.

64. Sullivan, MS: Back support mechanisms during manual lifting. Phys Ther 69:38, 1989.

65. Taylor, J, and Twomey, L: Sagittal and horizontal plane movement of the human lumbar vertebral column in cadavers and in living. Rheumatology Rehabilitation 19:223, 1980.

66. Taylor, JR, and Twomey, LT: Age changes in lumbar zygapophyseal joints. Spine 11(7):739, 1986.

67. Twomey, LT: A rationale for the treatment of back pain and joint pain by manual therapy. Phys Ther 72:885, 1992.

68. Twomey, LT: Commentary. Phys Ther 72:270, 1992.

69. Twomey, T, and Taylor, JR: Sagittal movements of the human lumbar vertebral column: A quantitative study of the role of the posterior vertebral elements. Arch Phys Med Rehabil 64:322, 1983.

70. Urban, L: The straight-leg-raising test: A review. Journal of Orthopaedic and Sports Physical Therapy 2:117, 1981.

71. Waddell, G: A new clinical model for the treatment of low back pain. Spine 12:632, 1987.

72. Wood, P: Applied anatomy and physiology of the vertebral column. Phys Ther 59:248, 1979.

73. Yasuma, T, et al: Histological development of intervertebral disc herniation. J Bone Joint Surg Am 68(7):1066, 1986.

Chapter

15

The Spine: Subacute, Chronic, and Postural Problems

In Chapter 14 basic spinal mechanics were reviewed and therapeutic exercise treatment interventions for spinal problems that have acute connective tissue, joint, and disk symptoms were described. Postural problems are often the underlying cause or may be the result of spinal injury. Musculoskeletal impairments from faulty posture or from injury include weak muscles, poor endurance in postural muscles, restricted joint range of motion, or restricted muscle flexibility. These impairments may limit the functional ability of the individual to perform repetitive activities or maintain sustained postures without causing reinjury or suffering painful symptoms. In addition, injured individuals may not be aware of their faulty posture or strength and flexibility problems, or they may not be aware of how to relieve stressful postures or minimize stressful activities.

This chapter describes common postural problems that underlie many subacute and chronic neck and back conditions. These problems need to be identified and therapeutic exercise intervention initiated as soon as possible following injury so that the patient learns safe movement patterns and learns how to progress exercises safely as injured or irritated tissues heal. This chapter describes therapeutic exercises used during the subacute and chronic stages of healing to regain flexibility, strength, and endurance for spinal stability and control. In addition, principles for progressing the patient to his or her maximum functional level are addressed. This includes modifying postural habits to relieve or prevent repetitive pain-producing stresses, developing a balance in length and strength of supporting muscles, and training the neuromusculoskeletal system to respond to the demands of the desired functional activities to prevent reinjury. The exercise techniques and principles of management described in this chapter can also be used for general stretching, strengthening, and conditioning programs as well as for the purpose of correcting postural problems before they cause injury.

OBJECTIVES

After studying this chapter, the reader will be able to:

1 Describe the dynamics of posture.
2 Identify characteristics of common postural deviations in each region of the spine.
3 Identify typical postural impairments as a result of spinal deviations.
4 Identify goals and techniques to use for treating postural impairments in the cervical, thoracic, and lumbar regions.
5 Establish a therapeutic exercise program to manage subacute and chronic musculoskeletal dysfunctions related to postural problems.

I. The Dynamics of Posture

A. Posture Defined

Posture is a "position or attitude of the body, the relative arrangement of body parts for a specific activity, or a characteristic manner of bearing one's body."[15]

1. Ligaments, fasciae, bones, and joints are inert structures that support the body, whereas muscles and their tendinous attachments are the dynamic structures that maintain the body in a posture or move it from one posture to another.
2. Gravity places stress on the structures responsible for maintaining the body upright in a posture. Normally, the gravitational line goes through the physiologic curves of the spinal column and they are balanced. If the weight in one region shifts away from the line of gravity, the remainder of the column compensates to regain equilibrium.

B. The Equilibrium of Posture[15,19]

For a weight-bearing joint to be stable, or in equilibrium, the gravity line of the mass must fall exactly through the axis of rotation, or there must be a force to counteract the force of gravity. In the body, the counter force is either muscle or inert structures. Upright posture usually involves a slight anterior-posterior swaying of the body of about 4 centimeters.[11]

In the standing posture, the following occur:

1. Ankle

The gravity line is anterior to the joint so it tends to rotate the tibia forward about the ankle. Stability is provided by the plantarflexor muscles, primarily the soleus muscle.

2. Knee

The normal gravity line is anterior to the joint, which tends to keep the knee in extension. Stability is provided by the anterior cruciate ligament, posterior capsule (locking mechanism of the knee), and tension in the muscles posterior to the knee (the gastrocnemius and hamstring muscles). The soleus provides active stability by pulling posteriorly on the tibia. With the knees fully extended, no muscle support is required at that joint to maintain upright posture, but if the knees flex slightly, the gravity line shifts posterior to the joint and the quadriceps femoris muscle must contract to prevent the knee from buckling.

3. Hip

The gravity line varies with the swaying of the body. When it passes through the hip joint, there is equilibrium, and no external support is necessary. When the gravitational line shifts posterior to the joint, some posterior rotation of the pelvis occurs, which is controlled by tension in the hip flexor muscles (primarily the iliopsoas). In relaxed standing, the iliofemoral ligament provides passive stability to the joint and no muscle tension is necessary. When the gravitational line shifts anteriorly, stability is provided by active support of the hip extensor muscles.

4. Trunk

Normally, the gravity line goes through the bodies of the lumbar and cervical vertebrae; then the curves are balanced. Some activity in the muscles of the trunk and pelvis help maintain the balance. As the trunk shifts, contralateral muscles contract and function as guy wires. Extreme or sustained deviations are supported by inert structures.

5. Head

The center of gravity of the head falls anterior to the atlanto-occipital joints. The posterior cervical muscles contract to keep the head balanced. In postures in which the head is forward, greater demand is placed on these muscles. At the extreme of flexion, tension in the ligamentum nuchae prevents further motion.

C. Etiology of Pain in Postural Problems

1. The ligaments, facet capsules, periosteum of the vertebrae, muscles, anterior dura mater, dural sleeves, epidural areolar adipose tissue, and walls of blood vessels are innervated and responsive to nociceptive stimuli.[14]
2. Endurance in muscles is necessary to maintain postural control. Sustained postures require continual small adaptations in the stabilizing muscles to support the trunk against fluctuating forces. Large repetitive motions also require muscles to respond to control the activity. In either case, as the muscles fatigue, the load is shifted to the inert tissues supporting the spine at the end-ranges. With the sustained load, creep and distention occur in the inert tissues, causing mechanical stress.
3. Mechanical stress to pain-sensitive structures, such as sustained stretch to ligaments or joint capsules or compression of blood vessels, causes distention or compression of the nerve endings, which leads to the experience of pain. This type of stimulus occurs in the absence of an inflammatory reaction. It is not a pathologic problem but a mechanical one because signs of an acute inflammation with constant pain are not present. Relieving the stress to the pain-sensitive structure relieves the pain stimulus, and the person no longer experiences pain.
4. If the mechanical stresses exceed the supporting capabilities of the tissues, breakdown will occur. If this occurs without adequate healing, overuse syndromes with inflammation and pain will affect function without an apparent injury. In addition, injuries occur more frequently when there is muscle fatigue. Relieving the mechanical stress along with decreasing the inflammation is important. Treatment intervention for acute symptoms is described in Chapter 14.

D. Pain Syndromes Related to Poor Posture

1. Postural fault and the postural pain syndrome

A **postural fault** is a posture that deviates from normal alignment but has no structural limitations. The **postural pain syndrome** refers to the pain that occurs from mechanical stress when a person maintains a faulty posture for a prolonged period; the pain is usually relieved with activity. There are no abnormalities in muscle strength or flexibility, but if the faulty posture continues, strength and flexibility imbalances will eventually develop.

2. Postural dysfunction

Postural dysfunction differs from the postural pain syndrome in that adaptive shortening of soft tissues and muscle weakness are involved. The cause may be prolonged poor posture habits, or it may be a result of contractures and adhesions formed during the healing of tissues after trauma or surgery. Stress to the shortened structures causes pain. In addition, strength and flexibility imbalances may predispose the area to injury or overuse syndromes that a normal musculoskeletal system could sustain.

3. Postural habits

Good postural habits in the adult are necessary to avoid postural pain syndromes and postural dysfunctions. Also, careful follow-up in terms of flexibility and posture training exercises is important following trauma or surgery to prevent dysfunctions from contractures and adhesions. In the child, good postural habits are important to avoid abnormal stresses on growing bones and adaptive changes in muscle and soft tissue.

II. Characteristics and Problems of Common Faulty Postures

A. Pelvic and Lumbar Region

1. Lordotic posture (Fig. 15–1A)

This posture is characterized by an increase in the lumbosacral angle (the angle that the superior border of the first sacral vertebral body makes with the horizontal, which optimally is 30 degrees), an increase in the lumbar lordosis, and an increase in the anterior pelvic tilt and hip flexion.[5] This is often seen with an increased thoracic kyphosis and forward head and is called a **kypholordotic posture.**[13]

a. *Potential sources of pain*
   (1) Stress to the anterior longitudinal ligament.
   (2) Narrowing of the posterior disk space and narrowing of the intervertebral foramen. This may compress the dura and blood vessels of the related nerve root or the nerve root itself, especially if there are degenerative changes in the vertebra or disk.[5]
   (3) Approximation of the articular facets. The facets may become weight bearing, which may cause synovial irritation and joint inflammation.

b. *Muscle imbalances observed*[13]
   (1) Tight hip flexor muscles (iliopsoas, tensor fasciae latae, rectus femoris) and lumbar extensor muscles (erector spinae)
   (2) Stretched and weak abdominal muscles (rectus abdominis, internal and external obliques)

Figure 15–1. (*A*) Lordotic posture characterized by an increase in the lumbosacral angle, an increased lumbar lordosis, an increased anterior tilting of the pelvis, and hip flexion. (*B*) Relaxed or slouched posture characterized by an excessive shifting of the pelvic segment anteriorly, resulting in hip extension, and shifting of the thoracic segment posteriorly, resulting in flexion of the thorax on the upper lumbar spine. A compensatory increased thoracic kyphosis and forward head placement are also seen. (*C*) Flat low-back posture characterized by a decreased lumbosacral angle, a decreased lumbar lordosis, and a posterior tilting of the pelvis. (*D*) Flat upper back and cervical spine characterized by a decrease in the thoracic curve, depressed scapulae, depressed clavicle, and an exaggeration of axial extension (flexion of the occiput on atlas and flattening of the cervical lordosis).

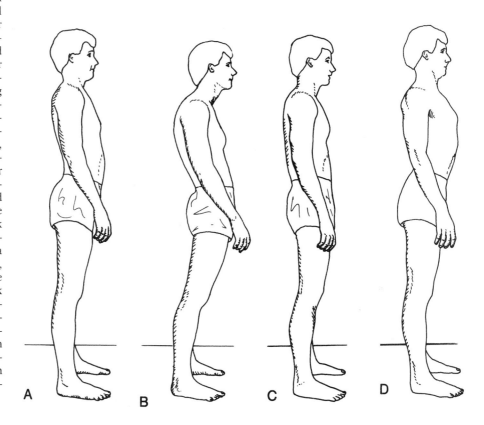

c. *Common causes*

Sustained faulty posture, pregnancy, obesity, weak abdominal muscles.

2. Relaxed or slouched posture (Fig. 15–1B)

This posture is also called **swayback**.[13] The amount of pelvic tilting is variable, but usually there is a shifting of the entire pelvic segment anteriorly, resulting in hip extension, and shifting of the thoracic segment posteriorly, resulting in flexion of the thorax on the upper lumbar spine. This results in an increased lordosis in the lower lumbar region, an increased kyphosis in the lower thoracic region, and usually a forward head. The position of the mid- and upper lumbar spine depends on the amount of displacement of the thorax. When standing for prolonged periods, the person usually assumes an asymmetric stance in which most of the weight is borne on one lower extremity, with periodic shifting of weight to the opposite extremity.

a. *Potential sources of pain*

(1) Stress to the iliofemoral ligaments, the anterior longitudinal ligament of the lower lumbar spine, and the posterior longitudinal ligament of the upper lumbar and thoracic spine. With asymmetric postures there is also stress to the iliotibial band on the side of the elevated hip. Other frontal plane asymmetrics may also be present; see Section II.D.

(2) Narrowing of the intervertebral foramen in the lower lumbar spine that may compress the blood vessels, dura, and nerve roots, especially with arthritic conditions.

(3) Approximation of articular facets in the lower lumbar spine.

b. *Muscle imbalances observed*

(1) Tight upper abdominal muscles (upper segments of the rectus abdominis and obliques), internal intercostal, hip extensor, and lower lumbar extensor muscles and related fascia

(2) Stretched and weak lower abdominal muscles (lower segments of the rectus abdominis and obliques), extensor muscles of the lower thoracic region, and hip flexor muscles

c. *Common causes*

As the name implies, this is a relaxed posture in which the muscles are not used to provide support. The person yields fully to the effects of gravity, and only the passive structures at the end of each joint range (such as ligaments, joint capsules, and bony approximation) provide stability. Causes may be attitudinal (the person feels comfortable when slouching), from fatigue (seen when required to stand for extended periods), from muscle weakness (the weakness may be the cause or the effect of the posture), or from a poorly designed exercise program (one that emphasizes thoracic flexion; see Chapter 21).

3. Flat low-back posture (Fig. 15–1C)

This posture is characterized by a decreased lumbosacral angle, a decreased lumbar lordosis, hip extension, and a posterior tilting of the pelvis.

a. *Potential sources of pain*

(1) Lack of the normal physiologic lumbar curve, which reduces the shock-absorbing effect of the lumbar region and predisposes the person to injury

(2) Stress to the posterior longitudinal ligament

(3) Increase of the posterior disk space, which allows the nucleus pulposus to imbibe extra fluid and, under certain circumstances, may protrude posteriorly when the person attempts extension (see Chapter 14)

b. *Muscle imbalances observed*

(1) Tight trunk flexor (rectus abdominis and intercostals) and hip extensor muscles

(2) Stretched and weak lumbar extensor and possibly hip flexor muscles

c. *Common causes*

Continued slouching or flexing in sitting or standing postures; overemphasis on flexion exercises in general exercise programs

B. Thoracic Region

1. Round back or increased kyphosis (see Fig. 15–1B)

This posture is characterized by an increased thoracic curve, protracted scapulae (round shoulders), and usually an accompanying forward head.

a. *Potential sources of pain*

(1) Stress to the posterior longitudinal ligament

(2) Fatigue of the thoracic erector spinae and rhomboid muscles

(3) Thoracic outlet syndrome (see Chapter 8)

(4) Cervical posture syndromes (see Section C)

   b. *Muscle imbalances observed*
      (1) Tight muscles of the anterior thorax (intercostal muscles), muscles of the upper extremity originating on the thorax, (pectoralis major and minor, latissimus dorsi, and serratus anterior), muscles of the cervical spine and head attached to the scapula (levator scapulae and upper trapezius), and muscles of the cervical region (see Section C)
      (2) Stretched and weak thoracic erector spinae and scapula retractor muscles (rhomboids and upper and lower trapezius)
   c. *Common causes*
      Similar to the relaxed lumbar posture or the flat low-back posture, continued slouching, and overemphasis on flexion exercises in general exercise programs

2. Flat upper back (Fig. 15–1D)

This posture is characterized by a decrease in the thoracic curve, depressed scapulae, depressed clavicle, and a flat-neck posture (see Section D). It is associated with an exaggerated military posture but is not a common postural deviation.
   a. *Potential sources of pain*
      (1) Fatigue of muscles required to maintain the posture
      (2) Compression of the neurovascular bundle in the thoracic outlet between the clavicle and ribs
   b. *Muscle imbalances*
      (1) Tight thoracic erector spinae and scapular retractors and potentially restricted scapular movement, which would decrease the freedom of shoulder elevation
      (2) Weak scapular protractor and intercostal muscles of the anterior thorax
   c. *Common cause*
      Exaggerating the upright posture

3. Scoliosis[4,6,8,12,16,25]

This usually involves the thoracic and lumbar regions. Typically, in right-handed individuals, there is a mild right thoracic, left lumbar S-curve, or a mild left thoraco-lumbar C-curve. There may be asymmetry in the hips, pelvis, and lower extremities.

   A **structural scoliosis** involves an irreversible lateral curvature with fixed rotation of the vertebrae (Fig. 15–2A). Rotation of the vertebral bodies is toward the convexity of the curve. In the thoracic spine, the ribs rotate with the vertebrae so that there is a prominence of the ribs posteriorly on the side of the spinal convexity and a prominence anteriorly on the side of the concavity. A posterior rib hump is detected on forward bending in a structural scoliosis (Fig. 15–2B).

   A *nonstructural scoliosis* is reversible and can be changed with forward or side bending and with positional changes such as lying supine or realignment of the pelvis by correction of a leg-length discrepancy or with muscle contractions. It is also called a **functional** or **postural scoliosis.**
   a. *Potential sources of pain*
      (1) Muscle fatigue and ligamentous strain on the side of the convexity
      (2) Nerve root irritation on the side on the concavity
   b. *Muscle imbalances*
      (1) Tight structures on the concave side of the curve.

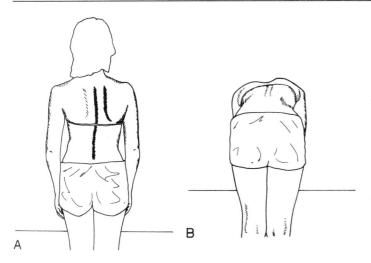

Figure 15–2. (*A*) Mild right thoracic left lumbar structural scoliosis with prominence of the right scapula. (*B*) Forward bending produces a slight posterior rib hump, indicating fixed rotation of the vertebrae and rib cage.

   (2) Stretched and weak structures on the convex side of the curve.
   (3) If one hip is adducted, the adductor muscles on that side will be tight and the abductor muscles will be stretched and weak. The opposite will occur on the contralateral extremity.[13]

c. *Common causes: structural scoliosis*
   Neuromuscular diseases or disorders (such as cerebral palsy, spinal cord injury, or progressive neurologic or muscular diseases), osteopathic disorders (such as hemivertebra, osteomalacia, rickets, or fracture), and idiopathic disorders in which the cause is unknown

d. *Common causes: nonstructural scoliosis*
   Leg-length discrepancy, either structural or functional; muscle guarding or spasm from a painful stimuli in the back or neck; and habitual or asymmetric postures

C. Cervical Region

1. Forward-head posture (see Fig. 15–1B)

This posture is characterized by increased flexion of the lower cervical and the upper thoracic regions, increased extension of the occiput on the first cervical vertebra, and increased extension of the upper cervical vertebrae. There also may be temporomandibular joint dysfunction with retrusion of the mandible.[22]

a. *Potential sources of pain*
   (1) Stress to the anterior longitudinal ligament in the upper cervical spine and posterior longitudinal ligament in the lower cervical and upper thoracic spine
   (2) Muscle tension or fatigue
   (3) Irritation of facet joints in the upper cervical spine
   (4) Narrowing of the intervertebral foramina in the upper cervical region, which may impinge on the blood vessels and nerve roots, especially if there are degenerative changes
   (5) Impingement on the neurovascular bundle from anterior scalene muscle tightness (see also thoracic outlet syndrome in Chapter 8)
   (6) Impingement on the cervical plexus from levator scapulae muscle tightness

     (7) Impingement on the greater occipital nerves from a tight or tense upper trapezius muscle, leading to tension headaches

     (8) Temporomandibular joint pain from faulty head, neck, and mandibular alignment and associated facial muscle tension

     (9) Lower cervical disk lesions from the faulty flexed posture

  b. *Muscle imbalances*

     (1) Tight levator scapulae, sternocleidomastoid, scalene, and suboccipital muscles. If the scapulae are elevated, there may also be tight upper trapezius muscles. With temporomandibular joint symptoms, the muscles of mastication may have increased tension.

     (2) Stretched and weakened anterior throat muscles (hyoid becomes fixed because of the stretched position) and lower cervical and upper thoracic erector spinae muscles.

  c. *Common causes*

    Occupational or functional postures requiring leaning forward for extended periods, relaxed postures, or the end result of a faulty pelvic and lumbar spine posture

2. Flat-neck posture (Fig. 15–1D)

This posture is characterized by a decreased cervical lordosis and increased flexion of the occiput on atlas (this is an exaggeration of axial extension). It may be seen with an exaggerated military posture (flat upper back). There may be temporomandibular joint dysfunction with protraction of the mandible.

  a. *Potential sources of pain*

     (1) Temporomandibular joint pain and occlusive changes

     (2) Decrease in the shock-absorbing function of the lordotic curve, which may predispose the neck to injury

     (3) Stress to the ligamentum nuchae

  b. *Muscle imbalances*

     (1) Short anterior neck muscles.

     (2) Theoretically, the levator scapulae, sternocleidomastoid, and scalene muscles become stretched and weakened.

  c. *Common causes*

    Exaggeration of the posture for extended periods of time. This posture is uncommon.

D. Frontal Plane Deviations From Lower Extremity Asymmetries

Any lower extremity inequality will have an effect on the pelvis that, in turn, affects the spinal column and structures supporting it. When dealing with spinal posture, it is imperative to assess lower extremity alignment, symmetry, foot posture, range of motion, and strength. See Chapters 11 to 13 for principles, procedures, and techniques for treating the hip, knee, ankle, and foot.

1. Characteristic deviations when standing with weight equally distributed to both lower extremities

  a. Elevated ilium on the long leg (LL) side, lowered on the short leg (SL) side

     (1) This puts the LL in hip adduction and the SL in hip abduction.

     (2) The sacroiliac (SI) joint on the LL side is more vertical; on the SL side it is more horizontal.

b. Side bending of the lumbar spine toward the LL side, coupled with rotation in the opposite direction

(1) This compresses the intervertebral disk on the LL side and distracts the disk on the SL side, as well as causes a torsional stress.

(2) There is extension and compression of the lumbar facets on the LL side (concave portion of curve) and flexion and distraction of the lumbar facets on the SL side (convex portion of curve).

(3) There is narrowing of the intervertebral foramina on the LL side.

c. The thoracic and cervical spine have a compensatory scoliosis in the opposite direction.

2. Potential sources of pain

a. Greater shear forces occur in the hip and SI joints on the LL side, which increases stress in the supporting ligaments and decreases the load-bearing surface within the joint. Degenerative changes occur more frequently in hips on the LL side.[9]

b. Stenosis in the lumbar intervertebral foramina on the LL side may cause vascular congestion or nerve root irritation.

c. Lumbar facet compression and irritation on the LL side.

d. Disk breakdown from torsional and asymmetric forces (see Chapter 14).

e. Muscle tension, fatigue, or spasm in response to asymmetric loading and response.

f. Lower extremity overuse syndromes.

3. Muscle imbalances

a. Tight hip muscles include adductors on the LL side and abductors on the SL side. There may also be asymmetric differences in the iliopsoas, quadratus lumborum, piriformis, erector spinae, and multifidus muscles, those on the concave side of the curve or LL side being tighter.

b. Stretched and weakened muscles include hip adductors on the SL side, abductors on the LL side, and, in general, muscles on the convex side of the curve.

4. Common causes

Asymmetry in the lower extremities may result from structural or functional deviations at the hip, knee, ankle, or foot. Common functional problems include unilateral flat foot and imbalances in the flexibility of muscles. The resulting asymmetric ground reaction forces transmitted to the pelvis and back may lead to tissue breakdown and overuse, particularly as a person ages, becomes overweight, or generally deconditions from inactivity.[20]

E. Summary of Common Impairments/Problems Associated With Postural Dysfunctions

1. Pain: from stress to sensitive structures and from muscle tension

2. Decreased range of motion: from flexibility imbalances

3. Muscle weakness and poor muscular endurance: from sustained faulty postures or disuse

4. Poor control of spinal mechanics and inadequate stabilization of the trunk: from imbalances in muscle length, strength, endurance, and coordination

5. Altered kinesthetic awareness of normal alignment and control: from prolonged faulty postural habits

6. Unable to manage posture and prevent pain: from lack of knowledge about healthy spinal mechanics

F. Common Impairments/Problems Following Injury During the Subacute Stage of Healing

Postural problems may be the underlying cause or may be the effect of an acute injury. For the patient who has sustained an acute injury, when the signs and symptoms of the inflammatory process are under control, progression through a program of nondestructive movement during the subacute stage prepares the tissue for rehabilitation training. Depending on the severity of injury the subacute stage usually lasts about 3 weeks (see Chapter 7). Care during this stage is critical because either the patient feels good and tends to overdo activities and reinjures the tissue or the patient is fearful and does not adequately resume safe movements and healing occurs with connective tissue restrictions. Either extreme will slow down the recovery process.

The following is a summary of impairments seen in the subacute stage of healing:

1. Pain: only when stress is placed on developing scar tissue near the end of the available range

2. Decreased range of motion: from the development of adhesions in the new scar tissue or development of contractures in tissues not moved through their range

3. Circulatory stasis: from decreased movement and swelling

4. Muscle weakness and poor muscular endurance: from reflex inhibition and disuse or from an underlying postural dysfunction

5. Poor control of spinal mechanics and inadequate stabilization of the trunk: from imbalances in muscle length, strength, endurance, and coordination

6. Fear of reinjury: from lack of knowledge of safe movement patterns

G. Common Impairments/Problems in the Chronic Rehabilitative Stage

A patient who has been treated through the acute and subacute phases of healing with appropriately graded exercises should have minimal impairments preventing common daily activities. Depending on the severity of injury, this takes approximately 3 to 6 weeks. There still will be some restricted flexibility and decreased muscle strength and endurance. For the individual who desires or requires an active lifestyle at a job, recreational activities, or athletic pursuits, additional training to strengthen muscles for advanced stabilization and control and to develop high-level endurance to safely meet the demands of the activity is necessary. Impairments in strength, endurance, timing, and skill will be related to the functional goals for the individual.

The following is a summary of impairments seen in the chronic rehabilitative stage:

1. Restricted flexibility: from any restrictive scar tissue or adhesions

2. Limited strength and endurance in postural and extremity muscles: with inability to maintain intense and repetitive activities or work

3. Slow, poorly coordinated, or guarded execution of skill activity

H. General Treatment Goals and Plan of Care

Treatment Goals	*Plan of Care*
1. Relieve pain and muscle tension.	1. External postural support if necessary. Muscle relaxation training. Education in safe movement.
2. Restore range of motion.	2. Specific stretching and flexibility exercises.
3. Restore muscle strength, endurance, and function.	3. Stabilization training. Specific resistive exercises. Endurance exercises. Functional control and retraining.
4. Retrain kinesthetic awareness and control of normal alignment.	4. Training and reinforcement techniques.
5. Patient involvement and education to manage posture to prevent recurrences.	5. Teach safe movement patterns and proper body mechanics. Teach patient preventive exercises and mechanics for relief of mechanical stress in daily activities. Teach relaxation exercises to cope with muscle tension. Instruct patient on how to modify environment: bed, chairs, car seats, work area.
6. Develop functional skills.	6. Activity training specific to desired functional outcome, emphasizing speed, timing, and endurance.

The following sections in the remainder of this chapter include procedures and techniques to meet the above goals and to fulfill the plan of care. The exercises are appropriate if, following a comprehensive assessment of the patient's history and clinical signs, it is determined that the patient's condition has progressed to the subacute stage after acute injury or disk derangement or that the presenting pain is due to the stresses of poor posture or related flexibility and strength losses. It is important to note that the following exercises are *not* listed as a protocol for treatment. Not all procedures are appropriate for all patients. A variety of exercises are described to deal with the impairments, allowing the therapist to make a careful selection of which ones best meet the goals for each patient at each stage of recovery.

III. Procedures to Relieve Pain From Stress and Muscle Tension

NOTE: These techniques are not appropriate to manage acute pain from inflammation, joint swelling, or disk derangements (see Chapter 14).

A. Muscle Relaxation Techniques

1. Active ROM

Whenever discomfort develops from maintaining a constant posture or from sustaining muscle contractions for a period of time, active range of motion in the opposite direction aids in taking stress off supporting structures, promoting circulation, and maintaining flexibility. All motions are performed slowly, through the full range, with the patient paying particular attention to the feel of the muscles. Repeat each motion several times.

a. *The cervical and upper thoracic region*

Position of patient: sitting, with arms resting comfortably on the lap, or standing. Instruct the patient to:

(1) Bend the neck forward and backward. (Backward bending is contraindicated with symptoms of nerve root compression.)

(2) Side bend the head in each direction, then rotate the head in each direction.

(3) Roll the shoulders; protract, elevate, retract, then relax the scapulae (in a position of good posture).

(4) Circle the arms (shoulder circumduction). This is accomplished with the elbows flexed or extended, using either small or large circular motions, with the arms pointing either forward or out to the side. Both clockwise and counterclockwise motions should be performed, but conclude the circumduction by going forward, up, around, and then back, so that the scapulae end up in a retracted position. This has the benefit of helping retrain proper posture.

b. *The lower thoracic and lumbar region*

Position of patient: sitting or standing. If standing, the feet should be shoulder-width apart, with the knees slightly bent. Have the patient place the hands at the waist with the fingers pointing backward. Instruct the patient to:

(1) Extend the lumbar spine by leaning the trunk backward (see Fig. 15–8B). This is particularly beneficial when the person must sit or stand in a forward-bent position for prolonged periods.

(2) Flex the lumbar spine by contracting the abdominal muscles, causing a posterior pelvic tilt; or if there are no signs of a disk problem, the patient can bend the trunk forward, dangling the arms toward the floor with the knees slightly bent. This motion is beneficial when the person stands in a lordotic or sway-back posture for prolonged periods.

(3) Side bend in each direction.

(4) Rotate the trunk by turning in each direction while keeping the pelvis facing forward.

(5) Stand up and walk around at frequent intervals when sitting for extended periods.

2. General conscious relaxation techniques

Relaxation for the entire body should be taught to a person who is generally tense (see Chapter 5).

3. Conscious relaxation training for the cervical region

As with general techniques, the specific techniques for this region develop the patient's kinesthetic awareness of a tensed or relaxed muscle and how to consciously reduce tension in the muscle. In addition, if done with posture training techniques in mind (see Section VI), the therapist can help the patient to recognize decreased muscular tension in which the head is properly balanced and the cervical spine is aligned in mid-position.

Position of patient: sitting comfortably with arms relaxed, such as resting on a pillow placed on the lap; the eyes are closed. The therapist is positioned next to the patient and uses tactile cues on the muscles and helps position the head as necessary. Instruct the patient to:

a. Use diaphragmatic breathing. He or she breathes in slowly and deeply through the nose, allowing the abdomen to relax and expand, then relaxes and allows the air to be expired through the relaxed open mouth. This breathing is reinforced after each of the following activities.

.b. Next, relax the jaw. The tongue rests gently on the hard pallet behind the front teeth with the jaw slightly opened. If the patient has trouble relaxing the jaw, have him or her click the tongue and allow the jaw to drop. Practice until the patient feels the jaw relax and the tongue rest behind the front teeth. Follow with relaxed breathing as in a.

c. Slowly flex the neck. As the patient does so, direct the attention to the posterior cervical muscles and the sensation of how the muscles feel. Use verbal cues such as, "Notice the feeling of increased tension in your muscles as your head drops forward."

d. Then slowly raise the head to neutral, inhale slowly, and relax. Help the patient position the head properly and suggest that he or she note how the muscles contract to lift the head, then relax once the head is balanced.

e. Repeat the motion; again direct the patient's attention to the feeling of contraction and relaxation in the muscles as he or she moves. Imagery can be used with the breathing such as "fill your head with air and feel it lift off your shoulders as you breath in, and relax."

f. Then go through only part of the range, noting how the muscles feel.

g. Next, just think of letting the head drop forward, then tightening the muscles (setting); then think of bringing the head back and then relax. Reinforce to the patient the ability to influence the feeling of contraction and relaxation in the muscles.

h. Finally, just think of tensing the muscles and relaxing, letting the tension go out of the muscles even more. Point out that he or she feels even greater relaxation. Once the patient learns to perceive tension in muscles, he or she can then consciously think of relaxing the muscles. Emphasize the fact that the position of the head also influences the muscle tension. Have the patient assume various head postures, then correct them until the feel is reinforced.

B. External Postural Support

Use of support such as a lumbar pillow while sitting or adaptations of a work station should be used to relieve sustained stressful postures.

C. Education

Demonstrate the relationship of the patient's faulty posture to the development of pain. Have the patient assume the faulty posture and wait until he or she experiences the stress. Direct the patient's attention to the position or activity when the stress or pain is felt and relate it to the posture. Then show the patient how to relieve the stress by changing postures or by using the techniques described in the previous sections (see also Section VI). Emphasize practicing posture correction procedures and relaxation techniques.

D. Modalities and Massage

Minimize or decrease use of modalities and massage once acute symptoms are under control so that the patient learns self-management through exercises, relaxation, and posture retraining and does not become dependent on external applications of interventions for comfort.

IV. Procedures to Increase the Range of Motion of Specific Structures

NOTE: To obtain an adequate stretch, apply the stretch force slowly and sustain it for at least 15 seconds. Release the force, then repeat three times. Re-evaluate to determine change, and decide whether to proceed with the same technique or to modify it.

A. Cervical and Upper Thoracic Region

1. **To stretch the anterior portion of the intercostal muscles and increase mobility of the anterior thorax**

   a. Position of patient: hook-lying, with hands behind head and elbows resting on the mat. To increase the stretch, place a pad lengthwise under the thoracic spine between the scapulae. Segmental breathing (Chapter 19) can also be used by having the patient start with the elbows together in front of the face, then inhaling as the elbows are brought down to the mat; holding; then exhaling as the elbows are brought together again.

   b. Position of patient: hook-lying with both arms elevated overhead. The patient attempts to keep the back flat on the mat while inhaling and expanding the anterior thorax.

   c. Position of patient: sitting on a firm, straight-back chair, with the hands behind the head. He or she then brings the elbows out to the side as the scapulae are adducted and thoracic spine extended (head held neutral, not flexed). To combine with breathing, have the patient inhale as he or she takes the elbows out to the side, and exhale as he or she brings the elbows in front of the face (see Figs. 19–14A and B).

2. **To stretch the scalene muscles**

   NOTE: Because these muscles are attached to the transverse processes of the upper cervical spine and the upper two ribs, they either flex the cervical spine or elevate the upper ribs when they contract bilaterally. Unilaterally, the scalenes side bend the cervical spine to the same side and rotate it to the opposite side.

   a. Position of patient: sitting. The patient first performs axial extension (tucks the chin and straightens the neck), then side bends the neck opposite and rotates it toward the tight muscles. The therapist stands behind the patient and stabilizes the upper ribs, with one hand over the top of the rib cage on the side of tightness, and stabilizes the head with the other hand around the side of the patient's head and face, holding the head against his or her trunk (Fig. 15–3). The patient inhales and exhales; the therapist then holds the ribs down as the patient inhales again. Repeat. This is a gentle contract-relax stretching maneuver.

   b. To perform the previous maneuver in a home program, the patient stands next to a table and holds onto its underside. He or she then positions the

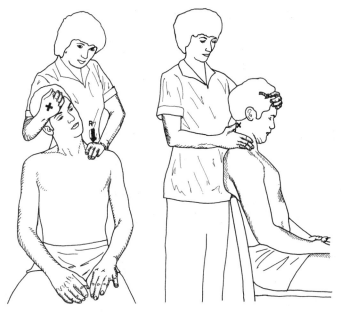

Figure 15–3.

Figure 15–4.

Figure 15–3. Unilateral active stretching of the scalenus muscles. The patient first performs axial extension, then side-bends the neck opposite, and rotates it toward the tight muscles. The therapist stabilizes the head and upper thorax as the patient breathes in, contracting the muscle against the resistance. As the patient relaxes, the rib cage lowers and stretches the muscle.

Figure 15–4. Stretching the short suboccipital muscles. The therapist stabilizes the second cervical vertebra as the patient slowly nods the head.

head as in a. To stretch, he or she leans away from the table, inhales, exhales, and holds the stretch position.

3. To stretch the short suboccipital muscles

a. Position of patient: sitting. The therapist identifies the spinous process of the second cervical vertebra and stabilizes it with his or her thumb or with the second metacarpophalangeal joint (and the thumb and index finger around the transverse processes) as the patient slowly nods, doing just a tipping motion of the head on the upper spine (Fig. 15–4). The therapist guides the movement by placing the other hand across the patient's forehead.

b. Position of patient: supine. The therapist sits on a stool at the head of the treatment table with forearms resting on the table. One hand stabilizes the C-2 vertebra by grasping the transverse processes between the proximal portions of the thumb and index finger, and the other hand supports the occiput. Nod the patient's head with the hand under the occiput to take up the slack of the suboccipital muscles, then ask the patient to roll the eyes upward. This will cause a gentle isometric contraction of the suboccipital muscles. After holding 6 seconds, ask the patient to roll the eyes downward. As the suboccipital muscles relax, take up the slack by passively nodding the head through any new range. Only motion between the occiput and C-2 should occur. The contraction is gentle in order to not cause overflow into the multisegmental erector spinae and upper trapezius muscles.

4. To stretch tight scapular and humeral muscles that affect posture

Shoulder girdle posture is directly related to cervical and thoracic posture. Techniques to increase flexibility in the shoulder and scapular muscles are described in Chapter 8. Of primary importance are the pectoralis major (see Fig. 8–18 to 8–20), pectoralis minor (see Fig. 8–21), levator scapulae (see Figs. 8–22 and 8–23), and shoulder internal rotator muscles (see Figs. 4–8 and 8–15).

5. **To increase general range of motion of the cervical spine and musculature**

   a. Inhibition techniques, as described in Chapter 5, can be used on any muscle group or motion. Suggested position for the patient is supine, with the therapist standing at the head end of the treatment table, supporting the patient's head in his or her hands.

   b. Traction techniques, as described in Chapter 16, can be used for the purpose of stretching the posterior ligaments, muscles, and the facet joint capsules. This is a nonspecific form of stretching.

6. **To stretch specific joint structures in the cervical spine**

   Joint mobilization and manipulation techniques can be used by those trained in the principles and maneuvers. They require advanced training and are beyond the scope of this text.

B. Mid and Lower Thoracic and Lumbar Regions

1. **To stretch the lumbar erector spinae muscles and soft tissue posterior to the spine (to increase trunk flexion)**

   Precaution: If flexion of the spine causes a change in sensation or causes pain to radiate down an extremity, reassess the patient's condition to determine if flexion is contraindicated.

   a. Position of patient: hook-lying. The patient first brings one knee and then the other toward the chest, clasps the hands around the thighs and pulls them to the chest, elevating the sacrum off the mat. This may be assisted by the therapist (Fig. 15–5).

   Precaution: Do not grasp around the tibia; it places stress on the knee joints as the stretch force is applied.

   b. Position of patient: cross-sitting. The patient places the hands behind the neck, adducts the scapulae, and extends the thoracic spine. This locks the thoracic vertebrae. He or she then leans the thorax forward onto the pelvis, flexing only at the lumbar spine. The therapist stabilizes the pelvis by pulling back on the anterior-superior iliac spines (Fig. 15–6).

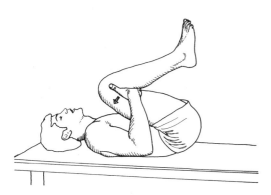

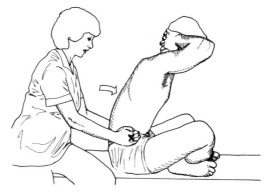

Figure 15–5. Self-stretching the lumbar erector spinae muscles and tissues posterior to the spine. The patient grasps around the thighs to avoid compression of the knee joints.

Figure 15–6. Stretching the lumbar spine, with the patient stabilizing the thorax in extension and the therapist stabilizing the pelvis.

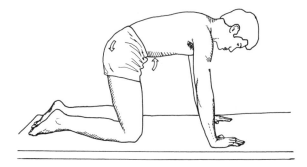

Figure 15–7. Active stretching of the lumbar spine. The patient tucks the abdomen in without rounding the thorax.

    c. Position of patient: on hands and knees. The patient is asked to tuck the abdomen in without rounding the thorax (concentrate on flexing the lumbar spine, not the thoracic spine), hold the position, then relax (Fig. 15–7). Repeat; this time bring the hips back to the feet, hold, then return to the hands and knees position (see Fig. 21–1A).

    d. Active trunk flexion exercises use the principle of reciprocal inhibition and can be used to help elongate tight lumbar extensor muscles.

  2. To stretch soft tissue anterior to the lumbar spine (to increase trunk extension)

    Precaution: Do not perform if extension causes a change in sensation or causes pain to radiate down an extremity (see Chapter 14).

    a. Position of patient: prone, with hands placed under the shoulders. The patient then extends the elbows and lifts the thorax up off the mat but keeps the pelvis down on the mat. This is a *prone press-up* (Fig. 15–8A). To increase the stretch force, the pelvis can be strapped to the treatment table. This exercise also stretches the hip flexor muscles and soft tissue anterior to the hip.

    b. Position of patient: standing, with the hands placed in the low-back area. He or she then leans backward and holds the stretch (Fig. 15–8B).

    c. Position of patient: on hands and knees. After the patient tucks the stomach

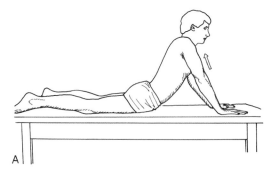
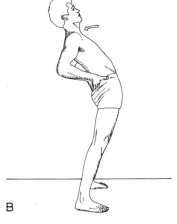

Figure 15–8. Self-stretching of the soft tissues anterior to the lumbar spine and hip joints with the patient (*A*) prone and (*B*) standing.

in, instruct to allow the spine to sag, creating lumbar extension. This can also be used to teach the patient how to control pelvic motion.

d. Any active trunk extension exercises as described in Section V following may be used as long as the exertion does not increase symptoms.

3. To stretch tight lower extremity musculature that affects posture

a. Hip muscles have a direct effect on spinal posture because of their attachment on the pelvis. See Chapter 11 for specific stretching techniques of these muscles.

b. Knee, ankle, and foot muscle-stretching techniques are described in Chapters 12 and 13.

C. To Increase Lateral Flexibility in the Spine

NOTE: Stretching has not been shown to correct or halt progression of a structural scoliosis. If these exercises are used for patients with structural scoliosis, they may be beneficial in gaining some flexibility prior to surgical fusion of the spine for correction of a scoliotic deformity. They may also be used to regain flexibility in the frontal plane when muscle or fascial tightness is present in functional scoliosis. All of the following exercises are designed to stretch tight structures on the concave side of the lateral curvature.

When stretching the trunk, it is necessary to stabilize the spine above and below the curve. If the patient has a double curve, one curve must be stabilized while the other is stretched.

1. Patient prone

a. Stabilize the patient at the iliac crest on the side of the concavity. Have the patient reach toward the knee with the arm on the convex side of the curve while stretching the opposite arm up and overhead (Fig. 15–9).

b. Patient stabilizes the upper trunk (thoracic curve) by holding onto the edge of the mat table with the arms. (No shoulder motion should occur.) The therapist lifts the hips and legs and laterally bends the trunk away from the concavity (Fig. 15–10).

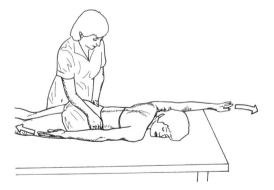

Figure 15–9. Stretching tight structures on the concave side of the thoracic curve. The patient has a right thoracic left lumbar curve. The therapist stabilizes the pelvis and lumbar spine while the patient actively stretches the thoracic curve.

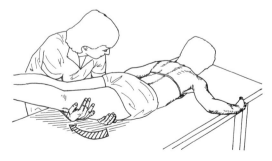

Figure 15–10. Stretching tight structures on the concave side of a left lumbar curve. The patient stabilizes the upper trunk and thoracic curve as the therapist passively stretches the lumbar curve.

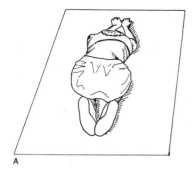
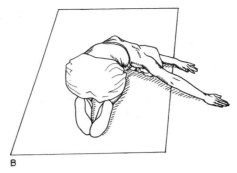

Figure 15–11. (*A*) Heel-sitting to stabilize the lumbar spine. (*B*) Tight structures on the concave side of a right thoracic curve are stretched by having the patient reach the arms overhead and then walk the hands to the right.

2. Patient heel-sitting (to stabilize the lumbar curve)

a. The patient leans forward so the abdomen rests on the anterior thighs (Fig. 15–11A), the arms are stretched overhead bilaterally, and the hands are flat on the floor.

b. Have the patient laterally bend the trunk away from the concavity by walking the hands to the convex side of the curve. Hold the position for a sustained stretch (Fig. 15–11B).

3. Patient side-lying on the convex side of the curve

NOTE: Stabilize the patient at the iliac crest. Do not allow the patient to roll forward or backward during the stretch.

a. Have the patient lie on a mat, top arm stretched overhead, with a rolled towel at the apex of the curve to neutralize the curve. Hold this position for a sustained period of time (Fig. 15–12).

b. Have the patient lie over the edge of a mat table, with a rolled towel at the apex of the curve and the top arm stretched overhead. Hold this head-down position as long as possible (Fig. 15–13).

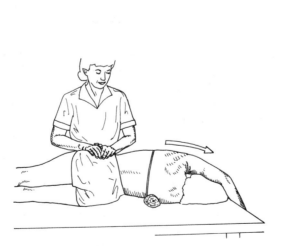
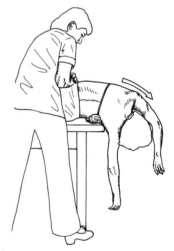

Figure 15–12. Stretching tight structures on the concave side of a right thoracic curve. The patient is positioned side-lying with a rolled towel at the apex of the convexity; the lumbar spine is stabilized by the therapist.

Figure 15–13. Side-lying over the edge of a mat table to stretch tight structures of a right thoracic scoliosis. The therapist stabilizes the pelvis.

    c. Segmental breathing is used to expand the lungs and derotate the ribs and vertebrae during unilateral stretching of the trunk. The patient concentrates on breathing in and expanding the ribs on the concave side of the trunk. Specific procedures for teaching breathing exercises are found in Chapter 19.

V. Procedures to Train and Strengthen Muscle Function and to Develop Endurance for Postural Control (Stabilization Exercises)[3,17,21,23,24,27]

A. General Guidelines

The primary functions of the muscles of the neck and trunk are to provide a stable base for the muscles of the extremities to execute their function and to support the trunk against the effects of gravity and other outside forces, that is, to maintain the desired postures. The trunk is not a rigid structure, though, and needs to be able to adapt to varying demands and postural requirements.

1. Training is initiated by teaching the patient *safe spinal ROM* in a variety of basic postures including supine, prone, side-lying, sitting, and standing. In addition to the basic patterns of ROM in the cervical spine, teach axial extension with chin tucking. In the lumbar spine, ROM is taught using pelvic tilting.

2. The patient then identifies the most comfortable position for the spine and muscles in whatever position is being used for the exercise. This is called **functional position** or **functional range**.[17] When their condition is not acute, most people find the mid-range to be their functional position. The mid-range is also called **resting position** or **neutral spine position**. It is important to recognize that this position or range is not static, nor is it the same for every person, and it may change as the tissues heal and nociceptive stimuli decrease.[17] The therapist directs the patient's awareness to the position of the spine and the feel of the muscles contracting while maintaining the position during the exercises.

3. Simple extremity motions are performed within the tolerance of the trunk or neck muscles to control the functional position. This causes an *isometric* or *stabilizing* contraction and is called **dynamic stabilization**.[3,17]

4. To safely develop *strength* and *endurance* in the stabilizing muscles, resistance is applied to the extremities, and repetitions of the motions are increased. The intent is to challenge the trunk muscles yet stay within their tolerance. Repetitions also help develop habit, so it is important to use careful instructions and feedback. Fatigue is determined by the inability of the trunk or neck muscles to stabilize the spine in its functional position.

    a. Begin at a resistance force that the patient can repeat for 30 seconds to 1 minute; progress to 3 minutes as tolerated.

    b. Progress by adding resistance or increasing the lever arm; initially reduce the time and again progress to doing the new activity to 3 minutes.

    c. Another way to develop endurance in the trunk muscles is to begin exercising at the most difficult level for that patient, then shifting to simpler levels of resistance as fatigue begins in order to keep moving. It is important that the patient does not lose control of the functional position.

5. Alternating isometric contractions between antagonists **(rhythmic stabilization)** also enhances stabilizing contractions. In addition, when performed sitting and standing, the alternating contractions are used to develop control of balance.

6. *Concentric and eccentric exercises* are incorporated into the program for strength and endurance control through the range of motion.

7. Muscles emphasized during the early training are those necessary for trunk support in the upright posture, for carrying out basic body mechanics, and for basic upper extremity lifting. Suggestions include trunk and cervical flexors and extensors, hip and knee extensors, shoulder and elbow flexors, and extensors and scapular retractors.

8. The patient is taught to control the functional position while moving from one position to another. This requires graded contractions and adjustments between the trunk flexors and extensors. It is termed **transitional stabilization** and requires greater awareness and concentration from the patient.[3,17] For example, any motion of the arms or legs away from the trunk tends to cause the spine to extend. The abdominals must contract to maintain the functional spinal position. Then as the arms or legs move anteriorward toward the center of gravity, the spine tends to flex. This requires the extensors to contract to maintain the functional position.

9. As the patient develops strength and control, *simple patterns of motion* are introduced toward the goal of developing safe body mechanics and movement. Suggestions include closed-chain partial squats and controlled lunges. During each exercise the functional position of the spine is maintained. Arm motions and weights are added as tolerated.

10. Once the patient learns control and develops strength and endurance in simple patterns, more *complex patterns with less support* are introduced, such as rotation and diagonal motions. Specific functional tasks are broken down into their basic components, learned, then integrated into the complex motion. Control, endurance, timing, and speed are each emphasized as the patient progresses toward the desired functional outcome.

11. The exercises described in this section are listed progressively from least difficult to more difficult. These are suggestions; creative adaptations should be considered to add variety and to meet the needs of individual patients. Begin at the level appropriate for the patient's strength and ability to control the motion without exacerbating symptoms. As the patient progresses, eliminate the simpler exercises and add more challenging ones. Many of the exercises can be used to train all of the regions of the spine because of the integrative nature of the activity.

12. Training follows stretching. If there is inadequate flexibility in the antagonistic muscles, the postural muscles cannot hold the parts in proper alignment.

B. Cervical and Upper Thoracic Region

1. To teach awareness of safe cervical range of motion

a. Position of patient: begin supine, progress to sitting and standing. The patient trucks the chin and attempts to flatten the neck against the mat through his or her comfortable range, relaxes, and attempts to find the functional position. If necessary, support the head as the patient moves through the range and place a small pillow under the head if the functional position is slightly forward.

b. Scapular and thoracic posture influences cervical range, so the patient is directed in protracting and retracting the shoulder girdle by rolling the shoulders forward, then pinching the scapulae together, and then finding the most comfortable position.

c. These motions are repeated every time a new position is assumed prior to beginning exercises for the region. See additional comments and suggestions in Section VI. Postural training is an integral part of the exercise program.

2. To train and strengthen muscles of axial extension and thoracic extension

NOTE: These exercises also bring in the lumbar extensors as stabilizers.

a. Position of patient: supine. The patient tucks the chin and attempts to flatten the neck against the mat while simultaneously adducting the scapulae. A stronger isometric contraction is simulated by pressing the head into the mat.

b. Position of patient: prone, with forehead on the treatment table and arms at the sides. The patient lifts the forehead off the plinth while keeping the chin tucked and maintaining the functional position (no head extension). This is a small motion (Fig. 15–14).

  Progress this exercise by having the patient lift the upper portion of the chest off the plinth. The arms can be kept at the sides or progressed to 90 degrees abduction or full elevation for increased resistance.

c. Position of patient: quadruped (hands and knees), over a padded stool or large gym ball. The patient tucks the chin and maintains the eyes focused toward the floor to maintain functional position. Arm motions are superimposed while the neck muscles stabilize the neck and head. Suggestions include reaching out to the side, reaching overhead, and swimming motions.

  Progress by having the patient lift weights in the hands while stabilizing the head and neck in this position Fig. 15–15).

d. Position of patient: sitting on chair or edge of a mat; progress to an unstable surface such as sitting on a large gym ball and eventually to standing. The patient assumes a neutral spinal posture and superimposes arm motions. Add resistance to the arms as tolerated. To emphasize the cervical and upper thoracic extensors, use motions such as pulling, horizontal abduction, and lateral rotation with scapular adduction against an elastic resistance or pulley force. Progress to patterns of motion that duplicate desired functional activities (see Figs. 8–32 and 15–28).

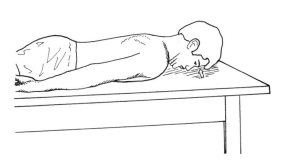

Figure 15–14. Axial extension exercises.

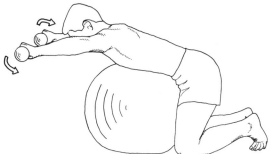

Figure 15–15. Developing cervical and upper thoracic stabilization. The patient maintains the head and neck in a neutral position while arm motions provide varying resistive forces. The gym ball provides an unstable surface requiring greater control.

NOTE: These exercises are also beneficial for lumbar stabilization.

e. Position of patient: standing. Place a basketball-sized inflatable ball between the back of the head and a wall. Maintain the position while moving the arms through various ranges of motion.

Progress by having the patient maintain the position while lifting free weights in the hands (Fig. 15–16).

3. To train and strengthen the cervical flexors

NOTE: Often with faulty forward-head postures the patient substitutes using the sternocleidomastoid (SCM) muscles to lift the head rather than the overstretched, weak, supra- and infrahyoid cervical flexors. To correct this muscle imbalance, use gentle motions with a lot of feedback.

a. Position of patient: supine. If the patient cannot tuck the chin and curl the neck to lift the head off the mat, begin the patient on a slant board or large wedged-shaped bolster under the thorax and head to reduce the effects of gravity. He or she practices tucking the chin and curling the head up. Use assistance until the correct pattern is learned (Fig. 15–17).

Progress by decreasing the angle of the board or wedge, then adding manual resistance if the patient does not substitute with the SCM.

b. Position of patient: standing with a basketball-sized inflatable ball between the forehead and a wall. He or she must keep the chin tucked and not go into a forward-head posture. The patient maintains the functional position while superimposing arm motions.

Progress by adding weights to the arm motions.

c. Position of patient: supine with the head over the edge of the mat, the neck maintained in a neutral functional position, and no support to the head. The

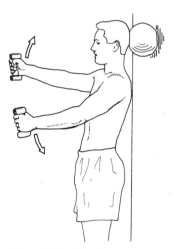

Figure 15–16. Strengthening the cervical and upper thoracic extensor muscles by maintaining control of the soft ball while varying resistance is applied through arm motions.

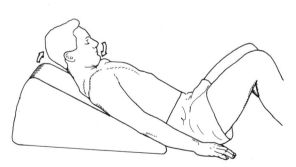

Figure 15–17. Training the short cervical flexors while deemphasizing the sternocleidomastoid for cervical flexion to regain a balance in strength for anterior cervical stabilization.

patient must be able to keep the neck in its safe functional position to perform this advanced stabilization exercise. He or she holds the position as tolerated. Progress by adding arm motions, then adding weights to the arm motions as tolerated.

d. The short neck flexors can also be trained while doing the prone-lying and quadruped position exercises for axial extension as previously described in Section 2 by having the patient squeeze a small towel roll under the chin to emphasize upper cervical flexion (nodding).

4. To strengthen the cervical muscles using manual resistance

Position of patient: supine. The therapist stands at the head end of the treatment table, supporting the patient's head for each exercise.

a. To apply manual resistance, place one hand on the patient's head to resist opposite the motion. Do not resist against the mandibule or the force will be transmitted to the temporomandibular joint. Resistance is given to isolated muscle actions or to general ranges of motion, whichever best gains muscle balance and function.

b. To provide isometric resistance, use the same procedure as in 2, except the intensity of resistance should prevent motion. The head can be placed in any position desired before applying the resistance. To avoid jerking the neck when applying or releasing the resistance, gradually build up the intensity, telling the patient to match your resistance; hold; then gradually release and, again, ask the patient to relax accordingly.

5. Self-resistance for isometric cervical exercises

Position of patient: sitting.

a. *Flexion.* The patient places both hands on the forehead and presses forehead into the palms in a nodding fashion but does not allow motion (Fig. 15–18A).

b. *Side-bending.* The patient presses one hand against the side of the head and

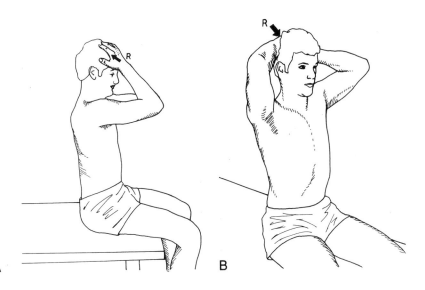

Figure 15–18. Self-resistance for isometric (*A*) cervical flexion and (*B*) axial extension.

A   B

attempts to side bend, trying to bring the ear toward the shoulder but not allowing motion.

c. *Axial extension*. The patient presses the back of the head into both hands, which are placed in the back, near the top of the head (Fig. 15–18B).

d. *Rotation*. The patient presses one hand against the region just superior and lateral to the eye and attempts to turn the head to look over the shoulder but does not allow motion.

6. Transitional stabilization for the cervical and upper thoracic regions

a. Position of patient: standing, with basketball-sized inflatable ball between the head and the wall. The patient rolls the ball along the wall, using the head. This requires the patient to turn the body as he or she walks along.

b. Position of patient: sitting on a large gym ball. The patient begins sitting, then walks the feet forward so that the ball rolls up the back and rests under the thorax (Figs. 15–19A and B). The head and neck are maintained in their functional position and the cervical flexors are emphasized. The person then walks the ball farther so that it rests under the head. The extensors are now emphasized (Fig. 15–19C). The patient walks the feet forward and backward, alternating stabilization between the flexors and extensors.

NOTE: This activity requires considerable strength in the cervical extensors to support the body weight and should be performed only in the rehabilitation phase when the patient has been properly progressed to tolerate the resistance.

Progress to advanced training by adding arm motions, then arm motions with weights in each of the positions.

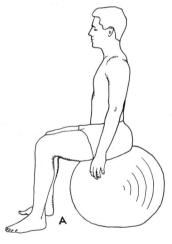

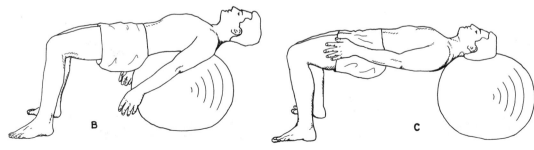

Figure 15–19. Advanced exercises for strengthening the cervical and upper thoracic flexors and extensors as stabilizers. Begin by (*A*) sitting on a large gym ball, then (*B*) walking forward while rolling the ball up the back. With the ball behind the mid-thoracic area, the cervical flexors must stabilize. Continue walking forward until the ball is (*C*) under the head; the cervical extensors now must stabilize. Walk back and forth between the two positions (*B* and *C*) to alternate control between the flexors and extensors. Progress by adding arm motions or arm motions with weights to increase resistance.

7. To train and strengthen muscles of the shoulder girdle that affect posture

See Chapter 8 for descriptions of shoulder girdle exercises. Emphasis is placed on the scapular retractors and shoulder lateral rotators.

C. Mid- and Lower Thoracic and Lumbar Regions

1. To teach awareness of safe lumbar range of motion

a. *Pelvic tilt*

Position of patient: hook-lying or supine. Teach the patient to perform a posterior pelvic tilt by slipping the hand under the low back and pushing the spine down on the hand. Use of the phrase "tuck your stomach in" may convey the idea for the correct motion. Then have the patient arch the back doing an anterior pelvic tilt. Repeat the posterior and anterior pelvic tilting until he or she can control the pelvic motion.

b. *Pelvic tilt; all fours*

Position of patient: on the hands and knees in the all-fours (quadruped) position. He or she practices controlling the pelvic tilt, rotating from an anterior tilt to a posterior tilt, as in Fig. 15–7, being sure motion is in the pelvis and lumbar spine, not in the thorax.

c. Practice tilting the pelvis through its pain-free range of motion in sitting, standing, and other functional positions. See additional suggestions for awareness and posture training in Section VI.

2. To train and strengthen the abdominal muscles as stabilizers of the trunk and pelvis and to increase muscular endurance for control

Progress to doing each exercise—or a combination of several exercises—initially for 1 minute; then progress for up to 3 minutes. Progress further by increasing resistance and then increasing speed.

a. Position of patient: supine with the pelvis and lumbar spine in its functional position. The patient sets the abdominals to hold the pelvis while arm and leg motions provide resistance.

(1) Alternately flex each arm overhead, progress by adding weights.

(2) Flex both arms simultaneously overhead; add weights.

(3) Affix elastic resistance or pulleys above the head; have the patient pull down against the resistance, alternating with one arm at a time or pulling down with both arms simultaneously. Progress by adding diagonal patterns (Fig. 15–20).

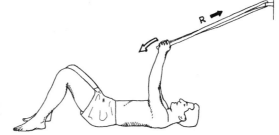

Figure 15–20. Developing the stabilizing action of the abdominal muscles by using pull-down activities against a resistive force from pulleys or elastic bands.

(4) Alternately bring one knee toward the chest and return; progress by alternately flexing, then extending, one leg, then the other. The opposite leg either remains extended on the mat or is in the hook-lying position so that only one leg is providing the resistance at a time. Progress by adding ankle weights (Fig. 15–21A).

(5) Progress to the 90–90 position (hips and knees each flexed to 90 degrees); alternately extend one leg, then the other (*modified bicycle exercise*, see Fig. 21–3). Begin with small motions; progress to larger motions as the patient demonstrates pelvic tilt stabilization. Progress by adding ankle weights.

(6) Flex one arm overhead while the opposite lower extremity extends; alternate (Fig. 15–21B). Progress by adding weights to the hands and ankles.

(7) To progress to a less stable surface, the patient can be positioned lying on a large gym ball under the thorax or neck (if the cervical stabilizers are strong), and all of the above exercises using arm and leg motions are repeated. (See Fig. 15–19.)

b. Position of patient: sitting. If necessary, begin with full support by having the patient sit with the back against a back rest on a chair; progress to sitting nonsupported on a stool, then to sitting on an unstable surface such as on a large gym ball. The patient sets the abdominal muscles to maintain the functional position of the spine.

(1) Alternately flex one arm overhead, then the other; then add resistance.

(2) Flex both arms overhead; then add resistance.

(3) Alternately lift one leg, then the other, using slight hip flexion and the knee in various degrees of extension, depending on control. Progress to lifting the opposite arm and leg simultaneously (Fig. 15–22).

(4) For advanced work lift both legs simultaneously, then all four extremities simultaneously.

c. Position of patient: kneeling or standing. He or she sets the abdominal muscles to maintain the functional position of the spine while performing these exercises.

NOTE: Progressing from sitting to kneeling to standing requires increased participation of more extremity muscles for stabilization at the hip, knee, and ankles and begins training for more functionally related weight-bearing activities.

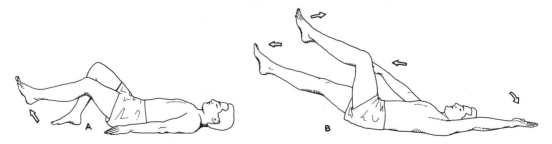

Figure 15–21. Developing abdominal strength as the muscles stabilize the spine in its functional position. (*A*) Light resistance is applied by flexing and extending one lower extremity while the other helps stabilize. (*B*) A strong controlling action in the abdominals is required when both upper and lower extremities are moving in alternating patterns.

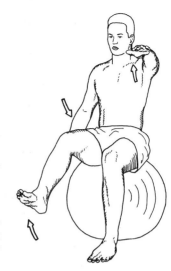

Figure 15–22. Strength, balance, and coordination are required to maintain spinal stabilization while sitting on a gym ball and moving the extremities. This activity is progressed by adding weights to the extremities.

(1) Set the abdominal muscles; then alternately lift one arm, then the other, overhead; lift both arms simultaneously. Add weights.

(2) Pulleys or elastic resistance is secured overhead or behind the patient. He or she sets the abdominals, then pulls down or forward with the arms (Fig. 15–23A). Various patterns such as shoulder extension, shoulder horizontal adduction, and diagonal extension patterns as well as unilateral or bilateral arm motions change the angle of pull and therefore change the pattern of stabilization required. It is more challenging if the patient keeps the elbows extended while going through the shoulder range of motion. These isometric exercises may be alternated with concentric and eccentric motions of the trunk flexors (Fig. 15–23B).

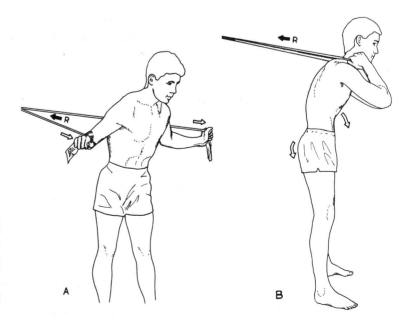

Figure 15–23. Using elastic resistance to train and strengthen the abdominal muscles in the upright position. (*A*) Isometrically setting the abdominals while the person brings the arms forward against the resistance. (*B*) Trunk flexion against resistance, emphasizing posterior pelvic tilt and approximating the ribs to the pubic bone.

3. To strengthen the abdominal muscles through the range of motion

a. Curl-ups

Position of patient: hook-lying, with the lumbar spine flat (posterior pelvic tilt). First, have the patient lift the head off the mat. This will cause a stabilizing contraction of the abdominal muscles. He or she progresses by lifting the shoulders until the scapulae and thorax clear the mat, keeping the arms horizontal (Fig. 15–24). The patient does not come to a full sit-up, because once the thorax clears the mat, the rest of the motion is performed by the hip flexor muscles. Further progress the difficulty of the curl-up by changing the arm position from horizontal to folded across the chest, then to behind the head. In all these activities, the low back should not arch; if it does, reduce the progression until the abdominals are strong enough to maintain lumbar flexion.

b. Curl-downs

If the patient is unable to perform the curl-up as in a, begin with curl-downs.

   Position of patient: starting in the hook-sitting or long-sitting position. The patient lowers the trunk only to the point where he or she can maintain a flat low back, then returns to the sitting position. Once the patient can curl-down full range, reverse and instruct to perform a curl-up.

c. Diagonal curl-ups

To emphasize the external oblique muscles, the patient performs a diagonal curl-up by reaching one hand toward the outside of the opposite knee while curling up, then alternating. Reverse the muscle action by bringing one knee up toward the opposite shoulder; then repeat with the other knee.

d. Double knee to chest

To emphasize the lower rectus abdominis and oblique muscles, have the patient set a posterior pelvic tilt, then bring both knees to the chest and return. Progress the difficulty by decreasing the angle of the hip and knee flexion (Fig. 15–25).

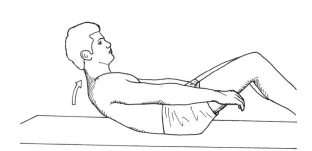

Figure 15–24. The curl-up exercise to strengthen the abdominal muscles. The thorax is flexed on the lumbar spine. The arms are shown in the position for least resistance. Progress by crossing the arms across the chest, then behind the head.

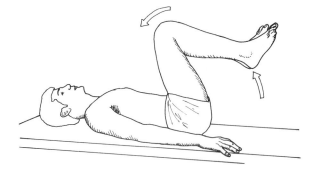

Figure 15–25. Strengthening the abdominal muscles by flexing the hip and pelvis on the lumbar spine. The legs are shown in the position for least resistance. Progress by decreasing the angle of hip flexion until the legs can be lifted with the knees extended.

e. Pelvic lifts

The patient begins with the hips at 90 degrees and knees extended. The patient performs a posterior pelvic tilt and lifts the buttock upward off the mat (small motion). The feet move upward toward the ceiling (Fig. 15–26). The patient should not push against the mat with the hands.

f. Bilateral straight-leg raising (SLR)

This is a progression in difficulty of the double knee-to-chest exercise. It should be undertaken only if the muscles are strong enough to maintain a posterior pelvic tilt. The patient begins with legs extended. The patient first performs a posterior pelvic tilt, then flexes both hips, keeping the knees extended. If the hips are abducted before initiating this exercise, greater stress is placed on the oblique abdominal muscles.

Precaution: The strong pull of psoas major causes shear forces on the lumbar vertebrae. If there is any low-back pain or discomfort, especially with spinal hypermobility or instability, this exercise should not be performed even if the abdominals are strong enough to maintain a posterior pelvic tilt.

g. Bilateral straight-leg lowering

This can be performed if the bilateral SLR is difficult. The patient begins with the hips at 90 degrees and knees extended. The patient lowers the extremities as far as he or she can while maintaining a flat back, then raises the legs back to 90 degrees. See precaution under f.

h. Concentric-eccentric resistance to trunk flexors

Position of patient: sitting or standing. Pulleys or elastic material is secured at shoulder level behind the patient.

(1) The patient holds the ends of the material with each hand. He or she then flexes the trunk, with emphasis on bringing the rib down toward the pubic bone and performing a posterior pelvic tilt, rather than hip flexion (see Fig. 15–23B).

(2) Diagonal motions are performed by bringing one arm down toward the opposite knee, with emphasis on moving the rib cage down toward the opposite side of the pelvis. Repeat the diagonal motion in the opposite direction.

(3) Progress the resistance as the patient's abdominal strength increases.

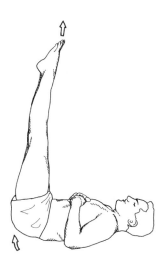

Figure 15–26. Pelvic lifts. Elevating the legs upward toward the ceiling by raising the buttock off the floor emphasizes strengthening the lower abdominal muscles.

4. **To train and strengthen the lumbar extensors as stabilizers of the trunk and to increase muscular endurance for spinal control**

   Progress endurance by increasing the time performing each exercise or combinations of exercises, initially for up to 1 minute, then progress to 3-minute bouts. Progress strength by adding resistance. Train using increased speed and complexity of movements.

   a. Position of patient: supine with the spine in its most comfortable functional position.
      (1) Pulleys or elastic resistance are secured to the foot of the treatment table or mat. The patient pulls up (flexion) with one arm, with both arms or alternating arms, and concentrates on maintaining the functional position of the spine.
      (2) Progress to include diagonal flexion patterns.

   b. Position of patient: all-fours (quadruped) position. If assistance is needed to stabilize the spine, the patient can be positioned over a padded stool, chair, or large gym ball. These exercises can also be performed prone, but the spine and hips are near the end-range of extension, so little motion is available. The prone position may be especially difficult in the early stages of healing or if there is significant hip or trunk flexor tightness. It is important to maintain the cervical spine in its functional position during these exercises. Having the patient tuck a small towel roll between the chin and neck emphasizes upper cervical flexion. If the patient is lying prone, a small roll under the forehead should be used so the head can be kept in alignment with space allowed for the nose.
      (1) Alternately lift one arm, then the other. Weights are added to the hands to increase resistance.
      (2) Alternately slide one leg posteriorly and return. If there is good spinal control, the patient lifts one lower extremity toward hip extension, returns it, and repeats with the other leg. The patient is cautioned to stabilize the pelvis. A rod or cane placed down the back provides a tactile cue for stabilization (Fig. 15–27A).
      (3) Progress by lifting the opposite arm and leg simultaneously, then alternate (Fig. 15–27B).
      (4) If supported by a stool or gym ball, the patient can lift both arms simultaneously and do swimming and reaching motions.

   c. Position of patient: sitting, with the spine in its functional position, facing a pulley or elastic resistance. Sitting on a large gym ball provides a less stable surface for balance training (Fig. 15–28A). When there is good stabilization, progress the patient to standing (Fig. 15–28B).

      Pull against the resistance with various patterns of upper extremity motion, including scapular retraction, shoulder horizontal abduction, abduction with external rotation, extension, and diagonal patterns.

5. **To train and strengthen the lumbar extensor muscle groups through the range of motion**

   a. Position of patient: supine, arms at the side. Instruct the patient to arch the back by pressing against the floor with the back of the neck and the sacrum (Fig. 15–29).
   b. Position of patient: prone, arms at the side. Have the patient tuck in the chin and lift the head. This brings in a stabilizing contraction of the lumbar exten-

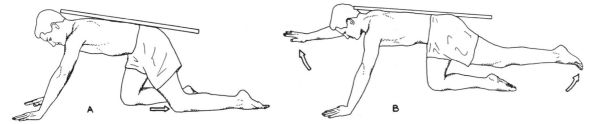

Figure 15–27. Quadruped exercises to develop control and strength in the spinal extensors. (*A*) Light resistance is applied by sliding one lower extremity outward while concentrating on controlling the spine. Balancing a rod on the back provides reinforcement that the trunk is not twisting. (*B*) Greater challenge is provided by lifting the opposite arm and leg simultaneously, then alternating extremities.

sor muscles. For greater range, have the patient lift the thorax as well as the head. (See Fig. 15–14.)

(1) To progress resistance, have the patient vary the arm position from resting at the side, to placing the hands behind the head, then to placing the arms in full elevation as he or she extends the spine. The lower extremities will need to be stabilized (Fig. 15–30).

(2) Leg lifts
   Position of patient: prone. Begin by lifting one leg several inches off the mat (hip extension), alternate with the other leg. Progress by lifting both legs simultaneously.

(3) Further progression can be accomplished by having the patient prone and lifting both elevated arms and extended legs simultaneously (Fig. 15–31).

(4) Resistance can be applied to any of the above exercises by having the patient hold weights in the hands or by strapping weights around the patient's legs.

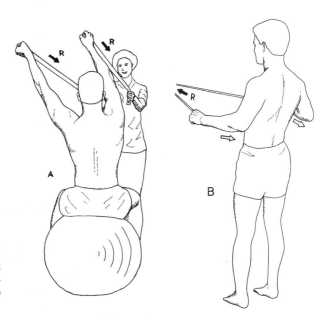

Figure 15–28. Using elastic resistance to train and strengthen the back extensor muscles to stabilize in the upright position (*A*) sitting on an unstable surface and (*B*) standing.

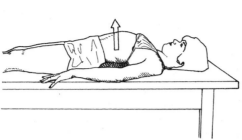

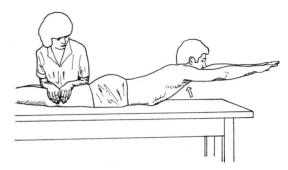

Figure 15–29. To strengthen the back extensors, have the patient arch the back while supine.

Figure 15–30. Strengthening the back extensors with the arms in position to provide maximum resistance. Additional resistance can be provided by holding weights in the hands.

   c. Position of patient: sitting or standing.
      (1) Resistance can be applied for concentric-eccentric extension exercises in the upright position by securing an elastic material at shoulder level in front of the patient. He or she holds on to the ends of the material, sets the pelvis, and extends the spine (Fig. 15–32). A boat-rowing motion with the arms also effectively stimulates the trunk extensors. Progress the exercise by increasing the grade of elastic resistance.
      (2) Rotation with extension
         Position of patient: standing. Use a pulley or elastic resistance secured under the foot or to a stable object opposite to the side being exercised. The patient pulls against the resistance, extending and rotating the back. Changing the angle of pull of the elastic material allows the therapist to re-create functional patterns specific to the patient's needs (Fig. 15–33).

6. To train and strengthen muscles of the lower extremity that affect posture

See Chapters 11 to 13.

D. Preparation for Functional Activities

NOTE: Many of the strengthening exercises described in the extremity chapters are appropriate to use in preparation for functional training. With postural problems and recovery from back or neck injuries it is critical to emphasize the functional spinal posture before and during total body exercises. Many of the stabilization and movement patterns described in the previous sections can also be progressed in intensity, repetitions, speed, and coordination to prepare for return to functional activities.

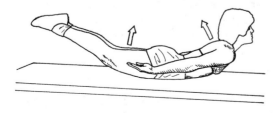

Figure 15–31. To strengthen the trunk and hip extensors, have the patient lift the trunk and legs off the mat simultaneously.

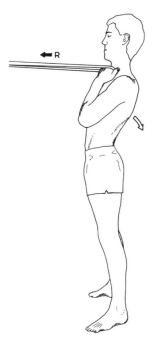

Figure 15–32. Using elastic resistance for concentric-eccentric back extension.

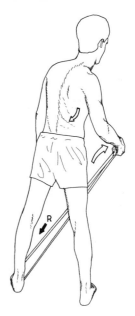

Figure 15–33. Rotation with extension strengthens the back extensors in functional patterns.

1. Modified bridging exercises

These require stabilization of the trunk flexors and extensors in conjunction with the gluteus maximus and quadriceps muscles. The abdominals function with the gluteus maximus to control posterior pelvic tilt, and the lumbar extensors stabilize the spine against the pull of the gluteus maximus.

a. Begin with the patient hook-lying. He or she maintains the functional spinal position while raising and lowering the pelvis, concentrating on flexing and extending at the hips, while not moving the spine (see Fig. 11–11).

b. Hold the bridge for isometric control.

   (1) Alternate arm motions; progress by adding weights to the hands.

   (2) Alternate lifting one foot, then the other by marching in place (Fig. 15–34A); progress by extending the knee as each leg is lifted. When the patient tolerates greater resistance, add ankle weights (Fig. 15–34B).

   (3) Abduct and adduct the thighs without letting the pelvis sag.

c. Progress by placing the feet on a stool, chair, or large gym ball and repeating the bridging activities.

2. Alternating isometric contractions (rhythmic stabilization)

The patient position begins supine and progresses to sitting on a stable surface, sitting on an unstable surface like a large gym ball, kneeling, and then standing.

a. The patient flexes the arm to 90 degrees and holds a rod or cane in both hands. The therapist also holds on to the rod and pushes and pulls while the patient isometrically holds against the resistance force (see Fig. 8–30). No movement should occur.

   (1) Initially the therapist provides verbal cues such as "pull against my resis-

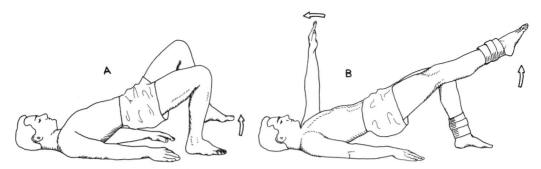

Figure 15–34. Holding a bridge to develop trunk control while superimposing extremity motions: (*A*) marching in place, (*B*) progressing to extending the extremities. Adding weights to the arms or legs requires greater strength and control.

tance but do not overpower me; feel your abdominal muscles contracting; now I'm pulling in the opposite direction; match the resistance and feel your back muscles contracting." Progress by shifting the resistance directions without the verbal cues and then by increasing speed.

(2) Once the patient learns to respond to the sagittal plane alternating resistance, the therapist provides side-to-side and rotating resistance.

b. Two canes or rods are used, one in each hand of the patient and one in each hand of the therapist. Alternating motions are resisted as described.

c. Patient supine with hips flexed around 90 degrees and knees fully flexed. The therapist provides resistance against the knees toward flexion, then extension or rotation, while the patient responds with alternating isometric contractions.

3. Push-ups with trunk stabilization

The patient begins prone on a large gym ball. He or she walks forward with the hands on the floor until just the thighs are supported by the ball, maintaining a stable spinal posture, and performs push-ups with the arms. To progress, walk out farther with the hands until just the legs are supported by the ball (Fig. 15–35).

4. Wall slides

The patient stands with the back to a wall and the spine held in its functional position. A towel placed behind the back makes the exercise easier. The exercise is more challenging if a large gym ball is placed between the back and the wall (see Fig. 11–15).

a. Slide down to a partial squat. Hold the position. Arm motions can be superimposed while holding the position. To progress, add weights.

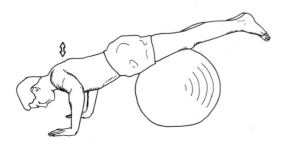

Figure 15–35. Push-up activities with the lower extremities balanced on a gym ball for strengthening the arms and developing trunk control.

b. Slide up and down repetitively, alternating arm motions with the sliding motions.

5. Partial lunges and partial squats

These exercises are described in Chapters 11 and 12. They are beneficial in strengthening total body movement in preparation for teaching body mechanics. Weights can be added to the upper extremities for resistance. In addition, arm motions are synchronized with the leg motions to develop coordination.

6. Walking against resistance

A pulley or elastic resistance is secured around the patient's pelvis with a belt, or the patient can hold the handle grips. The patient walks forward, backward, or diagonally against the resistive force. Emphasis is placed on spinal control.

Progress by having the patient push and pull weights with the upper extremities; emphasis is placed on maintaining the functional spinal position while the extremities are loaded.

7. Shifting weight and turning

The patient practices shifting weight forward/backward and side to side while maintaining the functional spinal position and absorbing the forces with the hips and knees. Turning is practiced by turning with small steps and rotating at the hips rather than the back. Instruct the patient to imagine two rigid poles connecting each shoulder to each hip that will not allow the spine to twist.

Progress by using weights.

8. Transitional stabilization activities

The patient learns to stabilize the spine against alternating trunk motions.
a. The patient begins in the quadruped position. He or she rocks back to resting the buttock on the heels, then shifts the body forward onto the hands in the press-up position. The patient concentrates on controlling the pelvis in its functional position rather than allowing full spinal flexion when rocking onto the heels or full spinal extension when shifting forward onto the extended upper extremities.
b. The patient begins standing. He or she then reaches downward while partially squatting. The tendency is for the spine to flex so the patient concentrates on maintaining a neutral spinal position with the spinal extensors. He or she then stands up and reaches overhead. This causes the spine to extend; the patient concentrates on using the trunk flexors to stabilize in the neutral position. Progress by lifting weights while controlling the functional posture of the spine.

E. Frontal Plane Strengthening Exercises

These exercises are used for general strengthening of the muscles that side bend the trunk. If there is a structural scoliosis, exercise alone has not been shown to halt or change the progression of the curve, but exercise used in conjunction with other methods of correction such as bracing has been shown to be beneficial.[1,2] When there is a scoliotic curve, the muscles on the convex side are usually stretched and weakened. The following exercises are described for use as strengthening exercises on the side of the convexity. Postural exercises for spinal control as described in Section V may be beneficial for general strengthening and conditioning when there is a scoliosis.

1. Patient standing. On the side of the concavity, the patient places one end of an elastic resistance under the foot and holds the other end in the hand. He or she then side bends the trunk toward the side of the convexity. This exercise can also be performed with a weight held in the hand on the side of the concavity.

2. Patient side-lying on the concave side of the curve with the lower arm folded across the chest; the therapist stabilizes at the iliac crest. Have the patient derotate the trunk and lift the head and shoulders (lateral trunk flexion) and slide the top arm down toward the knee (Fig. 15–36A). For greater range begin with the thorax over the side of the table.

     Progress the resistance by having the patient clasp hands behind the head and then laterally flex the trunk against gravity (Fig. 15–36B).

VI. Procedures to Retrain Kinesthetic and Proprioceptive Awareness for Posture Correction

A. Train Patient Awareness

Initially, normal alignment may be prevented because of tightness of soft tissue or malalignment of a vertebral segment, but developing patient awareness of balanced posture and its effects should begin early in the treatment program in conjunction with the stretching and muscle-training maneuvers.

B. Use Reinforcement Techniques During Treatment

1. Verbal reinforcement

As you interact with the patient, frequently interpret the sensations of muscle contraction and position that he or she should be feeling. This is done especially when teaching relaxation techniques (see Section III.A) and spinal control activities.

2. Visual reinforcement

Use mirrors so the patient can see how he or she looks, what it takes to assume good alignment, and then how it feels when properly aligned. Verbally reinforce what the patient sees.

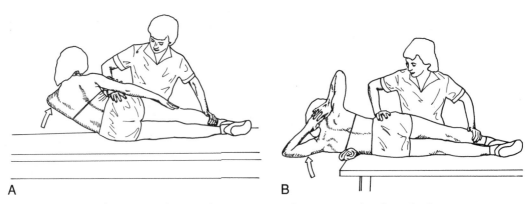

A   B

Figure 15–36. To strengthen weak structures on the convex side of a right thoracic curve, have the patient lie on the left side and lift the upper trunk off the mat (*A*) with the arms at the side and (*B*) with the arms overhead for greater resistance. With the thorax over the side of the table, greater range of motion is possible.

3. Tactile reinforcement

Help the patient position the head and trunk in correct alignment and touch the muscles that need to contract to move and hold the parts in place.

C. Teach Proper Movement and Balance Control

Isolate each imbalanced body segment and train the patient how to move that segment. If one region is out of alignment, it is likely that the entire spine is imbalanced to compensate, so total posture correction should be emphasized. Direct the patient's attention to the feel of proper movement and muscle contraction and relaxation. Use reinforcement techniques as described previously in Section B. It may be useful to have the patient assume an extreme corrected posture, then ease away from the extreme toward mid-position, then hold the corrected posture.

1. To train axial extension to decrease a forward-head posture

Position of patient: sitting or standing, with arms relaxed at the side. Lightly touch above the lip under the nose and ask the patient to lift the head up and away (Fig. 15–37A). Verbally reinforce the correct movement of tucking the chin in and straightening the spine, and draw attention to the way it feels. Have the patient move to the extreme correct posture, then return to mid-line.

2. To train scapular retraction

Position of patient: sitting or standing. For tactile and proprioceptive cues, gently resist movement of the inferior angle of the scapulae and ask the patient to pinch them together (retraction). The patient should not extend or elevate the shoulders (Fig. 15–37B).

3. To train control of the pelvic tilt and balance of the lumbar spine

Position of patient: sitting, then standing with the back against a wall. After the patient has learned pelvic tilt exercises, instruct to practice control of movement of the pelvis and lumbar spine by moving from extreme lordosis to extreme flat-

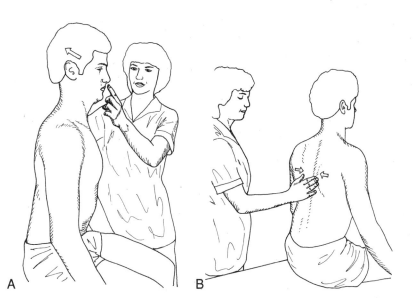

Figure 15–37. Training the patient to correct (*A*) forward head posture and (*B*) protracted scapulae.

A   B

back and then assuming a mild lordosis. Show that the hand should be able to easily slip between the back and the wall and that he or she can then feel the back with one side of the hand and the wall with the other side.

4. To train control of the thorax and thoracic spine

Position of patient: standing. The position of the thorax affects the posture of the lumbar spine and pelvis so that the feel of thoracic movement is incorporated in posture training for the lumbar spine. As the patient assumes a mild lordotic posture (as in 3), have him or her breathe in and lift the rib cage (extension). Guide to a balanced posture, not an extremely extended posture.

NOTE: It may be necessary to direct the patient's attention to the feel of shifting the thorax anteriorly and posteriorly and noting how it affects the lumbar spine. There is an important difference between standing with a lordotic posture (extreme lordosis in the lumbar spine with excessive anterior pelvic tilt) versus a relaxed posture (excessive extension in the lower lumbar spine with a rapid reversal into flexion in the upper lumbar spine and thorax). (See Section II of this chapter.) It is important to recognize the difference between these two postures. Often, because the excessive extension is noted in the lower lumbar segment in patients with slouched postures, the patient erroneously is placed on a flexion exercise and training program to flatten the low back.[5] This approach ignores or reinforces the already flexed posture of the thorax on the upper lumbar spine and tends to accentuate that problem, particularly because curl-up exercises are emphasized in the flexion routine. If the reader is confused with what has been described, try the following:

a. Stand; start with a normal lordotic. This requires elevation of the rib cage. Note that there is a mild anterior pelvic tilt and mild lumbar lordosis.

b. Now, tilt the pelvis anteriorly and assume an increased lordosis; note the associated hip flexion. This posture is, in fact, extreme, and some people demonstrate this as the source of their problems.

c. Now, again assume a mid-line normal lordotic posture (requiring tilting the pelvis posteriorly partway). From this normal posture, shift into a relaxed posture by allowing the pelvic segment to shift anteriorly and the rib cage to shift posteriorly and approximate the pelvis. Note the hips are now in extension with respect to the pelvis (not an anterior pelvic tilt), but the lower lumbar spine is in extension. The thorax is, in essence, flexed on the upper lumbar spine. Often, when in this posture, a person also shifts the weight onto one leg, thus adding asymmetry to the whole picture.

The point is that this relaxed posture should *not* be corrected with a total flexion approach as would be carried out with a lordotic postural problem. To emphasize curl-ups only perpetuates flexing the thorax on the upper lumbar spine; instead the motion needs to be extension. In the lower lumbar spine and hips, some flexion is necessary. Here, pelvic control with pelvic tilt exercises should be performed. For strengthening, active double knee-to-chest and modified bicycle exercises will emphasize flexion of the lower lumbar spine. Therefore, with this posture, a combined flexion-extension approach must be used in retraining for proper movement and control. The patient must learn to lift the rib cage and shift it anteriorly as the pelvis is shifted posteriorly, similar to taking a crooked stack of blocks and shifting it to straighten it. Telling the patient to think tall, breathe in to expand the anterior thorax, and lift the head may encourage the correct response. Additional verbal prompting to help the patient imagine and then re-create the correct posture may also help.

5. To teach awareness of the sensation of assuming a normal posture and developing spinal control

Position of patient: sitting. Instruct the patient to curl the entire spine by first flexing the neck, then the thorax, then the lumbar spine. Give cues for unrolling by first touching the lumbar spine as he or she extends it, then the thoracic spine as he or she extends it and takes in a breath to elevate the rib cage. Then direct attention to adducting the scapulae while you gently resist the motion, then lifting the head in axial extension while you give slight pressure against the upper lip. Verbally and visually reinforce the correct posture when it is obtained.

D. Demonstrate the Relationship of Faulty Posture to the Development of Pain

Have the patient assume the faulty posture and wait. When he or she begins to feel discomfort, point out the posture and then instruct to correct it and notice the feeling of relief. Many patients will not accept such a simple relationship between stress and pain, so draw their attention to noticing, throughout the day and after a night's rest, what posture they are in when pain comes on and how they can control it with the techniques they have been taught.

E. Reinforce Learning

It is not possible for a person to always maintain good posture. Therefore, to reinforce learning, teach the patient to use cues throughout the day to check posture. For example, instruct to check the posture every time he or she walks past a mirror, waits at a red light while driving a car, sits down for a meal, enters a room, or begins talking with someone. Find out what daily routines the patient has that could be used for reinforcement reminders; instruct to practice and report the results. Provide positive feedback as the patient becomes actively involved in the relearning process.

F. Postural Splints

If necessary, provide external support with a postural splint to prevent the extreme posture of round shoulders and protracted scapulae. It helps train correct muscle functioning by acting as a reminder for the patient to correct posture when he or she slouches. Also, by preventing the position of stretch from occurring, stretch weakness can be corrected.

VII. Procedures to Teach Management of Posture to Avoid Recurrences of the Problem

A. Body Mechanics

1. Have the patient practice lifting by stooping down to the object, bringing the object close to the body, setting the back in a functional or neutral position, then lifting with the hip and knee extensors.

a. Lifting with a neutral spinal posture provides greater stability to the spine[10] and uses both the ligamentous and muscular system to stabilize and control.[26]

b. Following back injury, the preferred lifting posture may have to be adapted, depending on the type of injury and the response of the tissues when stressed.[26]

c. When lifting with a flexed lumbar spine (posterior pelvic tilt), support for the spine is primarily from inert structures (ligaments, lumbodorsal fasciae, posterior annulus fibrosus, and facets); there is little muscle activity.

(1) This posture may be necessary when stooping to the floor. It may also be the posture of choice for a patient who has injured the back muscles because the muscles are "quiet" when the spine is in flexion.[26]

(2) Lifting with the lumbar spine in flexion may pose some problems. When lifting slowly with the lumbar spine in flexion, the load is maintained on the ligaments, and creep of the inert tissues occurs; this increases the chance of injury if the tissue is already weakened. In addition, with the muscles lengthened and relaxed, they may be at an unfavorable length-tension relationship to quickly respond with appropriate force to resist a sudden change in load. There is greater chance of ligamentous strain when a person lifts with a flexed spine.[10]

d. When lifting with an extended (lordotic) lumbar spine, the muscles supporting the spine are more active, which increases the compressive forces on the disk. This posture relieves stress on the ligaments, but for an individual whose back muscles fatigue quickly (in poor condition) this posture may jeopardize the spine when repeated lifts are performed because the ligaments are not taut and thus are not providing support.[26]

2. Have the patient practice carrying objects close to his or her center of gravity so he or she can feel the balance. When lifting, the closer the object is held to the center of gravity, the less stress is placed on the structures on the back and hip.

3. Have the patient practice shifting the load from side to side and turning. The action should be directed by the legs while the spine is kept stable with minimal trunk rotation.

4. Replicate the mechanics of the patient's job setting and practice safe mechanics.

B. Preventive Exercises

1. Review the following principles:
   a. Avoid any one posture for prolonged periods. If sustained postures are necessary, take frequent breaks and perform appropriate range of motion exercises at least every half hour. Finish all exercises by assuming a well-balanced posture.
   b. Avoid hyperextending the neck or being in a forward-head posture or forward-bent position for prolonged periods. Find ways to modify a task so it can be accomplished at eye level or with proper lumbar support.
   c. If in a tension-producing situation, perform conscious relaxation exercises.
   d. Use common sense and follow good safety habits.

2. Review flexibility and strengthening exercises appropriate for the patient to maintain adequate range of motion and develop adequate strength for good physical conditioning.

3. Review the relationship of posture and pain; when experiencing pain, check posture.

C. Adapt Environment

1. Review the patient's work and home environment.
    a. Chairs and car seats should have good lumbar support to maintain a slight lordosis. Use a towel roll or lumbar pillow if necessary.
    b. Chair height should allow knees to flex to take the pull off the hamstring muscles, support the thighs, and also allow the feet to rest comfortably on the floor.
    c. Desk or table height should be adequate to keep the person from having to lean over the work.
    d. Work and driving habits should allow frequent changing of posture. If normally sedentary, get up and walk every hour.
2. Review the patient's sleeping environment.
    a. Mattress needs to provide firm support to prevent any extreme stresses. If it is too soft, the patient sags and stresses ligaments; if it is too firm, some patients cannot relax.
    b. Pillows should be of a comfortable height and density to promote relaxation but should not place joints at an extreme position. Foam rubber pillows tend to cause increased tension in muscles because of the constant resistance they provide.
    c. Whether the person should sleep prone, side-lying, or supine is something that must be analyzed for each individual patient. Ideally, a comfortable posture is one that is mid-range and that does not place stress on any supporting structure. Pain that occurs in the morning is often related to sleeping posture; so, if this is the case, listen carefully to the patient's description of postures when sleeping and see if it relates to the pain. Then attempt to modify the sleep position accordingly.

VIII. Summary

The first section of this chapter has contained information on the dynamics of posture and characteristics and problems of common faulty postures and then has provided guidelines for developing exercise programs based on common problems found in postural pain syndromes and dysfunctions. The remainder of the chapter has described exercise progressions for stretching, strengthening, developing muscular endurance, and progressing to functional independence. Emphasis has been placed on developing a balance in length and strength of spinal musculature and learning control of the neck and trunk for stabilization during functional activities.

References

1. Blount, WP, and Blonske, J: Physical therapy in the nonoperative treatment of scoliosis. Phys Ther 47: 919, 1967.
2. Blount, WP, and Moe, JH: The Milwaukee Brace. Williams & Wilkins, Baltimore, 1980.
3. Bondi, BA, and Drinkwater-Kolk, M: Functional stabilization training. Workshop notes, Northeast Seminars, October 1992
4. Cailliet, R: Scoliosis. FA Davis, Philadelphia, 1975.
5. Cailliet, R: Low Back Pain Syndrome, ed 4. FA Davis, Philadelphia, 1988.
6. Cassella, MC, and Hall, JE: Current treatment approaches in the nonoperative and operative management of adolescent idiopathic scoliosis. Phys Ther 71:897, 1991.
7. Donaldson, WF: Scoliosis. In Ferguson, AB (ed): Orthopedic Surgery in Infancy and Childhood, ed 5. Williams & Wilkins, Baltimore, 1981.
8. Engler, GL: Scoliosis. In Nickel, VL (ed): Orthopedic Rehabilitation. Churchill-Livingstone, New York, 1982.
9. Friber, O: Clinical symptoms and biomechanics of lumbar spine and hip joint in leg length inequality. Spine 8:643, 1983.

10. Hart, DL, Stobbe, TJ, and Jaraiedi, M: Effect of lumbar posture on lifting. Spine 12:22, 1987.
11. Hellebrant, F, and Fries, E: The constancy of oscillograph stance patterns. Phys Ther Rev 22:17, 1942.
12. James, JIP: Scoliosis, ed 2. Churchill-Livingstone, London, 1976.
13. Kendall, F, McCreary, E, and Provance, PG: Muscles: Testing and Function, ed 4. Williams & Wilkins, Baltimore, 1993.
14. Lamb, C: The neurology of spinal pain. Phys Ther 59:971, 1979.
15. Lehmkuhl, LD, and Smith, LK: Brunnstrom's Clinical Kinesiology, ed 4. FA Davis, Philadelphia, 1983.
16. Lovell, WW, and Winter, RB (eds): Pediatric Orthopedics, ed 2. JB Lippincott, Philadelphia, 1986.
17. Morgan, D: Concepts in functional training and postural stabilization for the low-back injured. Topics in Acute Care and Trauma Rehabilitation 2:8, 1988.
18. Nemeth, G: On hip and lumbar biomechanics, a study of joint load and muscular activity. Scand J Rehabil Med (Suppl) 10:4, 1984.
19. Norkin, C, and Levangie, P: Joint Structure and Function: A Comprehensive Analysis, ed 2. FA Davis, Philadelphia, 1989.
20. Porterfield, JA: Dynamic stabilization of the trunk. Journal of Orthopaedic and Sports Physical Therapy 6:271, 1985.
21. Robinson, R: The new back school prescription: Stabilization training part I. Occup Med 7:17, 1992.
22. Rocobado, M: Temporomandibular Joint Dysfunctions. Workshop Notes, Cincinnati, 1979.
23. Saal, JA: The new back school prescription: Stabilization training part II. Occup Med 7:33, 1992.
24. Saal, JA: Dynamic muscular stabilization in the nonoperative treatment of lumbar pain syndromes. Orthop Rev 19:691, 1990.
25. Salter, RB: Textbook of Disorders and Injuries of the Musculoskeletal System, ed 2. Williams & Wilkins, Baltimore, 1983.
26. Sullivan, MS: Back support mechanisms during manual lifting. Phys Ther 69:38, 1989.
27. Sweeney, T: Neck school: Cervicothoracic stabilization training. Occup Med 7:43, 1992.

The Spine:
Traction Procedures

Traction is the "process of drawing or pulling."[24] When traction is used to draw or pull on the spinal column, it is called spinal traction. Traction is a therapeutic tool that falls in the realm of exercise because of its effects on the musculoskeletal system and use in stretching and mobilizing techniques.[12] Its mode of application is often through machines, although a therapist can apply traction to the joints of the spinal column through carefully applied manual and positional techniques. Its uses and applications are varied and subject to the patient's clinical response more than objective scientific argument for its success in decreasing symptoms. To date there are no randomized clinical studies strongly supporting or disproving the efficacy of traction for therapeutic intervention.[25]

Goals and plans of care for various posture and spinal problems are described in Chapters 14 and 15. In many instances, traction is a recommended procedure in the plan of care; therefore, the information in this chapter should be studied concurrently with the information in the previous two chapters for completeness.

OBJECTIVES

After studying this chapter, the reader will be able to:

1 Identify the effects of spinal traction.
2 Define the types of traction and how they are applied.
3 Identify the indications, limitations, contraindications, and precautions for the use of spinal traction.
4 Relate traction techniques for use within a total therapeutic exercise program.
5 Describe safety rules and procedures for mechanical and manual traction techniques.
6 Apply basic mechanical, positional, and manual traction techniques to the spine.

I. Effects of Spinal Traction[19]

A. Mechanical Elongation of the Spine[3,9,13,14,21,23]

1. The effect of elongation is mechanical separation of the vertebrae, which:

   a. Stretches the spinal muscles
   b. Tenses the ligaments and facet joint capsules
   c. Widens the intervertebral foramina
   d. Straightens the spinal curves
   e. Slides the facet joints
   f. Flattens a nuclear disk protrusion

2. Factors that influence the amount of vertebral separation

   a. Spinal position
      The greater the angle of flexion that the spine is placed in prior to the administration of traction, the greater the vertebral separation, especially the posterior aspect of the vertebral body.[5,20]

   b. Angle of pull
      The angle of pull of the traction force affects the amount of flexion of the spine.
      (1) In the cervical spine, the angle of pull creating the greatest posterior elongation is 35 degrees.[4]
      (2) In the lumbar spine, a harness that pulls from the posterior aspect of the pelvis rather than primarily from the sides is necessary to cause flexion of the spine.[21]

   c. Amount of force
      The effective force is influenced by the body position, weight of the part, friction of the treatment table, method of traction used, amount of patient relaxation, and the equipment itself. Generally, for vertebral separation:
      (1) In the cervical spine, under friction-free circumstances, a force of approximately 7 percent of the total body weight separates the vertebrae.[6] A minimum force of 11.25 to 13.5 kg (25 to 30 lb) is necessary to lift the weight of the head when sitting and to counteract the resistance of muscle tension. The greatest amount of separation occurs during the first few minutes of treatment at a given force.[8]
      (2) In the lumbar spine, a minimum friction-free force of half the body weight is necessary for mechanical separation.[6,11]

   d. Comfort and relaxation
      These are necessary for greatest benefit of vertebral separation.

B. Zygapophyseal (Facet) Joint Mobilization

1. Effects of mobilization from various positions and forces on the spine

   a. Sliding or translation of the facet surfaces
   b. Distraction or a separation of the facet surfaces
   c. Compression or an approximation of the facet surfaces

2. Factors that influence the direction the facet surfaces move

   a. Flexion of the spine
      Positioning the person in flexion causes a sliding of the articular surfaces be-

tween the facet joints. A longitudinal traction force reinforces the sliding effect and increases the amount of stretching that can be accomplished.

b. Side bending of the spine

Positioning the person in a side-bent position causes a sliding force between the articular facets on the convex side of the curve. Adding a longitudinal traction force increases the amount of stretching that can be accomplished on the convex side.

c. Rotation of the spine

Positioning the person in rotation causes a distraction of the facets on the side toward which the body of the superior vertebra is rotating and compression on the opposite side.[18,21,23]

C. Muscle Relaxation

1. Effects that occur with relaxation

a. Decreased pain from muscle guarding or spasm

b. Greater vertebral separation

2. Factors that influence the amount of relaxation

a. Position of patient

There is greater cervical muscle activity when sitting than when supine.[17] Subjectively, many patients report feeling more relaxed supine than sitting for cervical traction, and they have less tendency to deviate from the set position.[6,9] The patient needs to feel secure and well supported.[21]

b. Spinal position

Electrical activity in the upper trapezius muscle increases as the angle of application of cervical traction toward flexion increases; a lesser angle of pull results in greater relaxation.[7]

c. Duration of application

Both intermittent and continuous traction initially cause increased activity in the sacrospinalis muscles, but after 7 minutes, there is return of activity to near resting level.[10] In concluding a review of the literature, Harris states that 20 to 25 minutes of traction is necessary for muscle relaxation.[9]

d. Force

Muscle relaxation can be achieved at levels less than those needed for mechanical separation (4.5 to 6.75 kg, or 10 to 15 lb) in the cervical spine.[9]

D. Reduction of Pain

1. Effects that may result in inhibition or reduction of pain

a. Mechanical

(1) Movement of the region assists circulation and may help reduce stenosis from circulatory congestion, thus relieves pressure on dura, blood vessels, and nerve roots in the intervertebral foramina. Improving circulation may also help decrease the concentration of noxious chemical irritants.

(2) Separation of the vertebrae temporarily increases the size of the intervertebral foramina, which decreases pressure on an impinged nerve root.

(3) Tension on the facet joint capsule or distraction of the facet surfaces should release a meniscoid from an entrapment or extrapment.

(4) Mechanical stretching of tight tissue should increase the mobility of the

segment, thus decreasing pain from restricted movement or strain on tight tissues.

b. Neurophysiologic
   (1) Stimulation of mechanoreceptors may block the transmission of nociceptive stimuli at the spinal cord or brain stem level.
   (2) Inhibition of reflex muscles guarding will decrease the discomfort from the contracting muscles.

2. Factors that influence the amount of pain reduction

a. Position of the patient
   The patient is positioned for comfort and ease of application of the desired technique.

b. Spinal position
   (1) Acute stage. Usually the involved region of the spine is positioned so that the injured tissue is on a slack or in a pain-free position.
   (2) Subacute and chronic problems. Usually the spine is positioned with the involved segment, or the soft tissues related to the segment, on a stretch.

c. Force and duration
   (1) Acute stage. With injury and inflammation, only low-intensity oscillations (no stretch) for a short period should be used.
   (2) Subacute and chronic stage. The amount of force and duration of treatment can be progressively increased, depending on the goal for treatment, type of traction, condition being treated, and tolerance of the patient.
   (3) If a meniscoid is blocking motion, a stretch force is necessary to release the meniscoid tissue.

II. Definitions and Descriptions of Traction

A. Types of Application Defined

1. Static or constant traction

A steady force is applied and maintained for an extended time interval.

a. *Continuous or prolonged*
   A static traction in which the force is maintained for several hours to several days. Often it is applied in bed.
   (1) Only small amounts of weight can be tolerated.
   (2) It is ineffective in separating spinal structures and is primarily used for immobilization.

b. *Sustained*
   A static traction in which the force is maintained from a few minutes up to one-half hour.
   (1) It is useful as a prolonged stretch to spinal structures.
   (2) Stronger poundage than that used for continuous traction can be tolerated.

2. Intermittent

The force is alternately applied and released at frequent intervals, usually in a rhythmic pattern. Greater forces than that used for sustained traction can be tolerated by the patient.

B. Modes of Application

1. Mechanical

Various types of equipment are available for hospital, clinic, or home use, including motorized units, autotraction benches, and gravity traction frames. The motorized units usually have some form of objective indicator for measuring the amount of force applied.

2. Manual

Through positioning and handling, the therapist applies the traction force to the desired spinal segment. An objective measure of the amount of force cannot be made.

3. Positional

Through positioning, a sustained force on specific segments of the spinal column can be obtained. It may be asymmetric or symmetric.[18,21-23]

III. Indications for Spinal Traction[2,3,21,23]

A. Spinal Nerve Root Impingement

1. From a herniated nucleus pulposus

This condition requires enough traction force to cause vertebral body separation. The separation may have several effects on the bulging disk, including making the annular fibers and posterior longitudinal ligament taut, thus flattening the protrusion or decreasing the intradiskal pressure, thus the pressure on the bulge.[14] Traction time must be short because the pressure soon equalizes and pressure increases when the traction is released. To avoid the adverse effect from increased intradiskal pressure on release, the treatment times should be less than 10 minutes for sustained traction and less than 15 minutes for intermittent traction. Often, in the acute phase, intermittent traction is not well tolerated. Progression depends on the patient's response. When the symptoms are less irritable, higher forces applied intermittently are tolerated.

2. From spinal or foraminal stenosis caused by ligament encroachment, spondylosis, edema, or spondylolisthesis

Symptoms from these conditions can be temporarily relieved by applying enough force to separate the vertebrae and increase the size of the intervertebral foramina. If symptoms are highly irritable and large weights exacerbate the symptoms, gentle sustained traction may be tolerated initially (less than that required to separate the vertebrae for no more than 10 minutes). Progression depends on the patient's response. Change to intermittent traction when the patient's symptoms become predictable; greater forces can then be tolerated, allowing for vertebral separation.

B. Hypomobility of the Joints From Dysfunction or Degenerative Changes

Whenever range of motion is limited, spinal traction can be used to mobilize the joints, because the longitudinal force causes gliding of the facet surfaces. The primary disadvantage is that longitudinal spinal traction affects more than one joint, so it is a nonspecific form of stretching.

1. **To potentially localize the stretch force in the cervical spine**[12]

   a. Put the cervical spine in neutral to affect the upper segments.
   b. Put the cervical spine in flexion to affect the lower segments.

2. **To potentially localize the stretch force in the lumbar spine**[1]

   a. Put the lumbar spine in neutral to affect the lower segments.
   b. Put the lumbar spine and knees into flexion to affect the upper segments and lower thoracic region.

3. **To obtain unilateral effects**

   Position the spinal segment in a side-bending position or side bending with slight rotation before the traction force is applied. Positional traction is also used for this purpose.

   a. For maximum distraction of the facets on one side of the neck, the neck is side bent opposite and then rotated toward the side to be affected.
   b. For maximum sliding of the facets on one side, the neck is side bent and rotated opposite the side to be affected.
   c. For maximum sliding and distraction of the lumbar spine, the trunk is side bent opposite and then rotated toward the side to be affected.

4. **To achieve a stretch force**

   Vertebral separation must occur. Progress treatments depending on the patient's response.

5. ***Precaution:*** Use caution with degenerating joints; too much movement may increase their irritability. If traction causes increased pain or decreased range of motion, either too much traction force was used or it is inappropriate to continue as a method of treatment. Traction should not be used with potential instabilities from ligamentous necrosis in rheumatoid arthritis[16] or conditions in which there has been prolonged use of steroids.

C. Joint Pain From Symptomatic Facet Joints

1. **Acute stage**

   Small movements within the available range of motion are believed to stimulate mechanoreceptors and block pain perception at the spinal level[8,26] as well as to help maintain normal fluid exchange.[8,15] Gentle forces of intermittent traction may relieve pain; the forces should not cause vertebral separation and stretch any injured tissues.

2. **Chronic stage**

   Pain from hypomobility will require dosages that apply a stretch force to the limiting tissues. Patient tolerance will dictate whether to use higher dosages of intermittent or lower dosages of sustained or positional traction.

D. Muscle Spasm or Guarding

1. If the cause of the spasm or guarding is protrusion of the nucleus pulposus or is related to a facet problem, the cause of the problem should be treated, not just the muscle spasm.
2. With a soft tissue injury or torn muscle, the injured area should be kept in a shortened position during the acute phase of healing, then gradually lengthened as the scar becomes stable (see Chapter 7).

  a. Flexion of the spine places a stretch force on the posterior soft tissue structures and muscles of the spine and increases the amount of muscle contraction[7]; therefore, flexion should be avoided during the acute stage of healing.
  b. The spine is placed in a pain-free position.
  c. Usually a gentle intermittent traction is preferred following any acute injury when the extent of soft tissue injury is not known.
  d. If there is any exacerbation of symptoms, traction should not be given.

E. Meniscoid Blocking

A trapped meniscoid will block motion; frequently the patient is in a forward-bent position and cannot return to the upright position. Longitudinal traction will slide the facets and put tension on the joint capsule; positional traction will distract the joint surfaces as well as put tension on the joint capsule. Either one, applied at a high enough dosage to effect the desired facet motion, should release a trapped meniscoid.

F. Diskogenic Pain, Postcompression Fracture, and Other Conditions of the Spine

These conditions may respond to spinal traction. Begin with the spinal segment in a neutral or pain-free position. The symptoms should be monitored and adaptations made in the technique, depending on the patient's response.

IV. Limitations, Contraindications, and Precautions

A. Limitations of Traction

  1. The effect of vertebral separation is temporary, although the temporary relief may be enough to help break into a reflex pain cycle.
  2. No consistent protocols exist; rationale is hypothetical with inconsistent clinical results.[9,25] Personal experience and the patient's response dictate method, force, duration, and frequency of treatment.[2]
  3. The longitudinal traction force is nonspecific as to vertebral level. It affects the entire region.

B. Contraindications[9,21,23]

  1. Any spinal condition or disease process in which movement is contraindicated.
  2. Acute strains, sprains, and inflammation or any painful symptoms aggravated by initial traction treatments.
  3. Stretch forces to areas of spinal hypermobility.
  4. Rheumatoid arthritis of the cervical spine, in which potential necrosis of supporting ligaments could cause instability and subluxation or dislocation of a vertebra and spinal cord damage.[16]
  5. Any spinal condition in which structural integrity is compromised, such as spinal malignancy, osteoporosis, tumor, or infection.
  6. Pregnancy, uncontrolled hypertension, aortic aneurysm, severe hemorrhoids, cardiovascular disease, abdominal hernia, and hiatal hernia are contraindications for lumbar traction.

C. Precautions

1. Temporomandibular joint (TMJ) pain may be provoked with use of cervical halters, particularly when the chinstrap places a lot of force on the mandible. This occurs more often when the head is slightly flexed.[7] If pain increases in the TMJ, several alternatives are suggested:
   a. Use manual traction, thereby avoiding pressure under the mandible.
   b. Place cotton dental rolls between the back teeth; pressure under the chin from the traction strap will then cause a distraction of the TMJ.
   c. Use a cervical traction unit that does not require a chinstrap. Fixation comes from a strap secured across the patient's forehead and distraction from a pad under the occiput.[23]
2. Patients wearing dentures should not remove them, because the TMJ is forced into an abnormal resting position and can be traumatized with pressure from the chinstrap.
3. Some of the conditions listed under *Contraindications* may benefit from carefully applied traction. When mechanical traction is too forceful for the condition, manual or positional traction may be appropriate alternatives.
4. Patients with respiratory problems or those who develop claustrophobia when placed in the traction apparatus.

V. General Procedures

A. Determine Appropriateness for Choice of Traction by Testing With Manual Traction First

(See Sections VI and VII for techniques)
1. If the test traction relieves or reduces the symptoms, an initial treatment is given.
2. Conversely, if the test traction aggravates the symptoms, traction treatments should probably not be applied.
3. When evaluating, apply the traction force in various positions of flexion, extension, side bending, and rotation to find which position best reduces or relieves the symptoms. Use that position, if possible, for the initial treatment.
4. Re-evaluate the patient immediately afterward as well as the next day to determine whether traction should be modified or continued.

B. Determine if Manual, Positional, or Mechanical Traction Will Be Used

C. Position the Patient for Maximum Comfort and Relaxation

If using mechanical traction, secure the harnesses or halter to the patient and then attach it to the machine. Check to see that the rope pull is at the appropriate angle.

D. Determine Dosage and Duration

Refer to Section III for guidelines based on the patient's problem. To avoid treatment soreness:
1. The *dosage* chosen for the *initial treatment* should be less than that which would cause vertebral separation. Progression of poundage should be determined by the patient's response and the problem being treated.

2. The *duration* will depend on the type of traction (intermittent or sustained), the poundage used, the clinical condition of the patient, and the goals of the treatment.

E. Safety Rules for Mechanical Traction

1. Use only cables and ropes that are in good repair.
2. Secure the equipment so it will not move when the traction force is applied.
3. Check to see that the poundage dial is turned down to zero before setting up the patient or turning on the machine.
4. Periodically check the poundage calibration.
5. Use disposable tissue or gauze wherever the halters touch the patient's face, mouth, or hair. Disposable halters are available but are not easily adjusted to all patients.
6. Never leave the patient unattended while he or she is receiving traction unless he or she has some mechanism for deactivating the unit and some means to signal for assistance.

VI. Cervical Traction Techniques

A. Manual Traction

1. *Position of patient:* supine on the treatment table. The patient should be as relaxed as possible.
2. *Position of therapist:* standing at the head of the treatment table, supporting the weight of the patient's head in the hands. Hand placement depends on comfort. Suggestions include:
   a. Place the fingers of both hands under the occiput (Fig. 16–1A).
   b. Place one hand over the frontal region and the other hand under the occiput (Fig. 16–1B).

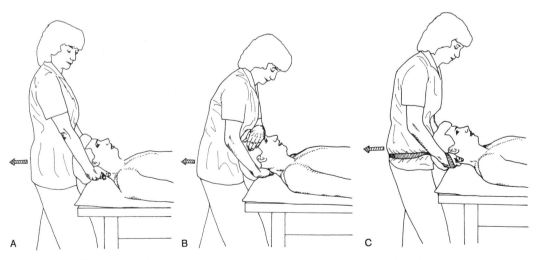

Figure 16–1. Manual cervical traction (*A*) with the fingers of both hands under the occiput, (*B*) with one hand over the frontal region and the other hand under the occiput, and (*C*) using a belt to reinforce the hands for the traction force.

    c. Place the index fingers around the spinous process above the vertebral level to be moved. This hand placement provides a specific traction only to the vertebral segments below the level at which the fingers are placed. A belt around the therapist's hips can be used to reinforce the fingers and increase the ease of applying the traction force (Fig. 16–1C).

3. When manual traction is used for evaluation, vary the patient's head position in flexion, extension, side bending, and side bending with rotation and apply a traction force in each position; note the patient's response.

4. When administering treatment, use the position that most effectively reduces or relieves the symptoms.

5. The therapist applies the force by fixing his or her arms isometrically, assuming a stable stance, and then leaning backward in a controlled manner. If a belt is used, the force is transmitted through the belt. If just the arm muscles are used to apply the force, the therapist tires quickly.

6. The force is usually applied intermittently, with a smooth and gradual building and releasing of the traction force. The intensity and duration are usually limited by the therapist's strength and endurance.

7. *Value of manual traction.*
    a. The angle of pull and head position can be controlled by the therapist.
    b. By placing the index fingers around specific spinous processes, the level of traction can be controlled to some degree.
    c. No stress is placed on the temporomandibular joint, as is frequently done with mechanical traction.

B. Positional Traction

1. *Position of patient:* supine on the treatment table.

2. *Position of therapist:* standing at the head of the treatment table, supporting the patient's head in his or her hands. Determine the segment to receive the majority of traction force and palpate the spinous process at that level.

3. *Procedure*[18]: Flex the head until motion of the spinous process just begins at the determined level. Support the head with folded towels at that level of flexion. Then side bend the head away from the side to be distracted until movement of the spinous process is felt at the desired level. Finally, rotate the head a few degrees toward the side to be distracted. Adjust the towel support to maintain this position for a low-intensity, sustained traction stretch to that facet joint and surrounding soft tissue.

4. *Value of positional traction:* The primary traction force can be isolated to a specific facet. This may be beneficial when selective stretching is necessary, as when the segment above or on the contralateral side is hypermobile and should not be stretched.

C. Mechanical Traction

1. Become familiar with the unit available by reviewing the manufacturer's directions. Learn the capabilities, limitations, and adjustments possible for the equipment.

2. *Position the patient for comfort.*
    a. Sitting

(1) This position uses less clinical space but requires more force to overcome muscle tension and accomplish separation of the vertebrae than does the supine position.[6]

(2) Use a comfortable chair with arm rests or place a pillow on the patient's lap for the arms to rest on.

(3) The height of the chair should support the thighs and allow the feet to rest comfortably on the floor or on a footstool.

  b. Supine (Fig. 16–2)

(1) This position requires less force to overcome muscle tension than sitting.

(2) This position tends to reduce the lordotic curve due to the force of gravity on the vertebrae.[6]

(3) Support the patient with pillows for maximum comfort.

(4) Depending on the angle of pull, friction of the head on the surface of the treatment table must be considered.

  c. Semireclining

(1) Use of a reclining chair or tilt table provides alternative positions to sitting or lying supine.

(2) Gravity may or may not have an influence, depending on angle of pull.

3. *Head position* for the patient is determined by the evaluation as well as the condition being treated.

  a. To obtain separation of the vertebrae, the head should be positioned in flexion up to 35 degrees; the greater the angle of neck flexion, the greater is the posterior elongation.[4]

  b. To obtain greater muscle relaxation, position the head closer to neutral.[7]

  c. To obtain unilateral effects, position the head in a side-bent position or in a position of side bending with slight rotation (as described in the positional traction section) before the traction is applied. Secure the patient's thorax with a strap so he or she is not realigned with the pull of the rope.

4. *Apply the head halter.*

  a. First, line the head halter with gauze or tissue.

  b. Adjust the halter to fit the patient comfortably. The major traction force must be against the occiput, not the chin, to minimize compression of the temporomandibular joint. Gauze may be placed between the teeth or padding under the chin to help absorb pressure.

  c. Do not remove dentures if the patient wears them or stress may be placed on the temporomandibular joints.

  d. Eyeglasses should be safely set aside.

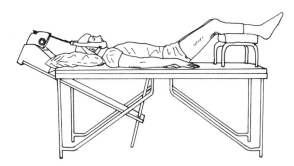

Figure 16–2. Mechanical traction to the cervical spine, with the patient supine.

    e. Attach the halter to the spreader bar of the traction unit; check that the patient is aligned for proper pull.

5. *Set controls.*

    a. The poundage dial should be set at zero before activating the unit.

    b. If the unit has off-on timers for intermittent traction, these should be set for the desired time intervals.

        (1) Only 7 seconds is needed for maximum separation at any one cycle, but such frequency tends to be irritating.

        (2) Suggested starting intervals are 30 seconds on, 30 seconds off or 1 minute on, 30 seconds off.

    c. Duration of treatment may be from 10 to 30 minutes for sustained or intermittent traction, depending on the patient's condition and goals for treatment.

6. *Activate the unit and gradually increase the force of traction.*

    a. To avoid treatment soreness, the first treatment should not exceed 10 to 15 lbs.

    b. Progression of dosage at succeeding treatments will depend on the goals and the patient's reaction.

7. *Safety*

Demonstrate to the patient how to turn the unit off if symptoms become worse.

8. *At the completion of treatment.*

    a. Turn all controls off and turn dial indicators back to zero. Remove the halter from the spreader bar, then remove the head halter.

    b. Re-evaluate the patient's condition. Be sure he or she does not feel dizzy or nauseated before leaving the treatment area.

    c. If the patient complains of headache, nausea, fainting, or increased symptoms during or following treatment, reduce the weight or length of treatment time at the next visit or discontinue treatments if the condition warrants.

D. Home Traction: Mechanical

1. Have the patient practice the traction set up under your supervision. Be sure he or she understands:

    a. What position and neck posture to use

        (1) With an over-the-door pulley system, sit facing the weight if the flexed position is to be used.

        (2) Sit facing away from the weight if the neutral or extended position is to be used. For the neutral position, the head should be directly under the pulley; for extension, the chair is moved forward.

        (3) If a supine position is desired, the head is usually positioned in flexion with the cervical halter attached to the pulley system; the weight of the body provides the counterforce.

    b. How to get comfortable

    c. How to apply and release the weights safely

2. Weight application varies. The most common method is with a weight pan or bag on a pulley system (Fig. 16–3). If the patient uses weights, have them on a chair or table next to him or her. Have the patient practice applying the weights so it is accomplished smoothly and safely.

3. Sustained traction (up to 30 minutes) using small amounts of weight (10 lbs) is easiest to apply. Intermittent traction requires that the patient lift the weight to take the force off the neck at frequent intervals. Assess both techniques to determine which one provides greater relaxation and relief of symptoms.

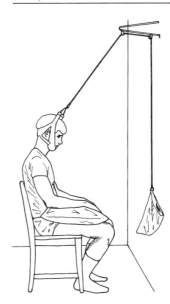

Figure 16–3. Home traction for the cervical spine using a bag of weights on a pulley system for the traction force with the patient positioned in flexion. For the neutral or extended position, the patient should sit under the pulley and face away from the weight.

E. Self-Traction

1. The patient is sitting or lying down. He or she is taught to place the hands behind the neck with the fingers interlocking; the ulnar border of the fingers and hands are under the occiput and mastoid processes. The patient then gives a lifting motion to the head. The head may be placed in flexion, extension, side bending, or rotation for more isolated effects. He or she may apply the traction intermittently or in a sustained manner.
2. Positional traction can also be used for self-traction. The patient learns to assume the position determined by the therapist as described in Section VI.B.

VII. Lumbar Traction Techniques

A. Manual Traction

1. Manual traction in the lumbar region is not as easily applied as in the cervical region because at least half the body weight must be moved and the coefficient of friction of the part to be moved must be overcome.
2. *Position of patient:* supine on a treatment table, preferably a split-traction table to minimize the resistance from friction.
3. *Position of therapist:* varies with the position of the patient's hips and lower extremities.
   a. With the lower extremities extended and the lumbar spine in extension, the therapist can exert a pull at the ankles.
   b. With the hips flexed to 90 degrees and the lumbar spine in flexion, the patient's legs are draped over the therapist's shoulders. The therapist then exerts the force with his or her arms wrapped across the patient's thighs.
   c. A pelvic belt with straps may be used.
4. When manual traction is used for evaluation, vary the amount of flexion, extension, or side bending and note the patient's response.
5. During treatment, use the spinal position that best reduces the patient's symptoms.

6. The therapist must use his or her entire body weight to effect any traction force. When applying a high-dosage traction force, the thorax is stabilized. Put a countertraction harness around the patient's rib cage and secure it to the head end of the table, or have a second person stabilize the patient by standing at the head end of the table and holding the patient's arms.

B. Positional Traction[18,21,23]

1. *Position of patient:* side-lying, with the side to be treated uppermost. A rolled blanket is placed under the spine at the level where the traction force is desired; this causes side bending away from the side to be treated and therefore an upward gliding of the facets (Fig. 16–4A).
2. *Position of the therapist:* standing, at the side of the treatment table facing the patient. Determine the segment to receive the majority of the traction force, and palpate the spinous processes at that level and the level above.
3. *Procedure*[18]: The patient relaxes in the side-bent position. Rotation is added to isolate a distraction force to the desired level. Rotate the upper trunk by gently pulling on the arm the patient is lying on while at the same time palpating the spinous processes with your other hand to determine when rotation has arrived at the level just above the joint to be distracted. Then flex the patient's uppermost thigh, again palpating the spinous processes until flexion of the lower portion of the spine occurs at the desired level. The segment at which these two opposing forces meet now has a maximum positional distraction force (Fig. 16–4B).
4. *Value of positional traction:* The primary traction force can be directed to the side on which symptoms occur or can be isolated to a specific facet and is therefore beneficial for selective stretching.

C. Mechanical Traction (Fig. 16–5)

1. Become familiar with the unit available by reviewing the manufacturer's operating instructions. The most effective traction is applied via a split-traction table, thus eliminating the need to overcome the coefficient of friction of half the patient's body weight.

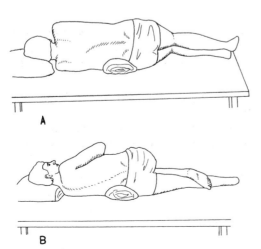

A

B

Figure 16–4. Positional traction for the lumbar spine. (*A*) Side bending over a 6- to 8-inch roll causes a longitudinal traction to the segments on the upward side. (*B*) Side bending with rotation adds a distraction force to the facets on the upward side.

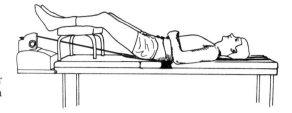

Figure 16–5. Mechanical traction to the lumbar spine in flexion using a split traction table with the patient supine.

2. *Apply the traction and countertraction harnesses.*
   a. Saunders recommends a heavy-duty traction harness made with a vinyl material that is attached directly to the patient's skin to avoid slippage.[21]
   b. The traction harness is applied over the pelvis so that the upper portion is secured above the crest of the ilium.
   c. The countertraction harness is used to keep the patient from slipping. It is attached around the lower rib cage.
3. *Position the patient either supine or prone.*
   a. The thorax should be on the stationary part of the table and the pelvis on the movable part (the movable part is kept locked until ready to activate the unit) so that the lumbar spine is positioned over the split in the table.
   b. Whether the spine is in flexion, extension, or side bending is determined by the evaluation and the patient's comfort and condition as well as the goals of the treatment.
   c. To obtain posterior separation of the vertebrae, the lumbar spine should be flexed (flattened).
      (1) When supine, the hips are flexed and the thighs rest on a padded stool.
      (2) When prone, several pillows are placed under the patient's abdomen.
4. *Attach the anchor straps.*
   a. The countertraction or stabilizing harness is secured to the head end of the traction table.
   b. The straps from the traction harness may attach to a spreader bar, which is attached to a traction rope.
   c. If unilateral traction is to be applied, attach only one anchor strap from the pelvic harness directly to the traction rope.[22]
   d. Check that the patient is aligned for proper pull, then take all the slack out of the straps.
5. *Set the controls.*
   a. Be familiar with the type of unit. Computer models may have options such as a progressive phase that will gradually increase the traction force at programmed intervals. Other units should be set at zero before activating the unit.
   b. If the unit has off-on timers for intermittent traction, set them for the desired time intervals.
   c. Set the duration of treatment. Duration may be up to 30 minutes for most mechanical units. The duration depends on the goals and the patient's condition and reaction to the traction.
6. *Unlock the split-traction table* so it will separate when the unit is activated.
7. *Activate the unit and gradually increase the force* (if the unit has not been preprogrammed to do so automatically).
   a. To avoid treatment soreness, the first treatment should not exceed half the patient's weight.

b. Progression of dosage at succeeding treatments will depend on goals and the patient's reaction.

8. *Safety*

Demonstrate to the patient how to turn the unit off if symptoms worsen while the unit is on. Make sure he or she has a signaling device to call for help if necessary.

9. *At the completion of the treatment:*

a. Turn all controls off and turn indicators back to zero.

b. Lock the split on the table before the patient attempts to get off.

c. Re-evaluate the patient; note any change in symptoms or range of motion.

D. Home Traction: Mechanical

1. A number of home traction units are available on the market. Choose one that best meets the goals for the patient. Set-up and instructions are specific to the design of each unit. Have the patient practice the traction set-up under your supervision. Be sure he or she understands:

a. Position

b. How to get comfortable

c. How to apply and release the traction force safely

2. Because most of the home units use body weight and position within a pulley system for the distraction force, sustained traction is most easily used. Determine a safe duration for the patient compatible with the goals for treatment.

E. Self-Traction: Manual

1. To separate the posterior segment of the lumbar spine, the patient is positioned supine. He or she then draws both knees up to the chest and holds them (grasping around the thighs). This can be undertaken intermittently by releasing the hold and bringing the legs partway down, then pulling them back up again (see Fig. 15–5).

   Precaution: Flexing the spine in this manner increases the intradiskal pressure; therefore, this technique should not be used to treat symptoms of an acute disk protrusion.

2. Positional traction can be used for self-traction. The patient learns to assume the position determined by the therapist as described in Section VII.B (see Fig. 16–4).

VIII. Summary

The basic concepts, indications, contraindications, and precautions of spinal traction have been described in this chapter, followed by procedural guidelines and techniques for applying cervical and lumbar traction with manual, positional, or mechanical techniques. Because spinal traction is just one technique for managing spinal and back problems, it has been suggested that this material be studied concurrently with the material in Chapters 14 and 15.

References

1. Broden, J: Manuell Medicin och Manipulation. Lakartidningen 63:1037, 1966. (As reported by Saunders, HD: Lumbar traction. Journal of Orthopaedic and Sports Physical Therapy 1:36, 1979.)

2. Cailliet, R: Neck and Arm Pain, ed 3. FA Davis, Philadelphia, 1991.

3. Cailliet, R: Low Back Pain Syndrome, ed 4. FA Davis, Philadelphia, 1988.

4. Colachis, S, and Strohm, B: A study of tractive forces and angle of pull on vertebral interspaces in the cervical spine. Arch Phys Med Rehabil 46:220, 1965.
5. Colachis, S, and Strohm, B: Effects of intermittent traction on separation of lumbar vertebrae. Arch Phys Med Rehabil 50:251, 1969.
6. Deets, D, Hands, K, and Hopp, S: Cervical traction: A comparison of sitting and supine positions. Phys Ther 57:255, 1977.
7. DeLacerda, F: Effect of angle of traction pull on upper trapezius muscle activity. JOSPT 1:205, 1980.
8. Grieve, G: Manual mobilizing techniques in degenerative arthrosis of the hip. Bull Orthop Sec APTA 2/1:7, 1977.
9. Harris, P: Cervical traction: Review of literature and treatment guidelines. Phys Ther 57:910, 1977.
10. Hood, C, et al: Comparison of electromyographic activity in normal lumbar sacrospinalis musculature during continuous and intermittent pelvic traction. Journal of Orthopaedic and Sports Physical Therapy 2:137, 1981.
11. Judovich, B: Lumbar traction therapy. JAMA 159:549, 1955.
12. Maitland, GD: Vertebral Manipulation, ed 5. Butterworth & Co, London, 1986.
13. Matthews, J: Dynamic discography: A study of lumbar traction. Ann Phys Med 9:275, 1968.
14. Mathews, J: The effects of spinal traction. Physiotherapy 58:64, 1972.
15. McDonough, A: Effect of immobilization and exercise on articular cartilage: A review of literature. Journal of Orthopaedic and Sports Physical Therapy 3:2, 1981.
16. Moneur, C, and Wiliams, HF: Cervical spine management in patients with rheumatoid arthritis. Phys Ther 68:509, 1988.
17. Murphy, MJ: Effects of cervical traction on muscle activity. Journal of Orthopaedic and Sports Physical Therapy 13:220, 1991.
18. Parris, S: Spinal Dysfunction: Etiology and Treatment of Dysfunction Including Joint Manipulation. Manual of Course Notes, Atlanta, 1979.
19. Pellecchia, GL: Lumbar traction: A review of the literature. Journal of Orthopaedic and Sports Physical Therapy 20:263, 1994.
20. Reilly, J, Gersten, J, and Clinkingbeard, J: Effect of pelvic-femoral position on vertebral separation produced by lumbar traction. Phys Ther 59:282, 1979.
21. Saunders, H: Lumbar traction. Journal of Orthopaedic and Sports Physical Therapy 1:36, 1979.
22. Saunders, H: Unilateral lumbar traction. Phys Ther 61:221, 1981.
23. Saunders, HD: Spinal traction. In Saunders, HD: Evaluation, Treatment and Prevention of Musculoskeletal Disorders. Viking, Minneapolis, 1985.
24. Taber's Cyclopedic Medical Dictionary, ed 17. FA Davis, Philadelphia, 1993.
25. van der Heijden, GJMG, et al: The efficacy of traction for back and neck pain: A systematic, blinded review of randomized clinical trial methods. Phys Ther 75:93, 1995.
26. Wyke, B: Neurological aspects of pain for the physical therapy clinician. PT Forum '82 (notes), Columbus, 1982.

Special Areas of Therapeutic Exercise

Principles of Exercise for the Obstetric Patient

CATHY J. KONKLER, BS, PT • CAROLYN KISNER, MS, PT

During and after pregnancy women present a unique challenge for the physical therapist. Pregnancy is a time of tremendous musculoskeletal, physical, and emotional change and yet is a condition of wellness. For many clients the therapist is usually able to assess and monitor the physical changes with the primary focus on maintaining wellness. The therapist is also able to assess and help the client with specific musculoskeletal complaints by incorporating the knowledge of injury and tissue healing with the knowledge of the changes from pregnancy. This chapter does not present a specific protocol of exercise for use with the pregnant or postpartum client; rather, it provides the reader with basic information about the physical changes of pregnancy as a foundation for the development of safe and effective exercise programs. The chapter also discusses modification of general exercises to meet the needs of the obstetric client and provides information to assist the reader in making decisions about exercises to include in an uncomplicated pregnancy exercise program. Cesarean delivery, high-risk pregnancy, and the special needs of clients with these conditions are discussed separately at the end of the chapter.

OBJECTIVES

After studying this chapter, the reader will be able to:

1 Identify the major stages and characteristics of pregnancy, labor, and delivery.
2 Describe the normal physiologic changes of pregnancy in the organ systems and musculoskeletal system.
3 Identify the common postural adjustments to pregnancy.
4 Define diastasis recti and its significance in pregnancy.
5 Describe the evaluation procedure for diastasis recti and corrective exercise for the condition.
6 Identify other pathologies of the musculoskeletal system caused by pregnancy.
7 Describe the structure, function, and significance of the pelvic floor.
8 Describe rehabilitation techniques for the pelvic floor.

9   Summarize the goals and guidelines of an obstetric exercise program for an uncomplicated pregnancy.

10   Identify absolute and possible contraindications to exercise in pregnancy.

11   Establish a safe therapeutic exercise program that addresses or modifies the changes of pregnancy and aids in preparation for labor.

12   Describe the maternal and fetal responses to exercise.

13   Define cesarean childbirth and high-risk pregnancy.

14   Identify exercise and rehabilitative goals for cesarean and high-risk clients.

15   Describe modifications or additions to exercise programs for the cesarean or high-risk client.

I. Overview of Pregnancy, Labor, and Delivery

A. Pregnancy (40 Weeks from Conception to Delivery)[4,16,35]

Pregnancy is divided into three trimesters.

1. Changes during the first trimester: weeks 0 to 12 of pregnancy

a. Implantation of the fertilized ovum in the uterus occurs 7 to 10 days after fertilization.

b. The mother may be nauseated or may vomit, is very fatigued, and will urinate more frequently because of pressure from the growing uterus.

c. The breast size may increase.

d. There is a relatively small weight gain of 0 to 1455 g (0 to 3 lb is normal).

e. Emotional changes may occur.

f. By the end of the 12th week, the fetus is 6 to 7 cm long and weighs approximately 20 g (2 oz). The baby now can kick, turn its head, and swallow and has a beating heart, but these movements are not yet felt by the mother.

2. Changes during the second trimester: weeks 13 to 26 of pregnancy

a. The pregnancy now becomes visible to others.

b. The mother begins to feel movement at around 20 weeks.

c. During this trimester, most women feel very good. Nausea and fatigue have usually disappeared.

d. By the end of the second trimester, the fetus is 19 to 23 cm (14 inches) in length and weighs approximately 600 g (1 to 2 lb).

e. The fetus now has eyebrows, eyelashes, and fingernails and would have a slight chance of surviving if born prematurely.

3. Change during the third trimester: weeks 27 to 40 of pregnancy (38 to 42 weeks is considered full term)

a. The uterus is now very large and has regular contractions, although these may only occasionally be felt.

b. Common complaints during the third trimester are frequent urination, back pain, leg edema and fatigue, round ligament pain, shortness of breath, and constipation.

c. By the time of birth, the baby will be 33 to 39 cm long (16 to 19 inches) and will weigh approximately 3400 g (7 lb, although a range from 5 to 10 lb is normal).

B. Labor[4,33,35]

1. Onset of labor

a. The exact mechanism for labor induction is not known.

b. Regular and strong involuntary contractions of the smooth muscles of the uterus are the primary symptom of labor.

c. True labor will produce palpable changes in the cervix.

   (1) *Effacement:* shortening or thinning of the cervix from a thickness of 5 cm, or 2 inches, before onset of labor to the thickness of a piece of paper (Fig. 17–1)

   (2) *Dilatation:* opening of the cervix from the diameter of a fingertip to approximately 10 cm, or 4 inches (Fig. 17–1)

2. Labor: stage 1

a. This is the cervical dilatation and effacement stage. At the end of this stage, the cervix is fully dilated and the baby is ready to be expelled from the uterus.

b. Stage 1 of labor is divided into three major phases.

   (1) *Cervical dilatation phase.* The cervix dilates from 0 to 3 cm (0 to 1 inch) and will almost completely efface. Uterine contractions occur from the top down, causing the cervix to open and pushing the fetus downward.

   (2) *Middle phase.* The cervix dilates from 4 to 7 cm (1 to 3 inches). Contractions are stronger and more regular.

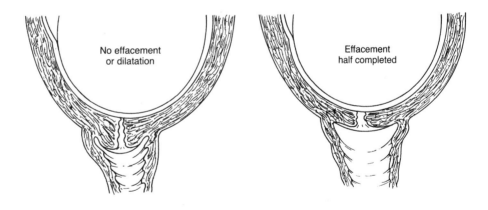

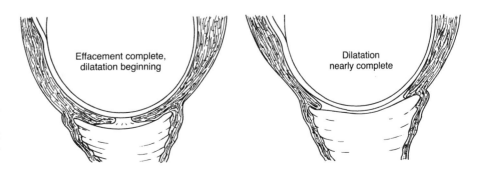

Figure 17–1. Effacement and dilatation of the cervix. (From Sandberg, E: Synopsis of Obstetrics, ed 10. CV Mosby, St Louis, 1978, p 192, with permission.)

(3) *Transition phase.* The cervix dilates from 8 to 10 cm (3 to 4 inches) and dilatation is complete. Uterine contractions are very strong and close together.

3. Labor: stage 2 (expulsion of the fetus)

a. Intra-abdominal pressure is the primary force expelling the fetus. This pressure is produced by voluntary contraction of the abdominals and diaphragm.

b. Fetal descent

Position changes (cardinal movements) by the fetus allow it to pass through the pelvis and be born (Fig. 17–2).

   (1) *Engagement.* The greatest transverse diameter of the fetal head passes through the pelvic inlet (the superior opening of the minor pelvis).

   (2) *Descent.* Continued downward progression of the fetus occurs.

   (3) *Flexion.* The fetal chin is brought closer to its thorax; this occurs when the descending head meets resistance from the walls and floor of the pelvis and the cervix.

   (4) *Internal rotation.* The fetus turns its occiput toward the mother's symphysis pubis when the fetal head reaches the level of the ischial spines.

   (5) *Extension.* The flexed fetal head reaches the vulva; the fetus extends its head, bringing the base of the occiput in direct contact with the inferior margin of the maternal symphysis pubis; this phase ends when the fetal head is born.

   (6) *External rotation.* The fetus rotates its occiput toward the mother's sacrum to allow the fetal shoulders to pass through the pelvis.

c. Expulsion

The fetal anterior shoulder passes under the symphysis pubis, and the rest of the body follows.

4. Labor: stage 3

a. *Placental stage* (expulsion of the placenta)

   (1) The uterus continues to contract and shrink following delivery; as the uterus decreases in size, the placenta detaches from the uterine wall, blood vessels are constricted, and bleeding slows. This can occur 5 to 30 minutes after fetal expulsion.

   (2) A hematoma forms over the uterine placental site to prevent further significant blood loss; mild bleeding persists for 3 to 6 weeks after delivery.

b. *Uterine involution*

The uterus continues to contract and decrease in size for 3 to 6 weeks following delivery; the uterus always remains a bit enlarged over its pre-pregnant size.

II. Anatomic and Physiologic Changes of Pregnancy*

A. Pregnancy Weight Gain

A pregnancy percent increase in total weight is normal. This is necessary to nourish the fetus. Weight gain is produced by (average figures):

---

*Refs. 3–5, 21, 26, 29, 31, 33, 35, 40.

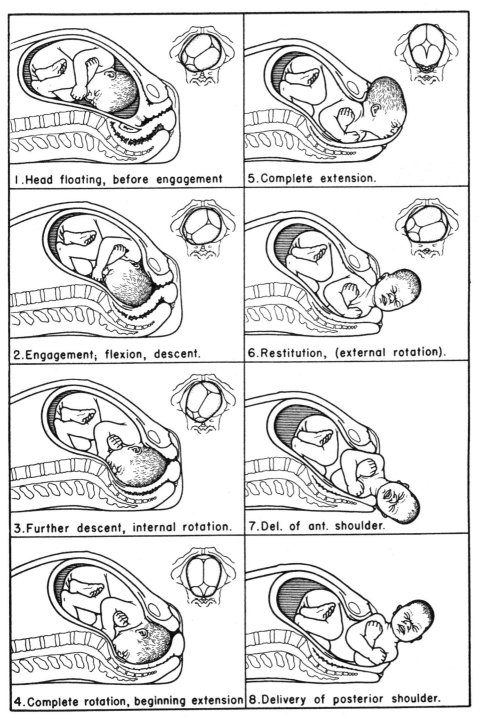

1. Head floating, before engagement

2. Engagement; flexion, descent.

3. Further descent, internal rotation.

4. Complete rotation, beginning extension

5. Complete extension.

6. Restitution, (external rotation).

7. Del. of ant. shoulder.

8. Delivery of posterior shoulder.

Figure 17–2. Principle movements in the mechanism of labor and delivery, left occiput anterior position. (From Pritchard, J, and MacDonald, P: Williams Obstetrics, ed 16. Appleton-Century Crofts, Norwalk, CT, 1980, with permission.)

Fetus	3.63–3.88 kg	(7.5–8.0 lb)
Placenta	0.48–0.72 kg	(1.0–1.5 lb)
Amniotic fluid	0.72–0.97 kg	(1.5–2.0 lb)
Uterus and breasts	2.42–2.66 kg	(5.0–5.5 lb)
Blood and fluid	1.94–3.99 kg	(4.0–7.0 lb)
Muscle and fat	0.48–2.91 kg	(1.0–6.0 lb)
	9.70–14.55 kg	(20.0–30.0 lb)

B. Organ Systems

1. Reproductive system

a. The uterus increases from a prepregnant size of 5 by 10 cm (2 by 4 inches) to 25 by 36 cm (10 by 14 inches).

b. The uterus increases 5 to 6 times in size, 3000 to 4000 times in capacity, and 20 times in weight by the end of pregnancy.

c. By the end of pregnancy, each muscle cell in the uterus has increased approximately 10 times its length prior to pregnancy.[40]

d. Once the uterus expands upward and leaves the pelvis, it becomes an abdominal organ rather than a pelvic organ.

2. Urinary system

a. The kidneys increase in length by 1 cm (0.5 inch).

b. Ureters enter the bladder at a perpendicular angle because of uterine enlargement. This may result in a reflux of urine out of the bladder and back into the ureter; therefore, there is an increased chance of developing urinary tract infections in pregnancy because of urinary stasis.

3. Pulmonary system

a. Edema and tissue congestion of the upper respiratory tract occur early in pregnancy because of hormonal changes.

b. There is upper respiratory hypersecretion (hormonally stimulated).

c. The subcostal angle progressively increases; the ribs flare up and out.

d. The anterior-posterior and transverse chest diameters each increase by 2 cm (1 inch).

e. Total chest circumference increases by 5 to 7 cm (2 to 3 inches) and does not always return to the prepregnant state.

f. Changes in rib position are hormonally stimulated and occur prior to uterine enlargement.

g. The diaphragm is elevated by 4 cm (1.5 inch); this is a passive change caused by the change in rib position.

h. The respiration rate is unchanged, but the depth of respiration increases.[33]

i. Tidal volume and minute ventilation increase, but total lung capacity is unchanged or slightly decreased.[33,40]

j. There is a 15 to 20 percent increase in oxygen consumption; a natural state of hyperventilation exists throughout pregnancy. This occurs to meet the oxygen demands of pregnancy.[33,40]

k. The work of breathing increases because of hyperventilation; dyspnea is present with mild exercise as early as 20 weeks into the pregnancy.[33,40]

4. Cardiovascular system

a. Blood volume progressively increases 35 to 50 percent (1.5 to 2 liters) throughout pregnancy and returns to normal by 6 to 8 weeks post-pregnancy.

b. Plasma increase is greater than red blood cell increase, leading to "physiologic anemia" of pregnancy, which is not a true anemia but is representative of the greater increase of plasma volume. The increase in plasma volume occurs as a result of hormonal stimulation to meet the oxygen demands of pregnancy.

c. Venous pressure in the lower extremities increases when standing as a result of increased uterine size and increased venous distensibility.

d. Pressure in the inferior vena cava rises in late pregnancy, especially in the supine position, because of compression by the uterus just below the diaphragm. In some women, the decline in venous return and resulting decrease in cardiac output may lead to symptomatic supine hypotensive syndrome.[12] The aorta is partially occluded in the supine position.

e. The heart size increases, and the heart is elevated due to the movement of the diaphragm.

f. Heart rhythm disturbances are more common in pregnancy.

g. Heart rate usually increases 10 to 20 beats per minute by full term and returns to normal levels within 6 weeks postpregnancy.

h. Cardiac output increases 30 to 60 percent in pregnancy and is most significantly increased when side-lying on the left. In this position, the uterus places the least pressure on the aorta.

i. Blood pressure decreases early in the first trimester. There is a slight decrease of systolic pressure and a greater decrease of diastolic pressure. Blood pressure reaches its lowest level approximately midway through pregnancy, then rises gradually from mid-pregnancy to reach the prepregnant level approximately 6 weeks postdelivery. Although cardiac output increases, blood pressure decreases because of venous distensibility.

5. Musculoskeletal system[26,31,40]

a. Abdominal muscles are stretched to the point of their elastic limit by the end of pregnancy.

b. Hormonal influence on the ligaments is profound, producing a systemic decrease in ligamentous tensile strength and an increase in mobility of structures supported by ligaments.

c. Joint hypermobility occurs as a result of ligamentous laxity and may predispose the patient to joint and ligamentous injury, especially in the weight-bearing joints of the back, pelvis, and lower extremities.

d. The pelvic floor muscles must withstand the weight of the uterus; the pelvic floor drops as much as 2.5 cm (1 inch).[31]

e. The pelvic floor may be stretched or incised or both during the birth process.

6. Thermoregulatory system[12]

a. During pregnancy basal metabolic rate and heat production increase.

b. An increase of 300 kilocalories per day is needed to meet the basic metabolic needs of pregnancy.

c. The fasting blood glucose level in pregnant women normally is lower than in nonpregnant women.

C. Mechanical Changes

1. Center of gravity

The center of gravity shifts upward and forward because of the enlargement of the uterus and breasts. This requires postural compensations for balance and stability.

2. Posture[26,31,40]

a. The shoulder girdle and upper back become rounded with scapular protraction and upper extremity internal rotation because of breast enlargement and postpartum positioning for infant care.
b. Cervical lordosis increases in the upper cervical spine, and forward-head posture develops to compensate for the shoulder alignment.
c. Lumbar lordosis increases to compensate for the shift in the center of gravity and the knees hyperextend, probably because of the change in the line of gravity.
d. Weight shifts toward the heels to bring the center of gravity to a more posterior position.
e. Changes in posture do not usually correct spontaneously after childbirth, and pregnant posture may be maintained as a learned posture. Carrying the infant in the arms can also perpetuate faulty posture.

3. Balance

With the increased weight and redistribution of body mass there are compensations to maintain balance.
a. The woman usually walks with a wider base of support.
b. Some activities such as walking, stooping, stair climbing, lifting, and reaching become difficult.
c. Some activities requiring fine balance and rapid changes in direction, such as aerobic dancing and bicycle riding, may become dangerous, especially during the third trimester.

III. Pregnancy-Induced Pathology

A. Diastasis Recti[2,6,19,26,31,33,40]

1. Definition

Separation of the rectus abdominis muscles in the mid-line at the linea alba. The etiology of pathology is unknown, but the continuity of the abdominal wall is disrupted (Fig. 17–3).

2. Incidence

Any separation larger than 2 cm is considered significant.[2,26]
a. The condition is not exclusive to childbearing women but is seen frequently in this population.
b. Diastasis recti possibly occurs in pregnancy as a result of hormonal effects on the connective tissue and the biomechanical changes of pregnancy. It causes no discomfort.[26]

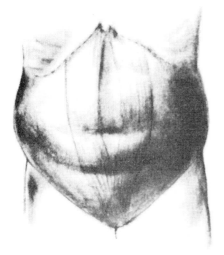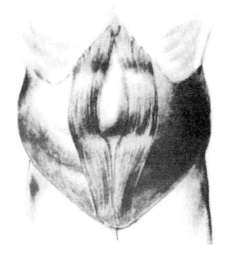

Figure 17–3. Diagramatic representations of diastasis recti. (From Biossonnault, JS, and Kotarinus, RK: Diastasis recti. In Wilder, E [ed]: Obstetric and Gynecologic Physical Therapy. Churchill-Livingstone, New York, 1988, p 397, with permission.)

    c. It is relatively uncommon in the first trimester, but the incidence increases as the pregnancy progresses, reaching a peak in the third trimester.

    d. It does not always spontaneously resolve following childbirth and may continue past the 6-week postpartum period.

    e. It can occur above, below, or at the level of the umbilicus but appears to be less common below the umbilicus.

    f. It appears to be less common in women with good abdominal tone prior to pregnancy.[2]

3. Significance

    a. The condition of diastasis recti may produce musculoskeletal complaints, such as low-back pain, possibly as a result of decreased ability of the abdominal musculature to control the pelvis and lumbar spine.

    b. In severe separations, the anterior segment of the abdominal wall is composed only of skin, fascia, subcutaneous fat, and peritoneum.[2,6,33] The lack of abdominal support provides less protection for the fetus.

    c. Severe cases of diastasis recti may progress to herniation of the abdominal viscera through the separation in the abdominal wall.

4. Diastasis recti test[2,5,6,10,26,40]

Patient position: hook-lying. Have the patient slowly raise her head and shoulders off the floor, reaching her hands toward the knees, until the spine of the scapula leaves the floor. The therapist places the fingers of one hand horizontally across the midline of the abdomen at the umbilicus (Fig. 17–4). If a separation exists, the fingers will sink into the gap. The diastasis is measured by the number of fingers that can be placed between the rectus muscle bellies. A diastasis can also present as a longitudinal bulge along the linea alba. Since a diastasis recti can occur above, below, or at the level of the umbilicus, it should be tested at all three areas.

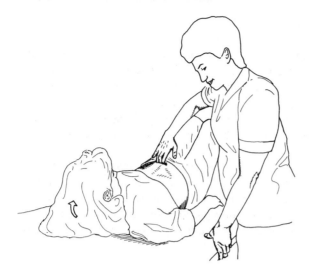

Figure 17–4. Diastasis recti test.

5. Treatment of diastasis recti

a. Test all pregnant clients for the presence of diastasis recti prior to performing abdominal exercises.

b. Perform corrective exercise for diastasis recti exclusive of other abdominal exercise until the separation is decreased to 2 cm or less (see Section V).[26] At that time, abdominal exercise can be resumed, but the integrity of the linea alba should be monitored to make sure the separation continues to decrease.

B. Low Back and Pelvic Pain[1,5,13,26,30,31,33,40]

1. Postural back pain: symptoms and treatment

a. Pain commonly occurs due to the postural changes of pregnancy, increased ligamentous laxity, and decreased abdominal function.

b. The symptoms of low back pain usually worsen with muscle fatigue from static postures or as the day progresses; symptoms are usually relieved with rest or change of position.

c. Low-back symptoms can be treated effectively with proper body mechanics, posture instructions, and improvement in work techniques[30] (see Chapter 15, see also Section V of this chapter). The use of deep-heating agents, electrical stimulation, and traction is generally contraindicated during pregnancy.

d. Usually back symptoms disappear following pregnancy if proper body mechanics are used during child care and daily activities.

e. Women who are physically fit generally have less back pain during pregnancy.[30]

2. Sacroiliac (posterior pelvic) back pain: symptoms and treatment

a. The incidence of pain in the posterior pelvis is unknown but appears to be fairly common in pregnancy. One study reported a four times greater incidence of posterior pelvic pain than low back pain in pregnant women.[30] Sacroiliac symptoms may be caused by ligamentous laxity coupled with postural adaptations.

b. Pain is usually localized to the posterior pelvis and is described as stabbing deep into the buttocks distal and lateral to L-5/S-1. Pain may radiate into the posterior thigh or knee but not into the foot.

    c. Symptoms include pain with prolonged sitting, standing, or walking; pain when climbing stairs or turning in bed; unilateral standing or torsion activities; pain that is not relieved by rest and frequently worsens with activity. There also may be pubic symphysis discomfort, subluxation, or both.[32]

    d. Use of external stabilization such as belts or corsets designed for use by pregnant women helps reduce the posterior pelvic pain, especially when walking.[30]

    e. Exercise must be modified so as to not aggravate the condition. Single-leg weight bearing should be avoided. Activities may need modification to minimize stresses on the symptomatic tissues, such as getting in and out of a car by keeping the legs together, then pivoting the legs and spine as a unit, side-lying with a pillow between the knees, and adapting sexual activities to avoid full range of hip abduction.

C. Varicose Veins[33]

1. Varicosities are aggravated in pregnancy by the increased uterine weight, venous stasis in the legs, and increased venous distensibility.
2. Occasionally, there may be a range of mild discomfort to severe pain in the lower extremities, especially when the legs are in the dependent position.
3. If there is discomfort, exercises may need to be modified so that minimal dependent positioning of the legs is required.
4. Elastic support stockings should be worn to provide an external pressure gradient against the distended veins, and the women should be encouraged to elevate the lower extremities as often as possible.

D. Pelvic Floor Dysfunction[7,17,26,33,38–41]

1. Structure of the pelvic floor (Fig. 17–5A)

The pelvic floor is a multilayered sheet of muscle stretched between the pubis and coccyx, forming the inferior support to the abdominopelvic cavity. The pelvic floor is pierced by the urethra, vagina, and rectum. The major muscle of the pelvic floor is the pubococcygeus muscle.

2. Functions of the pelvic floor

    a. Provides support for the pelvic organs and their contents
    b. Withstands increases in intra-abdominal pressure

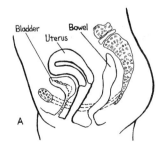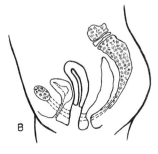

Figure 17–5. (*A*) Good pelvic floor support with a firm base, organs in place. (*B*) Inadequate support and the hammock stage, contents descended.

    c. Provides sphincter control of the perineal openings

    d. Functions in reproductive and sexual activities

3. Dysfunction

    a. Muscle and soft tissue laxity

       (1) The pelvic organs drop from their normal alignment because of increased pressure on the pelvic floor musculature, and organ prolapse may occur (Fig. 17–5B).

       (2) Urinary stress incontinence (involuntary urine loss with increases in abdominal pressure) may occur and worsen with subsequent pregnancies, increases in weight, or aging.

    b. Pelvic floor disruption

       (1) Episiotomy: an incision in the pelvic floor made during childbirth to enlarge the vaginal opening and allow faster delivery. It can produce prolonged pain, cause scarring, or become infected.

       (2) Tears and lacerations may occur during childbirth, particularly if the baby is large or if a forceps delivery is necessary.

    c. Hypertonicity: an increase in muscle tension or fascial tightness of the pelvic floor significant enough to impair normal sexual and elimination functions. This problem may occur as a result of improper postpartum healing and may be quite painful.[40]

4. Treatment techniques for pelvic floor dysfunction

    a. Therapeutic exercise techniques to the pelvic floor muscles are taught to improve control and for relaxation of the muscles (see Section V).

    b. Modalities such as superficial heat, ice, and massage may be used prenatally to relieve discomfort. Transcutaneous electrical stimulation or electrical muscle stimulation may also be used postpartum to modulate pain and to stimulate muscle contractions, respectively.

E. Joint Laxity[5,12,13,26,31,33,40]

1. Significance

    a. All joint structures are at increased risk of injury during pregnancy and during the immediate postpartum period.

    b. The tensile quality of the ligamentous support is decreased and, therefore, injury can occur if women are not educated regarding joint protection.

2. Treatment of joint laxity

    a. The woman is taught safe exercises to perform during the childbearing year, including modification of exercises to decrease excessive joint stress (see Section V).

    b. Non–weight-bearing or less stressful aerobic activities such as swimming, walking, or biking may be suggested, particularly for women who were exercising minimally before pregnancy.

IV. Effects of Aerobic Exercise During Pregnancy

A. Maternal Response to Aerobic Exercise[1,8,12,13,22,40]

1. Blood flow

Aerobic exercise does not reduce blood flow to the brain and heart. It does, however, cause a redistribution of blood flow away from the internal organs and possibly the uterus and toward the working muscles. This raises two concerns, that the reduction in blood flow may decrease the oxygen and nutrient availability to the fetus and that uterine contractions and preterm labor may be stimulated.[8] Stroke volume and cardiac output both increase with steady-state exercise. This coupled with increased blood volume and reduction in systemic vascular resistance during pregnancy may help offset the effects of the vascular shunting.[12]

2. Respiratory rate

The maternal respiration rate appears to adapt to mild exercise but does not increase proportionately with moderate and severe exercise when compared with a nonpregnant state. The pregnant woman reaches a maximum exercise capacity at a lower work level than a nonpregnant woman due to the increased oxygen requirements of exercise.

3. Hematocrit level

The maternal hematocrit level during pregnancy is lowered; however, it rises up to 10 percentage points within 15 minutes of beginning vigorous exercise. This condition continues for up to 4 weeks postpartum. As a result, cardiac reserve is decreased during exercise.[13]

4. Interior vena cava compression

Compression of the inferior vena cava by the uterus can occur after the fourth month of pregnancy, altering venous return and cardiac output. This has been suggested as a possible cause of **abruptio placentae,** or premature detachment of the placenta from the uterus.

5. Energy needs

Hypoglycemia occurs more readily during pregnancy; therefore, adequate carbohydrate intake is important for the pregnant woman who exercises.[12] A caloric intake of an additional 500 calories per day is necessary to support the energy needs of pregnancy and exercise, as opposed to only a 300-calorie-per-day increase for the sedentary pregnant woman.[1]

6. Core temperature

Vigorous physical activity and dehydration through perspiration can cause body core temperature to increase. This occurs in anyone who exercises. Concern has been expressed over this occurring in the pregnant woman because of the relationship of elevated core temperature to neural tube defects of the fetus. Studies report that during pregnancy the core temperature of physically fit women decreases during exercise. Apparently they have increased efficiency regulating their core temperature, and thus the thermal stress on the embryo and fetus is reduced.[9,12]

7. Uterine contractions

Norepinephrine and epinephrine levels increase with exercise. Norepinephrine increases the strength and frequency of uterine contractions. This may pose a problem for the woman at risk of developing premature labor.

8. Healthy woman response

Studies have shown that healthy women who continue to run throughout pregnancy deliver on the average of 5 to 7 days sooner compared with controls.[8,9]

Clapp[9] summarizes that, when evaluating runners, aerobic dancers, and controls, there were no differences between groups in premature labor (<37.5 weeks) or preterm premature rupture of the membranes and recommends that exercise, including weight bearing (even with ballistic motions such as with aerobic dancing), can be performed in mid and late pregnancy without risk of preterm labor or premature rupture of the membranes. The most recent statement by the American College of Obstetricians and Gynecologists also supports this.[12]

B. Fetal Response to Maternal Aerobic Exercise[9,12,18,22,40]

1. No conclusive human research has proved a detrimental fetal response to mild- or moderate-intensity maternal exercise. Recent studies suggest that even vigorous exercise does not have the detrimental effects on the fetus that once were feared, and therefore restrictions on exercise because of concerns for the effects on the embryo and fetus have been lessened.[9,12]

2. A 50 percent or greater reduction of uterine blood flow is necessary before fetal well-being is affected (based on animal research). No studies have documented such decreases in pregnant women who exercise, even vigorously. It is suggested that the cardiovascular adaptations in exercising women offset any redistribution of blood to muscles during exercise.[9,12]

3. Brief submaximal maternal exercise (up to 70 percent maternal aerobic power) does not adversely affect fetal heart rate.[12] The fetal heart rate (FHR) will usually increase 10 to 30 beats per minute at the onset of maternal exercise. Following mild to moderate maternal exercise, the FHR usually returns to normal levels within 15 minutes, but in some cases the FHR may remain elevated as long as 30 minutes following strenuous maternal exercise. Fetal bradycardia (indicating fetal asphyxia) during maternal exercise has been reported in the literature with the return to pre-exercise FHR levels within 3 minutes after maternal exercise, followed by a brief period of fetal tachycardia.[18] The healthy fetus appears to be able to tolerate brief episodes of asphyxia with no detrimental results.

4. The fetus has no mechanism such as perspiration or respiration by which to dissipate heat. But because physically fit women are able to dissipate heat and regulate their core temperature, this is no longer considered a reason to restrict exercise.[9,12]

5. Slight decrease in birth weight in the newborn of women who continue endurance exercises into the third trimester of pregnancy is reported on the average of 310 g. There is no change in head circumference or heel-crown length. The decreased weight is proposed to be the result of slightly earlier delivery and less body fat.[9]

V. Exercise During Pregnancy and Postpartum[13,14,26,29,31,32,40]

A. Potential Impairments/Problems of Pregnancy Summarized

1. Development of faulty postures
2. Upper extremity stresses caused by the physical changes of pregnancy and the muscular requirements of infant care
3. Changing body image
4. Altered circulation, varicose veins, lower extremity edema
5. Pelvic floor stress or trauma
6. Abdominal muscle stretch and trauma and diastasis recti

7. Decrease in cardiovascular fitness due to lack of knowledge about adequate and safe forms of exercise

8. Lack of knowledge about physical changes in pregnancy and childbirth, possibly increasing the chance that injury-inducing behaviors will occur

9. Inadequate relaxation skills, necessary for labor and delivery

10. Improper body mechanics

11. Development of musculoskeletal pathologies (described in Section III) associated with pregnancy

12. Lack of physical preparation (strength, endurance, relaxation) necessary for labor and delivery

13. Unsafe progression of postpartum exercise

B. General Goals and Plan for the Exercise Program

Goals	*Plan of Care*
1. Promote improved posture before and after pregnancy.	1. Posture evaluation. Exercises to stretch, train, and strengthen postural muscles. Posture awareness training.
2. Increase awareness of correct body mechanics.	2. Teach correct body mechanics in sitting, standing, lifting, and lying as well as transitions from one position to another.
3. Prepare the upper extremities for the demands of infant care.	3. Resistive exercises to appropriate muscles.
4. Promote increased body awareness and a positive body image.	4. Body awareness and proprioception activities. Posture reinforcement.
5. Prepare the lower extremities for the demands of increased weight bearing and circulatory compromise.	5. Evaluation of lower extremity status. Use of elastic support stockings. Stretching exercises to reduce cramping. Resistive exercises to appropriate muscles for strengthening. Evaluation for proper footwear.
6. Improve awareness and control of the pelvic floor musculature.	6. Teach awareness of pelvic floor muscle contraction and relaxation. Train and strengthen for muscle control.
7. Maintain abdominal function and prevent or correct diastasis recti pathology.	7. Evaluate and monitor diastasis recti. Teach appropriate exercises. Teach safe abdominal-strengthening exercises.
8. Promote or maintain safe cardiovascular fitness.	8. Instruct safe progression of aerobic exercise according to American College of Obstetricians and Gynecologists (ACOG) and American Physical Therapy Association (APTA) guidelines.
9. Provide information about the changes of pregnancy and birth.	9. Childbirth education classes.

Goals	*Plan of Care*
10. Improve relaxation skills.	10. Teach relaxation techniques.
11. Prevent problems associated with pregnancy (i.e., low back pain, pelvic floor weakness, decreased circulation).	11. Education about potential problems of pregnancy. Teach prevention techniques and appropriate exercises.
12. Prepare physically for labor, delivery, and postpartum activities.	12. Strengthen muscles needed in labor and delivery.
13. Provide education on safe postpartum exercise progression.	13. Postpartum exercise instruction.

C. Guidelines for Exercise Instruction*

1. Suggest each participant have a physical examination by a physician prior to engaging in an exercise program.
2. Each person should be individually evaluated prior to participation to screen for pre-existing musculoskeletal problems, posture, and fitness level. Exercise levels should not exceed prepregnancy levels.
3. Stretching exercises should be specific to a single muscle or muscle group and should not involve several groups at once. Asymmetric stretching or stretching multiple muscle groups can promote joint instability. Ballistic movements should be avoided.
4. No joint should be taken beyond its normal physiologic range.
5. Hamstring and adductor stretches should be used with caution. Overstretching of these muscle groups can increase pelvic instability or hypermobility.
6. Limit activities in which balancing or single-leg weight bearing is required, such as standing leg kicks. Besides possible loss of balance, these activities can promote sacroiliac or pubic symphysis discomfort.
7. It is suggested that supine positioning not exceed 5 minutes at any one time after the fourth month of pregnancy to avoid vena cava compression by the uterus. When supine, a small wedge or rolled towel placed under the right hip will lessen the effects of uterine compression on abdominal vessels and improve cardiac output by turning the patient slightly toward the left (Fig. 17–6).[1,29]
8. To avoid the effects of postural hypotension, rising from the floor to standing should be undertaken slowly.[13]
9. Discourage breath holding and avoid activities that increase the tendency toward the Valsalva maneuver, because this may lead to undesirable downward forces on the uterus and pelvic floor.

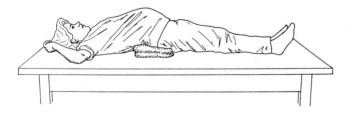

Figure 17–6. To prevent vena cava compressions when the patient is lying supine, a folded towel can be placed under the right side of the pelvis so the patient is tipped slightly to the left.

---

*Refs. 1, 12, 13, 23, 25, 26, 29, 31, 37.

10. Break frequently for fluid replenishment. The risk of dehydration during exercise is increased in pregnancy.
11. Encourage complete bladder emptying prior to exercise. A full bladder will place increased stress on an already weakened pelvic floor.
12. Include appropriate warm-up and cool-down activities.
13. Adapt or discontinue any exercise that causes pain.
14. When prone, avoid the knee-chest position with buttocks elevated above the chest level, especially in the postpartum client, because of the risk of air embolism.[23,25,27] A pregnant woman is at risk only if bleeding or other symptoms of early placental detachment are present. An air embolism can occur when the buttocks are elevated and the uterus moves superiorly. The pressure change causes air to be sucked into the vagina and uterus, where it can enter the circulatory system through the open placental wound.
15. Observe participants closely for signs of overexertion or complications. The following signs are reasons to discontinue exercise and contact a physician[13]:
    a. Pain
    b. Bleeding
    c. Shortness of breath
    d. Irregular heart beat
    e. Dizziness
    f. Faintness
    g. Tachycardia
    h. Back or pubic pain
    i. Difficulty in walking

D. Recommendations on Fitness Exercise[12]

NOTE: These recommendations are for pregnant women with no maternal or fetal risk factors and are adapted from the American College of Obstetricians and Gynecologists.[12]

1. Currently there are no data in humans suggesting that pregnant women need to decrease their intensity of exercise or lower their target heart rates but, because of decreased oxygen supply, they should modify the intensity according to their symptoms. When fatigued, a woman should stop exercising and never exercise to exhaustion.
2. It is preferable to exercise regularly at least 3 times per week rather than intermittently.
3. Non–weight-bearing aerobic exercises such as stationary cycling or swimming should be used to minimize the risk of injury but, if able, a woman may continue activities such as running and aerobic dancing.
4. If the woman cannot safely maintain balance because of the shifting and increasing weight, she should refrain from exercises that could result in falling and injury to herself or the fetus. She should also refrain from any activity that could result in abdominal trauma.
5. Adequate caloric intake for nutrition and adequate fluid intake and appropriate clothing for heat dissipation are critical.
6. Resumption of prepregnancy exercise routines during the postpartum period should be gradually resumed. Physiologic and morphologic changes of pregnancy continue for 4 to 6 weeks postpartum.

E. Contraindications to Exercise[1,3,12,13,27,29,31,40]

1. Absolute contraindications (see Section VII for more detail)

  a. Incompetent cervix; early dilatation of the cervix before the pregnancy is full term.

  b. Vaginal bleeding of any amount.

  c. Placenta previa: placenta is located on the uterus in a position where it may detach before the baby is delivered.

  d. Rupture of membranes: loss of amniotic fluid prior to the onset of labor.

  e. Premature labor: labor beginning prior to the 37th week of pregnancy.

  f. Maternal heart disease.

  g. Maternal diabetes or hypertension.

  h. Intrauterine growth retardation.[12]

2. Precautions to exercise

The woman with one or more of the following conditions may participate in an exercise program under close observation by a physician[1,3,13,27,29] and a therapist as long as no complications arise. Exercises may require modification.

  a. Multiple gestation (These infants are frequently born prematurely. Because some exercises may precipitate uterine contractions, these patients must be watched closely.[27])

  b. Anemia: reduction in the number of red blood cells, the amount of hemoglobin, or both (causes a reduction in the oxygen-carrying capacity of the blood)

  c. Systemic infection

  d. Extreme fatigue

  e. Musculoskeletal complaints and/or pain

  f. Overheating

  g. Phlebitis

  h. Diastasis recti

  i. Uterine contractions (lasting several hours after exercise)

F. Suggested Sequence for Exercise Class[1,31,40]

1. General rhythmic activities to "warm up"
2. Gentle selective stretching
3. Aerobic activity for cardiovascular conditioning (15 minutes or less)
4. Upper and lower extremity strengthening
5. Cool-down activities
6. Abdominal exercises
7. Pelvic floor exercises
8. Relaxation techniques
9. Educational information (as appropriate)
10. Postpartum exercise instruction (e.g., when to begin exercises, how to safely progress, precautions), as client may not be attending a postpartum class

G. Critical Areas of Emphasis and Selected Exercise Techniques[1,12,14,26,27,29,31]

1. Posture exercises

The growing fetus places added stress on postural muscles as the center of gravity shifts forward and upward and the body shifts to compensate and maintain stability. In addition, after delivery, activities involving holding and caring for the baby stress postural muscles. Muscles requiring emphasis for strengthening and stretching are listed. General exercise descriptions are listed in respective chapters. In addition, the following sections describe adaptations of exercises specific for the pregnant woman.

   a. *Stretching* (with caution)

     (1) Upper neck extensors and scalenes (Chapter 15).

     (2) Scapular protractors, shoulder internal rotators, and levator scapulae (Chapter 8).

     (3) Low back extensors (Chapter 15).

     (4) Hip adductors (Chapter 11). Caution: do not overstretch in women with pelvic instabilities.

     (5) Knee flexors (Chapter 12). Caution: do not overstretch in women with pelvic instabilities.

     (6) Ankle plantar flexors (Chapter 13).

   b. *Strengthening*

     (1) Upper neck flexors, lower neck and upper thoracic extensors (Chapter 15)

     (2) Scapular retractors and depressors (Chapter 8)

     (3) Shoulder external rotators (Chapter 8)

     (4) Trunk flexors (abdominals) (Chapter 15)

     (5) Hip extensors (Chapter 11)

     (6) Knee extensors (Chapter 12)

     (7) Ankle dorsiflexors (Chapter 13)

2. Abdominal muscle exercises*

As pregnancy progresses, the abdominals will not tolerate strenuous exercise. Therefore, exercise must be adapted to meet the needs of each individual. A check for diastasis recti must always be performed before initiating abdominal exercise. The following exercises progress from least to most strenuous.

   a. *Corrective exercises for diastasis recti* (Fig. 17–7)[5,26]

     (1) Head lift

       Position of woman: supine hook-lying with her hands crossed over midline at the diastasis to support the area. As she exhales, she lifts only her head off the floor or until the point just before a bulge appears. Her hands should gently pull the rectus muscles toward mid-line. Then have

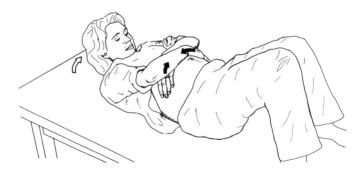

Figure 17–7. Corrective exercise for diastasis recti. The patient pulls with arms toward the mid-line.

---

*Refs. 2, 5, 6, 10, 11, 19, 24, 26, 34, 40.

the woman lower her head slowly and relax. This exercise emphasizes the rectus abdominus muscle and minimizes the obliques.

(2) Head lift with pelvic tilt

Patient position: supine hook-lying. If diastasis recti is present, the arms are crossed over the diastasis and pulled toward mid-line. She slowly lifts her head off the floor while performing a posterior pelvic tilt (see Chapter 15), then slowly lowers her head and relaxes. All abdominal contractions should be performed with an exhalation so that intra-abdominal pressure is minimized. Only this exercise and/or the head lift should be used until the separation is corrected to 2 cm, or 2 finger widths.[26]

b. *Leg sliding* (Figs. 17–8A and B)[26]

(1) Patient position: hook-lying with pelvis in posterior tilt. The woman holds the pelvic tilt as she first slides one foot along the floor until the leg is straight. She stops sliding the foot at the point in which she can no longer hold the pelvic tilt. Slowly she lifts the leg and brings it back to the starting position, then repeats with the other leg. Breathing should be coordinated with the exercise so that abdominal contraction occurs with exhalation.

(2) This exercise can be performed with both legs at the same time if abdominal muscles can maintain the pelvic tilt through the entire exercise.

c. *Quadruped pelvic tilt exercise*[5,10,11,24]

(1) Patient position: all-fours position on hands and knees. Instruct her to perform a posterior pelvic tilt. While keeping her back straight, she sucks the abdomen in and holds. Then she releases and performs an anterior tilt through partial range.

(2) For additional exercise, while holding the abdomen in and the back straight, laterally flex the trunk to the right (side bend to the right), looking at the right hip, then reverse to the left.

(3) Pelvic tilt exercises are practiced in a variety of positions, including side-lying and standing.

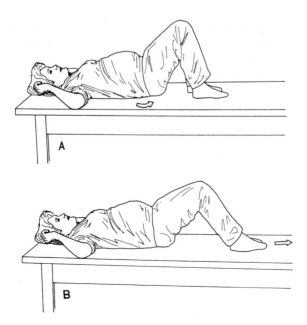

Figure 17–8. Leg sliding. (*A*) Supine hook-lying with posterior pelvic tilt. (*B*) Maintain pelvic tilt as the feet slide along the floor away from the body.

   d. *Trunk curls*

     (1) Curl-downs and curl-ups are classic abdominal exercises for rectus abdominis strengthening and can be used if tolerated and no diastasis recti is present. Protect the linea alba with crossed hands (Fig. 17–7) while performing trunk curls.

     (2) Diagonal curls are carried out to strengthen the oblique muscles. The woman lifts one shoulder toward the outside of the opposite knee as she curls up and down and protects the linea alba with crossed hands.

   e. *Resisted posterior pelvic tilt*

     (1) Pelvic lifts (see Fig. 15–26). The woman is supine with the lower extremities elevated to 90 degrees. She lifts the lower extremities upward as the pelvis comes up off the floor. When this exercise becomes difficult to accomplish during the third trimester as the uterus enlarges and pushes on the diaphragm, it should not be attempted. Once the woman learns pelvic tilt control postpartum, this exercise may be resumed.

     (2) Modified bicycle. The woman is supine with one lower extremity flexed and the other partially extended. The lower abdominals stabilize the pelvis against the varying weight of the lower extremities as they are flexed and extended in an alternating pattern as if cycling. The further the lower extremities extend, the greater the resistance. In order to not strain the back, the woman must keep it flat against the floor by controlling the arc of the cycling pattern (see Fig. 21–3).

     (3) Leg-lowering exercises cause excessive strain on the low back and should not be performed during pregnancy; they may be resumed postpartum. The legs should be lowered only through the range in which control of the posterior pelvic tilt and flattening on the low back is maintained. If low back strain is felt or the lumbar spine begins to arch, this exercise should not be performed. The pull of the psoas major may cause a shear force on the lumbar vertebrae and the supporting ligaments may be strained.

3. Stabilization exercises

   a. Exercise progressions for developing dynamic control of the pelvis and lower extremities as described in Chapter 15 should be initiated and progressed at the intensity the woman is able to safely control. These may be performed throughout the pregnancy and postpartum period.

   b. ***Precautions***

     (1) Because the trunk muscles are contracting isometrically while stabilizing, there is a tendency to hold the breath; this is detrimental to the blood pressure and heart rate. Caution the woman to maintain a relaxed breathing pattern and exhale during the exertion phase of each exercise.

     (2) If diastasis recti is present, adapt the stabilization exercises to protect the linea alba as described previously.

4. Pelvic motion training

These exercises are used to develop proprioceptive awareness and control of pelvic motions.

   a. *"Pelvic clock"*[15,24]

     Patient position: supine hook-lying. Instruct the woman to imagine her pelvis as the face of a clock. The top of the clock (12 o'clock) is the pubic symphysis and the bottom (6 o'clock) is the sacrum. She slowly rotates the pelvis in a clockwise motion, keeping the movement smooth, then reverses and rotates the pelvis smoothly in a counterclockwise direction.

b. *Pelvic clock progressions*

The exercise, once mastered, can also be performed in the side-lying, all-fours, sitting, or standing position.

5. Pelvic floor awareness training and strengthening

a. *Isometric exercises*

(1) Patient position: supine or side-lying positions are the easiest in which to begin; progress to sitting or standing.

(2) Instruct the woman to tighten the pelvic floor as if attempting to stop urine flow. Hold for 3 to 5 seconds and relax.[26,36] The bladder should be empty when performing this exercise.

(3) This training is valuable in preventing or treating incontinence and a "leaky bladder," which may occur with coughing, sneezing, laughing, or other straining activities. Instruct the woman to use this technique and practice sphincter control by attempting to stop her urine flow intermittently when using the bathroom.

(4) The pelvic floor muscles are highly fatigable. Contractions should not be held longer than 5 seconds and with a maximum of 10 repetitions per session.[26,36] When fatigued, substitution of the gluteals, abdominals, or hip adductors may occur.

b. *"Elevator" (graded isometric) exercise*

(1) Instruct the woman to visually imagine riding in an elevator. As the elevator goes from one floor to the next, contract the pelvic floor muscles a little more.

(2) Relax the muscles gradually, as if the elevator were descending one floor at a time.

6. Modified upper and lower extremity strengthening

As the abdomen enlarges, it becomes impossible to comfortably assume the prone position. Exercises that are usually performed in the prone position must be modified.

a. *Standing push-ups*[11,34]

Patient position: standing facing a wall, feet pointing straight forward, a shoulder-width apart, and approximately an arm-length away from the wall. The palms are placed on the wall at shoulder height. Have the woman slowly bend the elbows, bringing her face close to the wall, maintaining a stable pelvic tilt, and keeping the heels on the floor. Her elbows should be shoulder height. She then slowly pushes with her arms, bringing the body back to the original position.

b. *Hip extension*[10,11,26]

(1) Supine bridging (see Fig. 11–11)

(2) All-fours leg raising (Figs. 17–9A and B)

Patient position: on hands and knees (hands may be in fists or palms open and flat). Instruct the woman to first perform a posterior pelvic tilt, then slowly lift one leg, extending the hip to a level no higher than the spine while maintaining the posterior pelvic tilt. She then slowly lowers the leg and repeats with the opposite side. The knee may remain flexed or can be straightened throughout the exercise. Monitor this exercise and

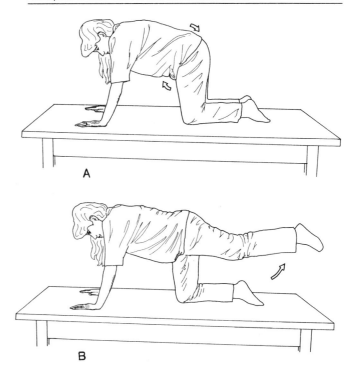

Figure 17–9. All-fours leg-raising. (*A*) Patient assumes quadruped position with posterior pelvic tilt. (*B*) Leg is raised only until it is in line with the trunk.

discontinue if there is stress on the SI joints or ligaments. If the woman cannot stabilize the pelvis while lifting the leg, have her just slide one leg posteriorly along the floor and return (see Fig. 15–27A).

c. *Modified squatting*

These exercises are used to strengthen the hip and knee extensors for good body mechanics and also to help stretch the peroneal area for flexibility during the delivery process.

(1) Instruct the woman to stand with feet a shoulder-width apart or wider, facing a counter, chair, or wall on which she can rest her hands for support. She slowly squats as far as is comfortable, keeping knees apart and over the feet and keeping the back straight. To protect her feet, she should wear shoes with good arch support. A woman with knee problems should perform only partial range of the squat.

(2) Wall slides. The woman stands with her back against a wall and her feet a shoulder-width apart. She slides her back down the wall as her hips and knees flex only as far as comfortable, then slides back up (see Fig. 11–15).

d. *Scapular retraction*

When scapular retraction exercises become difficult in the prone position, the woman should continue strengthening in the sitting position (see Fig. 8–32).

7. **Perineum and adductor flexibility**

In addition to the modified squatting exercises described above, these flexibility exercises prepare the legs and pelvis for childbirth.[5,10,26,31]

a. *Self-stretching*

The woman is positioned supine or side-lying and is instructed to abduct the hips and pull the knees toward the sides of her chest and hold the position for as long as comfortable (at least to the count of 10).

b. *Sitting*

Have the woman sit on a short stool with the hips abducted and feet flat on the floor.

8. Relaxation and breathing

Developing the ability to relax requires awareness of stress and muscle tension. Techniques of conscious relaxation allow the individual to control and cope with a variety of imposed stresses by being mentally alert to the task at hand while relaxing tense muscles that are superfluous to the activity. This is particularly important during labor and delivery when there are times that the woman should relax and allow the physiologic processes to occur without excessive tension in unrelated muscles.[27] Relaxation techniques for managing stress are described in Chapter 15. In addition, the following guidelines are suggested for the pregnant woman in preparation for labor and delivery.

a. *Mental imagery*

Use music and verbal guidance. Instruct the woman to concentrate on a relaxing mental image. Suggest that she focus on the image during the relaxation training so that the image can be called up to the conscious when recognizing the need to relax.

b. *Muscle setting*

(1) Have the woman lie in a comfortable position.

(2) Have her begin with the lower body. Instruct her to gently tighten and then relax first the muscles in the feet, then legs, thighs, pelvic floor, and buttocks.

(3) Next progress to the upper extremities and trunk, then to the head.

(4) Reinforce the importance of remaining awake and aware of the sensations of the muscles contracting and relaxing.

(5) Add deep, slow, relaxed breathing to the routine.

c. *Selective tension*

Progress the training by emphasizing awareness of muscles contracting in one part of the body while remaining relaxed in other parts. For example, while she is tensing the fist and upper extremity, the feet and legs should be limp. Reinforce the two sensations and the ability to control the tension and relaxation.

d. *Breathing*

General breathing techniques are described in Chapter 19. Slow, deep diaphragmatic breathing is the most efficient method for exchange of air to use with relaxation techniques and for controlled breathing during labor.

(1) The woman is taught to relax the abdomen during inspiration so that it feels as though the abdominal cavity is "filling up." During exhalation, the abdominal cavity becomes smaller; contraction of the abdominal muscles is not necessary with relaxed breathing.

(2) To avoid hyperventilation, avoid deep, rapid breathing. Caution the woman to decrease the intensity of the breathing if she experiences dizziness or feels tingling in the lips and fingers.

e. *Pelvic floor relaxation*[5,17,26]

(1) The woman is instructed to contract the pelvic floor as in the strengthening exercise, then allow total voluntary release and relaxation of the pelvic floor.

(2) This activity is coordinated with breathing. The woman is instructed to concentrate on a slow, deep breath and allow the pelvic floor to completely relax.

f. *Relaxation and breathing during labor*[27]

(1) *First stage.* Once labor begins, the contractions of the uterus progress. Relaxation during the contractions becomes more demanding. Provide the woman with suggested techniques to assist in relaxation.

(a) Have moral support from the father, family member, or special friend to provide encouragement and assist with comfort aids.

(b) Seek comfortable positions including walking or lying on pillows; include gentle motions such as pelvic rocking.

(c) Breathe slowly with each contraction; use the visual imagery and relax with each contraction. Some women find it helpful to focus their attention on some visual object. Other suggestions include singing, talking, or moaning during each contraction to prevent breath holding and encourage slow breathing.

(d) During the transition (near the end of the first stage) there is often an urge to push. Teach the woman to use quick blowing techniques, using the cheeks, not the abdominal muscles, to overcome the desire to push.

(e) Massage or apply pressure to any areas that hurt such as the low back. Using the hands may help distract the focus from the contractions.

(f) Apply local heat or cold to local symptoms; wipe off the face with a wet wash cloth.

(2) *Second stage.* Once dilation of the cervix has occurred, the woman may become active in the birth process by assisting the uterus during a contraction in pushing the baby down the birth canal.

(a) While bearing down, the woman takes in a breath, contracts the abdominal wall, and slowly breathes out. This will cause increased pressure within the abdomen along with relaxation of the pelvic floor.

Precaution: If the woman holds her breath, there will be increased tension and resistance in the pelvic floor. In addition, exertion with a closed glottis, known as the Valsalva maneuver, has adverse effects on the cardiovascular system.

(b) For maximum efficiency the woman should maintain relaxation in the extremities, especially the legs and perineum. Keeping the face and jaw relaxed assists with this.

(c) Between contractions, total body relaxation should be performed.

(d) As the baby is delivered, the woman should be instructed to just "let go" and breathe with light pants or groans to relax the pelvic floor as it stretches.

H. Exercises That Are Not Safe During Pregnancy

1. Bilateral straight-leg raising

This exercise typically places more stress on the abdominal muscles and low back than they can tolerate. It can cause back injury or diastasis recti and therefore should not be attempted.

2. "Fire hydrant" exercise

This exercise is performed on hands and knees. With the hip and knee flexed, the hip is abducted. If the leg is elevated too high, compression of the SI joint can occur. The exercise can be performed safely if hip abduction remains within the physiologic range (see Fig. 21–4). It should be avoided by any woman who has pre-existing SI joint symptoms.

3. All-fours hip extension

This exercise can be performed safely as explained earlier in this chapter (Fig. 17–9). It becomes unsafe and can cause low-back pain when the leg is elevated beyond the physiologic range of hip extension, causing the pelvis to tilt anteriorly and the lumbar spine to hyperextend.

4. Unilateral weight-bearing activities

Weight bearing on one leg (which includes slouched standing with the majority of weight shifted to one leg and the pelvis tilted down on the opposite side) during pregnancy can cause SI joint irritation and should be avoided by women with pre-existing SI joint symptoms. Unilateral weight bearing also can cause balance problems due to the increasing body weight and shifting of the center of gravity. This posture becomes a significant problem postpartum when the woman carries her growing child on one hip. Any asymmetries become accentuated and painful symptoms develop.

I. Exercise Critical to the Postpartum Period[1,26,40]

1. Uncomplicated vaginal delivery

Exercise can be started as soon after delivery as the woman feels able to exercise. All prenatal exercises can be performed safely in the postpartum period. Some exercises should be initiated as soon as possible after delivery.
  a. *Pelvic floor strengthening.* Exercises should be initiated as soon after the birth as possible. This exercise may increase circulation and aid healing.[26]
  b. *Diastasis recti correction.* Exercises should begin approximately 3 days after delivery and continue until correction to 2 cm is achieved. At that time, more vigorous abdominal exercise can be initiated. Until 3 days postdelivery, the abdominal musculature is too stretched to accurately test for diastasis recti. Therefore, the test should not be done until 3 days postdelivery.[26]
  c. *Aerobic and strengthening exercises.* As soon as the woman feels able, exercise can be resumed in a progressive program. A physical examination is suggested prior to the onset of vigorous exercise.

2. Precautions

  a. If bleeding increases or turns bright red, exercise should be postponed. The woman should rest more and allow a longer recovery time.
  b. Joint laxity may be present for some time after delivery, especially if the woman is breast-feeding. Precautions should be taken to protect the joints as described previously.
  c. Adequate warm-up and cool-down time is important.
  d. The prone knee-chest position should be avoided for at least 6 weeks postpartum because of the risk of air embolism (see Section V).

VI. Cesarean Childbirth[5,19,26-28,33,35]

A. Definition

Delivery of a baby through an incision in the abdominal wall and uterus rather than through the pelvis and vagina. General, spinal, or epidural anesthesia may be used.

B. Significance to Physical Therapists

1. Cesarean section is the single most common operation performed in the United States.[28]
2. The cesarean birth rate in the United States is 22.7 per 100 live births (1985); therefore, for those dealing with an obstetric population, the likelihood of treating a postcesarean patient is high.[28]
3. Women who have had cesarean deliveries still require pelvic floor rehabilitation. Many women experience a lengthy labor and trial pushing before a cesarean section is deemed necessary. Therefore, the pelvic floor musculature and tissues are not spared the stress of labor. Also, pregnancy itself creates significant stress on the pelvic floor musculature and tissues.
4. Rehabilitation of the patient who has had cesarean delivery is essentially the same as that of the patient who has had a vaginal delivery. However, a cesarean section is major abdominal surgery with all the risks and complications of such surgeries. The patient with a cesarean section will also require general postsurgical rehabilitation.
5. Many childbirth preparation classes do not adequately educate and prepare couples for the experience of a cesarean delivery. As a result, the patient with a cesarean section frequently feels as if her body has failed her, causing her to have more emotional changes than a woman who has experienced a more traditional delivery.

C. Impairments/Problems Summarized

1. Risk of pneumonia
2. Postsurgical pain and discomfort
3. Risk of vascular complications
4. Development of adhesions at incisional site
5. Faulty posture
6. Pelvic floor dysfunction
7. Abdominal weakness

D. General Treatment Goals and Plan of Care

Goals	*Plan of Care*
1. Improve pulmonary function and decrease the risk of pneumonia.	1. Breathing instruction. Coughing and/or huffing.[19,26]
2. Decrease incisional pain associated with coughing, movement, or breast feeding.	2. Postoperative TENS. Support incision with pillow when coughing or breast feeding. Incisional support with pillow or hands when exercising. Education regarding incisional care and risk of injury.

Goals	*Plan of Care*
3. Prevent postsurgical vascular complications.	3. Active leg exercises. Early ambulation.
4. Enhance incisional circulation healing; prevent adhesion formation.	4. Gentle abdominal exercise with incisional support. Scar mobilization and friction massage.
5. Decrease postsurgical discomfort from flatulence, itching, or catheter.	5. Positioning instruction, massage, and supportive exercises.
6. Correct posture.	6. Posture instruction.
7. Protected activities of daily living (ADL) to prevent injury.	7. Instruction in incisional splinting and positioning for ADL. Body mechanics instruction.
8. Prevent pelvic floor dysfunction.	8. Pelvic floor exercises.
9. Develop abdominal strength.	9. Abdominal exercises.

E. Suggested Activities for the Patient With a Cesarean Section[19,26]

1. Exercises

a. The woman should be instructed in all prenatal exercises as described in Section V.

b. The woman should be instructed to begin preventive exercises as soon as possible during the recovery period.

   (1) Initiate ankle pumping, active lower extremity range of motion, and walking to promote circulation and prevent venous stasis.

   (2) Initiate pelvic floor exercises to regain tone and control of the muscles of the perineum.

   (3) Deep breathing and coughing or huffing is used to prevent pulmonary complications (see 2 following).

c. Abdominal exercises need to be progressed more slowly. Check for diastasis and protect the area of the incision as with diastatic exercises. Initiate nonstressful muscle-setting technique and progress as tolerated.

d. Teach posture correction as necessary to retrain postural awareness and help realign posture in the nonpregnant state and to develop control of the shoulder girdle muscles as they respond to the increased stress of caring for the new baby.

e. Reinforce the value of deep diaphragmatic breathing techniques for pulmonary ventilation, especially when exercising, and relaxed breathing techniques to relieve stress and promote relaxation.

f. The woman should wait at least 6 to 8 weeks before resuming vigorous exercise. Emphasize the importance of progressing at a safe and controlled pace and not expecting to begin at her prepregnancy level.

2. Coughing or huffing

a. Coughing is difficult because of pain. An alternative is huffing.[26] A huff is a forceful outward breath using the diaphragm rather than the abdominals to push air out of the lungs. The abdominals are pulled up and in, rather than pushed out, causing decreased pressure in the abdominal cavity and less strain on the incision.

b. Huffing must be done quickly to generate sufficient force to expel mucus.

  c. Patient instructions

    (1) Support the incision with a pillow or the hands.

    (2) Say "ha" forcefully while pulling in the abdominal muscles.

3. Exercise to relieve intestinal gas pains[19,26]

  a. Abdominal massage or kneading while lying on the left side.

  b. Pelvic tilting and/or bridging (can be done in conjunction with massage).

  c. Bridge and twist. Maintain a position of bridging while twisting hips to the right and left. This position may also facilitate air embolism and should be used with caution in the early postpartum period.

  d. Partial abdominal curl-up.

4. Scar mobilization

Cross-friction massage should be initiated as soon as sufficient healing has occurred. This will minimize adhesions that may contribute to postural problems and back pain.

VII. High-Risk Pregnancy[3,20,21,31,33]

A. Definition

A pregnancy that is complicated by disease or problems that put the mother or fetus at risk for illness or death. Conditions may be pre-existing, be induced by pregnancy, or be an abnormal physiologic reaction during pregnancy.[20] The goal of medical intervention is to prevent preterm delivery, usually through use of bed rest, restriction of activity, and medications, when appropriate.

B. Conditions Considered High Risk

1. Preterm rupture of membranes

The amniotic sac breaks and amniotic fluid is lost prior to onset of labor. This can be dangerous to the fetus if it occurs before fetal development is complete. Labor may begin spontaneously after the membranes rupture. The chance for fetal infection also increases when the protection of the amniotic sac is lost.

2. Premature onset of labor

Labor that begins prior to 37 weeks of gestation or before completion of fetal development. Fetal life is endangered if delivery occurs too early.

3. Incompetent cervix

Painless dilatation of the cervix that occurs in the second trimester (after 16 weeks gestation) or early third trimester of pregnancy. This leads to premature membrane rupture and delivery of a fetus too small to survive.

4. Placenta previa

The placenta attaches too low on the uterus, near the cervix. As the cervix dilates, the placenta begins to separate from the uterus and may present before the fetus, thus endangering fetal life. Symptoms are intermittent, recurrent, painless bleeding that increases in intensity.

5. Pregnancy-related hypertension or pre-eclampsia

Characterized by hypertension, protein in the urine, and severe fluid retention. This can progress to maternal convulsions, coma, and death if it becomes severe (eclampsia). It usually occurs in the third trimester and disappears following birth. The cause is not understood.

6. Multiple gestation

More than one fetus forms. Complications of multiple gestation include premature onset of labor and birth, increased incidence of perinatal mortality, lower birth weight infants, and increased incidence of material complications (e.g., hypertension).

7. Diabetes

Maternal diabetes can be present before pregnancy or may occur as a result of the physiologic stress of pregnancy. Gestational diabetes (caused by pregnancy) usually disappears following pregnancy, but a greater tendency for development of the disease at some future time remains.

C. Impairments/Problems of the Bed-Bound Patient Summarized[31]

1. Joint stiffness and muscle aches
2. Muscle weakness and atrophy
3. Vascular complications
4. Decreased proprioception in distal body parts
5. Constipation due to lack of exercise
6. Postural changes
7. Boredom
8. Emotional stress; patient may be at risk of losing the baby
9. Guilt from the belief that some activity caused the problem or that the patient did not take good enough care of herself
10. Anxiety about her home situation or the impending birth

D. General Goals and Plan for Treatment of the Bed-Bound High-Risk Client[31]

Goals	*Plan of Care*
1. Decrease stiffness.	1. Positioning instructions. Facilitation of joint motion in available range.
2. Maintain muscle length and bulk and improve circulation.	2. Stretching and strengthening exercises within limits imposed by the physician.
3. Improve proprioception.	3. Movement activities for as many body parts as possible.
4. Improve posture within available limits.	4. Posture instruction, modified as necessary based on allowed activity level. Bed mobility and transfer techniques if able.
5. Relieve boredom.	5. Vary activities and positioning for exercises.

Goals	*Plan of Care*
6. Stress management and enhanced relaxation.	6. Relaxation techniques.
7. Prepare for delivery.	7. Childbirth education, breathing training, and exercises to assist and prepare for labor.
8. Enhance postpartum recovery.	8. Exercise instruction and home program for postpartum period. Body mechanics instruction.

E. Guidelines and Precautions[31]

1. All exercise programs for high-risk populations should be individually established based on diagnosis, limitations, physical therapy evaluation, and consultation with the physician. Activities must address patient needs but should not further complicate the condition.
2. The therapist should re-evaluate the patient after each treatment and note any changes.
3. The patient must be closely monitored during all activities.
4. Some exercises, especially abdominal exercises, may stimulate uterine contractions and, therefore, may need to be modified or discontinued.
5. A full bladder may stimulate uterine contractions. The patient should be encouraged to empty her bladder frequently.
6. Any uterine contractions, bleeding, or amniotic fluid loss must be monitored and reported.
7. No Valsalva maneuvers should be allowed. Any increases in intra-abdominal pressure should be avoided.
8. Exercises should be slow, smooth, and simple and should require minimal exertion.
9. It is necessary to develop good rapport with the patient; she must trust the therapist.
10. Many high-risk pregnancies result in cesarean deliveries, so the patient should be educated about cesarean delivery rehabilitation.
11. Incorporate maximum muscle activities into each movement.
12. Teach the patient self-monitoring techniques.

F. Suggestions for Exercise Programs With High-Risk Pregnancies[31]

1. Positioning instructions
a. Left side-lying to prevent vena cava compression, enhance cardiac output, and decrease lower extremity edema
b. Pillows to support body parts and enhance relaxation
c. Supine positioning for short periods, with a wedge placed under the right hip to decrease inferior vena cava compression (Fig. 17–6)
d. Modified prone positioning (side-lying, partially rolled toward prone, with pillow under abdomen) to decrease low-back discomfort and pressure

2. Range of motion instructions
a. Active range of motion (ROM) of all joints should be included.
b. Motions should be slow, nonstressful, and through the full range if possible.

    c. Teach in a gravity-neutral position if antigravity ROM is too stressful.

    d. The number of repetitions and frequency needs to be individualized to the woman's condition.

3. Suggested exercises

    a. Lying

        (1) Supine or side-lying with alternate knee to chest

        (2) Ankle pumping

        (3) Shoulder, elbow, and finger flexion and extension; reach to ceiling; arm circles

        (4) Unilateral straight-leg raise in supine or side-lying position

        (5) Bilateral active ROM in diagonal patterns for the upper and lower extremities

        (6) Lower extremity abduction and adduction

        (7) Pelvic tilt, bridging, gluteal setting

        (8) Abdominal exercises (check for diastasis); these should be very mild and closely monitored

        (9) Pelvic floor exercises

    b. Sitting (may not be allowed)

        (1) Feet dangling over edge of bed

        (2) Hip adductor and internal rotator stretch; tailor sitting

        (3) Upper extremity push-ups

        (4) Active ROM through diagonal patterns for upper and lower extremities

        (5) Ankle-pumping exercises

        (6) Alternate active ROM knee flexion and extension

        (7) Knee extension with ankle dorsiflexed to stretch hamstrings and heel cords

        (8) Arms reaching toward ceiling, then out to the side; arm circles added

        (9) Scapular retraction, with hands behind the head

       (10) Cervical ROM emphasizing flexion and lateral bending

    c. Ambulation (almost always contraindicated; when allowed, usually will be only to use bathroom)

        (1) Good posture in ambulation

        (2) Tip-toe or heel walking

        (3) Gentle, partial-range squatting to stretch quadriceps

        (4) Lower extremity rotation

4. Relaxation techniques (see Section V)

5. Bed mobility and transfer activities

    a. Moving up, down, side to side in bed.

    b. Rolling: incorporate neck and upper and lower extremities to aid movement.

    c. Supine to sitting, assisted by arms.

6. Preparation for labor

    a. Relaxation techniques

    b. Modified squatting: supine, sitting, or side-lying with knees to chest (see Section IV)

    c. Pelvic floor relaxation

    d. Breathing exercises

7. Postpartum exercise instruction (see Section V)

VIII. Summary

This chapter has provided an overview of pregnancy, labor, and delivery for therapists working with the obstetric patient. Specific anatomic and physiologic changes that occur during pregnancy have been enumerated. They included weight gain, changes in the organ systems, and postural changes. Certain pregnancy-induced pathologies including diastasis recti, low back pain, varicose veins, pelvic floor dysfunction, and joint laxity have been discussed and guidelines for treatment described. The maternal and fetal responses to aerobic exercise also have been discussed.

Specific exercises for pregnancy and the postpartum period have been outlined. Critical areas of emphasis for exercise, contraindications to exercise, and sequencing of exercise classes have been covered. Exercise guidelines and precautions for high-risk pregnancy and cesarean childbirth have been covered separately.

References

1. Artal, R, and Wiswell, R: Exercise in Pregnancy. Williams & Wilkins, Baltimore, 1986.
2. Boissonnault, J, and Blaschak, M: Incidence of diastasis recti abdominis during the childbearing years. Phys Ther 68:1082, 1988.
3. Boston Children's Medical Center and Feinbloom, R: Pregnancy, Birth and the Newborn Baby, ed 1. Dell Publishing, New York, 1979.
4. Boston Women's Health Book Collective: Our Bodies, Our Selves, ed 2. Simon & Schuster, New York, 1979.
5. Brewer, G: The Pregnancy After 30 Workbook, ed 1. Rodale, Emmaus, PA, 1978.
6. Bursch, S: Interrater reliability of diastasis recti abdominis measurement. Phys Ther 67:1077, 1987.
7. Chiarelli, P, and O'Keefe, D: Physiotherapy for the pelvic floor. Australian Journal of Physiotherapy 27:4, 1981.
8. Clapp, JF: A clinical approach to exercise during pregnancy. Clin Sports Med 13:443, 1994.
9. Clapp, JF: Exercise and fetal health. J Dev Physiol 15:9, 1991.
10. Dale, B, and Roeber, J: The Pregnancy Exercise Book. Pantheon Books, New York, 1982.
11. De Lyser, F: Jane Fonda's Workout Book for Pregnancy, Birth and Recovery. Simon & Schuster, New York, 1982.
12. Exercise During Pregnancy and the Postpartum Period. ACOG: An Educational Aid to Obstetrician-Gynecologists (Technical Bulletin No 189). Washington, DC, ACOG, 1994.
13. Exercise During Pregnancy and the Postnatal Period. ACOG Home Exercise Programs, Washington, DC, 1985.
14. Feigel, D: Evaluating Prenatal and Postpartum Exercise Classes. Bulletin of Section on Obstetrics and Gynecology, American Physical Therapy Association 7:12, 1983.
15. Feldenkrais, M: Awareness Through Movement: Health Exercises for Personal Growth, ed 1. Harper & Row, New York, 1972.
16. Flanagan, G: The First Nine Months of Life, ed 2. Simon & Schuster, New York, 1962.
17. Frahm, J: Strengthening the Pelvic Floor. Clinical Management in Physical Therapy 5:30, 1985.
18. Freyder, SC: Exercising while pregnant. Journal of Orthopaedic and Sports Physical Therapy Association 10:358, 1989.
19. Gent, D, and Gottlieb, K: Cesarean Rehabilitation. Clinical Management in Physical Therapy 5:14, 1985.
20. Gilbert, E, and Harman, J: High-Risk Pregnancy and Delivery, ed 1. CV Mosby, St Louis, 1986.
21. Ingalls, A, and Salerno, M: Maternal and Child Health Nursing, ed 5. CV Mosby, St Louis, 1983.
22. Jarski, RW, and Trippett, DL: The risks and benefits of exercise during pregnancy. J Fam Pract 30:185, 1990.
23. Knee-Chest Exercises and Maternal Death: Comments. Med J Aust 1:1127, 1973.
24. Mandelstam, D: The pelvic floor. Physiotherapy 64:8, 1978.
25. Markowiz, E, and Brainen, H: Baby Dance: A Comprehensive Guide to Prenatal and Postpartum Exercise. Prentice-Hall, Englewood Cliffs, NJ, 1980.
26. Nelson, P: Pulmonary Gas Embolism in Pregnancy and the Puerpurium. Obstet Gynecol Surv 15, 1960.
27. Noble, E: Essential Exercises for the Childbearing Years, ed 2. Houghton Mifflin, Boston, 1982.
28. Noble, E: Having Twins, ed 1. Houghton Mifflin, Boston, 1980.
29. Norwood, C: Cesarean Variations: Patients, Facilities or Policies. International Journal of Childbirth Education 1:4, 1986.
30. Ostgaard, HC, et al: Reduction of back and posterior pelvic pain in pregnancy. Spine 19:894, 1994.
31. Perinatal Exercise Guidelines. Section on Obstetrics and Gynecology, American Physical Therapy Association, 1986.
32. Physical Therapy Assessment and Treatment of the Female Patient. Obstetrical and Gynecological Implications, March 15–21, 1986. Sponsored by Programs in Physical Therapy, Northwestern University Medical School and Section on Obstetrics and Gynecology, American Physical Therapy Association.
33. Position Paper. Section on Obstetrics and Gynecology: Bulletin of Section on Obstetrics and Gynecol-

ogy, American Physical Therapy Association 8:6, 1984.

34. Pritchard, J, and MacDonald, P (eds): Williams' Obstetrics, ed 16. Appleton-Century-Crofts, New York, 1976.

35. Prudden, S, and Sussman, J: Pregnancy and Back-to-Shape Exercise Program. Workman Publishing, New York, 1980.

36. Sandberg, E: Synopsis of Obstetrics, ed 10. CV Mosby, St Louis, 1978.

37. Santiesteban, A: Electromyographic and dynamometric characteristics of female pelvic floor musculature. Phys Ther 68:344, 1988.

38. Shrock, P, Simkin, P, and Shearer, M: Teaching prenatal exercise: Part II—Exercises to think twice about. Birth Fam J 8:3, 1981.

39. Tchow, D, et al: Pelvic-floor musculature exercises in treatment of anatomical urinary stress incontinence. Phys Ther 68:652, 1988.

40. Wilder, E (ed): Obstetric and Gynecologic Physical Therapy: Clinics in Physical Therapy, Vol 20, ed 1. New York, Churchill-Livingstone, 1988.

41. Zacharin, RF: Pelvic Floor Anatomy and the Surgery of Pulsion Enterocele. Springer-Verlag/Wien, New York, 1985.

Management of Vascular Disorders of the Extremities

Vascular disorders, which cause disturbances of circulation to the extremities, can result in significant loss of function of either the upper or lower extremities. Disturbances of circulation may be caused by a number of acute or chronic medical conditions known as *peripheral vascular diseases* (PVDs). Peripheral vascular diseases can affect the arterial, venous, or lymphatic circulatory systems. Surgical procedures that interfere with the lymphatic system may also lead to vascular disorders. For example, surgical removal or radiation of lymphatic vessels is a part of some procedures for management of breast cancer. One or both may be necessary in the effective treatment of breast cancer but can also lead to chronic lymphedema of the upper extremity.

To contribute to the comprehensive evaluation and management of patients with peripheral vascular disorders, a therapist must have a sound understanding of the physical impairments associated with various arterial, venous, or lymphatic disorders. In addition, a therapist must be aware of the use and effectiveness, as well as the limitations, of therapeutic exercise in the evaluation and rehabilitation of patients with vascular disorders. Although therapeutic exercise is just one procedure used in the management of vascular disorders of the extremities, emphasis will be placed on this aspect of treatment when appropriate in this chapter.

OBJECTIVES

After studying this chapter, the reader will be able to:

1 Define common acute and chronic vascular disorders of the extremities that occur as a result of a variety of medical or surgical conditions and that affect the arterial, venous, and lymphatic circulatory systems.
2 Describe the primary and secondary impairments associated with specific disorders of the peripheral vascular system.
3 Explain the role of exercise in the evaluation and screening of patients with known or suspected vascular disorders affecting the extremities.
4 Describe the principles and effectiveness of therapeutic exercise for the rehabilitation of patients with specific vascular impairments.

5 Outline appropriate treatment goals and plan of care for patients with acute or chronic peripheral vascular disorders resulting in arterial, venous, or lymphatic circulatory dysfunction.

6 Describe the vascular, musculoskeletal, respiratory, and functional problems of patients after a mastectomy.

7 Outline the treatment goals and postoperative plan of care for a patient with a mastectomy.

8 Explain any precautions or contraindications to treatment of patients with vascular disorders.

I. Arterial Disorders

A. Types of Arterial Disorders

1. **Acute arterial occlusion**[11,17,20,26,38]

   a. Acute loss of blood flow to peripheral arteries may be caused by a thrombus (blood clot), embolism, or trauma to an artery.

   (1) The most common location of an arterial embolus is at the femoral-popliteal bifurcation, although an embolus can occur at other arterial bifurcations in the extremities.

   (2) Crush injuries to the vessels of the extremities can disrupt arterial blood flow and must be surgically repaired quickly to restore circulation and prevent tissue necrosis.

   b. An occlusion will result in absent or diminished pulses and complete or partial interruption of circulation to an extremity.

   c. The severity of the problem is dependent upon the location and size of the occlusion and the availability of collateral circulation.

   d. If little or no collateral circulation is available, an acute arterial occlusion will cause tissue ischemia and possibly gangrene of the distal limb.

2. **Chronic arteriosclerotic vascular disease (ASVD)**[11,17,20,26,38]

   a. Also called *arteriosclerosis obliterans* (ASO), *atherosclerotic occlusive disease*, or *progressive arterial occlusive disease* (PAOD), ASVD is the most common of all the arterial disorders affecting the lower extremities.

   b. Circulation progressively deteriorates because of narrowing, fibrosis, and occlusion of the large and medium arteries, usually in the lower extremities.

   c. This disease is most often seen in elderly patients and is commonly associated with diabetes mellitus.

3. **Thromboangiitis obliterans (Buerger's disease)**[10,11]

   a. This chronic disease, which predominantly is seen in young, male patients who smoke, involves an inflammatory reaction of the arteries to nicotine.

   b. It initially occurs in the small arteries of the feet and hands and progresses proximally and results in vasoconstriction, decreased arterial circulation to the extremities, ischemia, and eventual necrosis and ulceration of soft tissues.

   c. The inflammatory reaction and resulting signs and symptoms can be controlled if the patient stops smoking.

4. **Raynaud's disease (Raynaud's phenomenon)**[11,22,34]

   a. This functional arterial disease is caused by vasospasm, most often affecting the arterioles and small arteries of the fingers.

b. It is caused by an abnormality of the sympathetic nervous system and is usually seen in young adults.

c. Raynaud's disease is characterized by:

   (1) Sensitivity to cold
   (2) Blanching and cyanosis of the fingertips and nailbeds
   (3) Severe pain, sensory loss (tingling or numbness), and decreased function in the hands

d. Symptoms are slowly relieved by warmth.

B. Clinical Signs and Symptoms of Arterial Disease

1. Changes in skin color and temperature[11,17,20,25,26]

a. Pallor: a chalky, white color, blanching of the skin
b. Shiny and waxy appearance of the skin and decreased hair growth distal to the insufficiency
c. Decreased skin temperature
d. Dryness of the skin
e. Ulcerations, particularly at weight-bearing areas and bony prominences
f. Gangrene

2. Sensory disturbances[11,20,26,38]

a. Decreased tolerance to hot or cold temperatures
b. Paresthesia
   (1) Tingling and eventual numbness in the distal portion of the extremities
   (2) Susceptibility to wound infections after minor skin abrasions

3. Pain[11,17,26,28]

a. **Intermittent claudication** (exercise pain)
   (1) Exercise pain (muscle cramping) occurs when there is insufficient blood supply and ischemia in an exercising muscle.
   (2) Cramping occurs in musculature distal to the occluded vessel. The most common site of intermittent claudication is the calf muscle as the result of occlusion of the femoral artery. Exercise pain can also occur in the foot when the popliteal artery is occluded or, less commonly, in the buttock or low back if the iliac or aortic arteries are the sites of occlusion.
   (3) Pain slowly diminishes with rest.
   (4) Exercise tolerance progressively decreases, and ischemic pain occurs more readily as the disease progresses.

b. Pain at rest
   (1) A burning, tingling pain in the extremities occurs as a result of severe ischemia.
   (2) It frequently occurs at night because the heart rate and volume of blood flow to the extremities decreases with rest.
   (3) Partial or complete relief of pain may be achieved if the leg is placed in a dependent position, for example, over the edge of the bed.
   (4) Elevation of the limb will cause an increase in pain.

4. Paralysis[11,26]

a. Atrophy of muscles and eventual loss of motor function, particularly in the hands and feet, occurs with progressive arterial vascular disease.
b. Loss of motor function is compounded by pain, which further compromises functional capabilities.

C. Evaluation of Arterial Disorders[11,21,24-26]

To establish the type and current status of an arterial disease and to determine the effectiveness of any subsequent treatment, a complete evaluation of arterial blood flow is necessary. Some evaluation procedures and screening tests may be performed by the therapist; others are performed exclusively by the physician. An understanding of test procedures and their interpretation is important so the therapist can plan an effective treatment program.

1. **Palpation of pulses**
   a. The basis of any evaluation of the integrity of the arterial system is the detection of pulses in the distal portion of the extremities.
   b. Pulses are described as *normal, diminished,* or *absent.* Pulselessness is a sign of severe arterial insufficiency.
   c. The femoral, popliteal, dorsalis pedis, and posterior tibial pulses are commonly palpated in the lower extremity.
   d. The radial, ulnar, and brachial pulses are often palpated in the upper extremity.
   e. NOTE: Pulses are difficult to assess quantitatively. Other, more accurate and reliable noninvasive tests such as evaluation of blood flow by Doppler ultrasound supplement information gained from palpation of pulses.

2. **Skin temperature**
   a. Temperature of the skin can be grossly assessed by palpation. A limb with diminished arterial blood flow will be cool to the touch.
   b. If a discrepancy exists between an involved and an uninvolved extremity, a quantitative measurement of skin temperature should be made with an electronic thermometer.

3. **Skin integrity and pigmentation**
   a. Diminished or absent arterial blood flow to an extremity causes trophic changes in the skin peripherally.
   b. The patient's skin is dry and color is diminished (pallor). Hair loss and a shiny appearance to the skin also occur. Skin ulcerations may also be present.

4. **Test for rubor/reactive hyperemia**
   a. Changes in skin color that occur with elevation and dependency of the limb as the result of altered blood flow are evaluated.
   b. Procedure
      (1) The legs are elevated for several minutes above the level of the heart while the patient is lying supine.
      (2) Pallor (blanching) of the skin will occur in the feet within 1 minute or less if arterial circulation is poor.
      (3) The time necessary for blanching to develop is noted.
      (4) The legs are then placed in a dependent position, and the color of the feet is noted.
      (5) Normally, a pinkish flush appears in the feet after several seconds.
      (6) In occlusive arterial disease, a bright reddening or rubor of the distal legs and feet occurs.
      (7) The rubor may take as long as 30 seconds to appear.
   c. Alternate procedure
      (1) Reactive hyperemia can also be evaluated by temporarily restricting blood flow to the distal portion of the lower extremity with a blood pressure cuff.

(2) This restriction causes an accumulation of CO_2 and lactic acid in the distal extremity. These metabolites are vasodilators and affect the vascular bed of the blood flow–deprived area.

(3) When the cuff is released and blood flow resumes to the extremity, a normal hyperemia (flushing) of the extremity should occur within 10 seconds.

(4) In arteriosclerotic vascular disease it may take as long as 1 to 2 minutes for a flush to appear.

(5) NOTE: This method of assessing reactive hyperemia is quite painful and is not tolerated well in either normal individuals or patients with occlusive arterial disease.

5. Claudication time

a. An objective assessment of exercise pain (intermittent claudication) is performed to determine the amount of time a patient can exercise before experiencing cramping and pain in the distal musculature.

b. A common test is to have the patient walk at a slow predetermined speed on a level treadmill (1 to 2 mph). The time that the patient is able to walk before the onset of pain or before pain prohibits further walking is noted.[25,26]

c. This measurement should be taken to determine a baseline for exercise tolerance before initiating a program to improve exercise tolerance.

6. Doppler ultrasonography

a. This noninvasive assessment uses the Doppler principle to determine the relative velocity of blood flow in the major arteries and veins.[11,17,24,26]

b. A sound head, covered with coupling gel, is placed on the skin directly over the artery to be evaluated. An ultrasonic beam is directed transcutaneously to the artery.

c. Blood cells moving in the path of the beam cause a shift in the frequency of the reflected sound.

d. The frequency of the reflected sound emitted varies with the velocity of blood flow.

e. This information is transmitted visually, onto an oscilloscope or printed tape or audibly, via a loudspeaker or stethoscope.

f. Systolic pressure can also be measured at various points in arterial vessels.

NOTE: Although Doppler ultrasonic evaluations are not commonly performed by therapists, a recent study indicates that therapists who have been trained in the use of the technique have demonstrated competence and accuracy.[24]

7. Arteriography

a. This is an invasive procedure and is usually the last test to be performed. It is performed by a vascular surgeon prior to reconstructive vascular surgery.[9]

b. A radiopaque dye is injected in an artery.

c. A series of x-ray examinations are taken to detect any restriction of movement of the dye, indicating a complete or partial occlusion of blood flow.

d. Although this is an invasive procedure, it gives the most accurate picture of the location and extent of arterial obstruction.[9]

D. Treatment of Acute Arterial Occlusion

The treatment of acute arterial occlusion is often a medical or surgical emergency. The viability of the limb will depend on the location and extent of the occlusion and the availability of collateral circulation. Medical or surgical measures must be taken to reduce ischemia and restore circulation. The most common surgical treatment for an acute occlusion is a *thromboembolectomy*. If circulation cannot be significantly improved or restored, gangrene will develop in a very short time, and amputation of the extremity will be necessary.[11,17,20,26] ***Precaution:*** With an acute occlusion therapeutic exercise is contraindicated and the use of physical therapy procedures such as reflex heating is limited in the treatment of acute arterial occlusion.[11,17,20,22,26]

General Treatment Goals	*Plan of Care*
1. Decrease ischemia by restoration or improvement of blood flow.	1. Medical: bed rest; complete systemic anticoagulation therapy.
	Physical: reflex heating of the torso or opposite extremity.[11,22]
	Precautions: Local, direct heating of the extremity is *contraindicated*, because it can easily cause a burn to ischemic tissue. Use of support hose is also *contraindicated* as they may increase peripheral resistance to blood flow.
	Positioning the patient in bed, with the head slightly raised, will increase the blood flow to the distal portion of the extremity.[11,17,20,26]
	Thromboembolectomy and reconstructive arterial or bypass graft surgery are alternatives to nonoperative treatment.[11,17,20]
2. Protect the limb.	2. The limb must be protected from any trauma. Pressure on skin must be minimized by special mattresses, implementation of a turning schedule, and periodic repositioning of the patient.[11,20,26]
	Precaution: Avoid any pressure at the surgical site by restrictive clothing that could occlude blood flow.

E. Treatment of Chronic Arterial Disease[9,11,17,20,26,31,39]

Chronic arteriosclerotic vascular disease can often be conservatively treated by medical and physical means. Arteriosclerotic vascular disease does not usually require emergency medical or surgical care, except in the very advanced stages. Conservative measures are also useful in the management of thromboangiitis and Raynaud's disease.

In all cases, patients must be advised to stop smoking and alter their diet, including limitation or avoidance of salt, sucrose, and alcohol to lower their blood pressure, triglyceride, and cholesterol levels. These measures may not cure chronic arterial disorders but will minimize the risk factors.

Related medical disorders are also treated. Diabetes is commonly associated with chronic arteriosclerotic vascular disease and must be recognized and appropriately controlled. Hypertension is also managed with medication.

In patients with mild disease, a graded exercise program of walking or bicycling should be initiated to improve exercise tolerance and functional capacity in activities of daily living. A regular program of mild- to moderate-level exercise has been shown to decrease the occurrence of exercise pain (intermittent claudication).[11,12,20,31,33]

NOTE: Buerger or Buerger-Allen exercises, which were developed many years ago to progressively promote collateral circulation, involved a series of positional changes of the affected limb coupled with active ankle dorsiflexion and plantarflexion exercises.[10,17,20,43] Although these exercises are still occasionally included in some exercise programs for patients with peripheral vascular disease, there is little evidence that they are effective in improving blood flow to an extremity.[11,26] They are not advocated by the authors of this text.

Reconstructive vascular surgery, such as bypass grafts, may be indicated for patients with pain at rest. A graded exercise program after revascularization surgery may help maintain peripheral circulation. Patients with vasospastic disease may benefit from sympathetic blocks or sympathectomies to increase blood flow. If patients develop ulcerations and gangrene that cannot be treated medically or with conservative surgical procedures, amputation of the limb will be necessary.[9]

General Treatment Goals	*Plan of Care*
1. Improve exercise tolerance for ADL and decrease the incidence of intermittent claudication.	1. Regular, graded aerobic exercise program of walking or bicycling (see Chapter 4).
2. Improve vasodilation.	2. Vasodilation by iontophoresis.[1] Vasodilation by reflex heating.[1,22] NOTE: Although these physical measures have been advocated, their effectiveness is questionable.
3. Relieve pain at rest.	3. Sleep with the legs in a dependent position over the edge of the bed or with the head of the bed slightly elevated.
4. Prevent joint contractures and muscle atrophy, particularly if the patient is confined to bed.	4. Active or mild resistance range of motion exercises to the extremities.
5. Prevent skin ulcerations.	5. Patient education in the proper care and protection of the skin, particularly the feet. Proper shoe selection and fit. Avoid use of support hose.
6. Promote healing of any skin ulcerations that develop.	6. A wide variety of procedures for treating ischemic ulcers, including electrical stimulation and oxygen therapy, are used clinically.[11,27,38]

F. Principles and Procedures of a Graded Exercise Program for Patients With Chronic Arterial Insufficiency

1. Rationale for graded exercise[11,12,20,26,31]

a. During an active contraction of a muscle, blood flow temporarily decreases, but a rapid increase in blood flow occurs immediately after the muscle contraction.

b. After exercise is ended, there is a rapid decrease in blood flow during the first 3 to 4 minutes. This is followed by a slow decline to resting levels within 15 minutes.

c. With repeated, moderate-level exercise, blood flow in muscles can be increased 10 to 12 times the resting values for blood flow.

d. It has been suggested that regular daily exercise will increase walking endurance before the onset of exercise pain. Although it is questionable whether a regular graded exercise program improves collateral circulation in the extremities of humans with vascular disease, it has been demonstrated that exercise performed over time improves the efficiency of oxygen utilization in exercising muscles. This enables patients to tolerate exercise over a longer period and to walk longer distances before the onset of exercise pain.[11,26,31,33,39]

2. Procedure

a. The patient should be encouraged to walk or bicycle as far as possible, without causing intermittent claudication.

b. The graded endurance exercise should be carried out 3 to 5 days per week.

c. The patient should perform mild warm-up activities prior to initiating walking or bicycling. Warm-up activities could include static stretching of calf muscles and active isotonic pumping exercises of the ankle and toes.

d. See Chapter 4 for specific guidelines for establishing an aerobic exercise program.

3. *Precautions*

a. A maximum target heart rate should be established. A discussion of maximum target heart rate can be found in Chapter 4.

b. The patient should avoid exercising outside during very cold weather.

c. The patient must wear shoes that fit properly and will not cause skin irritations, blisters, or sores.

d. Patients with a history of cardiac disease must be monitored closely. An outline of these evaluation procedures can also be found in Chapter 4.

4. *Contraindications*

a. Graded ambulation or bicycling is discontinued if leg pain increases rather than decreases over time.

b. Patients with resting pain should not participate in an ambulation or a bicycling program.

c. Patients with ulcerations of the feet and wound or fungal infections should not participate in a walking program.

II. Venous Disorders

A. Types of Venous Disorders[11,18,20,26,36,37]

1. Acute thrombophlebitis

a. An acute inflammatory condition with occlusion of a superficial or deep vein by a thrombus.[11,18,36]

   (1) Superficial venous thrombosis
   If a blood clot is lodged in one of the superficial veins, the condition usually resolves without long-term complications.[11,18]

   (2) Deep venous thrombosis (DVT)

Thrombophlebitis of one of the deep veins can result in a pulmonary embolism and is life threatening.[11,18]

b. *Phlebothrombosis* is another term used to describe the occlusion of a vein by a blood clot.[21,37]

c. Acute venous disorders usually affect the lower extremities.

d. Risk factors associated with thrombophlebitis[11,37]:

 (1) Immobility and bed rest over a prolonged period

 (2) Obesity

 (3) Age of the patient (risk increases with age)

 (4) Orthopedic injuries

 (5) Postoperative patients

 (6) Congestive heart failure

 (7) Malignancy

 (8) Use of oral contraceptives

 (9) Pregnancy

2. Chronic venous disorders

a. *Varicose veins.*

b. *Chronic venous insufficiency.*

c. These chronic disorders are associated with venous hypertension and stasis in the lower extremities and inadequate return of blood to the heart.

 (1) The venous valves are not competent, and exercise no longer increases venous return.

 (2) Chronic venous insufficiency or development of a varicosity may follow an acute episode of thrombophlebitis.

B. Clinical Signs and Symptoms of Venous Disorders

1. Acute thrombophlebitis[11,18,25,26,36]

NOTE: Symptoms are most notable if a deep vein is involved.

a. Swelling of the extremity, most commonly seen with deep vein thrombosis

b. Pain

c. Tenderness of the calf muscles that increases when the ankle is dorsiflexed[25]

d. Inflammation and discoloration of the extremity

2. Chronic venous insufficiency[11,18,20,26]

a. Dependent edema

 (1) Associated with standing and sitting for prolonged periods of time.

 (2) Usually worse at the end of the day.

 (3) Edema decreases if the leg is elevated while the patient lies supine.

b. Aching or tiredness in the legs

c. Increased pigmentation and stasis of the limb

d. Skin ulcerations and secondary infection, which can lead to cellulitis

C. Evaluation of Venous Disorders

1. Phlebography[18,36]

a. A test used by the physician in addition to observation and the physical examination to diagnose venous disorders.

b. An invasive procedure similar to arteriography, using x-ray study and radiopaque dye injected into the venous system. The procedure is used to detect a venous thrombosis.

2. **Girth measurements of the extremity**[11,25,26]

   a. Circumferential measurements of the involved extremity are made to detect edema (or atrophy).
      (1) The girth of the involved extremity may be compared with the girth of the uninvolved extremity.
      (2) If consistent methods are used in taking measurements, the therapist can determine the effectiveness of treatment over time.
   b. One accepted method is to take circumferential measurements every 10 cm along the entire length of the extremity.

3. **Competence of the greater saphenous vein (percussion test)**[25,26]

   a. A test used for patients with varicose veins
   b. Procedure
      (1) Ask the patient to stand until the varicosities in the leg fill with blood.
      (2) Palpate a portion of the saphenous vein below the knee and then sharply percuss the vein above the knee.
      (3) If a thrust of blood is felt with the palpating finger below the knee, the valves are incompetent.

4. **Tests for possible deep venous thrombophlebitis**

   a. Homans' sign[25,26]
      (1) With the patient supine, forcefully dorsiflex the foot and squeeze the posterior calf muscles.
      (2) Many patients, but not all, with thrombophlebitis will experience significant pain in the calf muscles.
   b. Application of a blood pressure cuff around the calf[25]
      (1) Inflate the cuff until the patient experiences pain in the calf.
      (2) Patients with acute thrombophlebitis usually cannot tolerate pressures above 40 mm Hg.

D. Prevention of Thrombophlebitis[20]

1. Every effort should be made to *prevent* the occurrence of thrombophlebitis in patients at risk.
2. It is well established that venous return decreases with prolonged periods of bed rest.
3. Bed rest is the primary cause of acute postoperative thrombosis in the deep veins of the legs.
4. The risk of postoperative thrombophlebitis can be minimized by early ambulation and exercise, such as:
   a. Active pumping exercises (dorsiflexion, and circumduction of the ankle) performed regularly throughout the day while the patient is in bed
   b. Active or mild resistive range of motion to both lower extremities if the postoperative condition permits
   c. Daily passive ROM if active exercise is not possible because of a neuromuscular or medical condition
5. While the postoperative patient is resting in bed, the legs can be elevated periodically.

E. Treatment of Acute Thrombophlebitis[11,18,26]

Immediate medical management is essential in this life-threatening disorder. During the initial stages of treatment, the patient will be on complete bed rest and systemic anticoagulant therapy, and the involved extremity will be elevated. Movement of the extremity will cause pain and will increase congestion in the venous channels in the early inflammatory period.

NOTE: Passive or active range of motion exercises are contraindicated during this initial inflammatory period.

General Treatment Goals	*Plan of Care*
1. Relieve pain during the acute inflammatory period.	1. Application of moist heat, such as hot packs, to the entire length of the involved extremity.
2. In later stages, as the symptoms subside, regain functional mobility.	2. Graded ambulation with legs wrapped in elastic bandages or when pressure gradient support stockings are worn.
3. Prevent recurrence of the acute disorder.	3. The patient should avoid sitting or standing still for any length of time. Either resting with the legs elevated or walking is encouraged.

F. Treatment of Chronic Venous Insufficiency and Varicose Veins[11,18,20,26,28,30]

Patient education is primary in the treatment of these chronic disorders. The patient must be advised on how to prevent dependent edema, skin ulceration, and infections. The therapist may be involved in (1) measuring and fitting a patient for a pressure gradient support stocking; (2) teaching the patient how to put on the stocking before getting out of bed; (3) setting up a program of regular active exercise; and (4) teaching the patient proper skin care.

General Treatment Goals	*Plan of Care*
1. Increase venous return and reduce edema.	1. Individually tailored pressure-gradient support stockings should be worn during ambulation. Manual massage of the extremity in a distal to proximal direction. Use of intermittent compression pump. Regular ambulation, cycling, or an active exercise program. NOTE: Instruct the patient to elevate the lower extremities after graded ambulation until the heart rate returns to normal. Avoid prolonged periods of standing still and sitting with legs dependent. Elevation of the foot of the bed during rest.
2. Prevent skin ulcerations and wound infections.	2. Proper skin care.

III. Lymphatic Disorders

A. Disorders of the Lymphatic System: Possible Causes of Lymphedema[11,18,20,21,26,28,30]

1. A primary or congenital obstruction of the lymphatic system
2. An obstruction of the lymphatic system secondary to trauma or infection (cellulitis) of extravascular tissues
3. Chronic venous insufficiency
4. Surgical removal of lymphatic vessels
   a. The most common surgery in which lymph vessels are removed is the modified radical or radical mastectomy. Lymphedema may also develop as the result of radiation therapy to the area of the lymph nodes.
   b. The postoperative problems associated with mastectomy include more than just lymphedema of the upper extremity. For this reason, mastectomy will be covered separately and in detail in Section IV of this chapter.

B. Lymphedema: Background of the Problem[21]

1. **Lymphedema** is an excessive accumulation of extravascular and extracellular fluid in tissue spaces. It is caused by a disturbance of the water and protein balance across the capillary membrane.
   a. The lymphatic system is specifically designed to remove plasma proteins that filter into tissue spaces.
   b. Obstruction or removal of lymphatic vessels causes retention of proteins in tissue spaces.
   c. The increased protein concentration draws greater amounts of water into the interstitial space, leading to lymphedema.
2. Signs and symptoms of lymphatic disorders[11,20,21]:
   a. Lymphedema (painless swelling) of the distal extremity is most often seen over the dorsum of the hand or foot. *Pitting edema* indicates short-duration swelling, while *brawny edema* (hard edema) is associated with long-term venous insufficiency.
   b. Increased weight or heaviness of the extremity.
   c. Sensory disturbances (paresthesia) of the hand or foot.
   d. Stiffness of the fingers or toes.
   e. Tautness of skin.
   f. Susceptibility to skin breakdown.
   g. Decreased resistance to infection, causing frequent episodes of cellulitis.

C. Evaluation of Lymphatic Disorders[4,11,20]

1. Girth measurements of the extremity
2. Volumetric measurements of the extremity
   a. The involved extremity is immersed in a tank of water.
   b. The amount of water displaced as the extremity is lowered into the water is measured.
3. Palpation of the dependent limb to differentiate pitting edema from brawny edema with subcutaneous fibrosis

D. Treatment of Lymphedema[11,18,20,40]

The majority of patients seen by therapists in clinical settings have lymphedema secondary to obstruction of the lymphatic system from trauma, infection, radiation, or surgery. If a patient is at risk for developing lymphedema, *prevention* is the best goal.

To increase lymphatic drainage, the hydrostatic pressure of tissues must be increased. This is accomplished by external compression of the skin. Lymphatic and venous return can also be increased by elevation of the limb. Lymphedema caused by lymphatic disorders, such as lymphangitis and cellulitis, does not diminish as readily with elevation as does edema secondary to venous disorders.

General Treatment Goals	*Plan of Care*
1. Reduce lymphedema.	1. Intermittent mechanical compression with a pneumatic pump and sleeve or bag for several hours daily. Elevation of the extremity above the level of the heart (about 30 to 45 degrees) while sleeping and as often as possible during the day. Manual massage from distal to proximal along the length of the extremity. Isometric and isotonic pumping exercises of the distal muscles.
2. Prevent further edema.	2. Elastic support stocking or sleeve, individually measured and fitted to the patient. Regular elevation of the extremity. Avoidance of sources of increased load on the lymphatics such as: —static, dependent positioning of the limb —application of local heat —prolonged use of muscles for even light tasks —hot environments
3. Prevent infections and cellulitis.	3. Care of skin abrasions, small burns, and insect bites. Avoidance of harsh chemicals and detergents. Frequent application of moisturizers to the skin. Use of antibiotics.

IV. Mastectomy

According to the American Cancer society carcinoma of the breast is one of the most common forms of cancer in white females over the age of 40. It is also the leading cause of death in women between 40 and 60 years of age. About 1 out of 10 women will develop breast cancer sometime during her life.[3,32] Tumors that are detected early and are localized can be successfully treated by surgery, radiation therapy, chemotherapy, and hormone therapy. Although the use of surgical procedures, such as the lumpectomy and quadrectomy, is increasing, **mastectomy** (removal of the breast) is still the most common procedure in preventing the spread of breast cancer and in ensuring a high rate of survival.

After a mastectomy and the accompanying excision or radiation of adjacent axillary lymph nodes, a patient is at risk of developing upper extremity lymphedema, loss of shoulder motion, and limited functional use of the arm and hand. Axillary node dissection interrupts and slows the flow of lymph, which, in turn, can lead to lymphedema of the upper extremity. Radiation can cause fibrosis in the area of the axilla, which obstructs the lymphatic vessels and contributes to pooling of lymph in the arm and hand. Shoulder motion can become compromised as the result of incisional pain, delayed wound healing, and skin ulcerations associated with radiation therapy, and postoperative weakness of the muscles of the shoulder girdle. To prevent or minimize lymphedema and loss of upper extremity function, a comprehensive, postoperative plan of care that includes therapeutic exercise must be designed to meet the individual needs and goals of the patient who has undergone surgery and radiation therapy for breast cancer.

All therapists should be aware of Reach to Recovery, a one-to-one patient education program, sponsored by the American Cancer Society. Representatives of this program, most of whom are survivors of breast cancer, provide emotional support to the patient and family as well as current information on breast prostheses and reconstructive surgery.

A. Surgical Procedures[2,5,14,19,32]

1. Radical mastectomy

a. A radical mastectomy involves removal of the breast, the pectoralis muscles, chest fascia, and the ipsilateral axillary lymph nodes, as well as chemotherapy and radiation therapy to the involved area. Some of the nerve supply to the chest and shoulder musculature may also be disturbed.

b. Radical mastectomy was the treatment of choice until the 1970s, but it is performed only in advanced cases of breast cancer today.

c. Lymphedema, upper extremity weakness, and significant disfigurement result.

2. Modified radical mastectomy

a. The entire breast, fascia over the chest muscle, and axillary lymph nodes are removed.

b. The pectoralis muscles remain intact, which reduces cosmetic deformity and upper extremity weakness.

c. Radiation and chemotherapy may be necessary after surgery.

d. The modified radical mastectomy is used far more frequently today for most breast cancers than is the more severe radical mastectomy.

3. Simple mastectomy

a. A simple mastectomy involves surgical removal of the entire breast.

b. The lymphatic system and pectoralis muscles are preserved.

c. Postoperative radiation therapy is usually used to decrease the regional recurrence of the disease. Even though the lymphatic system remains intact, radiation may cause fibrosis in the lymph vessels and predispose the patient to the development of lymphedema.

4. Segmental mastectomy (quadrectomy) and lumpectomy

a. These procedures, which preserve a portion of normal breast tissue, are being increasingly used as an alternative to mastectomy.

  b. To minimize the risk of recurrence of the breast cancer, axillary lymph node dissection is often performed.
  c. Radiation therapy follows these procedures.
  d. The postoperative risk of developing lymphedema is similar to that of simple and modified radical mastectomies.

B. Postoperative Impairments and Problems*

1. Postoperative pain

  a. Incisional pain
    (1) A transverse incision across the chest wall is made to remove the breast tissue and underlying fascia on the chest musculature.
    (2) The sutured skin over the breast area may feel tight along the incision; movement of the arm pulls on the incision and is uncomfortable for the patient.
    (3) Healing of the incision may be delayed as the result of radiation therapy, which prolongs pain in the area of the incision.
  b. Posterior cervical and shoulder girdle pain[7]
    (1) Pain and muscle spasm may occur in the neck and shoulder region as a result of muscle guarding.
    (2) The levator scapulae, teres major and minor, and infraspinatus are often tender with palpation and can restrict active shoulder motion.
    (3) Decreased use of the involved upper extremity after surgery sets the stage for the patient to develop a chronic frozen shoulder and increases the likelihood of lymphedema in the hand and arm.

2. Lymphedema[2,5-8,14,19,35,41,42,45]

  a. Removal of the axillary chain of lymph nodes disrupts the normal circulation of lymph and causes swelling of the upper extremity.
  b. Radiation therapy may lead to the formation of scar tissue in the axilla, and sclerosis of vessels may occur as the result of chemotherapy; either can obstruct lymphatic vessels.
  c. Reduced use of the arm for functional activities and maintaining the arm in a dependent position also contribute to the development of postoperative lymphedema.
  d. Accumulation of extravascular and extracellular fluids in the upper extremity on the side of the surgery leads to:
    (1) Increased size of the extremity
    (2) Tautness of the skin and risk of skin breakdown and infection
    (3) Stiffness and decreased range of motion in the fingers
    (4) Sensory disturbances in the hand
    (5) Decreased function of the involved upper extremity

3. Chest wall adhesions[2,15,16,19,42]

  a. Restrictive scarring of underlying tissue on the chest wall can develop as the result of surgery, radiation fibrosis, or wound infection.
  b. Chest wall adhesions can lead to:
    (1) Increased risk of postoperative pulmonary complications

---

*Refs. 2, 6–8, 12, 14–16, 19, 29, 35, 41, 42, 44.

(2) Loss of ROM of the shoulder on the involved side

(3) Postural dysfunction

(4) Discomfort in the neck, shoulder girdle, and upper back

4. Weakness of the involved upper extremity[5,7,29]

a. Weakness of the horizontal adductors of the shoulder

(1) If a radical mastectomy is performed, the pectoralis major muscle is removed.

(2) This results in decreased strength and active motion of the upper extremity on the involved side on a permanent basis.

b. Weakness of the serratus anterior[7]

(1) In a modified radical and radical mastectomy, the axillary lymph nodes are removed. Lymph node dissection may also be performed with a segmental (partial) mastectomy or lumpectomy.

(2) The long thoracic nerve can be temporarily traumatized during axillary dissection and removal of the axillary lymph nodes.

(3) This results in weakness of the serratus anterior and compromised shoulder stabilization and function.

(4) Without the stabilization and upward rotation of the scapula that the serratus anterior normally supplies, active flexion and abduction of the arm will be limited.

(5) Faulty shoulder biomechanics and use of substitute motions with the upper trapezius and levator scapulae during overhead reaching activities can then cause subacromial impingement and resulting shoulder pain. This can be the precursor of a frozen shoulder.

c. Grip strength is often diminished as the result of lymphedema and secondary stiffness of the fingers.

5. Postural faults[2,5,7]

a. The patient may sit or stand with rounded shoulders and kyphosis because of pain, skin tightness, or psychological reasons. This contributes to faulty shoulder biomechanics and eventually restricts active use of the involved upper extremity.

b. Asymmetry of the trunk and abnormal scapular alignment may also occur as the result of a subtle lateral weight shift, particularly in a large-breasted woman.

6. Restricted shoulder motion[2,14–16, 19,42,44]

It is well documented that many patients experience some loss of shoulder motion after surgery and associated therapy for breast cancer. The following factors can potentially contribute to restricted ROM of the shoulder:

a. Incisional pain

b. Chest wall adhesions

c. Tenderness and muscle guarding of the shoulder girdle and posterior cervical musculature

d. Temporary or permanent weakness of muscles of the shoulder girdle

e. Rounded shoulders and trunk posture

f. Lymphedema

g. Decreased use of the involved hand and arm for functional activities

7. Psychological considerations[2,14,19,32,44]

a. A patient undergoing treatment for breast cancer experiences a wide variety of emotional and social issues. The needs and concerns of both the patient and the family must be considered. The patient and family members must cope with the potentially life-threatening nature of the disease as well as a difficult treatment regimen.

b. It is common for a patient to feel anxiety, agitation, anger, depression, a sense of loss and significant mood swings during treatment and recovery from breast cancer.

c. Besides the obvious physical disfigurement and altered body image associated with mastectomy, medications such as immunosuppressants and corticosteroids can also affect the emotional state of the patient.

d. Psychological manifestations affect physical well-being and can contribute to general fatigue, the patient's perception of functional disability, and motivation in treatment.

8. NOTE: It should be apparent that many of these clinical problems and potential impairments are interrelated and must be considered when a therapist develops a comprehensive postoperative plan of care for the patient.

C. Physical Therapy Treatment Goals and Plan of Care*

General Treatment Goals

1. Prevent postoperative pulmonary complications.
2. Prevent or minimize postoperative lymphedema.

3. Decrease lymphedema if or when it develops.

Plan of Care

1. Preoperative instruction in deep-breathing exercises and effective coughing (see Chapter 19).

2. Elevation of the involved upper extremity on pillows (about 30 degrees) while the patient is in bed or sitting in a chair.

   Wrapping the involved upper extremity with elastic bandages or wearing an elastic pressure-gradient sleeve.

   Pumping exercises of the arm on the side of the surgery.

   Early range of motion exercises and upper extremity ergometry.

   Precaution: Avoid static, dependent positioning of the arm.

3. Daily use of a mechanical pneumatic pressure pump for at least 1½ to 2 hours twice a day.

   Continual elevation of the involved upper extremity at night and use of an elastic sleeve during the day.

   Active use of the involved arm for light, functional activities.

   Distal to proximal massage while the arm is elevated.

*Refs. 2, 5–8, 14–16, 19, 23, 29, 35, 41, 42, 44, 45.

General Treatment Goals

4. Prevent postural deformities.

5. Prevent muscle tension and guarding in cervical musculature.

6. Maintain normal range of motion of the involved upper extremity.

7. Maintain or increase strength in the involved shoulder.

Plan of Care

4. Instruction in proper bed positioning preoperatively or on the first post-operative day, emphasizing mid-line and symmetric positioning of the shoulders and trunk.

    Carryover of symmetric posture to sitting and standing.

    Encourage the patient to assume an erect posture when sitting or standing to minimize a rounded shoulder posture.

    Posture training with an emphasis on scapular retraction exercises.

5. Active range of motion to the cervical spine to promote relaxation.

    Shoulder shrugging and shoulder circle exercises.

    Gentle massage to cervical musculature.

6. Active-assisted and active ROM exercises of the shoulder, elbow, and hand may be initiated as soon as possible but cautiously after surgery, usually on the first postoperative day. **NOTE:** Exercise may be initiated even when the drainage tubes and sutures are still in place.

    Precaution: Observe the incision and sutures carefully during exercises. Avoid any undue tension on the incision or blanching of the scar during shoulder exercises.

    "Gear-shift" exercises (see Fig. 8–9).

    Self-stretching to the shoulder with the involved arm supported on a table (see Figs. 8–14 through 8–17).

7. Isometric exercises to the shoulder musculature, initiated on the first post-operative day with the patient in bed.

    Closed-chain push-ups with the patient standing and leaning into a wall to strengthen the scapular stabilizers (see Fig. 9–29).

    Dynamic exercise against manual resistance may be initiated about 3 to 4 days postoperatively.

    Resistance may also be applied during open-chain shoulder exercise with a light hand-held weight (approximately 2 to 3 pounds) or a light-grade elastic resistance material.

General Treatment Goals

8. Improve exercise tolerance and sense of well-being and reduce fatigue.

9. Prepare the patient for active participation in a home program and possible participation in a cancer survivor support group.

Plan of Care

8. Graded low-intensity aerobic exercise program such as walking or cycling.

9. Patient education must be initiated on the first postoperative day. The expected hospital stay will be a few days to a week postoperatively.

NOTE: Although control of lymphedema and exercise are often suggested for patients who have undergone mastectomies, few studies have analyzed the effectiveness of specific rehabilitation procedures. In addition, some patients who have undergone mastectomies are not referred to physical therapy for participation in postoperative rehabilitation because of physicians' doubts of the benefits of therapy or concerns that early motion may increase the incidence of postoperative complications such as poor wound healing.[13,23]

The few studies that have been undertaken support the efficacy of a postoperative physical therapy program (consisting of active-assisted, active, and resisted ROM exercises; proprioceptive neuromuscular facilitation; functional activities; and hand and arm care) and its positive impact on postoperative ROM and functional use of the involved upper extremity. In these studies[15,41,42] the effectiveness of physical therapy (which generally involved early shoulder exercises) on the prevention or reduction of lymphedema was not consistently apparent. It should be noted that little, if any, description of activities that patients performed to prevent or decrease lymphedema was given in these studies. These studies also suggest that postoperative physical therapy does not prolong hospital stay or increase the incidence of postoperative complications.

V. Summary

An overview of peripheral vascular disease has been presented with specific discussion of arterial, venous, and lymphatic disorders. The signs and symptoms of acute and chronic vascular disorders have been outlined. Basic evaluation and diagnostic procedures used to assess vascular disorders have been briefly explained. Outlines of treatment goals and plan of care have been included for patients with acute or chronic arterial or venous disorders and lymphatic dysfunction. Because the postmastectomy patient is at risk for developing lymphedema and associated loss of function of the involved upper extremity, an expanded discussion of mastectomy and associated postoperative problems has been included in this chapter.

References

1. Abramson, DI: Physiologic basis for the use of physical agents in peripheral vascular disorders. Arch Phys Med Rehabil 46:216, 1965.
2. Adcock, JL: Rehabilitation of the breast cancer patient. In McGarvey, CL (ed): Physical Therapy for the Cancer Patient. Churchill-Livingstone, New York, 1990, pp. 67–84.
3. American Cancer Society: Cancer Facts and Figures, 1993. American Cancer Society, Atlanta, GA, 1993.
4. Beach, RB: Measurement of extremity volume by water displacement. Phys Ther 57:286, 1977.
5. Beeby, J, and Broeg, PE: Treatment of patients with radical mastectomies. Phys Ther 50:40, 1970.
6. Bertelli, G, et al: Conservative treatment of postmastectomy lymphedema: A controlled randomized trial. Am Oncology 2(8):575, 1991.
7. Bork, BE: Physical therapy for the post mastectomy patient. University of Iowa, Educational Program in Physical Therapy, 1980.
8. Brennan, MJ: Lymphedema following the surgical treatment of breast cancer: A review of pathophysiology and treatment. Journal of Pain and Symptom Management 7(2):110–116, 1992.
9. Burgess, EM: Amputations of the lower extremities. In Nickel, VL (ed): Orthopedic Rehabilitation. Churchill-Livingstone, New York, 1982.

10. Correlli, F: Buerger's disease: Cigarette smoker's disease may always be cured by medical therapy. J Cardiovasc Surg 14:28, 1973.

11. Eisenhardt, JR: Evaluation and physical treatment of the patient with peripheral vascular disorders. In Irwin, S, and Tecklin, JS (eds): Cardiopulmonary Physical Therapy, ed 3. Mosby–Year Book, St Louis, 1995, pp 215–233.

12. Ekroth, R, et al: Physical training of patients with intermittent claudication: Indications, methods, and results. Surgery 84:640, 1978.

13. Fell, TJ: Wound drainage following radical mastectomy. The effect of restriction of shoulder movement. Br J Surg 66:302, 1979.

14. Ganz, PA: Current issues in cancer rehabilitation. Cancer 65(Suppl 3):742–751, 1990.

15. Guttman, H, et al: Achievements of physical therapy in patients after modified radical mastectomy compared with quadrantectomy, axillary dissection and radiation for carcinoma of the breast. Arch Surg 125:389–391, 1990.

16. Hladiuk, M, et al: Arm function after axillary dissection for breast cancer: A pilot study to provide parameter estimates. J Surg Oncol 50(1):47–52, 1992.

17. Hurst, PAE: Peripheral vascular disease—Assessment and treatment. In Downie, PA (ed): Cash's Textbook of Chest, Heart and Vascular Disorders for Physiotherapists, ed 4. JB Lippincott, Philadelphia, 1987.

18. Hurst, PAE: Venous and lymphatic disease—Assessment and treatment. In Downie, PA (ed): Cash's Textbook of Chest, Heart and Vascular Disorders for Physiotherapists, ed 4. JB Lippincott, Philadelphia, 1987.

19. Kaplan, E, and Gumport, SL: Cancer rehabilitation. In Goodgold, J (ed): Rehabilitation Medicine. CV Mosby, St Louis, 1988, pp 289–292.

20. Kim, DJ, and Ebel, A: Therapeutic exercise in peripheral vascular disease. In Basmajian, JV, and Wolf, SL (eds): Therapeutic Exercise. Williams & Wilkins, Baltimore, 1990, p. 371.

21. Kottke, FJ: Common cardiovascular problems in rehabilitation. In Kottke, FJ, Stillwell, GK, and Lehmann, JF (eds): Krusen's Handbook of Physical Medicine and Rehabilitation, ed 3. WB Saunders, Philadelphia, 1982.

22. Lehmann, JF, and Delateur, BJ: Diathermy: Superficial heat and cold therapy. In Kottke, FJ, Stillwell, GK, and Lehmann, JF (eds): Krusen's Handbook of Physical Medicine and Rehabilitation, ed 3. WB Saunders, Philadelphia, 1982.

23. Lotze, MT, et al: Early versus delayed shoulder motion following axillary dissection. A randomized prospective study. Am Surg 193:288, 1981.

24. MacKinnon, JL: Study of Doppler ultrasonic peripheral vascular assessment performed by physical therapists. Phys Ther 63:30, 1983.

25. McCulloch, JM: Examination procedure for patients with vascular system problems. Clinical Management in Physical Therapy 1:17, 1981.

26. McCulloch, JM: Peripheral vascular disease. In O'Sullivan, SB, and Schmitz, TJ (eds): Physical Rehabilitation: Assessment and Treatment, ed 3. FA Davis, Philadelphia, 1994.

27. McCulloch, JM, Kloth, L, and Feedar, JA (eds): Wound Healing: Alternatives and Management, ed 2. FA Davis, Philadelphia, 1995.

28. McGarvey, CL: Pneumatic compression devices for lymphedema. Rehabil Oncol 10:16–17, 1992.

29. Neel, DI: Physical therapy following radical mastectomy. Phys Ther Rev 40:371, 1960.

30. Peters, K, et al: Lower leg subcutaneous blood flow during walking and passive dependency in chronic venous insufficiency. Br J Dermatol 124(2):177, 1991.

31. Ruell, PA, et al: Intermittent claudication. The effect of physical training on walking tolerance and venous lactate concentration. Eur J Appl Physiol 52:420, 1984.

32. Scanlon, EF: Breast cancer. In Holleb, AI, Fink, DJ, and Murphy, GP (eds): Clinical Oncology. American Cancer Society, Atlanta, GA, 1991.

33. Sidoti, SP: Exercise and peripheral vascular disease. Clinics Podiatr Med Surg 9(1):173, 1992.

34. Spencer-Green, G: Raynaud's phenomenon. Bull Rheum Dis 33:1, 1983.

35. Stillwell, GK, and Redford, JWB: Physical treatment of postmastectomy lymphedema. Proceedings of the Mayo Clinic 33:1, 1958.

36. Strandness, DE, Jr: Invasive and noninvasive techniques in the detection and evaluation of acute venous thrombosis. Vas Surg 11:205, 1977.

37. Vallbona, C: Bodily responses to immobilization. In Kottke, FJ, Stillwell, GK, and Lehmann, FJ (eds): Krusen's Handbook of Physical Medicine and Rehabilitation, ed 3. WB Saunders, Philadelphia, 1982.

38. Wagner, FW: The dysvascular lower limb. In Nickel, VL (ed): Orthopedic Rehabilitation. Churchill-Livingstone, New York, 1982.

39. Whitaker, R: Peripheral vascular disease—The place of physiotherapy. In Downie, PA (ed): Cash's Textbook of Chest, Heart and Vascular Disorders for Physiotherapists, ed 4. JB Lippincott, Philadelphia, 1987.

40. Wing, MT: Conservative management of peripheral edema. Phys Ther Forum 6:1, October 21, 1987.

41. Wingate, L: Efficacy of physical therapy for patients who have undergone mastectomies. Phys Ther 65:896, 1985.

42. Wingate, L, et al: Rehabilitation of the mastectomy patient: A randomized, blind, prospective study. Arch Phys Med Rehabil 70:21–24, 1989.

43. Wisham, LH, Abramson, AS, and Ebel, A: Value of exercise in peripheral arterial disease. JAMA 153:10, 1953.

44. Woods, EN: Reaching out to patients with breast cancer. Clinical Management in Physical Therapy 12:58–63, 1992.

45. Zeissler, RH, Rose, GB, and Nelson, PA: Postmastectomy lymphedema: Late results of treatment in 385 patients. Arch Phys Med Rehabil 53:159, 1972.

Chest Physical Therapy

Chest physical therapy is a multifaceted area of professional practice that deals with the evaluation and treatment of patients of all ages with acute or chronic lung disorders. It employs a wide range of therapeutic exercise and related modalities to effectively evaluate and treat the patient with cardiopulmonary dysfunction.[8,10]

The goals of chest physical therapy are to[8,10,16,18]:
1. Prevent airway obstruction and accumulation of secretions that interfere with normal respiration.
2. Improve airway clearance and ventilation through mobilization and drainage of secretions.
3. Improve endurance and general exercise tolerance.
4. Reduce energy costs during respiration through breathing retraining.
5. Prevent or correct postural deformities associated with respiratory disorders.
6. Promote relaxation.
7. Maintain or improve chest mobility.
8. Improve cough effectiveness.

Treatment settings vary widely. Inpatients may be treated in intensive care, chronic care, and postsurgical units; outpatients may be seen at home or followed in pulmonary clinics or rehabilitation centers.

OBJECTIVES

After studying this chapter, the reader will be able to:

1   Define chest physical therapy.
2   Identify the goals of chest physical therapy.
3   Summarize evaluation procedures pertinent to the assessment of the pulmonary patient.
4   Describe specific evaluation procedures.
5   Identify the goals, indications, and basic principles of breathing exercises and retraining.
6   Describe the procedures and a sequence for teaching a patient specific breathing exercises.
7   Describe the purpose and techniques of chest mobilization exercises.
8   Describe the normal cough mechanism.
9   Summarize factors that impair the cough mechanism.

10 Explain the procedure for teaching a patient an effective cough.
11 Summarize the goals, indications, and principles of postural drainage.
12 Describe the procedure, positions, and techniques of postural drainage.
13 Identify the precautions for and contraindications to postural drainage.

I. Review of Respiratory Structure and Function

A. The Thorax

1. Function

a. The main function of the thoracic cage is to protect the internal organs of respiration, circulation, and digestion.

b. The thoracic cage provides the site of attachment for the muscles of respiration to mechanically enlarge the thorax for inspiration or to compress the thorax for expiration.

c. It is also the site of attachment for upper extremity muscles, which function during lifting, pulling, or pushing activities. These activities are usually carried out in conjunction with inspiratory effort.

2. Skeletal structure

a. *Posterior*
The dorsal portion of the ribs articulate with the 12 thoracic vertebrae at the costotransverse and costovertebral joints.

b. *Anterior*
(1) First to 7th ribs articulate directly with the sternum via the costal cartilage.
(2) Eighth to 10th ribs have cartilaginous attachments to the rib above.
(3) Eleventh and 12th are floating ribs.

B. Muscles of Respiration[7–9,12,34,39,46]

1. Inspiration

a. *Diaphragm*
(1) The diaphragm is the major muscle of inspiration. During relaxed inspiration, it is the primary muscle responsible for movement of air.
(2) As it contracts, it moves caudally to increase the capacity of the thoracic cage.
(3) Nerve supply: phrenic nerve (C-3, C-4, C-5).

b. *External intercostals*
(1) The external intercostals act on inspiration. The internal and transverse intercostals participate minimally.
(2) Their function is to maintain the spaces between the ribs and to provide tone between the ribs with changes in intrathoracic pressure. During inspiration, the external intercostals also lift the ribs and increase the dimensions of the thoracic cavity in anteroposterior and transverse directions.
(3) Nerve supply: T-1 to T-12, respectively.

c. *Accessory muscles of inspiration*
The sternocleidomastoid (SCM), upper trapezius, and scalene muscles do not directly participate to move the ribs during resting inspiration. These muscles become increasingly active with greater inspiratory effort, which occurs frequently during strenuous physical activity. The accessory muscles of inspira-

tion may become the primary muscles of inspiration when the diaphragm is ineffective or weak as the result of chronic lung or neuromuscular diseases.

(1) The *SCM muscles* elevate the sternum to increase the anteroposterior (AP) diameter of the thorax. In patients with weakness of the diaphragm, the SCM muscles act as the primary muscles of inspiration. The nerve supply is cranial nerve XI and C-2 to C-3.

(2) The *upper trapezius* muscles elevate the shoulders and, indirectly, the rib cage during labored inspiration. They also fixate the neck so the scalenes have a stable attachment. Their nerve supply is cranial nerve XI.

(3) The *scalenes* participate minimally in normal resting inspiration to stabilize the first rib. During deep or pathologic breathing, the scalenes elevate the first two ribs and increase the size of the thoracic cavity if their superior attachments on the neck are fixed.

(4) During deep breathing, other muscles, such as the *serratus anterior* and the *pectoralis major and minor,* also act as muscles of inspiration by either elevating the ribs or pulling the ribs toward the arms through reverse muscle action when the upper extremities are fixed.

2. Expiration

a. *Relaxed expiration*

Expiration is a passive process when a person is at rest. When the diaphragm relaxes after a contraction, the diaphragm rises and the ribs drop. The elastic recoil of tissues decreases the intrathoracic area and increases intrathoracic pressure, which causes exhalation.

b. *Active expiration (controlled, forced, prolonged)*

Contraction of muscles, specifically the abdominals and the internal intercostals, causes active expiration.

(1) *Abdominals*

   (a) The rectus abdominis, the internal and external obliques, and the transverse abdominis contract to force down the thoracic cage and force the abdominal contents superiorly into the diaphragm. When the abdominals contract, the intrathoracic pressure increases and air is forced out of the lungs.

   (b) Nerve supply: T-10 to T-12.

(2) *Internal intercostals*

   (a) The internal intercostals primarily function during forceful expiration by depressing the ribs.

   (b) Nerve supply: T-1 to T-12, respectively.

C. Mechanics of Respiration[7-9,12,16,36,46]

1. Movements of the thorax during respiration

Each rib has its own pattern of movement, but generalizations can be made. The ribs attach anteriorly to the sternum (except 11 and 12) and posteriorly to the vertebral bodies, disks, and transverse processes, making a closed kinematic chain. The thorax enlarges in all three planes during inspiration.

a. Increase in the AP diameter.

(1) There is a forward and upward movement of the sternum and upper ribs. This is described as a *pump-handle* motion.

(2) The thoracic spine extends (straightens), enabling greater excursion of the sternum.

  b. Increase in the transverse (lateral) diameter.
    (1) There is an elevation and outward turning of the lateral (mid-shaft) portions of the ribs. This is described as a *bucket handle* motion.
    (2) The lower ribs (8 to 10), which are not attached directly to the sternum, also flair or open outward, increasing the subcostal angle. This is described as *caliper* motion.
    (3) The angle at the costochondral junction also increases, making the rib segments longer during inspiration.
  c. Increase in vertical dimension.
    (1) The central tendon of the diaphragm descends as the muscle contracts. This is described as a *piston action.*
    (2) Elevation of the ribs increases the vertical dimension of the thorax and improves the effectiveness of the diaphragm.
  d. At the end of inspiration, the muscles relax; elastic recoil causes the diaphragm to move superiorly. The ribs return to their resting position.

2. Movement of air: ventilation

  a. **Ventilation** is the mass exchange of gases to and from the body.
    (1) During inspiration, as the thorax enlarges, the pressure inside the lungs (alveolar pressure) becomes lower than the atmospheric pressure, and air rushes into the lungs.
    (2) At the end of inspiration, the muscles relax and the elastic recoil of the lungs pushes the air out, resulting in expiration.
    (3) The movement of air can be affected by breathing exercises.
  b. The term *ventilation* should not be confused with or used interchangeably with *respiration*, which involves the blood transport of gases to tissues and gaseous exchange between blood and tissues.

3. Compliance of the lungs

  a. Compliance refers to the distensibility (elastic recoil) of lung tissue or how easily the lungs inflate during inspiration.
  b. Normal lungs are very distensible (compliant).
  c. Compliance changes with age and the presence of disease.

4. Airway resistance

  a. The amount of resistance to the flow of air depends on:
    (1) The bifurcation and branching of airways.
    (2) The size (diameter) of the lumen of each airway. The diameter of the lumen can be decreased by:
      (a) Mucus or edema in the airways
      (b) Contraction of smooth muscles
    (3) The elasticity of the lung parenchyma.
  b. Normally, the airways widen during inspiration and narrow during expiration.
  c. As the diameter of the airway decreases, the resistance to airflow increases.
  d. In diseases that cause bronchospasm (asthma) or increased mucus production (chronic bronchitis), airflow resistance will be even greater than normal during expiration. Patients with these conditions will have great difficulty getting air out of their lungs during ventilation.

5. Flow rates

a. Flow rates indicate measurements of the amount of air moved in or out of the airways in a period of time. Flow rates, which are related to airflow resistance, reflect the ease with which ventilation occurs.

b. **Expiratory flow rate** is determined by the volume of air exhaled divided by the amount of time it takes for the volume of gas to be exhaled.

c. Flow rates will be altered as the result of diseases that affect the respiratory tree and chest wall. For example, in chronic obstructive lung disease, expiratory flow rate is decreased in comparison to normal. That is, it will take a prolonged period to exhale a specific volume of air.

D. Anatomy and Function of the Respiratory Tracts

1. Upper respiratory tract[8,12,16,35,39,42]

a. *Nasal cavity*

b. *Pharynx*

  (1) Function

    (a) Warms air to body temperature.

    (b) Filters and removes particles. Mucosal lining has cells that secrete mucus and cells that are ciliated. Cilia and mucosa trap particles. A sneeze removes large particles.

  (2) With illness and elevated body temperature

    (a) The mucous membrane tends to dry out, so the body secretes more mucus. This mucus dries out, and a cycle begins.

    (b) Action of the cilia is inhibited by drying of mucus.

    (c) The patient tends to breathe by mouth, which decreases the humidification of mucus and increases its viscosity.

c. *Larynx*

  (1) Extends from C-3 to C-6.

  (2) Controls airflow and, when it contracts rapidly, prevents food, liquids, or foreign objects from entering the airway.

2. Lower respiratory tract structure[8,12,16,39,42]: tracheobronchial tree (Fig. 19–1)

There are 23 generations (branchings) within the tracheobronchial tree.

a. *Trachea*

  (1) Extends from C-6 to the sternal angle (second rib, T-5), at which the trachea bifurcates

  (2) Passes in an oblique downward direction

  (3) Oval-shaped, flexible, cartilaginous tube

    (a) Supported by semicircular rings of cartilage.

    (b) The posterior wall is smooth muscle.

  (4) Contains an equal number of ciliated epithelial cells and mucus-containing goblet cells

b. *Mainstem bronchi: 2*

  (1) Right—almost vertical

  (2) Left—more oblique

c. *Lobar bronchi: 5*

  (1) Two mainstem bronchi divide into five lobar bronchi: three on the right and two on the left.

  (2) Mainstem and lobar bronchi have a great amount of cartilage.

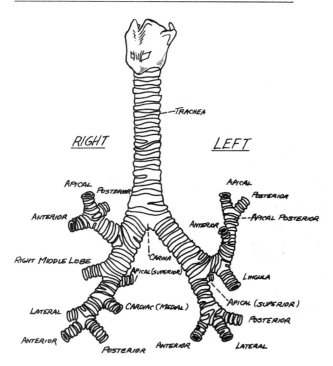

Figure 19–1. Lower respiratory tract—tracheobronchial tree. (From Frownfelter, DL: Chest Physical Therapy and Pulmonary Rehabilitation. Year-Book Medical Publishers, Chicago, 1987, p 26, with permission.)

    d. *Segmental bronchi: 18*
        (1) Lobar bronchi divide into 10 right segmental bronchi and 8 left segmental bronchi.
        (2) Segmental bronchi have scattered cartilage, smooth muscle, elastic fibers, and a capillary network.
        (3) The mainstem, lobar, and segmented bronchi have a mucous membrane essentially the same as the trachea.
    e. *Bronchioles*
        (1) Segmental bronchi divide into subsegmental bronchi and bronchioles, which have less and less cartilage and ciliated epithelial cells. These bronchioles divide into the *terminal bronchioles*, which are distal to the last cartilage of the tracheobronchial tree. Terminal bronchioles contain no ciliated cells.
        (2) Terminal bronchioles divide into *respiratory bronchioles* and provide a transitional zone between the bronchioles and alveoli. The respiratory bronchioles divide into alveolar ducts and alveolar sacs (Fig. 19–2). One duct may supply several sacs. The ducts contain smooth muscle, which narrows the lumen of the duct with contraction.
    f. *Alveoli*—approximately 300 million in the adult lung
        (1) Located in the periphery of the alveolar ducts and sacs.
        (2) Are in contact with capillaries (alveolar-arterial membrane).
        (3) Gas exchange occurs here.

3. Function of the tracheobronchial tree

    a. Conducts air to the alveolar system
    b. Helps with humidification and traps small particles to clean the air with the mucosal lining

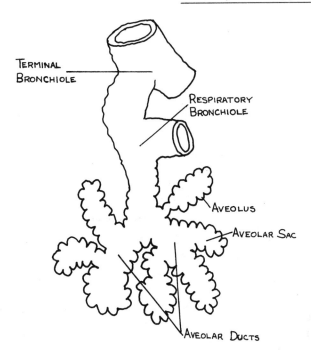

Figure 19–2. Bronchopulmonary segment.

    c. Moves mucus upward with the cilia
    d. Warms the air by the vascular supply
    e. Elicits the cough reflex because of the action of the chemical receptors

E. Anatomy of the Lungs (Fig. 19–3)[8,12,16,35,39,42]

  1. **Right lung**
    a. Three lobes—upper, middle, and lower
    b. Ten bronchopulmonary segments

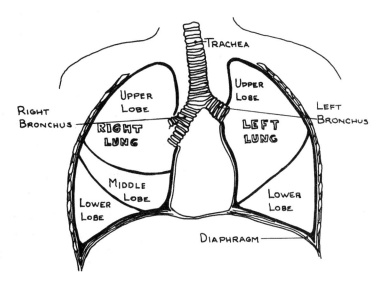

Figure 19–3. Structure of the right and left lungs.

2. **Left lung**
   a. Two lobes—upper and lower plus the lingula
   b. Eight bronchopulmonary segments
3. **Pleura**
   a. Viceral pleura—membrane that covers the lungs.
   b. Parietal pleura—membrane that covers the thoracic wall.
   c. A negative pressure in the minute space between the pleurae serves to keep the lungs inflated.
   d. Pleural fluid is found between the pleurae and lubricates the pleurae as they slide on each other during ventilation.

F. Lung Volumes and Capacities[62] (Fig. 19–4)

1. Pulmonary function tests that measure lung volumes and capacities are performed to evaluate the mechanical function of the lungs. Lung volumes and capacities are related to a person's age, weight, gender, and body position. A basic understanding of these tests will be useful for the therapist who is treating the patient with pulmonary dysfunction.
   a. **Total lung capacity (TLC)**
      (1) The total amount of air contained in the lungs after a maximum inspiration.
      (2) The TLC can be subdivided into four volumes: the tidal volume, inspiratory reserve volume, expiratory reserve volume, and residual volume.
      (3) Two or more lung volumes, when combined, are described as a capacity.
      (4) The vital capacity plus the residual volume equal the TLC.
      (5) TLC is approximately 6000 mL in a healthy young adult.
   b. **Tidal volume (TV)**
      (1) The amount of air exchanged during a relaxed inspiration followed by a relaxed expiration.
      (2) In a healthy, young adult, TV is approximately 500 mL per inspiration; approximately 350 mL of the tidal volume reaches the alveoli and participates in gas exchange (respiration).
   c. **Inspiratory reserve volume (IRV)**
      The amount of air a person can breathe in after a resting inspiration (approximately 3000 mL).
   d. **Expiratory reserve volume (ERV)**
      The amount of air a person can exhale after a normal resting expiration (approximately 1000 mL).

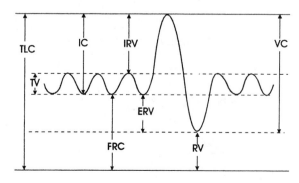

Figure 19–4. Normal lung values and capacities.

    e. **Residual volume (RV)**

       The amount of air left in the lungs after a maximum expiration (approximately 1500 mL).

    f. **Inspiratory capacity (IC)**

       The maximum amount of air a person can breathe in after a resting expiration (approximately 3500 mL).

    g. **Functional residual capacity (FRC)**

       The amount of air remaining in the lungs after a resting (tidal) expiration (approximately 2500 mL).

    h. **Vital capacity (VC)**

       The sum of the IC and the ERV. Vital capacity is measured by a maximum inspiration followed by a maximum expiration (approximately 4500 mL).

2. Effects of aging, body position, and disease on lung volumes and capacities.

    a. Vital capacity

       (1) Decreases with age

       (2) Decreases in the supine position as compared with erect (sitting or standing) posture

       (3) Decreases with restrictive and obstructive lung diseases

    b. Residual volume

       (1) Increases with age

       (2) Increases with obstructive lung diseases such as emphysema

G. Respiration

Respiration is a general term used to describe gas exchange within the body and can be categorized as either external respiration or internal respiration. Basic terms are described here but an in-depth discussion of respiratory physiology, including diffusion and perfusion, goes well beyond the scope of the text. The reader is referred to several references for further study.[8,12,13,16,19,21,35,41,57]

1. External respiration

    a. This term describes the exchange of gas at the alveolar capillary membrane and the pulmonary capillaries.

    b. When a person inhales and air is delivered to the alveoli via the tracheobronchial tree, oxygen diffuses through the alveolar wall and interstitial space and into the bloodstream through the pulmonary capillary walls. The opposite occurs with carbon dioxide transport.

2. Internal respiration

    a. This term describes the exchange of gas between the pulmonary capillaries and the cells of the surrounding tissues.

    b. Internal respiration occurs when oxygen in arterial blood diffuses from red blood cells into tissues requiring oxygen for function. The reverse occurs with carbon dioxide transport.

II. Evaluation in Chest Physical Therapy[14,16,22,24,43,63]

A. Purpose

1. To determine a patient's primary and secondary respiratory and ventilatory impairments that limit physical function

2. To determine a patient's suitability for participation in a pulmonary rehabilitation program
3. To develop an individualized treatment plan for the patient
4. To establish baseline information on the patient to measure a patient's progress and the effectiveness of the treatment
5. To determine when to discontinue the treatment
6. To plan and implement a home program

B. Background and Techniques of Evaluation for the Pulmonary Patient[14,16,22,24,54,63]

1. Interview with the patient and family

a. The evaluation process begins with an interview with the patient as well as family members if they are available. During the interview the therapist can identify the patient and/or family members' perception of any functional limitations and determine a patient's chief complaint and why the patient is seeking treatment.

b. In preparation for the interview, the medical history and diagnoses are obtained from the patient's medical record, if available, or more generally from the patient or family.

c. Relevant occupational and social history are obtained; particularly important are on-the-job physical demands, the environment of the workplace, as well as social habits such as smoking and drinking that affect a person's well-being.

d. Assessment of the home or family environment might include the patient's family responsibilities, the housing situation, and available family support systems.

2. General appearance of the patient

a. Vital signs
Check the heart rate, rate of respiration, and blood pressure of the patient prior to, during, and after treatment.

b. Observe the patient

(1) Level of awareness (level of consciousness)
Alert? Responsive? Lethargic? Cooperative? Oriented? Changes in levels of consciousness can occur if a patient becomes hypercarbic (increased P_{CO_2}) or hypoxic (decreased P_{O_2}).

(2) Color
Cyanotic peripherally? (Nail beds); Centrally? (Lips). Cyanosis occurs when a patient is hypoxic.

(3) Head and neck region

(a) Facial signs and expression (signs of respiratory fatigue or distress include nostrils flaring, focused or dilated pupils, sweating)

(b) Mouth or nose breathing

(c) Jugular vein engorgement (associated with increased venous pressure and a sign of right ventricular heart failure)

(d) Hypertrophy of accessory muscles of ventilation (use at rest is seen in patients with chronic lung disease or weakness of the diaphragm)

(e) Supraclavicular or intercostal retraction (indicates labored breathing)

(f) Pursed-lip breathing (use indicates difficulty with expiration and is often seen in patients with chronic obstructive lung disease)

    (4) Peripheral regions

        (a) Skin condition

        (b) Digital clubbing of the fingers (associated with chronic tissue hypoxia)

        (c) Edema (a sign of right ventricular failure)

    (5) Body type

        Obese, normal, cachectic (may suggest tolerance to exercise; marked obesity can alter breathing pattern)

3. Analysis of chest shape and dimensions and posture

    a. Symmetry of the chest and trunk

    Observe anteriorly, posteriorly, and laterally; the thorax and rib cage should be symmetrical.

    b. Mobility of the trunk

    Check active movements in all directions and identify any restricted spinal motions, particularly in the thoracic spine.

    c. Shape and dimensions of the chest

    The AP and lateral dimensions are usually 2:1.

    d. Common chest deformities

        (1) *Barrel chest:* The circumference of the upper chest appears larger than that of the lower chest. The sternum appears prominent and the AP diameter of the chest is greater than normal. Many patients with chronic obstructive pulmonary disorders, who are usually upper chest breathers, develop a barrel chest.

        (2) *Pectus excavatum* (funnel breast): The lower part of the sternum is depressed and the lower ribs flare out. Patients with this deformity are diaphragmatic breathers; excessive abdominal protrusion and little upper chest movement occur during respiration.

        (3) *Pectus carinatum* (pigeon breast): The sternum is prominent and protrudes anteriorly.

    e. Posture

        (1) Patients who have difficulty breathing as the result of chronic lung disease often lean forward on their hands or forearms when sitting or standing and stabilize and elevate the shoulder girdle (see Fig. 20–2) to assist with inspiration. This increases the effectiveness of the pectoralis and serratus anterior muscles to act as accessory muscles of inspiration by reverse action.

        (2) Note postural deformities such as kyphosis and scoliosis and postural asymmetry from thoracic surgery, which can restrict chest movements and ventilation.

4. Breathing pattern

    a. *Rate, regularity*, and *location* of respiration are noted at rest and with activity. The normal ratio of inspiration to expiration at rest is 1:2 and with activity, 1:1. Patients with chronic lung disease may have a ratio of 1:4 at rest, which reflects the difficulty these patients have with the expiratory phase of breathing. The normal sequence of inspiration is (1) the diaphragm contracts and descends and the abdomen (epigastric area) rises; (2) this is followed by lateral costal expansion as the ribs move up and out; and, finally, (3) the upper chest rises.

    b. In healthy individuals, the neck muscles (accessory muscles of inspiration) will act only during deep breathing.

c. *Abnormal breathing patterns*
   (1) **Dyspnea:** shortness of breath; distressed, labored breathing.
   (2) **Tachypnea:** rapid, shallow respiration; decreased tidal volume but increased rate; associated with restrictive or obstructive lung disease and use of accessory muscles of inspiration.
   (3) **Bradypnea:** slow rate with shallow or normal depth and regular rhythm; may be associated with drug overdose.
   (4) **Hyperventilation:** deep, rapid respiration; increased tidal volume and increased rate of respiration; regular rhythm.
   (5) **Orthopnea:** difficulty breathing in the supine position.
   (6) **Apnea:** cessation of breathing in the expiratory phase.
   (7) **Apneusis:** cessation of breathing in the inspiratory phase.
   (8) **Cheyne-Stokes:** cycles of gradually increasing tidal volumes, followed by a series of gradually decreasing tidal volumes, and then a period of apnea. This is sometimes seen in the patient with a severe head injury.

5. Palpation

a. *Symmetry of chest movement*
   Place your hands on the patient's chest and assess the excursion of each side of the chest during inspiration and expiration. Each of the three lobar areas can be checked.
   (1) To check *upper lobe expansion,* face the patient; place the tips of your thumbs at the midsternal line at the sternal notch. Extend your fingers above the clavicles. Have the patient fully exhale and then inhale deeply.
   (2) To check *middle-lobe expansion,* continue to face the patient; place the tips of your thumbs at the xyphoid process and extend your fingers laterally around the ribs. Again, ask the patient to breathe in deeply.
   (3) To check *lower lobe expansion,* place the tips of your thumbs along the patient's back at the spinous processes (lower thoracic level) and extend your fingers around the ribs. Ask the patient to breathe in deeply.
   (4) As the patient inhales and exhales, check the symmetry of movement of both sides of the chest.

b. *Depth of excursion*
   (1) Can be measured by taking the girth of the chest at three levels (axilla, xyphoid, and subcostal) during inspiration and expiration.
   (2) Can also be measured by placing both hands on the patient's chest and back as described. Note the amount of space between your thumbs after the patient takes a deep inspiration.

c. *Fremitus*
   (1) **Vocal (tactile) fremitus** is the vibration felt as the therapist palpates over the chest wall as a patient speaks. The procedure is used to assess the quality of the underlying tissues.
   (2) Procedure
       Place the palms of your hands lightly on the chest wall and ask the patient to speak a few words or repeat "99" several times.
   (3) Normally, fremitus is felt uniformly on the chest wall.
   (4) Fremitus is increased in the presence of secretions in the airways and decreased or absent when air is trapped as the result of obstructed airways.

d. *Chest wall pain*
   (1) Specific areas or points of pain over anterior, posterior, or lateral aspects of the chest wall can be identified with palpation.

     (2) *Procedure*

Firmly press against the chest wall with your hands to identify any specific areas of pain from musculoskeletal orgin. Ask the patient to take a deep breath and identify any painful areas of the chest wall.

     (3) **NOTE:** Chest wall pain of musculoskeletal origin often increases with direct point pressure during palpation or with a deep inspiration; chest pain caused by angina usually remains unchanged with palpation.

  e. *The mediastinum* (position of trachea)

     (1) The position of the trachea is normally oriented centrally in relationship to the suprasternal notch. The position of the trachea shifts as the result of asymmetrical intrathoracic pressures or lung volumes. For example, if the patient has had a lung removed (pneumonectomy), the lung volume on the operated side will decrease, and the trachea will shift toward that side. Conversely, if the patient has a hemothorax (blood in the thorax), intrathoracic pressure on the side of the hemothorax increases, and the mediastinum will shift away from the affected side of the chest.

     (2) *Procedure*

To identify a *mediastinal shift*, have the patient sit facing you with the head in mid-line and neck slightly flexed to relax the sternocleidomastoid muscles. With your index finger gently palpate the soft tissue space on either side of the trachea at the suprasternal notch. Determine whether the trachea is palpable at the mid-line or has shifted to the left or right.

6. Mediate percussion

  a. Definition

An evaluation technique designed to assess lung density, specifically air to solid ratio in the lungs.

  b. Procedure

Place the middle finger of the nondominant hand flat against the chest wall along an intercostal space. With the tip of the middle finger of the opposite hand tap firmly on the finger positioned on the chest wall. Repeat the procedure at several points on the right and left and anterior and posterior aspects of the chest wall.

  c. This maneuver produces a resonance; the pitch varies with the density of the underlying tissue.

  d. The sound will be dull and flat if there is a greater than normal amount of solid matter (tumor, consolidation) in the lungs in comparison with the amount of air.

  e. The sound will be hyperresonant (tympanic) if there is a greater than normal amount of air in the area (as in patients with emphysema).

  f. If asymmetrical or abnormal findings are noted, the patient should be referred to the physician for additional objective tests such as a chest x-ray.

7. Auscultation

  a. Definition

Listening to sounds within the body, specifically to breath sounds in an evaluation of the lungs.

  b. Breath sounds, normal and abnormal, occur because of movement of air in the airways during inspiration and expiration. A stethoscope is used to magnify these sounds. Breath sounds should be evaluated:

(1) To identify the areas of the lungs in which congestion exists and postural drainage should be performed

(2) To determine the effectiveness of any postural drainage treatment

(3) To determine whether or not the lungs are clear and whether or not postural drainage should be discontinued

c. Procedure

(1) Have the patient sit in a comfortable, relaxed position. Place the diaphragm of the stethoscope directly against the patient's skin along the anterior or posterior chest wall.

(2) Follow a systematic pattern (Figs. 19–5A and B) and place the stethoscope against specific thoracic landmarks (T-2, T-6, T-10) along the right and left sides of the chest wall.

(3) Ask the patient to breathe in deeply and out quickly through the mouth as you move the stethoscope from point to point.

(4) Note the quality, intensity, and pitch of the breath sounds.

d. Normal breath sounds are classified by:

(1) Location

(2) Pitch and intensity

(3) Ratio of sound heard on inspiration versus expiration

e. *Normal breath sounds*

(1) *Tracheal*

Loud, harsh, and very high pitched; heard only over the trachea. Tracheal breath sounds are heard equally during inspiration and expiration.

(2) *Bronchial*

Loud, hollow, and high-pitched; heard between the clavicles and at the manubrium anteriorly and between the scapulae posteriorly. These sounds are heard longer with the expiratory phase than with the inspiratory phase.

(3) *Bronchovesicular*

Softer, medium-pitched sounds; heard equally on inspiration and expiration only near the sternum, anteriorly, and between the scapulae, posteriorly.

(4) *Vesicular*

Soft, breezy but faint sounds; heard over most of the chest, except near the trachea and bronchi, and between the scapulae. These sounds are audible much longer on inspiration than on expiration.

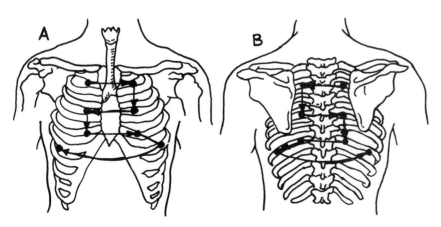

Figure 19–5. Pattern of specific thoracic landmarks for auscultation. The diaphragm of the stethoscope is placed along the right and left (*A*) anterior chest wall and the (*B*) posterior chest wall at T-2, T-6, and T-10. (From Frownfelter, DL: Chest Physical Therapy and Pulmonary Rehabilitation. Year-Book Medical Publishers, Chicago, 1987, p 135, with permission.)

NOTE: It is important that the therapist practice respiratory auscultation and be able to identify these normal breath sounds in normal individuals.

f. *Abnormal and adventitious (extra) breath sounds*

(1) Terminology used to describe abnormal and extra breath sounds is inconsistent. Terms used in this textbook are from guidelines for nomenclature proposed by the American Thoracic Society and the American College of Chest Physicians.[5,61]

(2) Breath sounds may be totally absent, indicating total obstruction of airways and lack of aeration, or may be diminished. This may be due to bronchospasm (in asthma) or collapse of an airway (**atelectasis,** emphysema) or blockage of airways with secretions (pneumonia).

(3) Adventitious breath sounds

(a) **Crackles**

Fine, discontinuous sounds (similar to the sound of bubbles popping or the sound of hairs being rubbed between your fingers next to your ear). Crackles, which can be fine or coarse, are heard primarily during inspiration as the result of secretions moving in the airways or in closed airways that are rapidly reopening. The former term for crackles was **rales.**

(b) **Wheezes**

Continuous high- or low-pitched sounds or sometimes musical tones heard during exhalation but occasionally audible during inspiration. Bronchospasm or secretions that narrow the lumen of the airways cause wheezes. The term previously used for wheezes was **rhonchi.**

8. Cough and sputum

a. An effective cough is sharp and deep. In the respiratory patient it may be superficial, soft, throaty, shallow, dry, or moist. If the cough is totally ineffective, suctioning may be indicated.

b. Sputum should be checked for:

(1) Color (clear, white, yellow, green, blood streaked). Clear secretions are normal. Yellow or green secretions indicate infection. The term used to describe blood-streaked sputum is **hemoptysis**.

(2) Consistency (viscous, thin, frothy).

(3) Amount.

9. Other areas of evaluation

a. Range of motion, particularly of the shoulders and trunk

b. Muscle strength

c. General endurance (see Chapter 4)

d. Functional independence

e. Pain

f. Use of assistive respiratory equipment

g. NOTE: In addition to the chest examination, other procedures such as evaluation of blood gases, radiographs, pulmonary function studies, graded exercise testing, and bacteriologic tests must also be performed for a complete assessment of the pulmonary patient.

III. Breathing Exercises

Breathing exercises are commonly incorporated into the overall pulmonary rehabilitation program of patients with acute or chronic pulmonary disorders. Breathing exercises are designed to retrain the muscles of respiration and improve or redistribute ventilation, lessen the work of breathing, and improve gas exchange and oxygenation. Active range of motion exercises to the shoulders and trunk also help expand the chest, facilitate deep breathing, and often stimulate the cough reflex.[15,16,18,26,33,43,49]

Research studies indicate that, although breathing exercises may affect and possibly alter a patient's rate and depth of ventilation, they may not necessarily have any impact on gas exchange at the alveolar level or on oxygenation.[8,23,33,56] Therefore, breathing exercises are only part of a treatment program designed to improve pulmonary status and to improve a patient's overall endurance and function in daily living activities. Depending on the patient's clinical problem, breathing exercises are often combined with medication, postural drainage, the use of respiratory therapy devices, and a graded exercise (conditioning) program.

A. Indications for Breathing Exercises

1. Acute or chronic lung disease
   a. Chronic obstructive lung disease
   b. Pneumonia
   c. Atelectasis
   d. Pulmonary embolism
   e. Acute respiratory distress
2. Pain in the thoracic or abdominal area because of surgery or trauma
3. Airway obstruction secondary to bronchospasm or retained secretions
4. Deficits in the central nervous system that lead to muscle weakness
   a. High spinal cord injury
   b. Acute, chronic, or progressive myopathic or neuropathic diseases
5. Severe orthopedic abnormalities, such as scoliosis and kyphosis, that affect respiratory function
6. Stress management and relaxation procedures

B. Goals of Breathing Exercises

1. Improve ventilation.
2. Increase the effectiveness of the cough mechanism.
3. Prevent pulmonary impairments.
4. Improve the strength, endurance, and coordination of respiratory muscles.
5. Maintain or improve chest and thoracic spine mobility.
6. Correct inefficient or abnormal breathing patterns.
7. Promote relaxation.
8. Teach the patient how to deal with shortness-of-breath attacks.
9. Improve a patient's overall functional capacity.

C. General Principles for Teaching Breathing Exercises

1. If possible, choose a quiet area for instruction in which you can interact with the patient with a minimum of distractions.
2. Explain to the patient the aims and rationale of breathing exercises specific to his or her particular impairments and functional limitations.

3. Have the patient assume a comfortable, relaxed position and loosen restrictive clothing.

    a. Initially, a hook-lying position in bed, with the head and trunk elevated approximately 45 degrees, is desirable. By totally supporting the head and trunk and by flexing the hips and knees and supporting the legs with a pillow, the abdominal muscles remain relaxed.

    b. Other positions such as supine, sitting, or standing may be used initially or as the patient progresses in treatment.

4. Observe and evaluate the patient's natural breathing pattern while at rest and with activity.

    a. Determine whether or not retraining is indicated.

    b. Determine the emphasis, either inspiratory or expiratory, that the breathing exercise program should take.

    c. Establish a baseline for assessment of change and progress in treatment.

5. If necessary, teach the patient relaxation techniques. This will relax the muscles of the upper thorax, neck, and shoulders to minimize the use of the accessory muscles of respiration. Pay particular attention to relaxation of the sternocleidomastoids, scalenes, upper trapezius, and levator scapulae.

6. Demonstrate the desired breathing pattern to the patient.

7. Have the patient practice the correct breathing pattern in a variety of positions at rest and with activity.

D. Precautions[8,16,18,33]

When teaching breathing exercises, be aware of the following precautions:

1. Never allow a patient to force expiration. Expiration should be relaxed and passive. Forced expiration only increases turbulence in the airways, which can lead to bronchospasm and increased airway restriction.

2. Do not allow a patient to take a very *prolonged* expiration. This causes the patient to gasp with the next inspiration. The patient's breathing pattern then becomes irregular and inefficient.

3. Do not allow the patient to initiate inspiration with the accessory muscles and the upper chest. Advise the patient that the upper chest should be relatively quiet during breathing.

4. Allow the patient to practice deep breathing for only three or four inspirations and expirations at a time to avoid hyperventilation.

E. Breathing Exercises and Methods of Instruction

All breathing patterns should be deep, voluntarily controlled, and relaxed, regardless of the pattern being taught to the patient.

1. Diaphragmatic breathing[8,16,18,20,23,26,33,59]

    a. The diaphragm controls breathing at an involuntary level, but a patient can be taught breathing control by correct use of the diaphragm and relaxation of accessory muscles.

    b. Diaphragmatic breathing exercises are designed to improve the efficiency of ventilation, decrease the work of breathing, increase the excursion (descent or ascent) of the diaphragm, and improve gas exchange and oxygenation. Diaphragmatic breathing exercises are also used to mobilize lung secretions during postural drainage.

c. Procedure

(1) Prepare the patient in a relaxed and comfortable position such as a semi-Fowler's position (reclined sitting), evaluate the breathing pattern, and demonstrate the correct method of diaphragmatic breathing.

(2) Place your hand(s) on the rectus abdominis just below the anterior costal margin (Fig. 19–6).

(3) Ask the patient to breathe in slowly and deeply through the nose. Have the patient keep the shoulders relaxed and upper chest quiet, allowing the abdomen to rise.

(4) Then tell the patient to slowly let all the air out using controlled expiration.

(5) Have the patient practice this three or four times and then rest. Do not allow the patient to hyperventilate.

(6) Have the patient place his or her own hand below the anterior costal margin and feel the movement (Fig. 19–7). The patient's hand should rise during inspiration and fall during expiration. By placing one hand on the abdomen, the patient can also feel the contraction of the abdominal muscles, which occurs with controlled expiration or coughing.

(7) After the patient understands and is able to breathe using a diaphragmatic pattern, suggest that he or she breathe in through the nose and out through the mouth.

(8) Practice diaphragmatic breathing in a variety of positions (sitting, standing) and during activity (walking and climbing stairs).

d. NOTE: The effect of diaphragmatic breathing exercises on ventilation, oxygenation, and excursion of the diaphragm in normal subjects and in patients with pulmonary disorders remains unclear.[8,26,33,64] Studies have both sup-

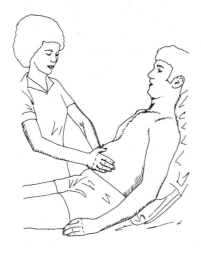

Figure 19–6. The semisitting position is a comfortable, relaxed position in which to teach diaphragmatic breathing.

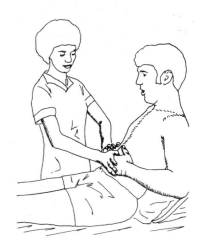

Figure 19–7. The patient places his or her own hands on the abdomen to feel the movement of proper diaphragmatic breathing. By placing the hands on the abdomen, the patient can also feel the contraction of the abdominals, which occurs with controlled expiration or coughing.

ported[23,45,47,48] and refuted[45,48] the positive impact of diaphragmatic breathing exercises on each of these areas of function. Diaphragmatic breathing exercises will continue to be an integral part of most chest physical therapy programs as research on the effects of diaphragmatic breathing continues.

2. Ventilatory muscle training[6,20,26,28,31,48]

The process of improving the strength or endurance of the muscles of breathing is known as *ventilatory muscle training* (VMT). This technique usually focuses on training the muscles of inspiration. VMT has been used in the treatment of patients with a variety of acute or chronic pulmonary disorders associated with weakness, atrophy, or inefficiency of the muscles of inspiration, specifically the diaphragm and external intercostals. With support from animal studies, it has been suggested that the principles of overload and specificity of training apply to skeletal muscles throughout the body, including the muscles of ventilation.

In humans, it is not feasible to evaluate morphologic or histochemical changes in the diaphragm that may occur as the result of strength or endurance training with invasive procedures. Instead strength or endurance changes must be assessed indirectly. Increases in respiratory muscle endurance have been measured by maximum voluntary ventilation and decreased diaphragmatic fatigue over time as reflected in decreased reliance on accessory muscles of inspiration. Respiratory muscle strength has been evaluated indirectly with measurements of inspiratory capacity and inspiratory mouth pressure using a spirometer.

Three forms of VMT involve weight training to strengthen the diaphragm, inspiratory resistance training, and incentive respiratory spirometry.

a. **Diaphragmatic training using weights** [3,15,17,26,30,33,58]
   (1) Have the patient assume a supine or slightly head-up position.
   (2) Be sure that the patient knows how to breathe in by primarily using the diaphragm.
   (3) Place a small weight (3 to 5 lb) over the epigastric region of the patient's abdomen.
   (4) Tell the patient to breathe in deeply while trying to keep the upper chest quiet. The resistance should not interfere with full excursion of the diaphragm and normal rise of the epigastric area.
   (5) Gradually increase the time that the patient breathes against the resistance of the weight. The weight can be increased when the patient can sustain the diaphragmatic breathing pattern without the use of accessory muscles of inspiration for 15 minutes.
   (6) Manual resistance or positioning can also be used to strengthen the diaphragm. In the head-down position the abdominal contents move superiorly and provide resistance to the diaphragm as it contracts and descends.[17,58]
   (7) **NOTE:** Although this method of strengthening the diaphragm is often suggested for patients with weakness, the results of a study of normal subjects indicate that the effectiveness of this method of strengthening is questionable.[37] In another study with patients with cervical level spinal cord injuries, abdominal weight training and inspiratory resistance training were both effective methods of ventilatory muscle training to improve respiratory muscle strength and endurance.[15] Further studies are warranted to determine the efficacy of abdominal weight training as well as other forms of VMT.

b. **Inspiratory resistance training***

   (1) Specifically designed breathing devices (resistors) are used for *inspiratory resistance training* to improve the strength and endurance of the muscles of inspiration and decrease the occurrence of inspiratory muscle fatigue.

   (2) Procedure

      (a) The patient inhales through a hand-held resistive training device that he or she places in the mouth. Inspiratory resistive training devices are narrow tubes of varying diameters that provide resistance to airflow during inspiration and therefore place resistance on inspiratory muscles to improve strength or endurance. The narrower the diameter of the airway, the greater the resistance.

      (b) The patient inhales through the tube for a specified period of time several times each day. The time is gradually increased to 20 to 30 minutes at each training session to increase inspiratory muscle endurance.

      (c) As the patient's strength and endurance improve, the diameter of the hand-held tube is decreased. The commercially available resistive devices have six different diameters to provide levels of resistance appropriate for each patient.

   (3) The effectiveness of inspiratory resistance training continues to be investigated. Some studies have shown that ventilatory muscle strength and endurance have improved as the result of this type of training, but other studies have shown that respiratory rate decreases and exercise tolerance increases over time.[3,11,31]

c. **Incentive respiratory spirometry**[20,33,58]

   (1) *Incentive spirometry* is a form of low-level resistance training that emphasizes sustained maximal inspiration. A synonymous term is *sustained maximal inspiratory maneuver*, which is performed with or without the use of a spirometer.[33] The patient inhales through a spirometer that provides visual or auditory feedback as the patient breathes in as deeply as possible. Incentive spirometry increases the volume of air inspired and has been used to prevent alveolar collapse in postoperative conditions and to strengthen weak inspiratory muscles in patients with neuromuscular disorders.

   (2) Procedure[16,58]

      (a) Place the patient in a comfortable position (supine or semiupright).

      (b) Have the patient take three to four slow, easy breaths.

      (c) Have the patient maximally exhale with the fourth breath.

      (d) Then have the patient place the spirometer in the mouth and maximally inhale through the spirometer and hold the inspiration for several seconds.

      (e) This sequence is repeated 5 to 10 times several times per day.

d. ***Precaution:*** Avoid prolonged periods of any form of resistance training for inspiratory muscles. Unlike muscles of the extremities, the diaphragm cannot totally rest to recover from a session of resistance exercises. Use of accessory muscles of inspiration (neck muscles) is a sign that the diaphragm is beginning to fatigue.[3,58]

---

*Refs. 1, 2, 6, 11, 15, 16, 28, 31, 33, 50, 51.

3. Segmental breathing[18,33,43,55,58]

It is questionable whether a patient can be taught to expand localized areas of the lung while keeping other areas quiet. It is known, however, that hypoventilation does occur in certain areas of the lungs because of pain and muscle guarding after surgery, atelectasis, and pneumonia. Therefore, there are certain instances when it will be important to emphasize expansion of problem areas of the lung and chest wall.

a. *Lateral costal expansion*

(1) This is sometimes called lateral *basal* expansion and may be done unilaterally or bilaterally.

(2) The patient may be sitting or in a hook-lying position.

(3) Place your hands along the lateral aspect of the lower ribs to fix the patient's attention to the areas at which movement is to occur (Figs. 19–8 and 19–9).

(4) Ask the patient to breathe out, and feel the rib cage move downward and inward.

(5) As the patient breathes out, place a firm downward pressure into the ribs with the palms of your hands.

(6) Just prior to inspiration, apply a quick downward and inward stretch to the chest. This places a quick stretch on the external intercostals to facilitate their contraction. These muscles move the ribs outward and upward during inspiration.

(7) Tell the patient to expand the lower ribs against your hands as he or she breathes in.

(8) Apply *gentle* manual resistance to the lower rib area to increase sensory awareness as the patient breathes in and the chest expands and ribs flare.

(9) Then, again, as the patient breathes out, assist by gently squeezing the rib cage in a downward and inward direction.

(10) The patient may then be taught to perform the maneuver independently. He or she may place the hand(s) over the ribs (Fig. 19–10) or apply resistance using a belt (Figs. 19–11A and B).

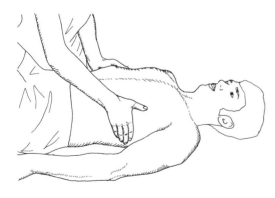

Figure 19–8. Bilateral lateral costal expansion—supine.

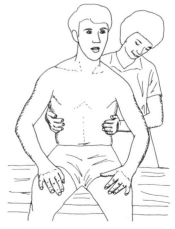

Figure 19–9. Bilateral lateral costal expansion—sitting.

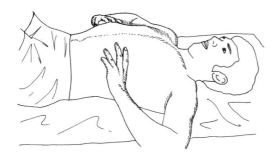

Figure 19–10. The patient applies his or her own manual pressure during lateral costal expansion.

b. *Posterior basal expansion*
  (1) Have the patient sit and lean forward on a pillow, slightly bending the hips.
  (2) Place your hands over the posterior aspect of the lower ribs.
  (3) Follow the same procedure as described above.
  (4) This form of segmental breathing is important for the postsurgical patient who is confined to bed in a semiupright position for an extended period of time. Secretions often accumulate in the posterior segments of the lower lobes.
c. *Right middle-lobe or lingula expansion*
  (1) Patient is sitting.
  (2) Place your hands at either the right or the left side of the patient's chest, just below the axilla.
  (3) Follow the same procedure as described for lateral basal expansion.
d. *Apical expansion* (Fig. 19–12)
  (1) Patient is sitting.
  (2) Apply pressure (usually unilaterally) below the clavicle with the fingertips.
  (3) This pattern is appropriate in an apical pneumothorax after a lobectomy.

4. Glossopharyngeal breathing[16,38,58]

a. Glossopharyngeal breathing is a means of increasing a patient's inspiratory capacity when there is severe weakness of the muscles of inspiration. It is taught

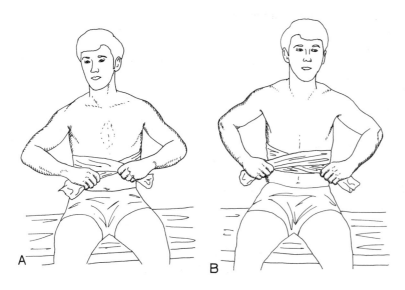

A   B

Figure 19–11. Belt exercises reinforce lateral costal breathing (*A*) by applying resistance during inspiration and (*B*) by assisting with pressure along the rib cage during expiration.

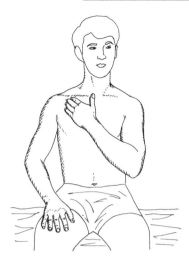

Figure 19–12. Segmental right upper lobe (apical) expansion.

to patients who have difficulty taking in a deep breath, for example, in preparation for coughing.

b. This type of breathing pattern was originally developed to assist postpolio patients with severe muscle weakness. Today, if it is used at all, it is most frequently taught to patients with high spinal cord injuries who can easily develop respiratory problems.[16,25,38]

c. Procedure

The patient takes in several "gulps" of air. Then the mouth is closed and the tongue pushes the air back and traps it in the pharynx. The air is then forced into the lungs when the glottis is opened. This increases the depth of the inspiration and the patient's vital capacity.[25]

NOTE: This technique is very difficult to teach and learn and will be a useful technique for only a limited number of patients.

5. **Pursed-lip breathing**[11,24,33,40]

a. Whether it is appropriate to teach pursed-lip breathing to a patient is debatable.

(1) Most therapist feel that gentle pursed-lip breathing with controlled expiration is a useful procedure, if it is performed appropriately. It is thought to keep airways open by creating a backpressure in the airways. It is taught to help a patient with chronic obstructive pulmonary disease (COPD) deal with attacks of shortness of breath.[16,33,43] Studies suggest that pursed-lip breathing decreases the respiratory rate, increases the tidal volume, and improves exercise tolerance.[11,33,40]

(2) Some patients spontaneously develop this pattern of breathing. If so, they should not be discouraged from using it.

(3) ***Precaution:*** The use of *forced* expiration during pursed-lip breathing must be avoided. Forceful or prolonged expiration while the lips are pursed can increase the turbulence in the airways and cause further restriction of the small bronchioles. For this reason, some therapists have suggested that patients may perform pursed-lip breathing inappropriately and, therefore, should not be taught this form of breathing.

(4) It is the opinion of the authors of this textbook that pursed-lip breathing (with passive expiration) is a valuable means of dealing with shortness of

breath attacks (dyspnea on exertion) and *should* be taught to patients with COPD.

b. Procedure

(1) Have the patient assume a comfortable position and relax as much as possible.

(2) Explain to the patient that expiration must be relaxed (passive) and that contraction of the abdominals must be avoided.

(3) Place your hand over the patient's abdominal muscles to detect any contraction of the abdominals.

(4) Instruct the patient to breathe in slowly and deeply.

(5) Then have the patient loosely purse the lips and exhale.

6. Preventing and relieving shortness of breath attacks

a. Many patients with COPD (emphysema and asthma, for example) may suffer from periodic attacks of dyspnea (shortness of breath), particularly with physical exertion or when in contact with allergens. Whenever a patient's normal breathing pattern is interrupted, shortness of breath can occur. It is helpful to teach patients to try to *prevent* shortness of breath attacks with *controlled breathing*, by *pacing activities*, and by becoming aware of what activity or situation causes dyspnea.

b. *Pacing* is the performance of functional activities, such as walking, stair climbing or work-related tasks, within the limits of a patient's breathing capacity.[8] Although some patients may intuitively understand to what limits functional activities can be pushed, other patients must be taught to recognize the early signs of dyspnea. If the patient becomes slightly short of breath, he or she must learn to stop an activity and use controlled, pursed-lip breathing until the dyspnea subsides.

c. Procedure

(1) Have the patient assume a relaxed, forward-bent posture (see Figs. 20–2, 20–3, and 20–4). This position stimulates diaphragmatic breathing (the viscera drops forward and the diaphragm descends more easily).

(2) Use bronchodilators as prescribed.

(3) Have the patient gain control of his or her breathing and reduce the respiratory rate by using pursed-lip breathing during expiration. Be sure that the patient does not use forceful expiration. Have the patient emphasize the expiratory phase of breathing.

(4) After each pursed-lip expiration, have the patient breathe in diaphragmatically, avoiding the use of accessory muscles.

(5) Have the patient remain in this posture and continue to breathe in as relaxed a manner as possible.

IV. Exercises to Mobilize the Chest

A. Definition

Chest mobilization exercises are any exercises that combine active movements of the trunk or extremities with deep breathing.

B. Goals

1. Maintain or improve mobility of the chest wall, trunk, and shoulders when it affects respiration. For example, a patient with tightness of the trunk muscles on one side of the body will not expand that part of the chest fully during inspiration. Exercises that combine stretching of these muscles with deep breathing will improve ventilation on that side of the chest.

2. **Reinforce or emphasize the depth of inspiration or controlled expiration.** For example, a patient can improve expiration by leaning forward at the hips or flexing the spine as he or she breathes out. This pushes the viscera superiorly into the diaphragm and further reinforces expiration.

C. Specific Exercises

1. **To mobilize one side of the chest**
    a. While sitting, have the patient bend away from the tight side to lengthen tight structures and expand that side of the chest during inspiration (Fig. 19–13A).
    b. Then, have the patient push the fisted hand into the lateral aspect of the chest, as he or she bends toward the tight side and breathes out (Fig. 19–13B).
    c. Progress by having the patient raise the arm on the tight side of the chest over the head and side bend away from the tight side. This will place an additional stretch on the tight tissues.

2. **To mobilize the upper chest and stretch the pectoralis muscles**
    a. While the patient is sitting in a chair with hands clasped behind the head, have him or her horizontally abduct the arms (elongating the pectoralis muscles) during a deep inspiration (Fig. 19–14A).
    b. Then, instruct the patient to bring the elbows together and bend forward during expiration (Fig. 19–14B).

3. **To mobilize the upper chest and shoulders**
    a. With the patient sitting in a chair, have him or her reach with both arms overhead (180 degrees bilateral shoulder flexion and slight abduction) during inspiration (Fig. 19–15A). Then have the patient bend forward at the hips and reach for the floor during expiration (Fig. 19–15B).

4. **To increase expiration during deep breathing**
    a. Have the patient breathe in while in a hook-lying position (hips and knees are slightly flexed) (Fig. 19–16A).

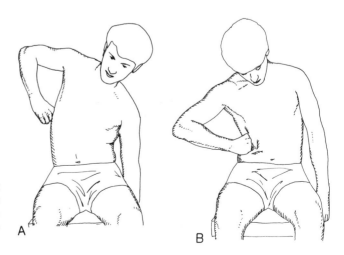

Figure 19–13. Chest mobilization during inspiration and expiration. To mobilize the lateral rib cage (*A*) have the patient bend away from the tight side during inspiration and (*B*) bend toward the tight side during expiration.

A   B

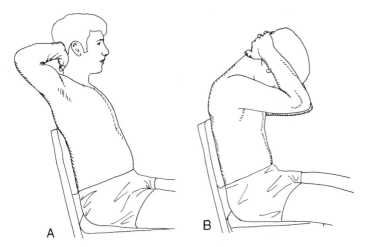

Figure 19–14. (*A*) A stretch is applied to the pectoralis muscles during inspiration and (*B*) the patient brings the elbows together to facilitate expiration.

    b. Then, instruct the patient to pull both knees to the chest (one at a time to protect the low back) during expiration (Figs. 19–16B and C). This pushes the abdominal contents superiorly into the diaphragm to assist with expiration.

5. Wand exercises (see Chapter 2) emphasizing shoulder flexion during inspiration may also be combined with breathing exercises.

D. Additional Activities

In addition to exercises specifically designed to mobilize the chest, the therapist may also instruct the patient in:

1. Posture correction

2. Manual stretching of the chest wall, trunk, and extremities

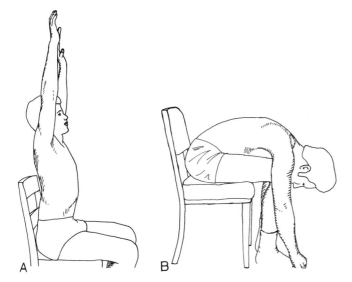

Figure 19–15. (*A*) Chest expansion is increased with bilateral movement of the arms overhead during inspiration. (*B*) Expiration is then reinforced by reaching the arms toward the floor.

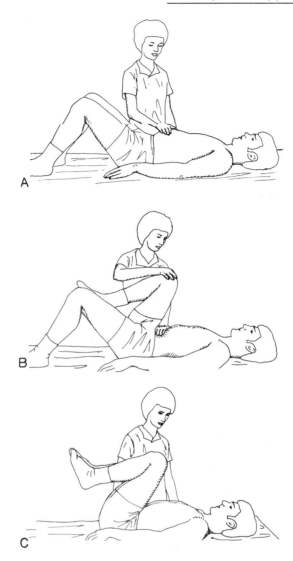

Figure 19–16. (*A*) Begin inspiration in the hook-lying position. (*B*) Bring one knee to the chest. (*C*) Then bring the other knee to the chest to assist expiration.

V. Coughing

An effective cough is necessary to eliminate respiratory obstructions and keep the lungs clear. It is an important part of treatment of patients with acute or chronic respiratory conditions.

A. The Cough Mechanism[16,32,52]

The following series of actions occur when a patient coughs:
1. Deep inspiration occurs.
2. Glottis closes and vocal cords tighten.
3. Abdominal muscles contract and diaphragm elevates, causing an increase in intrathoracic and intra-abdominal pressures.
4. Glottis opens.
5. Explosive expiration of air occurs.

B. The Normal Cough Pump

1. A cough may be reflexive or voluntary.
2. In the normal individual, the cough pump is effective to the seventh generation of bronchi. (There are a total of 23 generations of bronchi in the tracheo-bronchial tree.)
3. Ciliated epithelial cells are present up to the terminal bronchiole and raise secretions from the smaller to the larger airways in normal individuals.

C. Factors That Decrease the Effectiveness of the Cough Mechanism and Cough Pump[16,18,27,29,52]

1. Decreased inspiratory capacity because of

  a. Pain
    (1) Acute lung disease
    (2) Rib fracture
    (3) Trauma to the chest
    (4) Recent thoracic or abdominal surgery
  b. Specific muscle weakness that affects the diaphragm or accessory muscles of inspiration
    (1) High spinal cord injury
    (2) Anterior horn cell disease (Guillain-Barré syndrome)
  c. Depression of the respiratory center associated with general anesthesia or pain medication

2. Inability of the patient to forcibly expel air as the result of

  a. Spinal cord injury above T-12
  b. Myopathic disease and weakness such as muscular dystrophy
  c. Tracheostomy
  d. Critical illness that causes excessive fatigue
  e. Chest wall or abdominal incision

3. Decreased action of the cilia in the bronchial tree secondary to

  a. General anesthesia and intubation
  b. COPD (chronic obstructive pulmonary disease) such as chronic bronchitis, which is associated with a decreased number of ciliated epithelial cells in the bronchi
  c. Smoking

4. Increase in the amount or thickness of mucus caused by

  a. Cystic fibrosis
  b. Chronic bronchitis
  c. Pulmonary infections such as pneumonia
  d. Dehydration
  e. Intubation

D. Teaching an Effective Cough[16,18,43,52]

Because an effective cough is an integral aspect of airway clearance, a patient must be taught the significance of an effective cough, how to produce an efficient and controlled voluntary cough, and when to cough.

1. Evaluate the patient's voluntary or reflexive cough.

2. Place the patient in a relaxed and comfortable position for deep breathing and coughing.
   a. Sitting or leaning forward is usually the best position for coughing.
   b. The patient's neck should be slightly flexed to make coughing more comfortable.[52]
3. Teach the patient controlled diaphragmatic breathing, emphasizing deep inspiration.
4. Demonstrate a sharp, deep, double cough.
5. Demonstrate the proper muscle action of coughing (contraction of the abdominals).
6. Have the patient place the hands on the abdomen and make three *huffs* with expiration to feel the contraction of the abdominals (see Fig. 19–7).
7. Have the patient practice making a K sound to experience tightening the vocal cords, closing the glottis, and contracting the abdominals.
8. When the patient has put these actions together, instruct the patient to take a deep but relaxed inspiration, followed by a sharp double cough. The second cough during a single expiration is more productive.
9. Use an abdominal binder or glossopharyngeal breathing in selected patients with inspiratory or abdominal muscle weakness to enhance the cough, if necessary.
10. ***Precaution:*** Never allow the patient to suck air in by gasping, because it
    a. Increases the work (energy expenditure) of breathing and the patient fatigues more easily
    b. Tends to increase turbulence and resistance in the airways and may lead to increased bronchospasm (further constriction of airways)
    c. May push mucus or a foreign object deep into air passages

E. Additional Means of Facilitating a Cough[3,16,18,25]

1. Manual assisted cough[3,25,58]

   a. If the patient has abdominal weakness (for instance, as the result of a midthoracic or cervical spinal cord injury), manual pressure on the abdominal area will assist in developing greater intra-abdominal pressure for more forceful cough. Manual pressure can be applied by either the therapist or the patient.
   b. Procedure
      (1) Therapist assisted (Figs. 19–17 and 19–18)
         (a) With the patient in a supine position, the therapist places the heel of one hand on the patient's abdomen at the epigastric area just distal to the xyphoid process. The other hand is placed on top of the first, either keeping the fingers open or interlocking them.
         (b) After the patient inhales as deeply as possible, the therapist manually assists the patient as he or she attempts to cough. The abdomen is compressed with an inward and upward force, which pushes the diaphragm upward to cause a more forceful and effective cough.
         (c) This same maneuver can be performed with the patient in a chair. The therapist or family member can stand in back of the patient and apply manual pressure during expiration.
         (d) ***Precaution:*** Avoid direct pressure on the xyphoid process.
      (2) Self-assisted (see Fig. 19–18)
         (a) While the patient is in a sitting position, he or she crosses the arms across the abdomen or places the interlocked hands below the xyphoid process.

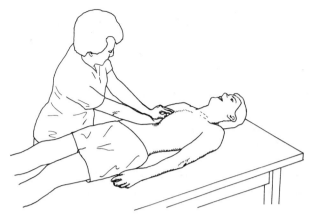

Figure 19–17. Therapist-assisted manual cough technique.

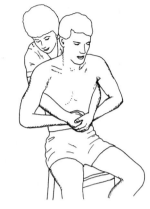

Figure 19–18. Therapist-assisted or self-assisted manual cough technique.

(b) After a deep inspiration, he or she pushes inward and upward on the abdomen with the wrists or forearms and simultaneously leans forward while attempting to cough.

2. Splinting[16,27,29]

If incisional pain from recent surgery is restricting the cough, teach the patient to splint over the incision.

a. Have the patient press the hands or a pillow firmly over the incision to support the painful area as he or she coughs (Fig. 19–19).

b. If the patient cannot reach the incision, the therapist should assist (Fig. 19–20).

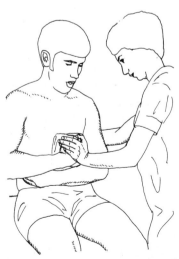

Figure 19–19. Splinting over an anterior surgical incision.

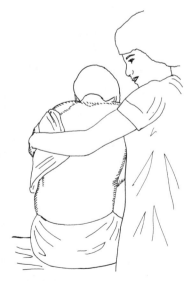

Figure 19–20. Splinting over a posterior lateral incision.

3. **Humidification**[16,52]

If secretions are very thick, work with the patient after humidification therapy or ultrasonic nebulizer (USN) therapy, both of which enhance the mucociliary transport system and facilitate a productive cough.

4. **Tracheal stimulation**[16,52]

Tracheal stimulation, sometimes called a *tracheal tickle*, may be used with infants or disoriented patients who cannot cooperate in the treatment.
   a. This is a somewhat uncomfortable maneuver, performed to elicit a reflexive cough.
   b. The therapist places two fingers at the sternal notch and applies a circular motion with pressure downward into the trachea to facilitate a reflexive cough.

F. Precautions

1. Avoid uncontrolled coughing spasms (*paroxysmal coughing*).
2. Avoid forceful coughing with patients who have a history of a cerebrovascular accident or aneurysm. Have these patients *huff* several times to clear the airways.
3. Be sure that the patient coughs while in a somewhat erect posture.

G. Suctioning: Alternative to Coughing

1. *Endotracheal suctioning* may be the only means of clearing the airways in patients who are unable to cough voluntarily or after reflex stimulation of the cough mechanism.
2. Suctioning is indicated in all patients with artificial airways.
3. The suctioning procedure will clear only the trachea and the mainstem bronchi.
4. ***Precaution:*** Only individuals who have been instructed in proper suctioning technique should use this alternative means of clearing the airways. Suctioning, if performed incorrectly, can introduce an infection into the airways or damage the delicate mucosal lining of the trachea and bronchi. Improper suctioning can also cause hypoxemia, abnormal heart rates, and atelectasis. A complete description of proper endotracheal suctioning technique is described in several references.[29,52]

VI. Postural Drainage

A. Definition

Postural drainage (bronchial drainage) is a means of mobilizing secretions in one or more lung segments to the central airways by placing the patient in various positions so that gravity assists in the drainage process.[4,8,16,18,59] When secretions are moved to the larger airways, they are then cleared by coughing or endotracheal suctioning. *Postural drainage therapy* also includes the use of manual techniques, such as percussion and vibration, as well as voluntary coughing.

B. Goals of Postural Drainage

1. **Prevent accumulation of secretions** in patients at risk for pulmonary complications. This may include:
   a. Patients with pulmonary diseases that are associated with increased production or viscosity of mucus, such as chronic bronchitis and cystic fibrosis

b. Patients who are on prolonged bed rest
c. Postsurgical patients who have received general anesthesia and who may have painful incisions that restrict deep breathing and coughing postoperatively
d. Any patient who is on a ventilator if they are stable enough to tolerate the treatment

2. Remove secretions already accumulated in the lungs of:
a. Patients with acute or chronic lung disease, such as pneumonia, atelectasis, acute lung infections, and COPD
b. Patients who are generally very weak or are elderly
c. Patients with artificial airways

C. Contraindications to Postural Drainage

1. Hemorrhage (severe hemoptysis)

a. Copious amounts of blood in the sputum.
b. NOTE: This is different from lightly blood-streaked sputum.

2. Untreated acute conditions

a. Severe pulmonary edema
b. Congestive heart failure
c. Large pleural effusion
d. Pulmonary embolism
e. Pneumothorax

3. Cardiovascular instability

a. Cardiac arrhythmia
b. Severe hypertension or hypotension
c. Recent myocardial infarction

4. Recent neurosurgery

Head-down positioning may cause increased intracranial pressure.

D. Manual Techniques Used During Postural Drainage Therapy[8,16,18,44,52,53,59]

In addition to the use of body positioning, deep breathing, and an effective cough to facilitate clearance of secretions from the airways, a variety of manual techniques are used in conjunction with postural drainage to maximize the effectiveness of the mucociliary transport system.[8,52] They include percussion, vibration, shaking, and rib springing. Findings from studies that have been implemented to evaluate the effectiveness of these manual techniques are inconsistent.[52]

1. Percussion

a. This technique is used to further mobilize secretions by mechanically dislodging viscous or adherent mucus from the lungs.
b. Percussion is performed with cupped hands (Fig. 19–21A) over the lung segment being drained. The therapist's cupped hands alternately strike the patient's chest wall in a rhythmic fashion (Fig. 19–21B). The therapist should try to keep shoulders, elbows, and wrists loose and mobile during the maneuver. Mechanical percussion is an alternative to manual percussion techniques.
c. Percussion is continued for several minutes or until the patient needs to alter position to cough.

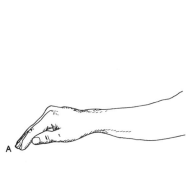
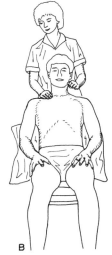
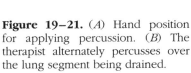

Figure 19–21. (*A*) Hand position for applying percussion. (*B*) The therapist alternately percusses over the lung segment being drained.

    d. This procedure should not be painful or uncomfortable. To prevent irritation to sensitive skin, have the patient wear a lightweight gown or shirt. Avoid percussion over breast tissue in women and over bony prominences.

    e. ***Relative contraindications***

      Prior to implementing percussion in a postural drainage program, the therapist must compare the potential benefits with the possible risks to the patient. In most instances, avoid the use of percussion

      (1) Over fractures, spinal fusion, or osteoporotic bone

      (2) Over tumor area

      (3) If a patient has a pulmonary embolus

      (4) If a patient has a condition in which hemorrhage could easily occur, such as in the presence of a low platelet count, or if a patient is receiving anticoagulation therapy

      (5) If a patient has unstable angina

      (6) If a patient has chest wall pain, for example, after thoracic surgery

2. Vibration

    a. The technique is used in conjunction with percussion in postural drainage. It is applied only during expiration as the patient is deep breathing to move the secretions to the larger airways.

    b. Vibration is applied by placing both hands directly on the skin and over the chest wall (or one hand on top of the other) and gently compressing and rapidly vibrating the chest wall as the patient breathes out (Fig. 19–22).

    c. Pressure is applied in the same direction as that in which the chest is moving.

    d. The vibrating action is achieved by the therapist's isometrically contracting (tensing) the muscles of the upper extremities from shoulders to hands.

3. Shaking

    a. Shaking is a more vigorous form of vibration applied during exhalation using an intermittent bouncing maneuver coupled with wide movements of the therapist's hands.

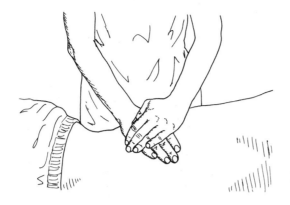

Figure 19–22. Hand placement for vibration during postural drainage.

b. The therapist's thumbs are locked together and the open hands are placed directly on the patient's skin and fingers are wrapped around the chest wall. The therapist simultaneously compresses and slakes the chest wall.

E. Postural Drainage Positions

1. Positions are based on the anatomy of the lungs and the tracheobronchial tree (see Figs. 19–1 and 19–3).
2. Each segment of each lobe is drained using the positions demonstrated in Figs. 19–23 to 19–34. The shaded area in each illustration indicates the area of the chest wall where percussion or vibration is applied.
3. The patient may be positioned on a
   a. Postural drainage table that can be elevated at one end
   b. Tilt table
   c. Reinforced padded table with a lift
   d. Hospital bed
4. A small child can be positioned on the therapist's lap.

F. Treatment Procedures for Postural Drainage

1. General considerations

a. Time of day
   (1) Never administer postural drainage directly after a meal.
   (2) Coordinate treatment with aerosol therapy. The philosophy varies.
       (a) Some therapists feel that aerosol therapy combined with humidification prior to postural drainage will help loosen secretions and increase the likelihood of productivity.
       (b) Others believe that aerosol therapy is best after postural drainage when the patient's lungs are clearer and maximum benefit can be gained from medication administered through aerosol therapy.
   (3) Choose a time (or times) of day that will be of benefit to the patient.
       (a) A patient's cough tends to be very productive in the early morning because of accumulation of secretions from the night before.
       (b) Postural drainage in the early evening will clear the lungs prior to sleeping and help the patient rest more easily.
b. Frequency of treatments will depend upon the pathology of the patient's condition.

RIGHT AND LEFT UPPER LOBES

Anterior apical segments

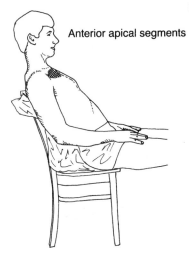

Figure 19–23. Percussion is applied directly under the clavicle.

Posterior apical segments

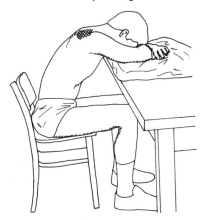

Figure 19–24. Percussion is applied above the scapulae. Your fingers curve over the top of the shoulders.

Anterior segments

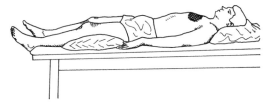

Figure 19–25. Percussion is applied bilaterally, directly over the nipple or just above the breast.

Posterior segment (left)

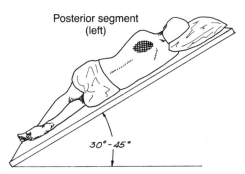

30° - 45°

Figure 19–26. Patient lies one-quarter turn from prone and rests on the right side. Head and shoulders are elevated 45 degrees or approximately 18 inches if pillows are used. Percussion is applied directly over the left scapula.

Posterior segment (right)

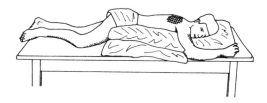

Figure 19–27. Patient lies flat and one-quarter turn from prone on the left side. Percussion is applied directly over the right scapula.

LINGULA

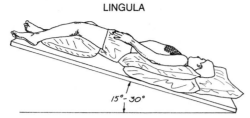

Figure 19–28. Patient lies one-quarter turn from supine on the right side, supported with pillows and in a 30-degree head-down position. Percussion is applied just under the left breast.

MIDDLE LOBE

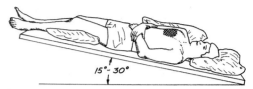

Figure 19–29. Patient lies one-quarter turn from supine on left side, supported with pillows behind the back, and in a 30-degree head-down position. Percussion is applied under the right breast.

RIGHT AND LEFT LOWER LOBES

Anterior segments

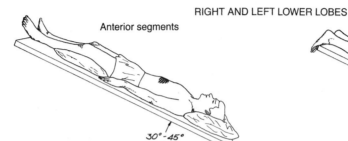

Figure 19–30. Patient lies supine, pillows under knees, in a 45-degree head-down position. Percussion is applied bilaterally over the lower portion of the ribs.

Posterior segments

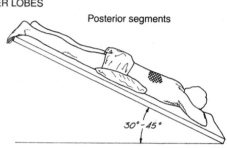

Figure 19–31. Patient lies prone, pillow under abdomen in a 45-degree head-down position. Percussion is applied bilaterally over the lower portion of the ribs.

Lateral segment (left)

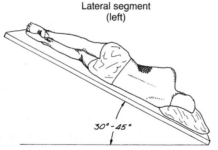

Figure 19–32. Patient lies on the right side in a 45-degree head-down position. Percussion is applied over the lower lateral aspect of the left rib cage.

Lateral segment (right)

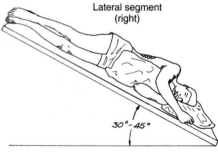

Figure 19–33. Patient lies on the left side in a 45-degree head-down position. Percussion is applied over the lower lateral aspect of the right rib cage.

Superior segments

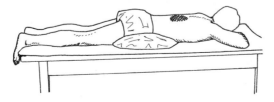

Figure 19–34. Patient lies prone, pillow under the abdomen to flatten the back. Percussion is applied bilaterally, directly below the scapulae.

(1) Thick, copious mucus: two to four times per day until lungs are clear
(2) Maintenance: one to two times per day to prevent further accumulation of secretions

2. Prepare the patient

a. Loosen tight or bulky clothing. It is not necessary to expose the skin. The patient may wear a lightweight shirt or gown.
b. Have a sputum cup or tissues available.
c. Have sufficient pillows for positioning and comfort.
d. Explain the treatment procedure to the patient.
e. Teach the patient deep breathing and an effective cough prior to beginning postural drainage.
f. If the patient is producing copious amounts of sputum, instruct the patient to cough a few times or have the patient suctioned prior to positioning.
g. Make any adjustments of tubes and wires, such as chest tubes, ECG wires, or catheters, so they remain clear during positioning.

3. Treatment sequence

a. Evaluate the patient (as outlined in Section II of this chapter) to determine which segments of the lungs should be drained.
   (1) Some patients with chronic lung diseases, such as cystic fibrosis, need to be drained in all positions.
   (2) Other patients may require drainage of only a few segments in which secretions have accumulated.
   (3) Check the patient's chart daily to determine his or her status.
   (4) Check the patient's vital signs, such as respiratory rate and pulse.
   (5) Evaluate breath sounds with a stethoscope.
b. Position the patient in the correct position for drainage. See that he or she is as comfortable and relaxed as possible.
c. Stand in front of the patient, whenever possible, to observe his or her color.
d. Maintain the desired position for at least 5 to 10 minutes if the patient can tolerate it, or as long as the position is productive.
e. Have the patient breathe deeply in a relaxed manner during drainage. Do not allow the patient to hyperventilate or become short of breath.
f. Apply percussion over the segment being drained while the patient is in the correct position.
g. Encourage the patient to take a deep, sharp double cough whenever necessary. It may be more comfortable for the patient to momentarily assume a semiupright position (resting on one elbow) and then cough.
h. If the patient does not cough spontaneously during positioning with percussion, instruct the patient to take several deep breaths and apply vibration during expiration. This may help elicit a cough.
i. If the patient's cough is not productive after 5 to 10 minutes of positioning, go on to the next position. Secretions that have been mobilized during a treatment may not be coughed up by the patient until 30 minutes to 1 hour after treatment.
j. The duration of any one treatment should not exceed 40 to 45 minutes, as the procedure is quite fatiguing for the patient.
   (1) Many patients need to be seen two or four times a day.
   (2) Schedule several treatment times if lungs are very productive or if any or all segments of both lungs must be drained.

4. Concluding the treatment

a. Have the patient sit up slowly and rest for a short while after the treatment. Watch for signs of postural hypotension when the patient rises from a supine position or from a head-down position to sitting.

b. Advise the patient that, even if the cough was not productive during treatment, it may be productive a short while after treatment.

c. Assess the effectiveness of the treatment and make appropriate notations in the patient's chart.

(1) Note the type, color, consistency, and amount of secretions produced.

(2) Note how the patient tolerated the treatment.

(3) Check the patient's vital signs after treatment.

(4) Auscultate over the segments that were drained and note changes in breath sounds.

(5) Observe the patient's breathing pattern to determine whether it is deeper, less rapid, more relaxed, or less labored.

(6) Check the symmetry of chest wall expansion.

5. Discontinue postural drainage

a. If chest x-ray is relatively clear

b. If patient is afebrile for 24 to 48 hours

c. If normal or near-normal breath sounds are heard with auscultation

d. If patient is on a regular home program

G. Modified Postural Drainage[16,18,52,60]

1. Rationale

Some patients who require postural drainage cannot assume or cannot tolerate the positions that are optimal for treatment. For example:

a. The patient with congestive heart failure may develop orthopnea (shortness of breath caused by lying flat).

b. The postneurosurgery patient may not be allowed to assume a head-down (Trendelenburg) position because this position causes increased intracranial pressure.

c. The postthoracic or postcardiac surgery patient may have chest tubes and monitoring wires that may limit positioning.

2. Procedure

The positions in which postural drainage is undertaken are modified to meet the patient's medical or surgical problems. This compromise, although not ideal, is better than not administering postural drainage at all.

H. Home Program of Postural Drainage

1. Postural drainage may have to be carried out on a regular basis at home for patients with chronic lung disease.

2. Patients need to be shown how to position themselves using inexpensive aids.

a. An adult may place pillows over hard wedges or stacks of newspapers to achieve the desired head-down positions in bed. A patient may also lean the chest over the edge of the bed, resting with the arms on a chair or stool.

b. A child may be positioned on an ironing board propped up against a couch.

3. A family member should be instructed in positioning and percussion to assist the patient when needed.

4. Guidelines and precautions, previously discussed, should be followed.

VII. Summary

In this chapter, a brief review of respiratory structure and function has been outlined. A review of the anatomy of the thorax, upper and lower respiratory tracts, and lungs has been followed by a discussion of the mechanics of breathing. Emphasis has been placed on discussing the musculature, chest movements, and mechanics of airflow that the therapist may affect during treatment. Evaluation procedures in chest physical therapy and an explanation of tests specific to chest assessment have been discussed. Overall goals of chest physical therapy and pulmonary rehabilitation have been summarized. Goals, procedures, and precautions for breathing exercises, chest mobility exercises, effective cough training, and postural drainage have then been discussed. The application of these chest physical therapy procedures are presented in Chapter 20 in conjunction with a discussion of common acute and chronic pulmonary disorders.

References

1. Aldrich, T: The application of muscle endurance training to the respiratory muscles in COPD. Lung 163:15, 1985.

2. Aldrich, T, and Karpel, J: Inspiratory muscle resistive training in respiratory failure. Am Rev Respir Dis 131:461, 1985.

3. Alvarez, SE, Peterson, M, and Lunsford, BA: Respiratory treatment of the adult patient with spinal cord injury. Phys Ther 61:1737, 1981.

4. American Association of Respiratory Care: AARC clinical practice guidelines: Postural drainage therapy. Respiratory Care 36:1418–1426, 1991.

5. American College of Chest Physicians and the American Thoracic Society Joint Committee on Pulmonary Nomenclature: Pulmonary terms and symbols. Chest 67:583, 1975.

6. Asher, MI, et al: The effects of inspiratory muscle training in patients with cystic fibrosis. Am Rev Respir Dis 126:855, 1982.

7. Basmajian, JV, and DeLuca, CJ: Muscles Alive, ed 5. Williams & Wilkins, Baltimore, 1985.

8. Brannon, FJ, et al: Cardiopulmonary Rehabilitation: Basic Theory and Application, ed 2. FA Davis, Philadelphia, 1993.

9. Campbell, E, Agostoni, E, and Davis J: The Respiratory Muscles. WB Saunders, Philadelphia, 1970.

10. Cardiopulmonary Section, American Physical Therapy Association: A statement: A definition of chest physical therapy. Cardiopulmonary Section Quarterly 4:15, Spring 1983.

11. Casiari, RJ, et al: Effects of breathing retraining in patients with chronic obstructive pulmonary disease. Chest 79:393, 1981.

12. Cherniak, RM, and Cherniak, L: Respiration in Health and Disease, ed 3. WB Saunders, Philadelphia, 1983.

13. Comroe, JH, et al: Physiology of Respiration. Year Book Medical Publishers, Chicago, 1974.

14. Crane, LD: The chest examination. Phys Ther Health Care 1:11, 1987.

15. Derrickson, J, et al: A comparison of two breathing exercise programs for patients with quadriplegia. Phys Ther 72:763–769, 1992.

16. Frownfelter, DL: Chest Physical Therapy and Pulmonary Rehabilitation, ed 2. Year Book Medical Publishers, Chicago, 1987.

17. Gaynard, P, et al: The effects of abdominal weights on diaphragmatic position and excursion in man. Clin Sci 35:589, 1968.

18. Glaskell, DV, and Webber, BA: The Brompton Hospital Guide to Chest Physiotherapy, ed 4. CV Mosby, St Louis, 1981.

19. Green, J: Fundamental Cardiovascular and Pulmonary Physiology, ed 2. Lea and Febriger, Philadelphia, 1987.

20. Gross, D: The effect of training on strength and endurance of the diaphragm in quadriplegia. Am J Med 68:27, 1980.

21. Harper, RW: A Guide to Respiratory Care: Physiology and Clinical Application. JB Lippincott, Philadelphia, 1981.

22. Hillegas, EA: Cardiopulmonary assessment. In Hillegas, EA, and Sadowsky, HS (eds): Essentials of Cardiopulmonary Physical Therapy. WB Saunders, Philadelphia, 1994.

23. Hughes, RC: Does abdominal breathing affect regional gas exchange? Chest 76:258, 1979.

24. Humberstone, N, and Tecklin, JS: Respiratory evaluation: Respiratory assessment and respiratory treatment. In Irwin, S, and Tecklin, J: Cardiopulmonary Physical Therapy, ed 3. Mosby-Year Book, St Louis, 1995.

25. Imle, PC: Physical therapy and respiratory care for the patient with acute spinal cord injury. Phys Ther Health Care 1:45, 1987.

26. Kigin, CM: Breathing exercises for the medical patient: The art and the science. Phys Ther 70:700–706, 1990.

27. Kigin, CM: Chest physical therapy for the postopera-

tive or traumatic injury patient. Phys Ther 61:1724, 1981.

28. Kim, MJ: Respiratory muscle training: Implications for patient care. Heart Lung 13:333, 1984.

29. Kuntz, WT: The acute care setting. In Hillegas, EA, and Sadowsky, HS (eds): Essentials of cardiopulmonary Physical Therapy. WB Saunders, Philadelphia, 1994.

30. Lane, C: Inspiratory muscle weight training and its effect on vital capacity of patients with quadriplegia. Cardiopulmonary Quarterly 2:13, 1982.

31. Leith, D, and Bradley, M: Ventilatory muscle strength and endurance training. J Appl Physiol 41:508, 1976.

32. Leith, DE: Cough. Phys Ther 48:439, 1968.

33. Levenson, CR: Breathing exercises. In Zadai, CC (ed): Pulmonary Management in Physical Therapy. Churchill-Livingstone, New York, 1992.

34. Luce, C: Respiratory muscle function in health and disease. Chest 81:82, 1982.

35. Martin, D, and Yountsey, J: Respiratory Anatomy and Physiology. CV Mosby, St Louis, 1988.

36. Mead, J, and Martin, H: Principles of respiratory mechanics. Journal of the American physical Therapy Association 48:478, 1968.

37. Merrick, J, and Axen, K: Inspiratory muscle function following abdominal weight exercise in healthy subjects. Phys Ther 61:651, 1981.

38. Metcalf, VA: Vital capacity and glossopharyngeal breathing in traumatic quadriplegia. Phys Ther 46:835, 1966.

39. Moore, K: Clinically Oriented Anatomy. Williams & Wilkins, Baltimore, 1980.

40. Meuller, RE, et al: Ventilation and arterial blood gas changes induced by pursed lip breathing. J Appl Physiol 28:784, 1970.

41. Nunn, K: Applied Respiratory Physiology. Butterworth, London, 1971.

42. Philo, R, et al: Guide to Human Anatomy. WB Saunders, Philadelphia, 1985.

43. Reinisch, E: Functional approach to chest physical therapy. Phys Ther 58:972, 1978.

44. Rochester, DF, and Goldberg, SK: Techniques of respiratory physical therapy. Am Rev Respir Dis 122:133, 1980.

45. Sackner, MA, et al: Distribution of ventilation during diaphragmatic breathing in obstructive lung disease. Am Rev Respir Dis 109:331, 1974.

46. Shaffer, T, Wolfson, M, and Bhutoni, VK: Respiratory muscle function: Assessment and training. Phys Ther 61:1711, 1981.

47. Shearer, MC, et al: Lung ventilation during diaphragmatic breathing. Phys Ther 52:139, 1972.

48. Smakowski, PS: Ventilatory muscle training. Part I:

The effectiveness of endurance training on rodent diaphragm. A scientific review of the literature from 1972–1991. Cardiopulmonary Physical Therapy Journal 4:2–3, 1993.

49. Sobush, DC: Breathing exercises: Laying a foundation for a clinical practice guideline. Cardiopulmonary Physical Therapy Journal 3:8–10, 1992.

50. Sobush, D, Dunning, M, and McDonald, K: Exercise prescription components for respiratory muscle training. Respiratory Care 34:30, 1985.

51. Sonne, L, and Davis, J: Increased exercise performance in patients with severe COPD following inspiratory resistive training. Chest 81:436, 1982.

52. Starr, JA: Manual techniques of chest physical therapy and airway clearance techniques. In: Zadai, CC (ed): Pulmonary Management in Physical Therapy. Churchill-Livingstone, New York, 1992.

53. Sutton, P, et al: Assessment of percussion vibratory shaking and breathing exercises in chest physiotherapy. Eur J Respir Dis 66:147, 1985.

54. Visich, R: Knowing what you hear: A guide to breath and heart sounds. Nursing 81:64, 1981.

55. Warren, A: Mobilization of the chest wall. In Hislop, H (ed): Chest Disorders in Children. Proceedings of a Symposium. American Physical Therapy Association, Washington, DC, 1968.

56. Watts, N: Improvement of breathing patterns. In Hislop, H (ed): Chest Disorders in Children. Proceeding of a Symposium. American Physical Therapy Association, Washington, DC, 1968.

57. West, JB: Respiratory Physiology: The Essentials. Williams & Wilkins, Baltimore, 1974.

58. Wetzel, J, et al: Respiratory rehabilitation of the patient with spinal cord injury. In Irwin, S, and Tecklin, J (eds): Cardiopulmonary Physical Therapy, ed 3. Mosby-Year Book, St Louis, 1995.

59. White, GC: Basic Clinical Competencies for Respiratory Care: An Integrated Approach. Delmar Albany, NY, 1988.

60. White, J, and Mawdsley, R: Effects of selected bronchial drainage positions on blood pressure of healthy human subjects. Phys Ther 63:325, 1983.

61. Wilkins, RL, et al: Lung sound nomenclature survey. Chest 98(4): 886–889, 1990.

62. Youtsey, J: Basic pulmonary function measurements. In Spearman, C (ed): Egan's Fundamentals of Respiratory Therapy, ed 4. CV Mosby, St Louis, 1982.

63. Zadai, CC: Comprehensive physical therapy evaluation: Identifying potential pulmonary complications. In Zadai, CC (ed): Pulmonary Management in Physical Therapy. Churchill-Livingstone, New York, 1992.

64. Zadai, CC: Physical therapy for the acutely ill medical patient. Phys Ther 61:1746, 1981.

Management of Obstructive and Restrictive Pulmonary Conditions

The intent of this chapter is to provide an overview of the clinical problems and major impairments as well as the goals and techniques of management of common pulmonary conditions. The two general classifications of pulmonary disorders that are discussed in this chapter are obstructive lung diseases and restrictive pulmonary disorders. The specific techniques of management of these conditions, such as evaluation procedures, breathing exercises, postural drainage, coughing, and mobility exercises for the trunk and thorax, have all been described and illustrated in Chapter 19. Guidelines for general conditioning and endurance training that are an integral part of a pulmonary rehabilitation program can be found in Chapter 4.

OBJECTIVES

After studying this chapter, the reader will be able to:

1 Define obstructive lung disease and restrictive lung disease.
2 Identify common causes of obstructive and restrictive lung diseases and disorders.
3 Summarize the general clinical problems/impairments found in patients with obstructive and restrictive lung diseases.
4 Identify general treatment goals and plan of care in obstructive and restrictive lung diseases.
5 Describe the clinical picture, summarize the clinical problems/impairments, and explain the goals and techniques of treatment of the following obstructive lung diseases: chronic bronchitis, emphysema, asthma, cystic fibrosis, and bronchiectasis.
6 Describe the clinical picture, summarize the clinical problems/impairments, and explain the goals and techniques of treatment of the following restrictive lung problems: post-thoracic surgery, atelectasis, and pneumonia.
7 Describe specific precautions in the treatment of each condition discussed.

I. Overview of Obstructive Lung Disease

A. Definition

Obstructive lung disease is a general term that refers to a number of chronic pulmonary conditions, all of which obstruct the flow of air in the respiratory tract and affect ventilation and gas exchange.[1,2,10,13,23] A number of specific diseases can be classified as obstructive in nature. Each disease has its unique features and is distinguished by the cause of the obstruction of airflow, the onset of the disease, the location of the obstruction, and the reversibility of the obstruction.

1. Specific obstructive pulmonary conditions[1,2,23]

    a. Chronic obstructive pulmonary disease (COPD)
        (1) Peripheral airway disease
        (2) Chronic bronchitis
        (3) Emphysema
    b. Asthma
    c. Cystic fibrosis
    d. Bronchiectasis
    e. Bronchopulmonary dysplasia

2. Terms synonymous with COPD

    a. COAD: chronic obstructive airway disease.
    b. COLD: chronic obstructive lung disease.
    c. NOTE: The term COPD is sometimes used to describe all chronic pulmonary diseases that have obstructive characteristics, not just chronic bronchitis, peripheral airway disease, and emphysema. In this text the term COPD will be used as described by the American Thoracic Society to refer only to chronic bronchitis, peripheral airway disease, and emphysema.[1]

B. Changes Associated with Obstructive Lung Disease[1,2,10,13,23]

1. Narrowing and obstruction of airways
2. Inflammation of the airways
3. Destruction of alveolar and bronchial walls
4. Increased production and retention of mucus
5. Abnormal pulmonary function tests (Fig. 20–1)
    a. Decreased vital capacity and expiratory reserve volume
    b. Increased residual volume
    c. Decreased expiratory flow rates

C. Impairments/Problems of Patients with Obstructive Diseases[2,4,10,13]

1. Dyspnea on exertion
Patients with obstructive diseases experience frequent episodes of shortness of breath with minimal physical activity.

2. Decreased exercise tolerance
Patients have a decreased capacity for exercise and inadequate endurance for daily activities.

3. Chronic, usually productive cough
Due to excessive production and chronic accumulation of pulmonary secretions, patients experience a chronic, usually productive cough.

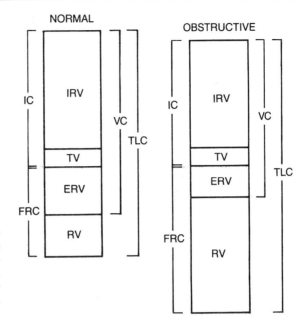

Figure 20–1. Normal lung volumes and capacities compared to abnormal lung volumes and capacities found in patients with obstructive pulmonary disease. (From Rothstein, J, Roy, A, and Wolf, SL: The Rehabilitation Specialist's Handbook. FA Davis, Philadelphia, 1991, p 604, with permission.)

4. **Frequent respiratory infections**
5. **Associated postural defects**

A more detailed explanation of specific obstructive lung diseases follows. Chronic bronchitis, peripheral airway disease and emphysema, asthma, cystic fibrosis, and bronchiectasis are discussed. The treatment goals and appropriate plan of care are then outlined.

II. Specific Obstructive Pulmonary Conditions

A. COPD: Peripheral Airway Disease, Chronic Bronchitis, and Emphysema

Peripheral airway disease, chronic bronchitis, and emphysema are classified as **chronic obstructive pulmonary diseases (COPD)**. Since these diseases are often closely related and often seen in conjunction with each other, the underlying goals and principles of treatment are similar.

1. **Peripheral airway disease: clinical picture[1,2]**

   a. Peripheral airway disease is characterized by inflammation, fibrosis, and narrowing of the small distal airways (less than 2 mm in diameter), specifically the terminal and respiratory bronchioles.

   NOTE: Peripheral airway disease is sometimes classified as a precursor to rather than a component of COPD.

   b. The inflammation of the small airways is associated with long-term exposure to pulmonary irritants, primarily cigarette smoke.

   c. The pathologic changes that occur in peripheral airway disease are:
   (1) Thickening of tissues and narrowing of the small peripheral airways
   (2) Hypertrophy of the smooth muscle of the airways
   (3) Negligible changes in pulmonary function tests

d. The patient experiences little to no signs or symptoms and no changes in functional capacity. Inflammation and early structural changes in the distal airways can be reduced or reversed by smoking cessation before the development of permanent airway changes associated with emphysema.

2. **Chronic bronchitis: clinical picture**[1,2,10,13]

   a. Chronic bronchitis is an inflammation of the bronchi that causes an irritating and productive cough that lasts at least 3 months and recurs over at least 2 consecutive years.

   b. This condition usually develops in heavy smokers. Factors other than smoking that may contribute, although to a lesser extent, to the development of chronic bronchitis are occupational exposure to vegetable and metal dusts and environmental pollution.

   c. The pathologic changes that occur in chronic bronchitis are[1]:
      (1) An increase in the number of mucus-producing goblet cells in the lining of the bronchial tree
      (2) A decrease in the number and action of the ciliated epithelial cells that mobilize and help clear secretions
      (3) A narrowing of airways because of chronic inflammation and partial obstruction of the bronchial tree and thickening of the lining

   d. General appearance of the patient
      (1) Chronic, productive cough
      (2) Cyanotic because of hypoxemia
      (3) Short of breath
      (4) Bloated and edematous because of venous stasis and right-side heart failure
      (5) Often overweight

3. **Emphysema: clinical picture**[1,2,4,23]

   a. Emphysema is a chronic inflammation, narrowing, thickening, and destruction of the respiratory bronchioles and alveoli. These airways become scarred, distorted, and kinked, and the alveoli lose their elastic recoil, then weaken and rupture. As a result, the patient experiences dyspnea and chronic obstruction of airflow during expiration, and air remains trapped in the lungs (residual volume increases). Over a period of years, severe chronic bronchitis and emphysema often lead to congestive heart failure and death.

   b. Emphysema is usually a condition that develops secondary to peripheral airway disease and chronic bronchitis. Although not as common, emphysema can also be a primary autoimmune disease characterized by a deficiency of the enzyme antitrypsin that can occur in nonsmokers.

   c. The pathologic changes that occur in emphysema are[1]:
      (1) An overinflation of the lungs and formation of pockets of air known as *bullae*. This causes an increase in the air space in the lungs.
      (2) Destruction of alveoli and loss of area in which effective gas exchange can occur.
      (3) Loss of elastic recoil of the peripheral lung tissues.

   d. General appearance of the patient
      (1) Chronic labored breathing and shortness of breath with supraclavicular or intercostal retractions
      (2) Pink and thin
      (3) Abnormal posture: forward head, rounded and elevated shoulders
      (4) Clubbing of fingers

(5) Excessive use and hypertrophy of accessory muscles and diminished diaphragmatic breathing during inspiration

(6) Use of pursed-lip breathing during expiration

(7) Increase in the AP diameter of the chest (barrel chest)

4. Impairments/problems of COPD summarized[1,2,4,13,20]

a. An increase in the amount and viscosity of mucous production.

b. A chronic, often productive cough.

c. Attacks of shortness of breath (dyspnea).

d. A labored breathing pattern that results in:

(1) Increased respiratory rate (tachypnea)

(2) Use of accessory muscles of inspiration and decreased diaphragmatic excursion

(3) Upper chest breathing

(4) Poor exchange of air in the lower lobes

e. Most difficulty during expiration; use of pursed-lip breathing.

f. Changes in pulmonary function.

(1) Increased residual volume

(2) Decreased vital capacity

(3) Decreased expiratory flow rates

g. Decreased mobility of the chest wall: a barrel chest deformity develops.

h. Abnormal posture: forward head and rounded and elevated shoulders.

i. Decrease in general endurance during functional activities.

5. General treatment goals and plan of care[2,10,13,23,26,27]

Treatment Goals

a. Decrease the amount and viscosity of secretions and prevent respiratory infections.

b. Remove or prevent the accumulation of secretions. (This is an important goal if emphysema is associated with chronic bronchitis or if there is an acute respiratory infection.)

c. Promote relaxation of the accessory muscles of inspiration to decrease reliance on upper chest breathing and to decrease muscle tension associated with dyspnea.

Plan of Care

a. Administration of bronchodilators, antibiotics, and humidification therapy.

If the patient smokes, he or she should be strongly encouraged to stop.

b. Deep and effective cough.

Postural drainage to areas where secretions are identified.

NOTE: Drainage positions may need to be modified if the patient is dyspneic in the head-down position.

c. Positioning for relaxation.

Relaxed head-up position in bed: trunk, arms, and head are well supported.

Sitting: leaning forward, resting forearms on thighs (Fig. 20–2).

Sitting: leaning forward against pillows on a table (Fig. 20–3).

Standing: leaning forward on an object, with hands on the thighs

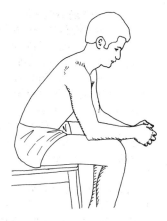

Figure 20-2. To relieve shortness of breath, the patient assumes a relaxed sitting position, leaning forward, resting the forearms on the thighs or on a pillow in the lap.

Treatment Goals

d. Improve the patient's breathing pattern and ventilation. Emphasize diaphragmatic breathing and *relaxed* expiration; decrease the work of breathing, rate of respira-

Plan of Care

(Fig. 20-4) or leaning backward against a wall.

Relaxation exercises for shoulder musculature: active shoulder shrugging followed by relaxation; shoulder and arm circles; horizontal abduction and adduction of the shoulders.

d. Breathing exercises: relaxed diaphragmatic breathing with minimal upper chest movement; lateral costal breathing; pursed-lip breathing (careful to *avoid forced* expira-

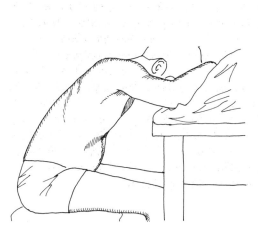

Figure 20-3. The patient can sit and lean forward on a pillow to relax and relieve a shortness of breath.

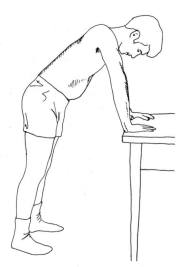

Figure 20-4. A patient can lean forward and support some weight on the arms while standing to relieve shortness of breath.

Treatment Goals	*Plan of Care*
tion, and the use of accessory muscles. Carry over controlled breathing to functional activities.	tion); inspiratory resistance exercises; practice controlled breathing during standing, walking, climbing stairs, and so on.
e. Minimize attacks of shortness of breath.	e. Have the patient assume a relaxed position (see Figs. 20–2 through 20–4) so the upper chest is relaxed and the lower chest is as mobile as possible.

Emphasize relaxed and controlled diaphragmatic breathing.

Have the patient breathe out as rapidly as possible *without forcing* expiration.

NOTE: Initially, the rate of respiration will be rapid and shallow. As the patient gets control of breathing, he or she will slow down the rate.

Administer supplemental oxygen in a severe attack, if needed.

f. Improve the mobility of the lower thorax.	f. Exercises for chest mobility, emphasizing movement of the lower rib cage during deep breathing (see Figs. 19–8 through 19–11).
g. Improve posture.	g. Exercises to decrease forward head and rounded shoulders (see Chapters 8 and 15).
h. Increase exercise tolerance.	h. Graded endurance and conditioning exercises (see Chapter 4).

NOTE: The efficacy of breathing exercises and general conditioning and its effect on lung function and respiratory muscle function in the patient with COPD is unclear. Little quantitative data are available to indicate that breathing retraining, abdominal muscle strengthening, or general conditioning exercises increase lung function. Patients with COPD who participate in a pulmonary rehabilitation program that includes aerobic conditioning exercises report a better level of general well-being, fewer episodes of dyspnea, decreased energy expenditure during physical activity, and a higher functional capacity. Chest physical therapy and a reconditioning program for the patient with COPD will not arrest the disease process or change lung function. Patients with mild to moderate COPD will benefit more from a conditioning program than will patients with late-stage disease.[3,4,12,15,20,26,27] Appropriate quantitative assessment prior to and after a patient has been involved in general conditioning will help to determine the effectiveness of the program.

B. Asthma

Asthma is an obstructive lung disease seen in young patients. It is related to hypersensitivity and reactivity of the trachea and bronchi and causes difficulties with respiration because of bronchospasm and increased production of mucus.[1,2,10,13,31]

1. Clinical picture[1,2,8,10,13,31]

a. The majority of patients with asthma are children.

b. Asthmatic attacks involve severe shortness of breath when the patient comes in contact with a specific allergen. An asthmatic attack may also be induced by vigorous physical activity (*exercise-induced asthma*). The patient has a very rapid rate of respiration and primarily uses accessory muscles for breathing. There are audible wheezes (rhonchi), and the patient feels severe tightness in the chest and may have a cough. Exhalation is incomplete or prolonged.

c. Pathologic changes

   (1) Severe spasm of smooth muscle of the bronchial tree.

   (2) Narrowing of airways.

   (3) Inflammation of the mucosal lining of the tracheobronchial tree and hypersecretion of mucus, which is usually sticky and therefore obstructive because of an increase in the size and number of goblet cells.

   (4) Severe asthma over a prolonged number of years can lead to emphysema.

d. General appearance of the patient

   (1) Labored breathing pattern and shortness of breath

   (2) Chronically fatigued

   (3) Often thin

   (4) Poor posture: rounded shoulders, forward head, and hypertrophy of accessory muscles

2. Impairments/problems summarized

a. Severe, episodic attacks of shortness of breath

b. Cough: usually unproductive during an asthmatic attack but productive later

c. Abnormal breathing pattern; overuse of accessory muscles, resulting in upper chest breathing and increased respiratory rate

d. Poor posture: rounded shoulders, forward head

3. General treatment goals and plan of care[2,8,10,13,23]

Treatment Goals	*Plan of Care*
a. Decrease bronchospasm.	a. Removal of allergen(s); bronchodilators.
b. Minimize attacks of shortness of breath and gain control of breathing.	b. Relaxation of upper chest and accessory muscles by positioning (see Figs. 20–2 through 20–4). Diaphragmatic breathing, emphasizing controlled but not forceful expiration. Use of pursed-lip breathing as needed. Use of controlled rate of breathing.
c. Mobilize and remove secretions *after* attack of shortness of breath.	c. Humidification of secretions with aerosol therapy. Effective coughing. Postural drainage (after, not during, the asthmatic attack, because it may increase bronchospasm).
d. Correct posture to decrease rounded shoulders and forward head.	d. Postural training (see Chapters 8 and 15).

Treatment Goals	*Plan of Care*
e. Gradually increase exercise tolerance and endurance for functional activities.	e. Avoid prolonged, vigorous physical activities. Encourage mild to moderate activities for short periods of time, followed by rest. Use controlled, paced breathing during exertion.

C. Bronchiectasis

Bronchiectasis is an obstructive lung disease characterized by permanent dilation of the medium-sized bronchi, usually the fourth to the ninth generations, and repeated infections in these areas.[1,2,13] The onset of bronchiectasis usually occurs in childhood and may be caused by a previous, necrotizing infection.

1. Clinical picture

  a. Severe infection of dilated, obstructed bronchioles.
  b. Productive cough with purulent sputum and hemoptysis.
  c. Pathologic changes:
    (1) Repeated infections of the lower lobes of the lungs in the dilated bronchi and bronchioles
    (2) Destruction of ciliated epithelial cells in infected areas
    (3) Accumulation of copious, purulent secretions
  d. If the infections are localized, a lobectomy may be indicated.

2. Impairments/problems summarized[2,13]

  a. Repeated infections of the affected lung area
  b. Accumulation of purulent secretions
  c. Productive cough
  d. Dyspnea

3. General treatment goals and plan of care[2,13,23]

Treatment Goals	*Plan of Care*
a. Clear the airways of secretions.	a. Effective, controlled cough. Postural drainage BID to QID during acute episodes.
b. Maintain appropriate level of hydration to thin secretions.	b. Eight to 10 glasses of water per day.
c. Prevent or control recurrent infections.	c. Home program of postural drainage to be carried on throughout life. Appropriate immunization and antibiotic therapy.

4. *Precautions*

  a. If *mild hemoptysis* (blood-streaked sputum) occurs, continue postural drainage but omit percussion for at least 24 hours.
  b. If *severe hemoptysis* (hemorrhage) occurs, discontinue postural drainage until advised by physician.

D. Cystic Fibrosis

Cystic fibrosis (CF) is a genetically based disease (autosomal recessive) that involves malfunction of the exocrine glands, leading to abnormal secretions in the body. The disease is characterized by a very high concentration of sodium and chloride in the sweat, diffuse lung disease, and malfunction of the pancreas. The disease must be managed throughout life with diet, pancreatic enzyme replacement, medication, and preventive chest physical therapy as soon as any symptoms are noted in the young child.

1. Clinical picture[7,8,29,31,32]

   a. Children with CF are usually small for their age because of pancreatic malfunction that leads to malabsorption of foods.
   b. The exocrine gland dysfunction within the pulmonary system leads to increased production of viscous mucus, which obstructs the airways. Chronic obstruction of the airways and pooling of secretions leave the child vulnerable to pulmonary infection.
   c. The child with CF has a chronic, productive cough and often exhibits dyspnea, tachypnea, and cyanosis.
   d. Expiratory flow rates decrease and residual volume increases over time due to hyperinflation of the lungs.
   e. Prognosis for survival has improved in the past 25 years. The average patient with CF now survives into the late 20s or early 30s. The digestive involvement can be effectively managed by diet and enzyme replacement therapy; pulmonary complications are eventually the cause of death.

2. Impairments/problems summarized[7,8,25,31]

   a. Increased production of viscous mucus throughout the lungs
   b. Periodic pulmonary infections
   c. Chronic cough
   d. Increased work of breathing and excessive use of accessory muscles of respiration
   e. Decreased exercise capacity and endurance for functional activities
   f. Possible problems of compliance with a life-long regimen of home postural drainage and prevention of lung infections

3. General treatment goals and plan of care[8,21,25,29-32]

Treatment Goals	*Plan of Care*
a. Prevent accumulation of secretions and pulmonary infection.	a. Daily home program of postural drainage, usually BID, if no acute pulmonary problems exist; use of bronchodilators.
b. Decrease viscosity of secretions.	b. Humidification, adequate hydration, and intermittent aerosol therapy.
c. Prevent use of accessory muscles of respiration.	c. Diaphragmatic breathing, lateral costal expansion, and inspiratory muscle strengthening. Daily practice and use of deep breathing during postural drainage is important. Emphasize *relaxed*

Treatment Goals	*Plan of Care*
	expiration so bronchospasm and air trapping does not occur.
d. Remove secretions during an acute infection.	d. Postural drainage QID or for longer periods of time, as needed. Appropriate use of antibiotics.
e. Increase exercise tolerance and endurance for functional activities.	e. Graded endurance and conditioning exercises (see Chapter 4).

NOTE: The key to successful preventive treatment of the complications of cystic fibrosis over many years is a consistent home program of postural drainage. This requires a supportive and cooperative family atmosphere.

III. Overview of Restrictive Lung Disorders

A. Definition

Restrictive lung disorders are characterized by the inability of the lungs to fully expand as the result of an extrapulmonary or pulmonary restriction.[2,6,12]
1. Tidal volume, inspiratory and vital capacities, and total lung capacity are all diminished.
2. The rate of respiration is usually increased (tachypnea).
3. In restrictive lung disorders, it is extremely difficult for the patient to take a deep inspiration.

B. Causes of Restrictive Lung Disorders[2,6,8,12]

1. Extrapulmonary restrictions

a. Pleural disease (pleural effusion)
b. Chest wall injury or stiffness
  (1) Chest wall pain, secondary to trauma, such as a penetrating wound to the thorax or a rib fracture, or to thoracic surgery
  (2) Structural abnormality (scleroderma, pectus excavatum)
  (3) Postural deformities (scoliosis, kyphosis, ankylosing spondylitis)
c. Respiratory muscle weakness
  (1) Neuromuscular disease or dysfunction (muscular dystrophy, anterior horn cell disease, parkinsonism)
  (2) CNS depression or injury (drug overdose, very high spinal cord injury)
d. Insufficient excursion of the diaphragm because of obesity or ascites

2. Pulmonary restrictions

a. Diseases of the lung parenchyma and pleura
  (1) Tumor
  (2) Interstitial pulmonary fibrosis
    (a) Silicosis
    (b) Asbestosis
    (c) Pneumonia
    (d) Sarcoidosis
    (e) Tuberculosis
  (3) Atelectasis
  (4) Pleural effusion
b. Disorders of cardiovascular origin

(1) Pulmonary edema

(2) Pulmonary embolism

   c. Inadequate or abnormal pulmonary development: hyaline membrane disease

   d. Normal aging

C. Changes Associated with Restrictive Disorders[2,6,8,12]

1. Decreased pulmonary compliance
   a. Chronic inflammation and fibrosis (thickening of the alveoli, bronchioles, or pleura)
   b. Decreased mobility of the chest wall
2. Abnormal lung volumes and capacities (Fig. 20–5)
3. Increased work of breathing
4. Decreased arterial blood gases (hypoxemia)
5. Pulmonary congestion

D. Impairments/Problems Of Patients With Restrictive Disorders[2,6,8,12]

1. Shortness of breath (dyspnea) and increased respiratory rate (tachypnea)
2. Inability to breathe in deeply
3. Increased use of accessory muscles of respiration
4. Ineffective, sometimes productive cough
5. Decreased thoracic mobility (primary or secondary)
6. Postural deviations
7. Respiratory muscle fatigue
8. General weakness and fatigue
9. Weight loss

IV. Specific Restrictive Pulmonary Conditions

A. Postthoracotomy

Patients with pulmonary or cardiac conditions that require surgical intervention are at high risk for restrictive pulmonary complications, such as atelectasis and pneumonia, after chest surgery. A **thoracotomy**, an incision into the chest wall, is required in a

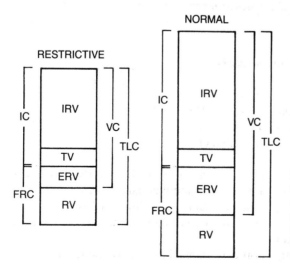

Figure 20–5. Normal lung volumes and capacities compared with abnormal lung volumes and capacities found in patients with restrictive pulmonary disorders. (From Rothstein, J, Roy, A, and Wolf, SL: The Rehabilitation Specialist's Handbook. FA Davis, Philadelphia, 1991, p 604, with permission.)

variety of pulmonary and cardiac surgeries. In addition to pulmonary complications, a thoracotomy predisposes the patient to postsurgical postural deviations. It has been recognized for many years that effective pulmonary hygiene, particularly in the early days after surgery, is an important adjunct to surgery. A carefully planned program of *preoperative* and *postoperative* chest physical therapy can minimize postsurgical complications and restore normal function for these patients.[6,10,18,22]

NOTE: Patients who undergo upper abdominal surgery also have a high risk of developing postoperative pulmonary complications. Postoperative pain is often greater after upper abdominal surgery than after thoracic surgery. This results in hypoventilation (vital capacity is decreased 55 percent for the first 24 to 48 hours after surgery) and an ineffective cough, which place the patient at risk for developing pneumonia or atelectasis.[6,18] A postoperative program of chest physical therapy has also been shown to be beneficial for these patients.[18,22,24,33]

1. Pulmonary surgery[6,18,24]

  a. Reasons for surgery
    (1) Malignant or benign tumors
    (2) Lung abscess
    (3) Bronchiectasis
    (4) Tuberculosis
    (5) Abnormalities of the pleura
  b. Types of surgery
    (1) **Lobectomy**
       Removal of one or more lobes of the lungs, usually as the result of carcinoma
    (2) **Pneumonectomy**
       Removal of an entire lung
    (3) **Segmental resection**
       Removal of a segment of a lobe of the lung, usually for benign tumors, or diseased tissue secondary to bronchiectasis or tuberculosis
    (4) **Pleurectomy**
       An incision into the pleura

2. Cardiac surgery (open heart surgery)[6,10,17,18,24]

  a. Reasons for surgery
    (1) Coronary artery disease
    (2) Cardiac valve insufficiency and stenosis
    (3) Aneurysm
    (4) Congenital abnormalities of the heart
       (a) Atrial or ventricular septal defects (ASD or VSD)
       (b) Patent ductus arteriosus (PDA)
    (5) Arrhythmias requiring a cardiac pacemaker
  b. Types of surgery
    (1) Open heart procedures, which have been performed since the 1950s, require extracorporeal perfusion (total cardiopulmonary bypass using the heart-lung bypass pump). Open heart surgery procedures include:
       (a) Aortocoronary bypass surgery, which constitutes 50 percent of all open heart surgical procedures
       (b) Replacement of the mitral, aortic, or tricuspid valves of the heart

(c) Repair of atrial and ventricular septal defects and patent ductus arteriosus

(d) Commissurotomy: splitting or cutting of the commissures of a valve secondary to valvular stenosis

(e) Aneurysmectomy: cutting, approximation, and resuturing of a cardiac aneurysm

(f) Pacemaker implantation

(2) Heart transplantation surgery

3. Factors that increase the risk of pulmonary complications and restrictive lung dysfunction after pulmonary or cardiac surgery[6,11,16,18,19,24]

The postthoracotomy patient experiences considerable chest pain, which leads to chest wall immobility, poor lung expansion, and an ineffective cough. Pulmonary secretions also tend to be greater than normal postoperatively. Therefore, the patient is more likely to accumulate pulmonary secretions and develop secondary pneumonia or atelectasis. The factors that increase postoperative pulmonary complications are:

a. General anesthesia

(1) Decreases the normal ciliary action of the tracheobronchial tree

(2) Depresses the respiratory center of the central nervous system, which causes a shallow respiratory pattern (decreased tidal volume and vital capacity)

(3) Depresses the cough reflex

b. Intubation (insertion of an endotracheal or nasogastric tube)

(1) Causes muscle spasm and immobility of the chest

(2) Irritates the mucosal lining of the tracheobronchial tree, which causes an increase in the production of mucus

(3) Decreases the normal action of the cilia in the tracheobronchial tree, which leads to pooling of secretions

c. Incisional pain

(1) Causes muscle splinting and decreases chest wall compliance, which, in turn, causes a shallow breathing pattern. Lung expansion is restricted and secretions are not adequately mobilized.

(2) Restricts a deep and effective cough. The patient usually has a weak, shallow cough that does not effectively mobilize and clear secretions.

d. Pain medication

Although pain medication administered postoperatively tends to diminish incisional pain, it also

(1) Depresses the respiratory center of the central nervous system

(2) Decreases the normal ciliary action in the bronchial tree

e. General inactivity and bed rest postoperatively cause secretions to pool, particularly in the posterior basilar segments of the lower lobes.

f. General weakness and fatigue decrease the effectiveness of the cough.

g. Other risk factors not directly related to the surgery include:

(1) The patient's age (over age 50)

(2) History of smoking

(3) History of COPD or restrictive pulmonary disorder due to neuromuscular weakness

(4) Obesity

(5) Poor mentation and orientation

4. Impairments/problems of the postthoracotomy patient summarized[5,6,10,17,18,22,24]

a. Poor lung expansion or an inability to take a deep inspiration because of incisional pain

b. Decreased effectiveness of the cough because of incisional pain and irritation of the throat from intubation

c. Possible accumulation of pulmonary secretions either preoperatively or postoperatively

d. Decreased chest wall and upper extremity mobility

e. Poor postural alignment because of incisional pain or chest tubes

f. Increased risk of deep vein thrombosis and pulmonary embolism because of extracorporeal perfusion (in the open heart surgery patient) or bed rest and inactivity postoperatively

g. General weakness, fatigue, and disorientation

5. Preoperative evaluation and treatment

a. A thorough preoperative evaluation of the patient who is to undergo either pulmonary or cardiac surgery is an essential component of a comprehensive plan of care. It should include an evaluation of[6,17,18,24,28]:

(1) Breathing pattern, respiratory rate, and heart rate

(2) Effectiveness and productivity of the cough

(3) Accumulation of secretions and the possible need for postural drainage

(4) Range of motion, particularly of the shoulders

(5) Posture and alignment of the trunk

b. Preoperative treatment and patient education

The preoperative period is an ideal time to prepare the patient physically and psychologically for surgery and to teach the patient activities that will be carried out in the early postoperative days. Instructions or treatment should include:

(1) A general explanation of what to expect postoperatively, such as the location of the incision, incisional pain, the placement and function of chest tubes, endotracheal intubation, intravenous tubes, Foley catheter, an arterial line, or cardiac electrodes and monitor

(2) Breathing exercise instruction with an emphasis on deep inspiration using:

(a) Diaphragmatic breathing with sustained maximal inspirations

(b) Lateral and posterior basal breathing

(3) Incentive spirometry or inspiratory resistance training as an adjunct to deep-breathing exercises

(4) Effective cough instruction and an explanation of splinting techniques

(5) Removal of any accumulated secretions with full or modified postural drainage

(6) Lower extremity exercise to maintain circulation and prevent deep vein thrombosis or pulmonary embolism

(7) Postural alignment in bed

6. Thoracic surgery: postoperative considerations[5,6,11,16,24]

The patient who has undergone a thoracotomy for a pulmonary or cardiac condition will usually be hospitalized for approximately 1 week. In addition to the primary pulmonary or cardiac problem such as a malignant tumor, lung abscess, or coronary artery disease, the patient may also have related cardiopulmonary problems such as angina, congestive heart disease, chronic bronchitis, or emphysema.

The patient with a long history of cardiac disease may also have preoperative pulmonary conditions such as hypoxemia, dyspnea on exertion, orthopnea, or pulmonary congestion. If this is the case, the postoperative rehabilitation may be longer and more complicated.

Most patients undergoing pulmonary surgery will have a large posterolateral, lateral, or anterolateral chest wall incision. A standard posterolateral approach (Fig. 20–6), for example, is performed by incising the chest wall along the intercostal space that corresponds to the location of the lung lesion. The incision divides the trapezius and rhomboid muscles posteriorly and the serratus anterior, latissimus dorsi, and external and internal intercostals laterally.

Postoperatively, the incision is quite painful, and the potential for pulmonary complications is significant. Many patients, quite understandably, complain of a great deal of shoulder soreness on the operated side. Loss of range of shoulder motion and postural deviations are possible because of the disturbance of the large arm and trunk musculature during surgery.

The most common incision used with cardiac surgery is a *median sternotomy.* A large incision extends along the anterior chest from the sternal notch to just below the xyphoid. The sternum is then split and retracted so that the chest cavity can be exposed. After the completion of the surgical procedure, the sternum is closed with stainless steel sutures. Postoperatively there is actually less incisional pain after a median sternotomy than after a posterolateral thoracotomy, but deep breathing and coughing are still painful. After a median sternotomy a patient tends to exhibit rounded shoulders and is at risk for developing tightness of the pectoralis muscles bilaterally.

Extracorporeal perfusion by means of a heart-lung bypass pump is required during open heart surgery. Although development of the heart-lung bypass pump in the 1950s has revolutionized cardiac surgery, extracorporeal circulation also puts the patient at further risk of developing postoperative pulmonary or circulatory complications. Pulmonary hypoxia occurs as circulation to the heart and lungs is bypassed. Microemboli in the pulmonary vascular system occur more frequently with extracorporeal perfusion.

During cardiac surgery, an endotracheal tube is put in place and remains in place 1 day postoperatively so that the patient can be mechanically ventilated for the first 24 hours. The patient's cardiac status is constantly monitored postoperatively by an ECG.

After a thoracotomy or median sternotomy, one or two chest drainage tubes are put in place at the time of surgery to prevent a **pneumothorax** or a **hemothorax**. While these tubes are in place, crimping, clamping, or traction on the tubes must be avoided during postoperative treatment.

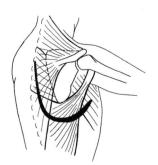

Figure 20–6. A posterolateral approach commonly used in thoracic surgery incises and divides the trapezius, rhomboid, latissimus dorsi, serratus anterior, and internal and external intercostal muscles.

The patient will fatigue easily in the first few postoperative days, so treatment sessions should be short but frequent, usually QID. The duration and intensity of treatment should be slowly and gradually increased during the patient's hospital stay.

Check the patient's chart regularly to note any day-to-day changes in vital signs, temperature, and laboratory test results. Always monitor vital signs such as heart rate and rhythm, respiratory rate, and blood pressure prior to, during, and after every treatment session.

7. General treatment goals and plan of care*

Postoperative Goals

a. Ascertain the status of the patient before each treatment.

b. Promote relaxation and relieve postoperative pain.

c. Maintain adequate ventilation and re-expand lung tissue to prevent atelectasis and pneumonia.

d. Assist in the removal of secretions.

Plan of Care

a. Evaluate color, respiratory rate, heart rate, breath sounds, sputum, drainage into chest tubes, and orientation.

b. Position the patient in a semi-Fowler's position (head of bed elevated to 30 degrees and hips and knees slightly flexed). This position reduces traction on the thoracic incision.

Coordinate treatment with administration of pain medication.

c. Begin deep-breathing exercises on the day of surgery as soon as the patient is conscious; diaphragmatic breathing; segmental expansion.

Add incentive spirometry or inspiratory resistance exercises to improve inspiratory capacity.

Emphasize a deep inhalation followed by a 3- to 5-second hold and then a relaxed exhalation.

Continue deep-breathing exercises postoperatively, with 6 to 10 consecutive deep breaths per hour, until the patient is ambulatory.

d. Begin deep, effective coughing as soon as the patient is alert and can cooperate.

Precaution: Adequately splint over the incision with your hand or a pillow to minimize incisional pain (see Figs. 19–19 and 19–20).

Encourage early mobilization, i.e., moving in bed, sitting up, and standing and walking.

*Refs. 2, 6, 9, 16–19, 22, 24, 26, 33, 34.

Treatment Goals

Plan of Care

Initiate modified postural drainage, *if necessary;* modified postural drainage may be necessary several days after surgery if secretions accumulate. If x-ray examinations and breath sounds are normal and if the patient can breathe deeply and cough effectively, postural drainage will not be necessary.

Precautions: Modify the postural drainage positions in which the patient is placed to minimize stress to the incision. The head-down position should be avoided until the chest tubes are removed. Take great care when turning the patient (use a logroll). Be sure to avoid traction or pressure on chest tubes and avoid percussion near the site of the incision.

e. Begin active exercises to the lower extremities, with emphasis on ankle pumping exercises on the first day after surgery.

Continue leg exercises until the patient is allowed out of bed and is ambulatory.

e. Maintain adequate circulation in the lower extremities to prevent deep vein thrombosis and pulmonary embolism.

f. Begin relaxation exercises to the shoulder area on the first postoperative day. These can include shoulder shrugging or shoulder circles.

Initiate active-assistive range of motion to the shoulders, being careful not to cause pain.

f. Maintain range of motion in the shoulders.

NOTE: Reassure the patient that gentle movements will not disturb the incision.

Progress to active shoulder exercises on the succeeding postoperative days to the patient's tolerance until full active range of motion has been achieved.

Precaution: In a patient with a lateral incision, to prevent dislodging a chest tube, limit shoulder flexion on the operated side to 90 degrees for several days until the chest tube is removed.

Treatment Goals	*Plan of Care*
g. Prevent postural defects.	g. Reinforce symmetric alignment and positioning of the trunk on the first postoperative day when the patient is in bed.
	NOTE: The patient will tend to lean toward the side of the incision.
	Instruct the patient in symmetric sitting posture when he or she is allowed to sit up in a chair or at the side of the bed.
h. Restore exercise tolerance.	h. Begin a progressive and graded ambulation or stationary cycling program as soon as chest tubes are removed and the patient is allowed to be out of bed.

B. Pneumonia

Pneumonia is an inflammation of the lung parenchyma, characterized by consolidation and exudation, and is caused by a bacterial or viral infection of the lower respiratory tract.[2,6,10,14] Chest physical therapy, when applied appropriately and in conjunction with antibiotics and respiratory modalities, can be an important aspect of the overall treatment of the patient with pneumonia. Patients with obstructive lung disease, such as chronic bronchitis, emphysema, and cystic fibrosis; patients who have recently undergone surgery; comatose patients; and patients with artificial airways are at particular risk for developing pneumonia. Whenever possible, chest physical therapy should be used to *prevent* pneumonia in these patients.

1. **Classifications of pneumonia**
   a. By anatomic location
      (1) *Bronchopneumonia*
          Inflammation of the bronchial tree.
          (a) Common in the postoperative patient, especially those with a history of chronic bronchitis.
          (b) Characterized by a productive cough and copious amounts of purulent sputum. There is usually no pain with deep inspirations or cough and no consolidation or pleural effusion.
          (c) Early and vigorous chest physical therapy is indicated.
      (2) *Acute lobar pneumonia*
          Inflammation of an entire lobe or lobes of the lung, often caused by a pneumococcal infection.
          (a) Not common today because of effective chemotherapy.
          (b) Characterized by fever and pulmonary consolidation; dyspnea; a nonproductive cough in the early stages; and acute and localized chest pain with deep inspiration or cough. In the later stage when pain and fever subside and consolidation decreases, the cough becomes productive and rust-colored sputum is produced.
          (c) In the early acute stage, chest physical therapy should consist of deep, relaxed breathing, localized to the area of involvement, to mobilize se-

cretions. The patient may be assisted with IPPB therapy during breathing exercises. Percussion should not be performed because of pain.

      (d) In the later stages, when the cough becomes productive and pain decreases, postural drainage with percussion may be performed over the affected areas.

  (3) *Segmental pneumonia*

    Localized to one or two small segment(s) of a lobe.

b. By causal organism

  (1) *Viral pneumonia*

    (a) Fever, dyspnea, and a chronic, nonproductive cough.

    (b) Chest physical therapy includes deep-breathing exercises.

    (c) Postural drainage with percussion is not undertaken because secretions are not present.

  (2) *Bacterial pneumonia*

    Often named by the organism: pneumococcus, streptococcus, or staphylococcus organisms.

    (a) Fever, dyspnea, tachypnea, and a productive cough with rust-colored sputum are present.

    (b) Chest physical therapy is initiated early and vigorously, with emphasis on deep breathing, postural drainage with percussion, and frequent positional changes.

2. General treatment goals and plan of care[2,6,10,14]

Treatment Goals	Plan of Care
a. Control the infection.	a. Use of appropriate medications, usually antibiotics.
b. Maintain or improve ventilation.	b. Deep-breathing exercises, localized to the area of involvement. Oxygen therapy and temporary use of mechanical ventilation. Frequent positional changes of the patient in and out of bed.
c. Mobilize secretions when consolidation and pain decrease and the cough becomes productive.	c. Postural drainage with percussion and vibration to the affected areas. Effective cough: ensure that the cough is deep and controlled. Assisted coughing techniques when necessary. Adequate humidification.

3. Precautions

a. Postural drainage should be used only for patients with increased mucus production, accumulated secretions, and a productive cough.

b. Percussion and vibration should not be used in patients who are experiencing a great deal of pleural pain with coughing or with deep inspirations.

C. Atelectasis

Atelectasis is a restrictive lung dysfunction in which lobes or segments of a lobe of a lung have collapsed. Lung tissue can collapse because of an increase in pressure on the lungs from a pneumothorax, hemothorax, or increased pleural fluid. Airway obstructions from abnormal secretions and tumor can cause collapse of lung tissue distal to the obstruction.[13,35]

1. Clinical picture and impairments/problems summarized

    a. Absent breath sounds over the collapsed lung area.

    b. Tachypnea; cyanosis.

    c. Decreased chest movement over the affected area.

    d. Atelectasis is prone to develop in patients with accumulated secretions and a poor cough after intubation and thoracic surgery.

2. General treatment goals and plan of care

Treatment Goals	*Plan of Care*
a. Reinflate collapsed areas of the lung.	a. Postural drainage with percussion and vibration for removal of secretions.
b. Increase inspiratory capacity.	b. Segmental breathing with emphasis over collapsed areas. Splinting to decrease pain if present. Initiate incentive spirometry with deep inspirations followed by a 3- to 5-second hold.

V. Summary

This chapter has provided general information on obstructive and restrictive lung disorders and diseases. The causes and physical impairments associated with obstructive diseases, such as chronic bronchitis, emphysema, asthma, cystic fibrosis, and bronchiectasis, have been outlined. The causes and physical impairments of patients with selected restrictive lung disorders and dysfunction have also been discussed. Particular emphasis has been placed on the respiratory and physical problems of the patient who has undergone thoracic or cardiac surgery.

An outline of the goals of treatment and guidelines and precautions for therapeutic management have also been given. The reader is referred to Chapter 19 for specific details of chest physical therapy procedures, such as breathing exercises, postural drainage, and exercises for thoracic mobility.

References

1. American Thoracic Society: Standards for the diagnosis and care of patients with chronic obstructive pulmonary disease (COPD) and asthma. Am Rev Respir Dis 136:225–244, 1987.
2. Brannon, FJ, et al: Cardiopulmonary Rehabilitation. Basic Theory and Application, ed 2. FA Davis, Philadelphia, 1993.
3. Busch, AJ, and McClements, JD: Effects of supervised home exercise program on patients with severe chronic obstructive pulmonary disease. Phys Ther 68:469, 1988.
4. Casciari, RJ, et al: Effects of breathing retraining in patients with chronic obstructive pulmonary disease. Chest 79:393, 1981.
5. Clough, P: Physical therapy management of the postthoracotomy shoulder. Cardiopulmonary Section Quarterly, American Physical Therapy Association 3:7, 1982.
6. Clough, P: Restrictive lung dysfunction. In Hillegass, EA, and Sadowsky, HS (eds): Essentials of Cardiopulmonary Physical Therapy. WB Saunders, Philadelphia, 1994.
7. Davis, PB: Cystic fibrosis. A major cause of obstructive airway disease in the young. In Cherniak, NS

(ed): Chronic Obstructive Pulmonary Disease. WB Saunders, Philadelphia, 1991.

8. DeCesare, JA, Graybill-Tucker, CA, and Gould, AL: Physical Therapy for the child with respiratory dysfunction. In Irwin, S, and Tecklin, JS (eds): Cardiopulmonary Physical Therapy, ed 3. Mosby-Year Book, St Louis, 1995.

9. Dull, JL, and Dull, WL: Are maximal inspiratory breathing exercises or incentive spirometry better than early mobilization after cardiopulmonary bypass? Phys Ther 63:655–659, 1983.

10. Glaskell, DV, and Webber, BA: The Brompton Hospital Guide to Chest Physiotherapy, ed 4. CV Mosby, St Louis, 1981.

11. Gless Williams, et al: Thoracic and Cardiovascular Surgery, ed 4. Appleton-Century-Crofts, New York, 1983.

12. Gold, W: Restrictive lung disease. Journal of the American Physical Therapy Association 48:455, 1968.

13. Hammon, WE: Pathophysiology in chronic pulmonary disease. In Frownfelter, D (ed): Physical Therapy and Pulmonary Rehabilitation, ed. 2. Year Book Medical Publishers, Chicago, 1987.

14. Hobson, L: Viral and bacterial pneumonia. In Frownfelter, D (ed): Chest Physical Therapy and Pulmonary Rehabilitation, ed 2. Year Book Medical Publishers, Chicago, 1987.

15. Hodgkins, JE: The scientific status of chest physiotherapy. Respiratory Care 26:657, 1981.

16. Horwath, PT: Care of the Cardiac Surgery Patient. Wiley, New York, 1984.

17. Howell, S, and Hill, JD: Chest physical therapy procedures in open heart surgery. Phys Ther 58:1205, 1978.

18. Imler, PC: Physical therapy for patients with cardiac, thoracic or abdominal conditions following surgery or trauma. In Irwin, S, and Tecklin, JS (eds): Cardiopulmonary Physical Therapy, ed 3. Mosby-Year Book, St Louis, 1995.

19. Kigin, CM: Physical therapy for the postoperative or traumatic injury patient. Phys Ther 61:1724, 1981.

20. Lane, C: COPD: The effects of training. Cardiopulmonary Section Quarterly, Journal of the American Physical Therapy Association 1:2, 1980.

21. Orenstein, DM, and Nixon, PA: Exercise in cystic fibrosis. In Torg, JS, Welsh, RP, and Shephard, RJ (eds): Current Therapy in Sports Medicine, Vol 2. BC Decker, Toronto, 1990.

22. Perlstein, MF, and Matthews, F: Cardiovascular and thoracic surgery. In Frownfelter, D (ed): Chest Physical Therapy and Pulmonary Rehabilitation, ed 2. Year Book Medical Publishers, Chicago, 1987.

23. Petty, T: Diagnosis and treatment of chronic obstructive pulmonary disease. Chest 97:1S–33S, 1990.

24. Sadowsky, HS: Thoracic surgical procedures, monitoring and support equipment. In Hillegass, EA, and Sadowsky, HS (eds): Essentials of Cardiopulmonary Physical Therapy. WB Saunders, Philadelphia, 1994.

25. Sawyer, E, and Clanton, TL: Improved pulmonary function and exercise tolerance with inspiratory muscle conditioning in children with cystic fibrosis. Chest 104:1490–1497, 1993.

26. Shaffer, T, Wolfson, M, and Bhutoni, VK: Respiratory muscle function, assessment and training. Phys Ther 61:1711, 1981.

27. Simpson, L: Effect of increased abdominal muscle strength on forced vital capacity and forced expiratory volume. Phys Ther 63:334, 1983.

28. Stein, M, and Cassara, FL: Preoperative pulmonary evaluation and therapy for surgery patients. JAMA 211:787, 1962.

29. Tecklin, J, and Holsclaw, D: Cystic fibrosis and the role of the physical therapist in its management. Phys Ther 53:386, 1973.

30. Tecklin, J, and Holsclaw, DS: Evaluation of bronchial drainage in patients with cystic fibrosis. Phys Ther 55:1081, 1975.

31. Tecklin, J: Pediatric Physical Therapy, ed 2. JB Lippincott, Philadelphia, 1994.

32. Tecklin, J: Physical therapy for children with chronic lung disease. Phys Ther 61:1774, 1981.

33. Thomas, JA, and McIntosh, JM: Are incentive spirometry, intermittent positive pressure breathing and deep breathing exercises effective in the prevention of postoperative pulmonary complications after upper abdominal surgery? A systematic overview and meta-analysis. Phys Ther 74:3–10, 1994.

34. Vraciu, JK, and Vraciu, R: Effectiveness of breathing exercises in preventing pulmonary complications following open heart surgery. Phys Ther 57:1367, 1977.

35. Whol, ME: Atelectasis. Journal of the American Physical Therapy Association 48:472, 1968.

Critical Analysis of Exercise Programs

When establishing a balanced exercise program, two concerns should be addressed: what goals and kinds of exercise make up a well-designed program, and do the proposed exercises safely and effectively accomplish the intended goals? The patient's condition; age; any previous injuries, deformities, or dysfunctions; and any potential risks from diseases should be taken into account.

Information about exercise routines is found everywhere: in popular magazines, in sports and health magazines and journals, on television and videotapes, and in books. These routines are designed by anyone, from the physician to the shapely movie personality, either with or without consultation from someone trained in safe exercise techniques. Well-intended people advise others in exercise routines to stretch, tone, strengthen, prepare for this or that, slim down, or build up. Most people have at one time or another become involved in a supervised exercise program, perhaps at school or at a health club or YMCA. Today, with the popularity of aerobic conditioning and exercise programs, many people with good intentions try various forms of exercising without adequate preparation or guidance only to find that they develop back, leg, or joint pain; muscle strain; or simple muscle soreness from overexercising or exercising improperly. They either become discouraged and feel defeated or they persevere and injure themselves. Why this happens can be traced to the observation that some of the exercises chosen are not biomechanically safe for the strength, flexibility, or endurance level of the person doing the exercise or they are the wrong exercises to accomplish the intended purpose.

This chapter is designed to help the reader critically analyze commonly used exercises in terms of how they can be used to evaluate problems and then be adapted to accomplish a desired goal. The intent is not to describe the ideal exercise protocol—there is no such thing—but to help the reader recognize that to accomplish an exercise goal as safely as possible, exercises have to be adapted to the individual level of the person involved and must be balanced with other appropriate exercise activities.

OBJECTIVES

After studying this chapter, the reader will be able to:

1 Look at specific activities used for testing and determine whether they are evaluating appropriate factors safely and correctly.

2 Look at specific exercises and determine whether they are safely accomplishing the intended goals.

3 Identify misconceptions in common exercises and exercise programs.

I. Designing an Exercise Program: Why Exercise?

There are many reasons for exercising. One general reason is to improve or maintain physical well-being. Other reasons could be to prepare for an upcoming athletic event, to relieve anxiety, to build up strength, to slim down, or simply to enjoy the social interaction with others who also exercise. Whatever the reason, it is important to choose an exercise program that best meets the needs of the individual. The intended purpose or goals for the program need to be identified. Common goals are to:

Increase strength (see Chapter 3).

Increase endurance (see Chapter 4).

Increase flexibility (see Chapter 5).

Increase skill in an activity. This includes coordination, agility, balance, timing, and speed.

II. Establishing a Baseline by Which Improvement Can Be Measured

Realistic testing can serve as a motivational tool when progress is noted. Therapists routinely use manual muscle testing[1,2,5,10] and other objective forms of testing such as tensiometer readings and isokinetic torque output readings to obtain a baseline of muscle strength. Goniometric measurements are taken to obtain an objective baseline of range of motion and flexibility.[9,10] These testing procedures have been standardized and are commonly accepted as reliable indicators of change and are not discussed here. Other tests commonly used in group exercise programs are not as objective and can be misleading. Tests used for physical fitness and conditioning programs need to be scrutinized by asking the following questions:

Does the test in fact test the intended muscle or function?

Will the test grade improve as muscle function improves?

Is the test biomechanically safe?

A. To Test Strength

A method typically used is to repeat a strenuous activity until the person tires. Improvement in strength is noted as the number of repetitions increases. This is a satisfactory method of testing strength as long as it is recognized that endurance is also related to the number of repetitions performed. In addition, the test should have various grades of difficulty so that the person can be tested at a level in which at least one repetition can be accomplished safely and correctly. Then, as ability improves, progress is noted first by the increased number of repetitions, then by progression to the next level of difficulty at a lower number of repetitions.

1. In popular exercise programs, strength is usually tested by having the subjects perform an activity that uses the body weight as resistance.

a. Sit-ups and straight-leg lifts are used to test abdominal muscle strength.

b. Push-ups and chin-ups are used to test arm muscle strength.

c. Prone-lying chest and leg lifts are used to test back muscle strength.

d. Jumping activities are used to test leg strength.

e. Throwing a ball is used to test arm strength.

2. If the above activities are not performed correctly, they can be biomechanically unsafe, or they may not test the muscles intended. If continued as an exercise, the appropriate muscle will not be strengthened, or supporting structures will be stressed and damaged. Also, if the person is unable to perform a test, progress cannot be measured in the early stages of the program; a simpler form of the test needs to be used. Other activities than the ones listed here may also be used to test strength, but just these will be analyzed to illustrate what needs to be considered when choosing an activity for testing.

a. *Analysis of sit-ups (curl-ups) as a test of abdominal strength*

(1) To isolate the abdominal muscles as trunk flexors, the person must curl the trunk, not arch the back, and needs to come up no further than clearing the thorax from the floor. Once the thorax clears the floor, the rest of the motion is hip flexion, using primarily the action of the hip flexor muscles.[4] If the back is allowed to arch, a sit-up is possible without abdominal muscle participation through reverse muscle action of the iliopsoas (hip flexor) muscles. In addition, fixating the feet and sitting up through full range encourage reverse muscle action of the hip flexors rather than contraction of the abdominals to perform the motion and, therefore, should not be performed when testing abdominal strength.

(2) The hips and knees are placed in a partially flexed position to release the stretch on the iliopsoas and sartorius muscles, allowing the pelvis to rotate posteriorly as the abdominals contract.[4] This does not inhibit or decrease the action of the hip flexors, as commonly believed.

(3) The position of the arms and hands will vary the resistance and thus the difficulty of the activity. The easiest position is with the hands alongside the trunk; next in difficulty is with the hands across the chest; the most difficult is with the hands behind the head. If the person cannot curl up with the arms at the side, note how far he or she can curl (just the head; the head and shoulders; or the head, shoulders, and upper thorax).

(4) The person should not use momentum by throwing the arms or jerking the trunk when curling up.

b. *Analysis of bilateral straight-leg raising as a test for abdominal strength*

(1) To test the strength of the abdominal muscles in this activity, the back must be kept flat and not allowed to arch.[4] If the back arches, it means the abdominal muscles are not strong enough to stabilize the pelvis and lumbar spine against the pull of the iliopsoas muscles. Raising and lowering of the legs can be accomplished purely by the iliopsoas muscles. Individuals with a hypermobile or unstable low-back region may complain of low back pain even if the pelvis is stabilized by the abdominals because of the shear force on the vertebrae from the pull of the psoas major muscle. This is an unsafe test or exercise for these people. Placing the hands under the pelvis to help stabilize assists the abdominals and thus eliminates the validity of this test.

(2) Maximum resistance from the legs occurs when the legs are horizontal (just off the floor).

(3) To use this activity as a test of lower abdominal strength, begin with the re-

sistance from the legs in the least stressful position by having both hips flexed to 90 degrees and the knees extended; instruct the person to maintain the back flat against the exercise mat as the legs are slowly lowered. When the back begins to arch, the angle of the legs with respect to the floor should be noted as the maximum resistance tolerated by the abdominals.[4]

(4) An alternative test for lower abdominal muscle strength is to perform repetitive posterior pelvic tilts while the extremities are held vertical at 90 degrees (see Fig. 15–26). The lower abdominals are required to lift the weight of the legs through the pelvic range of motion rather than stabilize against the long lever arm of the leg weight as in the straight-leg raise test. The test is scored by the number of repetitions completed.

c. *Analysis of push-ups as a test of upper extremity strength*

(1) To effectively perform a push-up, the individual must have not only adequate upper extremity strength but also strength in the trunk, hip, and knee muscles to maintain a rigid structure to lift. If the person can maintain the trunk and lower extremities in line, then the triceps and pectoralis major muscles become the prime movers in this activity. This activity can be modified to allow the knees to bend so that not as much weight needs to be lifted.

(2) The main problem with this activity as a test is that many people cannot maintain the isometric hold in the trunk and lower extremities or do not have enough strength in the arms to perform even one push-up. Therefore, it is difficult or impossible to measure progress in the weaker individual, and this becomes a test of only those who already are in a state of fitness. An easier level would be to have the subject perform push-ups against a wall or a bar placed at shoulder level. To progress the difficulty (resistance), move the feet further away from the wall or lower the bar, until eventually the subject is near horizontal and can be tested by pushing up from the floor.

(3) The position of the hands with respect to the shoulders also affects the difficulty of this activity. It is more difficult to perform with the hands placed directly under the shoulders than with the hands out to the side. For consistency, the hands should always be placed in the same position.

d. *Analysis of pull-ups or chin-ups as a test of strength in the arms*

(1) This test requires the shoulder extensor, elbow flexor, and finger flexor muscles to lift the body weight. If the activity is performed with the forearms supinated, elbow flexion primarily occurs from action of the biceps brachii muscle; if performed with the forearms pronated, the biceps lose their functional advantage and the flexion primarily is from action of the brachialis muscles.

(2) Either one of these positions is difficult for the less-trained individual; for those not able to perform even one pull-up, a simpler test needs to be defined. A modified pull-up requires use of an adjustable bar. The easiest position would be with the bar at the shoulder height of the subject. The person holds onto the bar and leans backward, keeping the feet on the floor; then he or she pulls the body toward the bar until the chest touches it and then lowers the body to the starting position. To progress the difficulty of the activity, the bar is lowered and the subject hangs the extended body below the bar, the feet remaining on the floor. As strength improves, the

subject can then be tested in the standard pull-up position in which the entire body weight is lifted.

e. *Analysis of prone chest lifts for testing strength of the back extensors*

   (1) With the subject lying prone and with the hands behind the head, he or she can extend the spine only if someone holds down the legs, or else both legs and thorax will lift from the floor, making it a difficult activity.

   (2) With the legs stabilized, most people are able to lift the chest off the floor; if the person is quite weak, the test is made easier by placing the arms alongside the trunk rather than behind the head. This activity requires strength in the neck and thorax extensors as well as scapula adductors to hold the upper spine and shoulders in position while the lower back is extending. Weakness in any one of these areas will make this test difficult.

f. *Analysis of prone leg lifts for testing strength of the back extensors*

   (1) To perform this test, someone must hold down the subject's thorax, or it too will lift from the floor, making it a difficult activity.

   (2) This activity requires strength in the hip extensor muscles to keep the hip extended. It may be difficult to perform if the back extensors are weak because of the long lever arm that the legs provide. For someone who cannot perform it, the resistance of the lever arm is reduced by flexing the knees.

g. *Analysis of vertical or long jumping activities as a test of leg strength*

   (1) To jump, the subject must have strength in the ankle plantarflexing gastrocnemius and soleus muscles.

   (2) Whether the subject is allowed to take a running start before jumping needs to be consistent, because running provides additional momentum to the body.

   (3) Testing should include all the antigravity muscles in the entire lower extremity such as performing step-ups. This test requires use of the quadriceps for knee extension and the gluteus maximus and hamstring muscles for hip extension. To prevent extraneous substitute movement when lifting the trailing leg, the heel and toe should leave the ground at the same time, and when placing the lead foot down while descending, the heel should be placed down before the toes. Also, to avoid the effects of momentum, excessive trunk movements should not be allowed.

h. *Analysis of throwing a ball as a test of arm strength*

   (1) This activity requires the subject to have not only strength in the upper extremity but also coordination of trunk and lower extremity motions as well as skill for proper timing in release and follow-through. An imbalance in muscle strength or flexibility of the shoulder and trunk could also affect proper execution. As a result, measurement of the distance a ball is thrown may not give a realistic picture of arm strength.

   (2) The subject should receive training for properly coordinated execution of this activity if it is going to be used as a measure of strength.

B. To Test Flexibility

The motion should be performed without bouncing; the subject should sustain the position for several seconds. Usually greater flexibility occurs after warming the tissues. For consistency and safety, 15 minutes of light activity should precede flexibility testing.

1. In popular exercise programs, flexibility is usually tested with one activity—forward bending and attempting to touch the toes while sitting or standing. Its purpose is to test back and hamstring muscle length. Because this activity is so commonly used both as a test and as an exercise, its faults will be discussed, with emphasis on alternative ways of measuring flexibility more accurately.

   a. Bending forward and touching the toes can be accomplished if the low back, hamstrings, or upper back is overflexible, even if one of the other regions is tight. Also, disproportionate length between arms, trunk, and legs can make this activity easier for some and more difficult for others. The only way to discern the region of tightness is to observe the contour of the back and position of the pelvis. This is usually not done in group exercise programs and usually can be performed only by someone trained to recognize the variations in movement of body parts. The common criterion is how close to the floor a person can get the fingers, not which region of the back or legs is most flexible or tight. The danger is that, if toe touching is used as an exercise, the overflexible region will continue to remain hypermobile in compensation for the tight region, so the less flexible part may not increase in flexibility. If the subject performs toe touching while long-sitting, there is a tendency to also flex the thoracic spine excessively.

   b. There is a belief that young people lose their flexibility because of a soft life and are no longer able to touch their toes.[11] In a classic article, this problem is discussed by Kendall, who states:

      > There is a period between the years of ten and fourteen when a majority of children may not be able to touch the toes with knees straight. The inability to successfully perform this feat apparently results from a discrepancy between leg and trunk length during this growth period. To encourage or force children to accomplish this feat may be harmful in the sense that undue flexibility of the back may result.[4]

      The long bones grow rapidly during puberty; the flexibility of muscles lags behind.[6] To excessively stretch the muscles when they are already undergoing lengthening because of the rapid growth of the bones may also lead to weakness in the overstretched muscles. Or possibly, the tendon may elongate and the muscle tissue may not adapt, resulting in a weakened muscle.[3]

   c. *To realistically test the flexibility of the hamstrings*
      The pelvis should be stabilized and one leg tested at a time. The subject should lie supine, keep one leg extended on the floor, and lift the other leg, keeping the knee straight to the point at which pulling is felt in the posterior thigh. This is termed unilateral straight-leg raising. The ankle is allowed to plantarflex to minimize the pull of the gastrocnemius muscle posterior to the knee.

   d. *To test the flexibility of the low-back region*
      (1) The subject flexes the hips and knees and "sits on the heels" with the legs under the trunk and places the arms overhead on the floor (Fig. 21–1A). Besides the back extensors, this also tests the flexibility of the quadriceps femoris, gluteus maximus, and shoulder extensor muscles.
      (2) If the person cannot perform the test because of knee pain, an alternative is to stabilize the pelvis by sitting with the legs crossed. He or she stabilizes the upper back in extension by placing both hands behind the head and bringing the elbows out to the side. He or she then bends forward, flexing only the low back, and does not allow the thorax to curl.

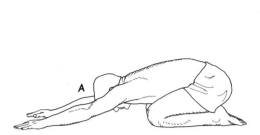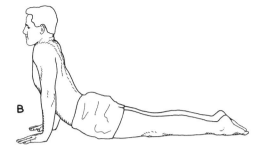

Figure 21–1. (*A*) Test position to observe flexibility in the low back, gluteus maximus, quadriceps femoris, and shoulder extensor muscles. (*B*) Test position to observe flexibility of trunk and hip flexors. The individual moves from position *A* to *B* and returns to position *A*. Smoothness of motion is observed in addition to flexibility.

2. Other tests of flexibility should also be performed, particularly to regions that tend to become tight from faulty postures or muscle imbalances. Suggestions include:
    a. *Flexibility of the scapular protractors*
       Test to determine whether or not the person can lie supine with hands behind the neck and then lower the elbows to the exercise mat.
    b. *Flexibility of the short upper neck extensors*
       Test to determine whether or not the person can lie supine and almost flatten the cervical spine against the exercise mat.
    c. *Flexibility of the trunk and hip flexors*
       Test to determine whether or not the person can lie prone, then press the thorax upward (as in a push-up) while keeping the pelvis on the floor. The hands should be placed under the shoulders, not out to the side or forward (Fig. 21–1B).
    d. *Flexibility of the ankle plantarflexors*
       Test to determine how far the person can dorsiflex the ankles while sitting with the knees extended.

C. To Test Endurance

1. To test local muscle endurance

High repetitions of a movement without resistance are repeated until the muscles fatigue. The number of repetitions is counted.

2. To test cardiovascular endurance

The simplest method is to have the patient perform a controlled repetitive total body activity for a period of time and to check the heart rate. As endurance for performing that activity improves, the resting heart rate will decrease. Because of potential physical risks, the reader is referred to the complete procedures and precautions discussed in Chapter 4.

3. In some testing procedures, speed is used to measure endurance.

Speed may have some effect on endurance, but skill, agility, and coordination are also necessary for performing an activity with speed, and, therefore, it is not a true indicator of endurance.

D. To Test Skill

Skill encompasses coordination, agility, balance, timing, and speed. Often, speed is used as the measure of ability to perform a skilled activity, implying that the faster one can do an activity, the more skillful he or she is. This is not easily resolved because it holds true for some skills but not others. Prior to testing, the person should have adequate instruction and should practice so that he or she knows what is required in the skill.

III. Establishing Realistic Goals

Review the results of the testing procedures to determine the goals of the exercise program. In other words, what muscles need to be strengthened, what regions need to be stretched, does endurance need to be improved, or do functional activities and skills need to be developed or improved? The goals then can give a realistic picture of what exercises need to be included in the program. Exercises used to accomplish the goals need to be scrutinized with the following questions:

Is the proposed exercise able to meet the goal?

If the exercise cannot meet the goal, what is the best and safest way to do so?

Are there any problems with the individual that will require special precautions or modifications of the exercises?

A. Exercises to Increase Strength

Many of the activities used to test strength can also be used as exercises to increase strength, either by increasing the number of repetitions or increasing the resistance. When weights are not available for increasing the resistance, as is the case in many group exercise classes, resistance can be increased by increasing the lever arm of the moving part. Examples of this include moving the arms farther away from the axis of motion, as occurs with the curl-up activity (Section I.A.2.a) or changing the angle of the body with respect to gravity as described with the pull-up activity (Section I.A.2.d).

1. Common errors in strengthening programs

a. The activity required is too strenuous.

Most exercises require that some muscles act as stabilizers for part of the body as other muscles do the intended motion. Either one or both muscle groups may be strengthened with the activity (the stabilizers, through isometric holding; the prime movers, through the isotonic activity). If any or all involved muscle groups are too weak to carry out the intended function, strain can occur. Begin exercises at a resistance level at which *all* the muscle groups can function properly. For example:

(1) *Bilateral straight-leg raising*

This activity requires that the abdominal muscles be strong enough to stabilize the pelvis (keep the back flat) against the pull of the hip-flexing iliopsoas muscles. The extended legs provide a long lever arm, and thus the hip flexors must contract forcefully to lift them. If the abdominals are not strong, they cannot stabilize against the strong hip flexor pull; the pelvis will be pulled anteriorly and the lumbar spine will arch. This causes back strain. If the subject cannot perform the straight leg-lowering test (see Section I.A.2.b) and keep the back flat, he or she should *not* perform straight leg-lifts as an exercise. Modifications include performing the straight leg-lowering activity only to the point at which the back begins to arch (as described in the testing section) or shortening the lever arm of the resistance by bending the hips and knees and doing knee-to-chest exercises. As strength in the stabilizing action of the abdominals improves, less and less bend in the hips and knees is used.

(2) *Scissors*

This activity is performed with the person supine and legs held extended several inches above the exercise mat. The person then abducts and adducts the legs, mimicking a scissors motion. The mechanics of the activity are similar to straight-leg raising in that it requires a strong abdominal muscle contraction to stabilize the pelvis against the pull of the hip flexor muscles, which, in this case, must contract strongly to hold the legs off the ground. There is no resistance to the abductor and adductor muscles, because the legs move parallel to the ground. To stabilize the pelvis, the person is often instructed to place the hands under the pelvis. This defeats the intent of strengthening the abdominals, because they then do not have to work. To modify this exercise if the person does not have strength in the abdominals to stabilize the pelvis (cannot perform the straight-leg-lowering test), begin with the hips flexed 90 degrees and perform the scissoring with the legs in this position of least resistance. Progress by gradually lowering the legs to an angle just before the back begins to arch and scissor in that position, keeping the back flat.

(3) *Curl-ups*

This activity requires that the abdominal muscles pull the thorax toward the pelvis to flex the lumbar spine. The abdominal muscles function only in the first third of the range of sitting up. Full sit-ups serve no additional benefit but may have some detrimental effects such as increasing intradiskal pressure, especially if the sit-up is performed with the hips and knees flexed.[7] If the abdominal muscles are not strong enough the person arches the back to lock the spine and lifts the trunk by flexing the pelvis on the femurs (reverse muscle action of the hip flexors).[5] If the subject cannot perform a curl-up with the hands behind the head, begin at an easier level, for example, with the arms at the side. If he or she still cannot curl up, instruct to begin strengthening by just lifting the head (this sets the abdominals), progress with lifting the head and shoulders (arms at the side of the trunk), then the head, shoulders, and thorax. Eventually progress by moving the arms across the thorax, then behind the neck. Do not allow momentum to occur by jerking of the arms. The jerking of the arms could also cause neck pain. This exercise should also include diagonal motions of the trunk to recruit the oblique abdominals muscles. See Chapter 15 for additional suggestions and precautions for strengthening the abdominal muscles.

b. There is an overemphasis on exercises that perpetuate faulty postures.

(1) *Flexion exercises*

Examples are exercise programs that primarily consist of flexion activities (curling the trunk, flexing the hips, flexing the shoulders, and protracting the scapulae) without including a comparable number of exercises to extend the trunk, hips, and shoulders and retract the scapulae. To have a well-balanced program, for every flexion exercise there should be an extension exercise in the same region. For example, for every curl-up exercise, perform a lumbar extension exercise; for every push-up exercise, perform a shoulder abduction, scapular retraction exercise; for every hip flexion exercise, perform a hip extension exercise (see Chapters 8 through 13 and 15 for exercise suggestions).

(2) *Inverted bicycle*

This popular exercise is performed by the subject starting supine, then rolling up onto the shoulders so that the feet are up in the air. The weight of the inverted body is borne on the upper thoracic and cervical spine (Fig. 21–2). Once in this position, the person attempts to balance while flexing and extending the lower extremities in a reciprocal manner. Problems with this exercise include the position itself, which places the head in a forward-head posture. The body weight becomes a strong stretch force into flexion on the upper thoracic region, a region that frequently tends to be flexed from faulty posture. The flexed and inverted position compresses the lungs and heart, decreasing their potential effectiveness. It is questionable whether the benefits of this exercise outweigh the combined negative effects on the neck and upper back posture, circulation, and respiration. To adapt this exercise to meet various goals:

(a) If balance is the purpose, use of a balance beam in the upright position is safer.

(b) If improving strength in the trunk muscles is the purpose, a number of exercises are safer and more effective, such as appropriately graded curl-ups, leg lifts, and prone extension. A *modified bicycle* exercise is another alternative. The subject lies supine and maintains a posterior pelvic tilt while the lower extremities are flexed and extended in a reciprocal pattern (Fig. 21–3). The amount of hip extension allowed depends on the strength of the abdominal muscles and their ability to stabilize the pelvis and keep the back flat.

(c) If relieving circulatory stress in the legs is the purpose, lying supine with just the legs elevated is safer. Various motions of the feet and legs can be added to the elevated legs.

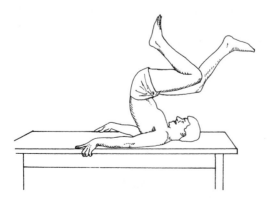

Figure 21–2. A poorly designed exercise. The inverted bicycle exercise accentuates the faulty postures of forward head and round upper back and compresses the thorax.

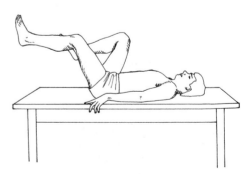

Figure 21–3. The modified bicycle exercise can be used to strengthen the abdominal muscles if the back is kept flat while the hips and knees are flexed and extended.

(d) If coordination of the lower extremities is the purpose, performing the modified bicycle is safer.

c. Differentiation is not made between the discomfort of fatigue and strain.

(1) This may result in damage to the part that is being strained. The cliché *"No pain, no gain"* is often misunderstood and, therefore, abuse to vulnerable tissue occurs. To develop strength, the muscles need to be exercised to near fatigue, but once fatigued, the subject begins substituting and therefore can strain a poorly stabilized part or develop an overuse syndrome. If straining occurs, the activity is either too difficult to begin with or the muscles involved are fatigued and can no longer perform the function properly.

(2) Another cliché is *"going for the burn."* With muscle fatigue comes a burning sensation. Some people design exercises that cause a "burn" with fewer repetitions to feel challenged. An example is "the crunch," an abdominal exercise in which the curl-up is combined with a dynamic posterior pelvic tilt (such as bringing knees to chest). It is important to note that the burn is experienced earlier in this activity than with a simple curl-up because both ends of the rectus abdominus are moving toward the center simultaneously and the muscle reaches active insufficiency. The demand on the muscle is in a nonfunctional range for most people so that, even though a burn is felt, the muscle is not being challenged in a range in which it can develop its strongest contraction (which would be mid-range). This is similar to exercising the hamstrings by extending the hip and simultaneously flexing the knee, an activity that causes hamstring cramping.

d. The original design of the exercise is altered or exaggerated.

This is sometimes done with the idea of progressing the exercise by making it more difficult. The result places stresses on supporting tissues. For example:

(1) *Fire hydrant*

This exercise, if performed properly, should strengthen the gluteus maximus muscle. The individual is on the hands and knees in the all-fours position, then extends and externally rotates the thigh, keeping the knee flexed. The subject should keep the pelvic tilt neutral (requiring good pelvic stability) and stop the motion at the end of the range of hip extension (Fig. 21–4). Instead, individuals often challenge themselves to see how high they can kick the leg, causing locking of the hip joint ligaments and capsule and the transmission of stresses to the sacroiliac (SI) joint and lumbar spine. If momentum is also a part of the exercise routine, the uncontrolled forces cause additional stress to the SI and lumbar spinal joints and sup-

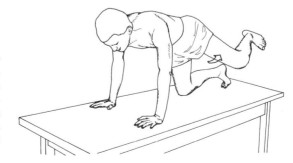

Figure 21–4. The fire hydrant is a potentially damaging exercise. To do this exercise correctly, the subject must stabilize the pelvis midrange, then stop the extension, external rotation motion when the hip has completed its range. The leg should not be "kicked as high as possible," or stress to the hip, sacroiliac joint, and lumbar spine results.

porting tissues. If a person exaggerates this motion or has SI or low-back problems, he or she should not perform this exercise.

(2) *Side-lying abduction*

For effective strengthening of the prime mover for hip abduction, the gluteus medius, the individual is side-lying, with the bottom leg flexed for stability. The top leg should be extended in line with the trunk and kept neutral to rotation; then abduction against gravity is performed. The range of abduction is approximately 30 to 45 degrees.[9] To exaggerate this exercise, individuals usually roll the pelvis backward and kick the leg upward with excessive flexion and rotation while abducting the hip. This substitutes action of the tensor fasciae latae muscle, which, through its attachment on the iliotibial band, can lead to increased tension in the band and lateral knee pain. Tightness in this muscle can lead to faulty mechanics when running and, therefore, should not be emphasized over the gluteus medius.

e. Some exercises are biomechanically unsafe because of the extreme forces placed on vulnerable structures.

It is worthy to repeat that many of the aforementioned exercises, when performed incorrectly or excessively, are unsafe or at least may precipitate musculoskeletal problems. Examples of exercises that are biomechanically unsafe include:

(1) *Bridging with full body weight on the head and feet*

To assume this bridging position, the individual begins supine with hips and knees flexed so that the feet are on the floor, and then lifts the body weight upward, pressing the head and feet into the floor so that only the head and feet are supporting the body. This position results in extreme pressure on the cervical spine and has the potential to cause damaging compressive forces on the disks.[8] This exercise has been safely modified by having the individual press upward with the feet and upper back (see Fig. 11–11), thus keeping all forces off the vulnerable neck structures yet obtaining the benefit of strengthening the hip and spinal extensors. The neck musculature is then exercised separately. Additional strengthening can be performed using a gym ball (see Fig. 15–19c).

(2) *Duck waddle and deep-knee bends*

Squatting full range so that the knees are maximally flexed, then shifting weight from side to side (often done with children when mimicking animals) causes excessive stress to the structures at the knee. The ligaments are strained, the menisci are maximally compressed between the tibia and femur, and the patella is maximally compressed against the femur, predisposing the articular cartilage to damaging forces. Highly trained or elite athletes and dancers may progressively work into this activity because of the requirement for performance,[8] but for the recreational athlete or untrained individual, the structures have not been appropriately trained to respond to the excessive forces. Modification of the exercise is to perform partial squats, going through only partial range of hip and knee flexion while standing, thus exercising the quadriceps femoris and hip extensor muscles through a functional range and in a functional pattern.

(3) In summary, any exercise can become biomechanically unsafe if performed by an individual unprepared for the activity or performed by an individual with predisposing musculoskeletal dysfunctions or diseases. (Refer to ap-

propriate chapters throughout this book for detailed explanations and precautions.)

2. Suggestions for a safe strengthening program

a. First, identify which muscle groups need strengthening and choose exercises that, when properly executed, will strengthen the appropriate muscles.

b. Begin each exercise at a level safe for the individual. If straining is necessary to complete the exercise, it is probably too difficult and should be simplified with less exercise resistance.

c. When fatigue occurs, do not push to the point of straining.

d. Balance each exercise between antagonistic muscle groups and include each region of the body.

e. Perform each exercise in a biomechanically correct manner so that the muscles to be strengthened are performing the prime motion or the stabilization.

f. If there is poor posture and flexibility, strengthen the muscles antagonistic to the tight muscles.

g. Warm up the muscles to be strengthened with light repetitive activity for 15 minutes. If antagonistic muscles are tight, stretch them after the warm-up, prior to strengthening, so that the full range of motion can be used during the resistance exercises. Finish the strengthening program by again stretching each muscle group.

h. The speed of the motion can vary and will depend on the purpose of the exercise. (See Chapter 3 for discussion on specificity of exercises.)

B. Exercises to Increase Flexibility

1. Common errors in flexibility programs

a. Improper emphasis

Stretching routines may emphasize regions that are already flexible and neglect regions that are tight from faulty postures. Total body stretching, such as toe touches, may maintain or overstretch a mobile area and not affect a tight area and therefore not satisfactorily meet the goal. See discussion in the testing section on toe touching (Section II.B).

b. Flexibility imbalances

In areas in which there is a strength imbalance between antagonistic muscle groups, there tends to also be a flexibility imbalance. Just as flexion exercises tend to be overemphasized in strengthening programs, extensors tend to be overstretched in flexibility programs.

c. Use of ballistic stretch

Ballistic stretching can be dangerous. It can cause tearing of soft tissue and may increase tone in the muscles to be stretched.

d. Exercise pain

The phrase *"No pain, no gain"* is often used inappropriately as the guideline for intensity of stretch. An effective stretching or flexibility routine should not cause pain or excessive stress to tissues. For an effective stretch, there should be a "pulling" sensation in the tight tissue. A low-intensity prolonged stretch is more effective and longer lasting than a high-intensity quick stretch. Refer to Chapter 5 for additional information.

e. Faulty biomechanics

Some popular stretching exercises do not respect the biomechanics of the region. Whenever abnormal stresses are placed on supporting tissue or joint structures, the exercise should be modified. Some examples include:

(1) *Locking the intermediate joint with forward bending or push-ups*

When performing any forward-bending exercises, individuals have a tendency to lock their knees. This stresses the posterior capsule and anterior cruciate ligaments and over time can lead to genu recurvatum. The knees should be slightly bent, or unlocked, whenever performing forward-bending exercises. Similarly, with push-ups, locking the elbow stresses the joint.

(2) *Hurdler's stretch*

When the hurdler's stretch position is assumed for the purpose of stretching the hamstring and rectus femoris muscles, excessive stress is placed on the medial capsule and medial collateral ligaments of the knee that is placed behind the individual. The hurdler's position can effectively be used to stretch the rectus femoris muscle as described in Chapter 11 (see Fig. 11–2), but alternative positions are recommended for hamstring stretches, such as unilateral straight-leg raising. By lying supine and lifting one lower extremity to the point of stretch, the individual can support the knee with the hands. An effective stretch can occur even with the knee slightly flexed.

(3) *Gastrocsoleus stretch*

An easy and apparently effective way to stretch the plantarflexors is by standing with the leg to be stretched placed behind the individual. The individual then shifts the weight forward onto the leg in front, keeping the heel of the hind foot on the floor. If the knee is kept straight, the gastrocnemius is stretched; if the knee is bent, the soleus is stretched. The major problem occurs when this exercise is performed without good arch support or barefooted and when the foot is turned slightly outward. The forces are transmitted to the ligamentous structures supporting the arch and may lead to a hypermobile foot. When performing this stretch, keep the shoes on and modify this exercise by turning the foot inward prior to the stretch; this will lock the bones of the foot and provide stability of the arch. (See Chapter 13 for additional information.)

2. Suggestions for a safe flexibility program

a. If a subject is excessively mobile in a segment or region of the body, selectively stretching tight structures is safer than total body stretching. Isolate stretching of the hamstring, the low back, and the upper back muscles as described in the testing section (Section II.B). Other suggestions for self-stretching techniques are found for each region of the body in Chapters 8 through 13 and in Chapter 15.

b. Maintain a balance in flexibility between antagonistic muscle groups. If there is decreased flexibility because of poor posture, emphasize stretching the tight muscles. Typically, they are the hip flexors, trunk flexors, shoulder flexors, and scapular protractors.

c. Use a sustained stretch rather than bouncing or ballistic stretches. Maintain each position approximately 10 seconds or longer.

d. Stretching (flexibility exercises) should be used prior to and after a strengthening or conditioning program.

e. Do not stress joints and ligaments at the end of the range; protect vulnerable joints.

f. Warm up the tissues prior to stretching with gentle rhythmic activities.

C. Exercises to Increase Endurance

1. Suggestions for a safe muscle endurance program

a. For local muscle endurance, an exercise is performed with many repetitions and minimal resistance to the point of muscle fatigue. When signs of fatigue occur, do not push to the point of straining the supporting tissue.

b. Increased muscle endurance is a by-product of increased strength when repetitions of motion are used.

c. Do not sacrifice musculoskeletal safety for the sake of endurance. Maintain sound biomechanical principles.

2. Suggestions for a safe cardiovascular endurance program

Chapter 4 describes aerobic conditioning principles and procedures. Specific precautions and suggestions for medical conditions are also explained.

a. Establish the target heart rate and maximum heart rate.

b. Warm up gradually for 5 to 10 minutes; include stretching and repetitive motions at slow speeds, gradually increasing the effort.

c. Increase the pace of the activity so that the target heart rate can be maintained for 20 to 30 minutes. Examples include fast walking, running, bicycling, swimming, cross-country skiing, and aerobic dancing.

d. Cool down for 5 to 10 minutes with slow, total body repetitive motions and stretching activities.

e. The aerobic activity should be three to five times per week.

f. To avoid injuries from stress, use appropriate equipment, such as correct footware, for proper biomechanical support. Avoid running, jogging, or aerobic dancing on hard surfaces such as asphalt and concrete.

g. To avoid overuse syndromes to structures of the musculoskeletal system, proper warm-up and stretching of muscles to be used should be performed. Progression of activities should be within the tolerance of the individual. Overuse commonly occurs when there is an increase in time or effort without adequate rest (recovery) time between sessions. Increase repetitions or time by no more than 10 percent per week.[8] If pain begins while exercising, heed the warning and reduce the stress.

h. Individualize the program of exercise. All people are not at the same fitness level and therefore cannot perform the same exercises. Any one exercise has the potential to be detrimental if attempted by someone not able to execute it properly. Begin at a safe level for the individual and progress as the individual meets the desired goals.

D. Exercises to Increase Skill

1. Skill includes coordination, agility, balance, timing, and speed.

2. The skill needs to be identified and analyzed and broken into the components that make up the action. The action may require strength, flexibility, and endurance as a base before the skill can be properly executed. Exercises that replicate the motion, velocity, and position then follow. Ultimately, the skill must be practiced for timing and form.

E. Re-evaluate at Frequent Intervals to See if the Baseline Has Changed

Use the same testing procedures for consistency in interpreting the results. If there is no change, either the exercises are not being carried out properly or they are not appropriate. As improvement occurs, the satisfaction of improved function is immeasurable.

IV. Summary

Popular exercise programs may be the precipitating factor in musculoskeletal complaints, not because exercising should not be done, but because the exercises are performed improperly or for the wrong purpose. This chapter has outlined an approach for analyzing and choosing safe testing and exercising procedures and has cited several commonly misunderstood and misused tests and exercises as examples.

References

1. Clarkson, HM, and Gilewich, GB: Musculoskeletal Assessment: Joint Range of Motion and Manual Muscle Strength. Williams & Wilkins, Baltimore, 1989.
2. Daniels, L, and Worthingham, C: Muscle Testing Techniques of Manual Examination, ed 5. WB Saunders, Philadelphia, 1986.
3. Gossman, M, Sahrmann, S, and Rose, S: Review of length associated changes in muscle. Phys Ther 62:1799, 1982.
4. Kendall, F: A criticism of current tests and exercises for physical fitness. Journal of the American Physical Therapy Association 45:187, 1965.
5. Kendall, F, McCreary, E, and Provance, PG: Muscles: Testing and Function, ed 4. Williams & Wilkins, Baltimore, 1993.
6. Kendall, H, and Kendall, F: Normal flexibility according to age groups. J Bone Joint Surg Am 30:690, 1948.
7. Liemohn, W, Snodgrass, L, and Sharpe, G: Unresolved controversies in back management—A review. Journal of Orthopaedic and Sports Physical Therapy 9:239, 1988.
8. Lubell, A: Potentially dangerous exercises: Are they harmful to all? Phys Sports Med 17:187, 1989.
9. Norken, C, and White, DJ: Measurement of Joint Motion: A Guide to Goniometry. FA Davis, Philadelphia, 1985.
10. Palmer, ML, and Epler, M: Clinical Assessment Procedures in Physical Therapy. JB Lippincott, Philadelphia, 1990.
11. Schultz, P: Flexibility: Day of the static stretch. The Physician and Sports Medicine, 7:109, 1979.

Glossary

abruptio placentae. Premature detachment of the placenta from the uterus

accessory movement. Movement within a joint and surrounding soft tissues that is necessary for normal range of motion but cannot be voluntarily performed

accommodating resistance exercise. A term used synonymously with **isokinetic exercise**

active inhibition. A type of stretching exercise in which there is reflex inhibition and subsequent elongation of the contractile elements of muscles

adaptation. The ability of an organism to change over time in response to a stimulus

adenosine triphosphate (ATP). A high-energy compound from which the body derives energy

adhesions. Abnormal adherence of collagen fibers to surrounding structures during immobilization, following trauma, or as a complication of surgery, which restricts normal elasticity of the structures involved

aerobic exercise. Submaximal, rhythmic, repetitive exercise of large muscle groups, during which the needed energy is supplied by inspired oxygen

aerobic system. An aerobic energy system in which ATP is manufactured when food is broken down

airway resistance. The resistance to the flow of air in the lungs offered by the bronchioles

amniotic fluid. The liquid contained in the amniotic sac. The fetus floats in the fluid, which serves as a cushion against injury and helps maintain a constant fetal body temperature

anaerobic exercise. Exercise that occurs without the presence of inspired oxygen

anaerobic glycolytic system (lactic acid system). An anaerobic energy system in which ATP is manufactured when glucose is broken down to lactic acid

apnea. Cessation of breathing

apneusis. The cessation of breathing during the inspiratory phase of respiration

arteriosclerosis obliterans (ASO). See **arteriosclerotic vascular disease**

arteriosclerotic vascular disease (ASVD). Progressive narrowing, loss of elasticity, fibrosis, and eventual occlusion of the large and middle-sized arteries, usually in the lower extremities

arteriovenous oxygen difference (a-$\bar{v}O_2$ difference). The difference between the oxygen content of arterial and venous blood

arthritis. Inflammation of the structures of a joint

arthrodesis. Surgical fusion of bony surfaces of a joint with internal fixation such as pins,

727

nails, plates, and bone grafts; usually done in cases of severe joint pain and instability in which mobility of the joint is a lesser concern

arthroplasty. Any reconstructive joint procedure, with or without a joint implant, designed to relieve pain and/or restore joint motion

arthroscopy. Examination of the internal structures of a joint by means of an endoscopic viewing apparatus inserted into the joint

arthrotomy. Surgical incision into a joint

asthma. An obstructive lung disease seen in young patients, associated with a hypersensitivity to specific allergens and resulting in bronchospasm and difficulty in breathing

atelectasis. Collapse or incomplete expansion of the lung

ATP-PC system. An anaerobic energy system in which adenosine triphosphate (ATP) is manufactured when phosphocreatine (PC) is broken down

atrophy. The wasting or reduction of size of cells, tissues, organs, or body parts

auscultation. Listening to heart or lung sounds within the body, usually with a stethoscope

balance. The ability to maintain the body's center of gravity over the base of support

bradypnea. Slow rate of respiration; depth either shallow or normal

bronchiectasis. A chronic obstructive lung disease characterized by dilation and repeated infection of medium-sized bronchioles

Buerger's disease. See **thromboangiitis obliterans**

bursitis. Inflammation of a bursa

capsular pattern. A pattern of limitation, characteristic for a given joint, that indicates that a problem exists with that joint

cardiac output. The volume of blood pumped from a ventricle of the heart per unit of time; the product of heart rate and stroke volume

cardiovascular endurance. The ability of the lungs and heart to take in and transport adequate amounts of oxygen to the working muscle, allowing activities that involve large muscle masses to be performed over long periods of time

chondromalacia patellae. Deterioration of the articular cartilage at the posterior aspect of the patella

chondroplasty. A débridement procedure to repair joint cartilage, usually at the patellofemoral joint; also called abrasion arthroplasty

chronic bronchitis. An inflammation of the bronchi that causes an irritating, productive cough that lasts up to 3 months and recurs over at least 2 consecutive years

chronic obstructive pulmonary disease (COPD). A term used to describe a variety of chronic lung conditions such as chronic bronchitis, emphysema, and peripheral airway disease

chronic pain syndrome. Used to describe patients with long-standing low back pain who have developed illness behavior and hopelessness. There is no longer a direct relationship between the pain and the apparent disability, and treatment of the painful symptoms usually does not change the condition. The patient may require psychological and sociological intervention and behavior modification techniques

circuit training. A training program that uses selected exercises or activities performed in sequence

closed-chain exercise. Exercise in which the distal end of the segment is fixed to a supporting surface as the trunk and proximal segments move over the fixed part. This includes functional exercises, especially for the lower extremities, in which the foot is stabilized on the ground and the muscles control the hips, knees, and ankles in activities such as squatting, climbing steps, and getting in and out of a chair

clubbing, digital. Broadening or thickening of the soft tissues of the terminal phalanges of the fingers and toes, often seen in persons with chronic pulmonary disease

compression dressing. A sterile bandage applied around or over a new surgical incision to compress the wound site and promote healing

concentric exercise. An overall shortening of the muscle occurs as it generates tension and contracts against resistance

conditioning. An augmentation of the energy capacity of the muscle through an exercise program

continuous training. A training program that uses exercise over a given duration without rest periods

contracture. Shortening or tightening of the skin, fascia, muscle, or joint capsule that prevents normal mobility or flexibility of that structure

contusion. Bruising from a direct blow, resulting in capillary rupture

coordination. Using the right muscles at the right time with correct intensity. Coordination is the basis of smooth and efficient movement, which often occurs automatically

crackles. Fine or coarse lung sounds heard with a stethoscope primarily during inspiration and caused by movement of secretions in the small airways of the lungs; also referred to as **rales**

cumulative trauma disorder. Musculoskeletal symptoms from excessive or repetitive motion causing connective tissue or bony breakdown. Initially, the inflammatory response from the microtrauma is subthreshold but eventually builds to the point of perceived pain and resulting dysfunction. Syndromes include shin splints, carpal tunnel, bursitis, tendinitis, cervical tension, thoracic outlet, tennis elbow, and marching fracture. Also known as cumulative trauma syndrome, repetitive strain injury, and **overuse syndrome**

cyanosis. A bluish appearance of skin and mucous membranes due to insufficient oxygenation of the blood

cystic fibrosis. A genetically-based disease that involves malfunction of the exocrine glands and leads to chronic lung infections and pancreatic dysfunction

deconditioning. A change that takes place in cardiovascular, neuromuscular, and metabolic functions as a result of prolonged bed rest or inactivity

degenerative joint disease (DJD). See **osteoarthritis**

delayed-onset muscle soreness (DOMS). Exercise-induced muscle tenderness or stiffness that occurs 24 to 48 hours after vigorous exercise

derangement (disk protrusion). Any change in the shape of the nucleus pulposus of the intervertebral disk that causes it to protrude beyond its normal limits

disability. The inability to undertake normal activities of daily living (ADL) as a result of physical, mental, social, or emotional impairments

diagnosis. The recognition or the determination of the cause and nature of a pathologic condition

dislocation. Displacement of a part, usually the bony partners within a joint

distensibility. The ability of an organ or tissue to be stretched out or enlarged

distraction. A pulling apart or separation of joint surfaces

dorsal clearance. Surgical removal of diseased synovium from the extensor tendons of the fingers and wrist

dynamic stabilization. An isometric or stabilizing contraction of trunk or proximal girdle muscles to maintain control of the functional position in response to imposed fluctuating forces through the moving extremities

dynamometer. A device that quantitatively measures muscle strength

dysfunction. A loss of function as a result of adaptive shortening of soft tissues and loss of mobility

dyspnea. Shortness of breath; labored, distressed breathing

eccentric exercise. Overall lengthening of the muscle occurs as it develops tension and contracts to control motion against the resistance of an outside force; negative work is done

efficiency. The ratio of work output to work input

elasticity. The ability of soft tissue to return to its original length after a stretch force has been released

embolus. A thrombus, or clot of material, that has been dislodged and transported in the blood stream from a larger to a smaller vessel, resulting in occlusion of the vessel

emphysema. A chronic obstructive pulmonary disease that is characterized by inflammation, thickening, and deterioration of the respiratory bronchioles and alveoli

end-feel. The quality of feel the evaluator experiences when passively applying pressure at the end of the available range of motion

endurance. The ability to resist fatigue

endurance, general (total body). The ability of an individual to sustain low-intensity exercises, such as walking, jogging, or climbing, over an extended period

endurance, muscular. The ability of a muscle to perform repeated contractions over a prolonged period

energy systems. Metabolic systems involving a series of chemical reactions resulting in the formation of waste products and the manufacture of adenosine triphosphate (ATP). The systems include the ATP-PC (adenosine triphosphate-phosphocreatine) system, the anaerobic glycolytic system, and the aerobic system

ergometer. An apparatus, such as a stationary bicycle or treadmill, used to quantitatively measure the physiologic effects of exercise

exercise bouts. The number of sets of a repetition maximum performed during each exercise session

exercise duration. The total number of days, weeks, or months during which an exercise program is performed

exercise frequency. The number of times exercise is performed within a day or within a week

exercise load. The amount of weight used as resistance during an exercise

exercise prescription. Individualized exercise program involving the duration, frequency, intensity, and mode of exercise

expiratory flow rate. The volume of air exhaled per unit of time

expiratory reserve volume (ERV). The maximum amount of air an individual can exhale after a normal, relaxed expiration

extension bias. Describes the preferred position of spinal extension (lordosis) in which the patient's symptoms are decreased. Usually the symptoms increase in spinal flexion

extensor lag. The range of active knee extension is less than the range of passive extension of the knee, usually the result of inhibition or dysfunction of the quadriceps mechanism; synonymous with **quadriceps lag**

extrapment. A tissue trapped on the outside of a structure unable to assume its normal relationship. When a meniscoid tissue becomes trapped outside a zygapophyseal joint as the surfaces slide together, the motion is blocked and tension is placed on the capsular tissue

extrusion. A protrusion of the nucleus pulposus of the intervertebral disk in which the nuclear material ruptures through the outer annulus and lies under the posterior longitudinal ligament

fast-twitch (FT) fiber. A skeletal muscle fiber with a fast reaction time that has a high anaerobic capacity and is suited for phasic muscle activity

fatigue, general (total body). The diminished response of a person during prolonged physical activity, such as walking or jogging, that may be due to a decrease in blood sugar (glucose) levels, a decrease in glycogen stores in muscle and liver, or a depletion of potassium, especially in the elderly

fatigue, local (muscle). A diminished response of the muscle due to a decrease in energy stores, insufficient oxygen, and a buildup of lactic acid; protective influences from the central nervous system; or a decrease in the conduction of impulses at the myoneural junction

fetus. The developing embryo in the uterus from 7 to 8 weeks after fertilization until birth

fitness. A general term indicating a level of cardiovascular functioning that results in heightened energy reserves for optimum performance and well-being

flat low-back posture. A posture characterized by decreased lumbosacral angle, decreased lumbar lordosis, and posterior tilting of the pelvis

flexibility. The ability of muscle and other soft tissue to yield to a stretch force

flexibility exercise. A general term used to describe exercises performed by a person to passively or actively elongate soft tissues without the assistance of a therapist

flexion bias. Describes the position of spinal flexion in which the patient's symptoms are lessened. Usually the symptoms are provoked in spinal extension

forward head posture. A posture characterized by an increased flexion of the lower cervical and upper thoracic regions, increased extension of the occiput on the first cervical vertebra, and increased extension of the upper cervical vertebrae

fremitus, vocal or tactile. The vibration that can be felt on the chest wall as a person speaks

functional excursion. The distance a muscle can shorten after it has been stretched to its maximum length

functional exercise. Exercise that mimics functional activities but is performed in a controlled manner

functional limitation. A limitation from an impairment that is not disabling yet interferes with normal function

functional position. The position or range of motion in which the patient experiences the greatest comfort or least amount of stress on the tissues in the region. It may also be referred to the **resting position** or neutral position. The position is not static and may change as the patient's condition changes

functional residual capacity. The amount of air remaining in the lungs after a resting expiration

functional skills. Motor skills that are necessary to independently perform activities or tasks of daily living; refined movements requiring coordination, agility, balance, and timing

ganglion (pl., ganglia). A ballooning of the wall of a joint capsule or tendon sheath

gestation. The period of development from the time of fertilization to birth (pregnancy)

glossopharyngeal breathing. A type of breathing exercise used to increase a patient's inspiratory capacity by gulping in air

glycogen. The storage form of carbohydrates in the body, found predominantly in the muscles and the liver

handicap. The social disadvantage resulting from an impairment or disability that prevents or limits persons in their occupation, environment, or social setting

hemarthrosis. Bleeding into a joint, usually from severe trauma

hemoptysis. The expectoration of blood or blood-streaked sputum from the bronchial tree and lungs

hemothorax. A collection or effusion of blood in the pleural cavity

herniation. Abnormal protrusion of an organ or other body structure through a defect or natural opening in a covering membrane, muscle, or bone

hyperplasia. An increase in the number of fibers or cells

hypertrophy. An increase in the cross-sectional size of a fiber or cell

hyperventilation. An increase in the rate and depth of respiration above a level necessary for normal ventilatory function

impairment. Any loss or abnormality of psychological, physiologic, or anatomic structure or function. It limits or changes an individual's ability to perform a task or activity

incentive spirometry. A form of inspiratory muscle training in which the patient inhales maximally and sustains the inspiration

inspiratory capacity. The amount of air a person can inhale after a resting expiration

inspiratory reserve volume (IRV). The maximum amount of air a person can inhale after a relaxed inspiration

inspiratory resistance training. A method of strengthening the muscles of inspiration

intermittent claudication. The cramping of muscles after short periods of exercise; often seen in patients with occlusive arterial disorders

intermittent traction. A traction force that is alternately applied and released at frequent intervals, usually in a rhythmic pattern

interval training. A training program that alternates bouts of heavy work with periods of rest or light work

intrinsic muscle spasm. The prolonged contraction of a muscle in response to the local circulatory and metabolic changes that occur when a muscle is in a continued state of contraction

intubation. Insertion of a tube, such as an endotracheal or nasogastric tube, into the body

involution. The progressive contraction of the uterus following childbirth, returning the organ to near its prepregnant size

isokinetic exercise. A form of active-resistive exercise in which the speed of movement of the limb is controlled by a preset rate-limiting device

isometric (static) exercise. A form of exercise in which tension develops in the muscle but no mechanical work is performed. There is no appreciable joint movement, and the overall length of the muscle remains the same

isotonic (dynamic) exercise. A form of exercise involving the concentric or eccentric muscular contractions that result in movement of a joint or body part against a constant load

joint mobilization. Passive traction and/or gliding movements applied to joint surfaces that maintain or restore the joint play normally allowed by the capsule, so that the normal roll-slide joint mechanics can occur as a person moves

joint play. Capsular laxity or elasticity that allows movements of the joint surfaces. The movements include distraction, sliding, compression, rolling, and spinning

kypholordotic posture. A posture characterized by an exaggerated thoracic kyphosis and lumbar lordosis, and usually forward head

kyphosis. A posterior convexity in the spinal column. A posterior curve is primary because it is present at birth and remains in the thoracic and sacral regions of the spine

kyphotic posture. A posture characterized by an exaggerated posterior curvature of the thoracic spine; syn: **humpback, round back**

labor. The physiologic process by which the uterus contracts and expels the products of conception after 20 or more weeks of gestation

load-resisting exercise. Any exercise in which a load or a weight producing an external force resists the internal force generated by a muscle as it contracts

lobectomy. Surgical removal of a lobe of a lung

lordosis. An anterior convexity in the spinal column. An anterior curve is secondary or compensatory and occurs in the cervical and lumbar spinal regions as the spine of a young child adapts to the upright position

lordotic posture. A posture characterized by an increase in the lumbosacral angle, causing an increased lumbar lordosis, anterior pelvic tilt, and hip flexion

lung compliance. Refers to the distensibility or elastic recoil of lung tissue

lymphedema. Excessive accumulation of extravascular and extracellular fluid in tissue spaces

manipulation. A passive movement using physiologic or accessory motion, which may be applied with a thrust or when the patient is under anesthesia. The patient cannot prevent the motion

mastectomy. Removal of a breast

maximal aerobic power (max $\dot{V}o_2$). The maximal volume of oxygen consumed per unit of time

maximal heart rate reserve (HRR). The difference between the resting heart rate and the maximal heart rate

mediastinal shift. Asymmetric positioning of the trachea, palpable at the suprasternal notch

meniscectomy. An intra-articular procedure at the knee by which the meniscus (fibrocartilage) is removed surgically

metabolic equivalent (MET). The amount of oxygen required per minute under quiet resting conditions; equal to 3.5 milliliters of oxygen consumed per kilogram of body weight per minute

mobilization. Passive stretching movements performed by a therapist at a speed slow enough that the patient can stop the movement

multiple-angle isometrics. The application of resistance at multiple points in the ROM to isometric muscle contractions

muscle-setting exercise. A form of isometric exercise but one not performed against any appreciable resistance; gentle static muscle contractions used to maintain mobility between muscle fibers and to decrease muscle spasm and pain

muscle soreness, acute. Pain or tenderness in muscle that occurs during strenuous exercise as the muscle fatigues

muscle soreness, delayed-onset. See **delayed-onset muscle soreness**

muscle spasm. See **intrinsic muscle spasm**

non–weight-bearing bias. Describes the preferred position in which the patient's symptoms are lessened when in non–weight-bearing positions such as lying down or in traction or when reducing spinal pressure by leaning on the upper extremities (using arm rests to unweight the trunk), by leaning the trunk against a support, or when in a pool. The condition is considered gravity sensitive because the symptoms are worsened when standing, walking, running, coughing, or similar activities that increase spinal pressure

occlusion. Closure or obstruction of a vessel such as an artery or vein

open-chain exercise. Exercise in which a distal segment of the body moves freely in space

orthopnea. Difficulty breathing while lying supine

osteoarthritis (degenerative joint disease). A chronic degenerative disorder primarily affecting the articular cartilage with eventual bony overgrowth at the margins of the joints

osteoporosis (bone atrophy). A condition of bone that leads to a loss of bone mass, a narrowing of the bone shaft, and widening of the medullary canal

osteotomy. The surgical cutting and realignment of bone to correct deformity and reduce pain

outcome measure. An activity that is objectively documented and is part of the goal for therapeutic intervention

overload. Stressing the body or parts of the body to levels above that normally experienced

overpressure. A stretch force applied to soft tissues at the end of the ROM

overstretch. A stretch beyond the normal range of motion of a joint and the surrounding soft tissues

overtraining. A term synonymous with **overwork**

overuse syndromes. See **cumulative trauma disorders**

overwork. A phenomenon that causes temporary or permanent deterioration of strength as a result of exercise, most often observed clinically in patients with nonprogressive lower motor neuron diseases who participate in excessively vigorous resistance exercise programs. Also known as **overtraining**

oxygen deficit. The time period during exercise in which the level of oxygen consumption is below that necessary to supply all the ATP required for the exercise

oxygen transport system ($\dot{V}o_2$). Composed of stroke volume, heart rate, and arterial–mixed venous oxygen difference

pallor. Chalky white appearance or blanching of the skin

paresthesia. Abnormal sensation perceived as burning or prickling

pathologic fracture. A fracture that occurs as the result of minor stresses to bone already weakened by disease (osteoporosis)

pendulum (Codman's) exercises. Self-mobilization techniques that use the effects of gravity to distract the humerus from the glenoid fossa and gentle pendulum motions to move the joint surfaces

percussion. A technique used with postural drainage to mobilize secretions by mechanically dislodging viscous or adherent secretions in the lungs

percussion, mediate. A technique used to assess the air to solid ratio in the lungs

peripheral airway disease. An early form of obstructive lung disease characterized by inflammation, fibrosis, and narrowing of the small airways.

phlebitis. Inflammation of a vein

phosphocreatine (PC). Creatine phosphate; an energy-rich compound that plays a critical role in providing energy for muscular contraction

physiologic movement. Movement that a person normally can carry out, such as flexion, extension, rotation, abduction, and adduction

plasticity. The quality of soft tissue that allows it to maintain a lengthened state after a stretch force has been removed

pleural effusion. The presence of fluid in the pleural cavity

pleurectomy. An incision into the pleura

plyometric training. High-intensity, high-velocity resistance exercise characterized by a resisted eccentric muscle contraction followed by a rapid concentric contraction and designed to increase muscular power and coordination also known as **stretch-shortening drills**

pneumonectomy. Surgical excision of lung tissue. In some instances, the term denotes removal of an entire lung

pneumonia. An inflammation of the lungs characterized by consolidation and exudation; often caused by a bacterial or viral infection

pneumothorax. The presence or accumulation of air in the pleural cavity

postural drainage. A means of clearing the airways of secretions by placing the patient in various positions so that gravity will assist in the flow of mucus

postural dysfunction. A faulty posture in which adaptive shortening of soft tissues and muscle weakness has occurred

postural fault (postural pain syndrome). A posture that deviates from normal alignment but has no structural limitations

posture. A position or attitude of the body, the relative arrangement of body parts for a specific activity, or a characteristic manner of bearing one's body

power. Work per unit of time (force $\times$ distance/time) or force times velocity

progressive resistance exercise (PRE). An approach to exercise whereby the load or resistance to the muscle is applied by some mechanical means and is quantitatively and progressively increased over time

prolapse. A protrusion of the nucleus pulposus that is still contained by the outer layers of the annulus

pulmonary edema. An infiltration of fluid (serum) in the lungs

pumping exercises. Active repetitive exercises, usually of the ankles or wrists, performed to maintain or improve circulation in the extremities

Q angle. The angle formed by intersecting lines drawn from the anterior-superior iliac spine through the mid-portion of the patella and from the anterior tibial tuberosity through the mid-patella. The norm is 15 degrees

quadriceps lag. A term synonymous with **extensor lag**

rales. A term used synonymously with **crackles**

range of motion (ROM). The amount of angular motion allowed at the joint between any two bony levers

range of motion, active. Movement within the unrestricted ROM for a segment that is produced by an active contraction of the muscles crossing that joint

range of motion, active-assistive. A type of active ROM in which assistance is provided by an outside force, either manually or mechanically, because the prime-mover muscles need assistance to complete the motion

range of motion, passive. Movement within the unrestricted ROM for a segment that is produced entirely by an external force. There is no voluntary muscle contraction

Raynaud's disease. A functional vasospasm of the small arteries, particularly in the hands, caused by an abnormality of the sympathetic nervous system

reflex muscle guarding. The prolonged contraction of a muscle in response to a painful stimulus. Guarding ceases when the pain is relieved but may progress to muscle spasm

reflux. A backward or return flow of urine back toward the kidneys from the bladder

relaxation. A conscious effort to relieve tension in muscles

relaxed (slouched) posture. Also called **sway back posture**. A posture characterized by a shifting of the pelvic segment anteriorly, resulting in hip extension, and shifting of the thoracic segment posteriorly, resulting in flexion of the thorax on the upper lumbar spine. An increased lordosis in the lower lumbar region, an increased kyphosis in the thoracic region, and a forward head are usually observed with relaxed posture

repetition maximum (RM). The greatest amount of weight a muscle can move through the range of motion a specific number of times in a load-resisting exercise routine

residual volume (RV). The amount of air that is left in the lungs after a maximum expiration

resistance exercise. Any form of active exercise in which a dynamic or static muscular contraction is resisted by an outside force

resistance exercise, manual. A type of active exercise in which resistance is provided by a therapist or other health professional to either a dynamic or static muscular contraction

resistance exercise, mechanical. A type of active exercise in which resistance is applied through the use of equipment or mechanical apparatus

resistance exercise, variable. A form of isotonic exercise carried out using equipment that varies the resistance to the contracting muscle throughout the ROM

respiration, external. The exchange of gas at the alveolar capillary membrane and the pulmonary capillaries

respiration, internal. The exchange of gas between the pulmonary capillaries and the cells of the surrounding tissues

resting position. The position of the joint in which there is maximum laxity in the capsule and surrounding structures

rheumatoid arthritis. A chronic joint disease that is often systemic; characterized by inflammation of the synovial membrane, with periods of exacerbation and remission

rhonchi. The former term used to describe wheezes

rhythmic stabilization. A form of isometric exercise in which manual resistance is applied to one side of a proximal joint, then to the other; no movement occurs and the individual stabilizes against the antagonistic forces

round-back posture. A posture characterized by an increased thoracic curve, protracted scapulae, and a forward head

rubor. Redness of the skin associated with inflammation

scaption. Elevation of the humerus in the plane of the scapula that is 30 to 45 degrees anterior to the frontal plane; also called scapular plane abduction

scoliosis. An abnormal lateral curvature of the vertebral column

scoliosis, functional. A nonstructural reversible lateral curvature of the spine, also called nonstructural or postural scoliosis

scoliosis, structural. An irreversible lateral curvature of the spine with fixed rotation of the vertebrae

selective tension. The administration of specific tests in a systematic manner to determine whether the site of a lesion is in an inert structure (joint capsule, ligament, bursa, fascia, dura mater, or dural sheath around nerve roots) or in a contractile unit (muscle with its tendons and attachments)

self-mobilizing. Techniques whereby the patient is taught to apply joint mobilization techniques to restricted joints using proper gliding techniques

self-stretching. Techniques whereby the patient is taught to stretch a joint or soft tissue passively by using another part of the body for applying the stretch force

setting exercise. See **muscle-setting exercise**

short-arc extension (terminal extension) exercise. Active or active-resisted extension of a joint through the final degrees of its range of motion; most often applied to the knee from 35 degrees flexion to full extension

slow-twitch (ST) fiber. A skeletal muscle fiber with a slow reaction time and a high aerobic capacity, suitable for tonic muscle activity

specificity of training. The principle underlying the development of a training program for a specific activity or skill and the primary energy systems involved during performance

sprain. Severe stress, stretch, or tear of soft tissues such as joint capsule, ligament, tendon, or muscle

stability. The synergistic coordination of muscle contractions around a joint that provides a stable base for movement

stabilization exercise. A form of exercise designed to develop control of proximal areas of the body in a stable, symptom-free position in response to fluctuating resistance loads. Exercises begin very easy so that control is maintained, and they progress in duration, intensity, speed, and variety. Often called dynamic stabilization exercise

static traction. A steady traction force applied and maintained for an extended time interval. It may be continuous (prolonged) or sustained

steady state. Pertaining to the time period during which a physiologic function remains at a constant value

strain. Overstretching, overexertion, overuse of soft tissue; tends to be less severe than a sprain; occurs from slight trauma or unaccustomed repeated trauma of a minor degree. This term also refers to the amount of deformation that occurs in tissues when a stress is applied

strength. The force output of a contracting muscle. It is directly related to the amount of tension a contracting muscle can produce

stress. A load or force applied to tissues per unit area

stress testing. A multistage test that determines the cardiovascular functional capacity of the individual

stretch-shortening drills. A term synonymous with **plyometric training**

stretch weakness. The weakening of muscles that are habitually kept in a stretched position beyond their physiologic resting length

stretching. Any therapeutic maneuver designed to lengthen (elongate) pathologically shortened soft tissue structures and thereby to increase range of motion

stretching, cyclic. A repeated passive stretch usually applied by a mechanical device

stretching, passive. A type of mobility exercise in which manual, mechanical, or positional stretch is applied to soft tissues and in which the force is applied opposite to the direction of shortening

stretching, selective. The process of stretching some muscle groups while selectively allowing others to become tight to improve function in a patient with paralysis

stretching, self. See **self-stretching**

stroke volume. The amount of blood pumped out of the ventricles with each contraction (systole)

subluxation. An incomplete or partial dislocation that often involves secondary trauma to surrounding soft tissue

suspension. A technique that is used to free a body part from the resistance of friction by suspending the part in a sling attached to a rope that is fixed either above the center of gravity or above the axis of the joint

sway back posture. See **relaxed (slouched) posture**

synovectomy. Surgical removal of the synovium (lining of the joint) in patients with chronic joint swelling

synovitis. Inflammation of a synovial membrane; an excess of normal synovial fluid within a joint or tendon sheath

target heart rate. A predetermined heart rate to be obtained during exercise

tendinitis. Scarring or calcium deposits in a tendon

tendinosis. Degeneration of a tendon from repetitive microtrauma; collagen degeneration without inflammation

tenosynovectomy. Surgical removal of proliferated synovium from tendon sheaths

tenosynovitis. An inflammation of the synovial sheath covering a tendon

tenovaginitis. A thickening of a tendon sheath

terminal extension. See **short-arc extension**

thoracotomy. Any surgical cutting of the chest wall

thromboangiitis obliterans (Buerger's disease). An inflammatory reaction and subsequent vasospasm of the arteries as a result of exposure to nicotine

thrombophlebitis. An inflammatory occlusion of a deep or superficial vein with a thrombus

thrombosis. The formation of a clot in a blood vessel

thrombus. A blood clot

tidal volume (TV). The amount of air that a person breathes in and breathes out during a relaxed inspiration and expiration

tight weakness. The weakening of a muscle that has been kept in a habitually shortened position. It may test strong in the shortened position but tests weak as it is lengthened

total lung capacity (TLC). The total amount of air in the lungs; the vital capacity plus the residual volume

traction. The process of drawing or pulling

transfer of training. Carryover of the effects of an exercise program from one mode of exercise or performance to another. Also known as cross-training

transitional stabilization. A stabilization technique whereby the functional position of the spine is stabilized by the trunk muscles while the body moves from one position to another. This requires graded contractions and adjustments between the trunk flexor and extensor muscles

Valsalva maneuver. An expiratory effort against a closed glottis

vasoconstriction. Narrowing of a blood vessel because of contraction of smooth muscle in the walls of the vessels, resulting in a decrease in blood flow

velocity spectrum rehabilitation. Isokinetic exercises performed over a wide range of exercise speeds

ventilation. The movement or mass exchange of air in and out of the body; also referred to as **external respiration**

vibration. A technique of rapid shaking with small amplitude used with postural drainage to mobilize secretions

vital capacity (VC). The greatest amount of air that a person can inspire and expire

wheezes. Abnormal breath sounds heard during exhalation characterized by high- or low-pitched sounds or musical tones; also called **rhonchi**

Index

Numbers followed by an "f" indicate a figure; numbers followed by a "t" indicate a table.

Abdominal muscle(s)
  exercises in pregnancy, 613–615,
    613–615f
  testing strength of
    with bilateral straight-leg raising,
      713–714
    with sit-ups, 713
  training and strengthening of, 557–561,
    557–561f
Abrasion arthroplasty, of knee, 425, 436
  indications for, 438
  postoperative management of, 439
  procedures for, 438
Abruptio placentae, 607
AC joint. *See* Acromioclavicular joint
AC procedure(s). *See* Agonist contraction
  procedure(s)
Accessory movement(s), in joint
  mobilization, 184
Accessory muscles of inspiration, 650–651
Accommodating resistance exercise(s), 68
Acetabulum, 387
Achilles tendon, 473
  complete rupture of
    indications for surgery in, 487
    postoperative management of,
      487–488
    surgical procedures for, 487
  tendinitis of, 482
Acromioclavicular (AC) joint, 275
  hypomobility of, 286
  joint mobilization techniques for,
    anterior glide, 205, 206f
  joint problems
    functional limitations/disabilities in,
      286
    impairments/problems in, 286
    nonoperative management of, 286
    related diagnoses and etiology of
      symptoms in, 285–286
    surgical management of, 286–287

  overuse syndromes of, 285
  subluxations or dislocations of, 286
Actin, 147, 147f
Active inhibition, 19
  agonist contraction, 160, 164
  definition of, 145, 159
  of extensor carpi radialis brevis muscle,
    344–345
  of hamstring muscles, 454
  hold-relax procedure, 159–160, 163
    with agonist contraction, 160,
      163–164
    precautions for, 163–164
  of quadriceps femoris muscle, 454–455
  techniques of, 163–165
Active insufficiency, 24
Active-resistive training, 84
Acute lobar pneumonia, 707–708
Adaptation, 114
  aerobic exercise program in coronary
    disease, 134
Adaptive shortening. *See* Contracture
Adductor pollicis muscle, self-stretching of,
  380
Adhesion(s), 146, 239
Adhesive capsulitis. *See* Frozen shoulder
Adjusted working weight, 90
Aerobic energy system, 116
Aerobic exercise(s)
  age differences and
    child, 137–138
    older adult, 139–141
    young adult, 138–139
  cardiovascular changes due to
    with exercise, 129
    at rest, 129
  cardiovascular response to, 119
  in chronic illness and deconditioning,
    134–135
  in coronary disease, 131–134
  in disability and functional limitations, 135

  duration of, 125
  efficiency of, 118
  energy expenditure in, 116–117
  energy systems in, 115–116
  fitness testing of healthy subjects for, 120
  frequency of, 125–126
  intensity of, 116, 124
    exercise heart rate, 124
    maximum heart rate, 124
    overload principle in, 124
    specificity principle in, 125
  metabolic changes due to
    with exercise, 130–131
    at rest, 130
  mode of, 126
  multistage testing for, 122, 123f
  oxygen consumption in, 120
  physiologic response to, 118–120, 118f
  in postpartum period, 620
  in pregnancy
    fetal response to, 608
    maternal response to, 606–608
  problems, goals, and plan of care in,
    135–137
  program for
    circuit training in, 128
    circuit-interval training in, 127–128
    continuous training in, 127
    cool-down period in, 128–129
    determinants of, 123–124
    exercise period in, 127–128
    interval training in, 128
    warm-up period in, 126–127
  recruitment of motor units, 116
  respiratory changes due to
    with exercise, 130
    at rest, 130
  respiratory response to, 119
  reversibility principle of, 126
  stress testing in convalescing and at-risk
    individuals, 121–122, 121f

Aerobic exercise(s) (*continued*)
  terminology in
    adaptation, 114
    conditioning, 113–114
    deconditioning, 114, 115f
    endurance, 113
    fitness, 112–113, 112f
    maximal oxygen consumption, 113
    myocardial oxygen consumption, 114
  thermoregulation in, 607
Aerobic power, 58
Afterload, 114
Age/aging
  aerobic exercise and, 137–141
  changes in collagen with, 155
  intervertebral disk problems and, 507
  lung volumes and capacities and, 657
  role in chronic pain and inflammation, 254
Agonist contraction (AC) procedure(s), 160, 164
Air embolism
  in postpartum period, 620
  in pregnancy, 611
Airway resistance, 652
All-fours hip extension, 620
All-fours leg raising, 616–617, 617f
Alveolus, 654
Anaerobic ability, at different ages, 138
Anaerobic glycolytic system, 115–116
Anaerobic power, 58
Anconeus muscle, 335
Anesthesia, general, 702
Aneurysmectomy, 702
Ankle. *See also* Achilles tendon
  arthrodesis of, 479–481
  balance exercises for, 493–494, 493f
  bones of, 228f
  closed-chain exercises for, 492–493, 493f
  flexibility imbalances in, 488–494
  functional relationships of ankle and foot, 473
  in gait, 474–475, 477
  joint mobilization techniques for
    subtalar joint, 229–230f, 230–231
    talocrural joint, 227–230, 228–229f
  joint problems
    acute and subacute problems, management of, 477
    functional limitations/disabilities in, 477
    impairments/problems in, 476–477
    nonoperative management of, 476–478
    related diagnoses in, 476
    subacute and chronic problems, management of, 477–478
  joints of, 228f, 470–472
  ligament tears, surgical repair of
    indications for, 485
    long-term results of, 487
    postoperative management of, 486–487
    procedures for, 486
  manual resistance exercises for
    dorsiflexion and plantarflexion, 82, 82f
    inversion and eversion, 83

  motions of
    primary plane, 470
    triplanar, 470
  muscle function in, 473–475
  nerves of, 475
  open-chain exercises for, 491–492, 492f
  overuse syndromes
    acute phase, management of, 484
    impairments/problems in, 483
    related diagnoses and etiology of symptoms in, 482–483
  plantarflexors, testing flexibility of, 717
  postimmobilization stiffness in, 476
  posture and, 532
  range of motion exercises for
    dorsiflexion, 39, 39f
    plantarflexion, 39
    self-assisted, 44, 46f
  resistance exercises for, 492, 492f
  self-stretching of muscles of, 489–490
    evertor muscles, 490
    plantarflexors, 489, 490f
  sprain of
    functional limitations/disabilities in, 484–485
    impairments/problems in, 484
    mechanisms and sites of injuries in, 484
    nonoperative management of, 485
  strengthening muscles of, 488–494
  stretching for
    dorsiflexion with knee extended, 179
    dorsiflexion with knee flexed, 179
    inversion and eversion, 180
    plantarflexion, 179
  total ankle joint replacement, 479–480
  training and strengthening muscles of postural control, 490–494, 491–493f
  traumatic soft tissue injuries to, 484–488
Ankle joint. *See* Talocrural joint
Annulus fibrosus, 497–498, 500
Anterior cruciate ligament
  deficiency of, 413
  injury to, 441
    nonoperative management of, 441–442
  intra-articular reconstruction of
    graft material for, 442–444
    indications for, 443
    postoperative management of, 444–447
    procedures for, 443–444
Anterior tibialis muscle, in shin splints, 483
Aortocoronary bypass surgery, 701
Apnea, 660
Apneusis, 660
Arm, range of motion exercises for, self-assisted, 43, 44f
Arterial disorder(s)
  acute occlusion, 630
    treatment of, 633–634
  chronic disease
    exercise program for, 635–636
    treatment of, 634–635
  clinical signs and symptoms of, 631
  evaluation of, 632–633
  types of, 630–631

Arteriography, 633
Arteriosclerosis obliterans, 630
Arteriosclerotic vascular disease, chronic, 630, 634–635
Arteriovenous oxygen difference, at different ages, 137–141
Arthritis. *See* Osteoarthritis; Rheumatoid arthritis
Arthrodesis, 268–269, 394
  at ankle and foot, 478–479
    indications for, 480
    postoperative management of, 481
    procedures for, 481
  of knee, 425
  of shoulder
    indications for, 290
    long-term results of, 290–291
    postoperative management of, 290
    procedures for, 290
Arthrokinematics, 184–190
Arthroplasty, 269–270
  abrasion, 425, 436
  excision. *See* Excision arthroplasty
  interpositional, 269–270
  material used in, 270
  metacarpophalangeal implant, 366–368
  proximal interphalangeal implant, 368–370
  total ankle joint replacement, 479–480
  total elbow replacement, 340–342
  total joint replacement, 270
  total knee replacement, 427–431
  total wrist replacement, 364–366
Arthroscopic procedure(s), 265–266
  portals in, 266
Arthrotomy, 266
Assessment. *See* Patient evaluation, assessment in
Asthma, 695–697
  airway resistance in, 652
  clinical picture in, 696
  exercise-induced, 696
  impairments/problems in, 696
  treatment goals and plan of care in, 696–697
Astrand-Rhyming test, 113
Atelectasis, 663, 699
  clinical picture in, 709
  impairments/problems in, 709
  treatment goals and care plan in, 709
Atherosclerotic occlusive disease, 630
ATP-PC energy system, 115
Atrophy, muscle, 14, 148
Auscultation, in evaluation for chest physical therapy, 661–663, 662f
Autogenic inhibition, 159–160
Autogenic relaxation, 166
Autorange, 158

Back
  flat upper, 535f, 537
  pain in pregnancy, 604–605
  testing strength of back extensors
    with leg lifts, 715
    with prone chest lifts, 715

Back-to-Work Clinic, 106f
Bacterial pneumonia, 708
Balance
    definition of, 21
    exercises to develop, 21
    goal of therapeutic exercise, 20–21
    hip in, 392
    knee in, 464
    in pregnancy, 602
    strengthening ankle and foot, 493–494,
        493f
Balance board, 101, 412, 491, 493, 493f
Balance training, 412
Ballistic stretching, 156
BAPS system, 101
Barbell(s), 95
Barrel chest, 659
Bed rest, 638
    prolonged, 14, 26, 114, 115f, 143
Biceps brachii muscle, 334–335
    range of motion exercise for, 32, 32f
    stretching of, 319
Bicipital tendinitis, 291
Bicycle (exercise equipment), 100, 101f
Bicycle exercise(s)
    inverted, 720–721, 720f
    modified, 720–721, 720f
Biofeedback, 20, 165
Biologic fixation, 395
Blood flow, during exercise, 17, 606–607
Blood pressure, 114
    at different ages, 138
    in pregnancy, 601
    response to exercise, 119
    training effects on, 129
    Valsalva maneuver and, 59–60
Body mechanics, 571–572
Bone malalignment, 254
Boutonnière deformity, 359
Brachialis muscle, 334
    myositis ossificans of, 342
Brachioradialis muscle, 334
Bradypnea, 660
Brawny edema, 640
Breaking strength, 151, 151f
Breath sound(s), 661–663, 662f
    abnormal and adventitious, 663
    absence of, 663
    bronchial, 662
    bronchovesicular, 662
    normal, 662–663
    tracheal, 662
    vesicular, 662
Breathing exercise(s)
    diaphragmatic breathing, 665–667, 666f
    diaphragmatic training using weights,
        667
    glossopharyngeal breathing, 670–671
    goals of, 664
    incentive respiratory spirometry, 668
    indications for, 664
    inspiratory resistance training, 668
    precautions in, 665
    in pregnancy, 618–619
    preventing/relieving shortness of breath,
        672
    pursed-lip breathing, 671–672

    segmental breathing, 669–670, 669–671f
    teaching of, 664–665
    ventilatory muscle training, 667–672
Breathing pattern
    abnormal, 660
    rate, regularity, and location of
        respiration, 659
Bridging exercise, 410–411, 411f, 565, 566f
    with full body weight on head and feet,
        722
    supine, 616
Brief repetitive isometric exercise (BRIME),
        92
BRIME. See Brief repetitive isometric
        exercise
Brodex system, 105
Bronchiectasis
    clinical picture in, 697
    impairments/problems in, 697
    treatment goals and plan of care in, 697
Bronchiole, 654
Bronchitis, chronic. See Chronic bronchitis
Bronchopneumonia, 707
Bronchospasm, 663
Bronchus
    lobar, 653
    mainstem, 653
    segmental, 654
Bruce protocol, 122
Bucket-handle motion, of thorax, 652
Buerger's disease. See Thromboangiitis
        obliterans
Buerger-Allen exercise(s), 635
Bulla, 692
Bursitis, 238
    ischiogluteal, 402
    psoas, 401
    of shoulder, 291
    trochanteric, 401
Buttock region
    nerves in, 392
    referred pain into, 392

Calcaneal nerve, 475
Calcaneocuboid joint, 472
Calcaneofibular ligament, tears of,
        485–487
Caliper motion, of thorax, 652
Can-Do Exerciser, 101
Cardiac output, 17, 601
    at different ages, 137–141
    response to exercise, 119
    training effects on, 129
Cardiac rehabilitation, 131–134
Cardiac reserve, 17
Cardiac surgery, 701–702. See also
        Postthoracotomy patient
Cardiovascular system
    adaptation to training stimulus, 114
    changes with aerobic exercise
        with exercise, 129
        at rest, 129
    determination of cardiovascular fitness,
        120
    endurance, 113

    adaptive changes leading to increased
        endurance, 17
    suggestion for safe program, 725
    testing of, 717
    evaluation of, 8
    during exercise, 17
    increased fitness as goal of therapeutic
        exercise, 16–18
    precautions for resistance exercises,
        59–60
    in pregnancy, 601
    response to aerobic exercise, 119
Care plan. See Plan of care
Carpal tunnel syndrome
    etiology of symptoms of, 372
    functional limitations/disabilities in, 372
    impairments/problems in, 372
    nonoperative management of, 373
    postoperative management of, 373
Carpometacarpal joint, thumb, 212f,
        354–355
    joint mobilization techniques for,
        361–362
        glides, 217, 218f
        for thumb joint, 216–217, 218f
        traction, 216–217, 216f, 218f
        volar glide, 216
    replacement of
        indications for, 370
        postoperative management of,
            370–371
        procedures for, 370
Case history, 5
Cementless fixation, 395
Center of gravity, in pregnancy, 602
Cerebral palsy, 14
Cervical collar, 523
Cervical region
    increasing range of motion in, 545–547,
        546f
    manual resistance exercises for, 555
    postural problems in, 535f, 538–539
    relaxation training for, 543–544
    self-resistance for isometric exercises for,
        555f, 556
    stabilization exercises for, 552–557,
        553–556f
    tension headache, 526
    torticollis, 525–526
    training and strengthening muscles of
        axial extension, 553–554, 553–554f,
            569, 569f
        flexion, 554–555, 554f
    transitional stabilization of, 555–556, 556f
Cervical scoliosis. See Torticollis
Cervical spine
    dynamic support for, 503–504, 504f
    muscle and soft tissue lesions of
        acute phase, management of, 523
        site of injury, 522
        subacute and chronic phase,
            management of, 525
    range of motion of, 547
    range of motion exercises for, 543
        extension (backward bending or
            hyperextension), 41
        flexion (forward bending), 40

Cervical spine (*continued*)
    lateral flexion (side bending), 41
    rotation, 41, 41f
    safe range, 552–553
    rheumatoid arthritis of, 519
    stretching of, 547
    traction for
        home program, 586, 587f
        manual, 583–584, 583f
        mechanical, 584–586, 585f
        positional, 584
        self-traction, 587
Cervix. *See* Uterine cervix
Cesarean childbirth
    coughing or huffing after, 622–623
    definition of, 621
    exercises after, 622
    impairments/problems after, 621
    intestinal gas pains after, 623
    scar mobilization after, 623
    significance to physical therapists, 621
    treatment goals and plan of care after,
        621–622
Chest
    barrel, 659
    depth of excursion of, 660
    pectus carinatum, 659
    pectus excavatum, 659
    symmetry of movement of, 660
Chest lift, prone, testing strength of back
    extensors, 715
Chest mobilization exercise(s)
    definition of, 672
    goals of, 672–673
    increasing expiration during deep
        breathing, 673–674, 675f
    mobilization of one side of chest, 673,
        673f
    mobilization of shoulders, 673, 674f
    mobilization of upper chest, 673, 674f
    wand exercises, 674
Chest physical therapy, 649–687
    breathing exercises. *See* Breathing
        exercise(s)
    chest mobilization exercises, 672–674,
        673–675f
    coughing, 675–679
    evaluation for, 658–663
        appearance of patient, 658–659
        auscultation, 661–663, 662f
        breathing patterns, 659–660
        chest shape, 659
        cough and sputum, 663
        interview with family, 658
        mediate percussion, 661
        palpation, 660–661
        posture of patient, 659
        purpose of, 657–658
    postthoracotomy, 700–707
    postural drainage, 679–687, 681–684f
Chest wall
    adhesions in mastectomy, 643–644
    incisions in, 704, 704f
    injury or stiffness of, 699
    pain over, 660–661
Cheyne-Stokes respiration, 660
Child, aerobic exercise in, 137–138

Chin-up(s), as test of upper extremity
    strength, 714–715
Cholesterol, blood, 131
Chondromalacia patellae, 431
Chondroplasty, knee, 425, 436
    arthroscopic, 425
    indications for, 438
    postoperative management of, 439
    procedures for, 438
Chronic bronchitis, 679, 690–695
    airway resistance in, 652
    clinical picture in, 692
Chronic illness, aerobic exercise program
    in, 134–135
Chronic obstructive pulmonary disease
    (COPD), 690–695
    clinical picture in, 691–693
    expiratory flow rate in, 653
    impairments/problems in, 693
    terms synonymous with, 690
    treatment goals and plan of care in,
        693–695, 694f
Cilia, respiratory, 676
Circuit training, 128
Circuit weight training, 91
Circuit-interval training, 128
Claudication. *See* Intermittent claudication
Clavicle
    elevation and rotation with humeral
        motion, 277
    surgical resection of, 286–287
Claw fist, 362
Claw hand, 382
Claw toe, 476
Clinical evaluation. *See* Patient evaluation,
    clinical
Closed-chain exercise(s), 68, 88–89
    for ankle and foot, 492–493, 493f
    for elbow, 350
    for hip, 412, 413f
    for knee, 456, 461
        dynamic, 462–464, 463f
        isometric, 461–462
    protected, 248
    for shoulder, 324
Closed-chain resistance device(s),
    101–102, 103f
Codman's exercise. *See* Pendulum
    exercise(s)
Collagen
    changes affecting stress-strain response,
        154–155
    effect of age on, 155
    effect of corticosteroids on, 155
    effect of immobilization on, 154–155
    effect of inactivity on, 155
    in intervertebral disks, 498
    in remodeling process, 154, 242–243
Collagen disease, 143
Collagen fiber, 152–153, 153f
    interpretation of stress-strain curve,
        153–154
Commissurotomy, 702
Common peroneal nerve, 475
Compliance, with exercise program, 13
Compliance, of lungs, 652
Component motion(s), 184

Compression, 150, 189
    joint, in patient evaluation, 7
Concentric exercise(s)
    delayed-onset muscle soreness and, 64
    isotonic, 67
Concentric isotonic contraction, 159
Conditioning, 113–114, 124
Conditioning program, 17–18
    for knee, 464
Connective tissue
    composition of, 152, 153f
    mechanical characteristics of, 150–155
    mobility of, 18
Connective tissue disease. *See* Collagen
    disease
Continuous passive motion, 52–53, 244
    benefits of, 53
    equipment for, 53, 54f
    procedure in, 53
Continuous training, 127–128
Contractile tissue. *See* Muscle
Contract-relax technique, 159
Contracture, 18, 24–25, 143, 238, 253
    adhesions and, 146
    definition of, 145
    irreversible, 146
    myostatic, 146
    pseudomyostatic, 146
    surgical release of, 267
Contusion, 238
    of spine, 521–525
Convalescing individual, stress testing in,
    121–122, 121f
Convex-concave rule, 187, 187f, 197
Cool-down period, 64, 128–129
Coordination
    definition of, 20–21
    exercises to develop, 21
    goal of therapeutic exercise, 20–21
COPD. *See* Chronic obstructive pulmonary
    disease
Coronary bypass surgery, aerobic exercise
    program in, 131–134
Coronary disease, aerobic exercise
    program in, 131–134
    adaptive changes in, 134
    arm vs. leg exercises, 133–134
    in-patient phase of, 131
    out-patient phases of, 132–133, 132f
Corset, 523
Corticosteroid, 155
Cough/coughing
    after cesarean childbirth, 622–623
    cough mechanism, 675
    in evaluation for chest physical therapy,
        663
    factors that decrease effectiveness of,
        676
    humidification and, 679
    manual assisted, 677–678, 678f
    in obstructive lung disease, 690
    paroxysmal, 679
    precautions for, 679
    self-assisted, 677–678, 678f
    splinting over incision, 678, 678f
    teaching effective cough, 676–677
    tracheal stimulation to induce, 679

Cough pump, 676
Coxa valga, 388
Coxa vara, 388, 390
Crackles, 663
Creep, 152, 154
Cross training, 66
Cruciate ligament. *See* Anterior cruciate
    ligament; Posterior cruciate ligament
Cryostretching, 165
Cuff weight, 95, 96f
Cumulative trauma disorder, 238, 253
Curl-down(s), 560
Curl-up(s), 560, 719
    diagonal, 560
    as test of abdominal strength, 713
Cybex II+ system, 105, 105f
Cycle ergometer test, 113
Cyclic loading, 154
Cyclic stretching, 158
Cystic fibrosis, 679
    clinical picture in, 698
    impairments/problems in, 698
    treatment goals and plan of care in,
        698–699

Daily adjustable progressive resistance
    exercise (DAPRE), 90
DAPRE. *See* Daily adjustable progressive
    resistance exercise
Deconditioning, 114, 115f
    aerobic exercise program in, 134–135
Deep-knee bend(s), 722
Degenerative joint disease. *See*
    Osteoarthritis
DeLorme technique, of isotonic resistance
    exercises, 89–90
Deltoid muscle
    function of, 278
    strengthening of, 321–323, 322f
    stretching of, 319–320
Dermatomyositis, 143
Diabetes, in pregnancy, 624
Diagnosis, 9, 10t
Diaphragm, 650–651
Diaphragmatic breathing, 665–667, 666f
    using weights, 667
Diastasis recti
    correction after vaginal delivery, 620
    corrective exercises for, 613–614, 613f
    definition of, 602, 603f
    incidence of, 602–603
    significance of, 603
    test for, 603, 604f
    treatment of, 604
Digit(s). *See* Finger(s); Toe(s)
Disability
    aerobic exercise program in, 135
    definition of, 4, 10t
    identification of, 11
    tests to document, 9
Disease, definition of, 10t
Diskogenic pain, 508, 581
Dislocation, 238
    of shoulder. *See* Shoulder, dislocations
        of

Distraction, 189–190
    joint, in patient evaluation, 7
DOMS. *See* Muscle soreness, delayed-onset
Doppler ultrasonography, in arterial
    disorders, 633
Double knee to chest, 560, 560f
Drawer test, 223–224, 224f
Duck waddle, 722
Dumbbell(s), 95, 96f
Dynamic flexibility, 144
Dynamic splint, 157, 158f
Dynamic stabilization, 72
    of spine, 551
Dynasplint, 157, 158f
Dysfunction, 238
Dyspnea, 660, 690

Eagle Fitness System, 98–99, 100f
Eccentric exercise(s), 69–71, 248
    delayed-onset muscle soreness and, 64
    isotonic, 67
    precautions for, 70–71
    for shoulder, 328
Eccentric isokinetic training, 94
Edema. *See* Lymphedema
Elastic limit, 150, 151f
Elastic range, 150, 151f
Elastic resistance material, 96–97, 101–102
Elasticity, of soft tissue, 147–148
Elastin fiber, 152
Elbow
    bones of, 208f
    capsule of, 333
    closed-chain exercises for, 350
    extensor muscles of, 334–335
    flexibility imbalances in, exercises for,
        347–350
    flexor muscles of, 334
    functional training and conditioning for,
        350
    golfer's, 343
    joint mobilization techniques for
        humeroradial articulation, 209–210,
            210–211f
        humeroulnar articulation, 207–209,
            208–209f
        radioulnar articulation, 211–212,
            211–212f
    joint problems
        acute, management of, 337
        functional limitations/disabilities in,
            336–337
        impairments/problems in, 336
        nonoperative management of,
            336–339
        related diagnoses and etiology of
            symptoms in, 336
        subacute and chronic, management
            of, 337–339
        surgery and postoperative
            management of, 339–342
    joints of, 208f, 333–334
    manual resistance exercises for, flexion
        and extension, 77–78, 78f
    mechanical resistance exercises for, 346,
        346f

myositis ossificans about, 342
nerves around, 335–336
overuse syndromes
    acute, management of, 344
    etiology of symptoms of, 343
    functional limitations/disabilities in,
        344
    impairments/problems in, 343
    related diagnoses in, 343
    subacute or chronic, management of,
        344–347
pulled, 338
pushed, 338
range of motion exercises for
    flexion and extension, 31, 32f
    overhead pulleys, 48
    self-assisted, 43
    wand exercises, 46
resistance exercises for, 344–347,
    345–346f
    flexion, 348–349, 349f
    pronation and supination, 349
self-stretching for, 345, 345f
strengthening muscles of, 347–350
    extensors, 348–349, 349f
    flexors, 348, 349f
    supinators and pronators, 349
stretching for, 347–348
    extension, 171, 171f, 348
    flexion, 171, 171f, 347–348
    supinators and pronators, 348
tennis, 343
total elbow arthroplasty, 340–342
Electrocardiogram, exercise, 121, 121f
Emotional stress, spinal problems and,
    522
Emphysema, 690–695
End-feel, 6
    abnormal, 6
Endotracheal intubation, 702–703
Endotracheal suctioning, 679
End-plate, cartilaginous, of intervertebral
    disks, 498
End-range isometric contraction, 159
Endurance. *See also* Cardiovascular system;
        General body endurance; Muscular
        endurance
    definition of, 113
    goal of therapeutic exercise, 16–18
    guidelines for developing, 17–18
    of knee, 464
    for postural control, 551–571
    resistance exercises to increase, 58
    of shoulder, 328
    suggestions for safe program
        cardiovascular endurance, 725
        muscle endurance, 725
    testing of, 717
    types of, 16–17
Endurance limit, 152
Energy expenditure
    in aerobic exercise, 116–117, 607
    daily, 117f
Energy system
    aerobic, 116
    anaerobic glycolytic, 115–116
    phosphagen (ATP-PC) system, 115

Environment
  adaptations of
    to prevent postural problems, 573
    to prevent spinal problems, 524
  factors in chronic pain and
    inflammation, 254
Epicondylitis
  lateral, 343
  medial, 343
Erector spinae muscle(s), 501f, 502–503
  stretching of, 547–548, 548f
Excision arthroplasty, 269, 478
  with implant, 269
  for metatarsalgia
    indications for, 481–482
    postoperative management of, 482
    procedures for, 482
Exercise bicycle, 100, 101f
Exercise bout(s), 85–86
Exercise duration, 86
Exercise frequency, 86
Exercise load, 84–85
Exercise pressor response, 119
Exercise program
  critical analysis of, 711–726
  designing of, 712
  development of, 4–13, 4f
  establishing baselines to measure
    improvement against, 712–718
  establishing goals for, 718–726
  reasons for, 712
  re-evaluation to see if baseline has
    changed, 726
Exercise tolerance, decreased, 690
Exercise-induced asthma, 696
Expiration
  muscles of, 651
  relaxed, 651
Expiratory flow rate, 653
Expiratory reserve volume, 656, 656f
Extension exercise(s), balancing with
  flexion exercises, 719–720
Extensor carpi radialis brevis muscle, 335
  active inhibition of, 344–345
Extensor carpi radialis longus muscle, 335
Extensor carpi ulnaris muscle, 335
Extensor communis muscle, self-stretching
  of, 381
Extensor digitorum longus muscle, 474
Extensor digitorum muscle, 335
  range of motion exercises for, 35, 36f
Extensor hallucis longus muscle, 474
External oblique muscle, 501f, 651
Extracorporeal circulation, 703
Extrapment, 518
Extremity, girth measurements of, 638, 640

Facet joint(s), spine, 499
  lesions of
    acute lesions, management of,
      520–521
    diagnoses in, 519–520
    functional limitations/disabilities in,
      520
    impairments/problems in, 519–520
    pathology of, 517–518

subacute and chronic lesions,
  management of, 521
traction in, 521
mechanical relationships to
  intervertebral disk, 518
mobilization using spinal traction,
  576–577
pain from, spinal traction in, 580
Failure, stress-strain curve, 151, 151f, 154
Fascitis, plantar, 483
Fast-twitch fiber, 116
Fat, body, 131
Fatigue, 152
  associated with specific diseases, 60–61
  general muscular (total-body), 60
  local muscle, 60
  in resistance exercises, 60–61
Femoral head, 387
Femur, motions of, 387
Femur, proximal, fracture of, 399–401
  closed reduction of, 400
  extracapsular, 400
  intracapsular, 400
  open reduction and internal fixation of,
    400–401
  postoperative management of, 400–401
Fencer's squat posture, 404, 405f
Fetus, response to maternal aerobic
  exercise, 608
Fibroblast(s), 240–242
Fick equation, 113
Finger(s)
  joint mobilization techniques for,
    361–362
    carpometacarpal joints, 216–217, 216f,
      218f
    intermetacarpal joints, 216, 216f
    interphalangeal joints, 217–218, 219f
    metacarpophalangeal joints, 217–218,
      219f
  manual resistance exercises for, 79, 79f
  metacarpophalangeal implant
    arthroplasty, 366–368
  proximal interphalangeal implant
    arthroplasty, 368–370
  range of motion exercises for
    interphalangeal joint, 34–35, 35f
    self-assisted, 44
  stretching for
    interphalangeal joints, 173–174
    metacarpophalangeal joints, 173
    specific extrinsic and intrinsic muscles,
      174
Finger ladder exercise, 47, 47f
Fire hydrant exercise, 620, 721–722, 721f
Fist
  claw, 362
  full, 362
  sublimis, 362
Fitness, 112–113, 112f
  exercises during pregnancy, 611
  goals for nation, 112f
Flaccid paralysis, 62
Flat foot. See Pes planus
Flat low-back posture, 535f, 536
Flat-neck posture, 535f, 539
Flexibility

common errors in program for
  exercise pain, 723
  faulty biomechanics, 724
  flexibility imbalances, 723
  improper emphasis, 723
  use of ballistic stretch, 723
definition of, 144
dynamic, 144
exercises for, 19, 145
goal of therapeutic exercise, 18–19
passive, 144
of soft tissue, 18–19
suggestions for safe program, 724–725
testing of, 715–717
Flexion exercise(s), balancing with
  extension exercises, 719–720
Flexor carpi radialis muscle, 335
Flexor carpi ulnaris muscle, 335
Flexor digitorum longus muscle, 474
Flexor digitorum profundus muscle, 335
  range of motion exercises for, 35, 36f
  self-stretching of, 381, 381f
Flexor digitorum superficialis muscle, 335
  self-stretching of, 381, 381f
Flexor hallucis longus muscle, 474
Flexor superficialis muscle, range of
  motion exercises for, 35, 36f
Foot
  arthrodesis at, 480–481
  balance exercises for, 493–494, 493f
  bones of, 470
  closed-chain exercises for, 492–493, 493f
  excision arthroplasty for metatarsalgia,
    481–482
  flexibility imbalances in, 488–494
  functional relationships of ankle and
    foot, 473
  in gait, 474–475, 477
  joint mobilization techniques for
    intertarsal joints, 231–232, 231f
    tarsometatarsal joints, 231–232, 231f
  joint problems
    acute and subacute problems,
      management of, 477
    functional limitations/disabilities in,
      477
    impairments/problems in, 476–477
    nonoperative management of,
      476–478
    related diagnoses in, 476
    subacute and chronic problems,
      management of, 477–478
  joints of, 470–472
  motions of
    primary plane, 470
    triplanar, 470
  muscle function in, 473–475
  nerves of, 475
  open-chain exercises for, 491–492, 492f
  overuse syndromes
    acute phase, management of, 484
    impairments/problems in, 483
    related diagnoses and etiology of
      symptoms in, 482–483
    subacute and chronic phases,
      management of, 484
  postimmobilization stiffness in, 476

pronation of, 470
referred pain in, 475
resistance exercises for, 492, 492f
self-stretching of muscles of, 489–490
    evertor muscles, 490
strengthening muscles of, 488–494
supination of, 470
training and strengthening muscles of
    postural control, 490–494, 491–493f
traumatic soft tissue injuries to, 484–488
Foraminal stenosis, 579
Forearm. *See also* Elbow
    flexibility imbalances in, exercises for,
        347–350
    joint problems
        acute problems, management of, 337
        functional limitations/disabilities in,
            336–337
        impairments/problems in, 336
        nonoperative management of,
            336–339
        related diagnoses and etiology of
            symptoms in, 336
        subacute and chronic problems,
            management of, 337–339
        surgery and postoperative
            management of, 339–342
    joints of, 333–334
    manual resistance exercises for,
        pronation and supination, 78, 78f
    overuse syndromes
        acute, management of, 344
        etiology of symptoms of, 343
        functional limitations/disabilities in,
            344
        impairments/problems in, 343
        related diagnoses, 343
        subacute or chronic, management of,
            344–347
    pronator muscles of, 335
    range of motion exercises for
        pronation and supination, 33, 33f
        self-assisted, 43, 44f
    strengthening muscles of, 347–350
    stretching muscles of, 347–348
        supination or pronation, 171–172
    supinator muscles of, 335
Forefoot, 470
Forward bending, as test of flexibility,
    716
Forward-head posture, 535f, 538–539, 569,
    569f
Fracture
    clinical considerations in
        after immobilization, 262
        during immobilization, 261
    pathologic, 62, 400
    of proximal femur, 399–401
    of spine, 581
    stress, 152, 154
    treatment considerations during
        immobilization, 261
Free weights, 95–96, 96f, 104
    patient position for, 102, 102–103f
Fremitus, 660
Frozen shoulder, 279–280
Full fist, 362

Full-arc exercise(s), 88
    for knee, 459–460
Functional excursion, 24
Functional immobility, as indication for
    joint mobilization, 191
Functional limitation(s)
    aerobic exercise program in, 135
    clinical evaluation of, 5–9
    definition of, 4, 10t
    identification of, 11
    tests to document, 9
Functional outcome, goals for, 11–12
Functional patterning, 54
Functional position
    in acute problems of spine, 504–505
        extension bias, 505
        flexion bias, 505
        non–weight-bearing bias, 505
    in postural problems, 551
Functional range. *See* Functional position
Functional residual capacity, 656f, 657
Functional scoliosis, 537, 549
Functional skill(s)
    definition of, 21
    exercises to develop, 21
    goal of therapeutic exercise, 20–21
Funnel breast, 659

Gait
    ankle and foot in, 474–475, 477
    hip in, 390
    knee in, 420–421
    muscle control during, 390
    orthopedic problems and, 390–391
Ganglion, 238
Gastrocnemius muscle, 420–421, 532
    stretching of, 404
Gastrocsoleus muscle
    in shin splints, 483
    stretching of, 724
Gear-shift exercise(s), 309–310, 310f
General anesthesia, 702
General body endurance, 16–17
    guidelines for developing, 17–18
General muscular (total-body) fatigue, 60
General relaxation, 166
Genu recurvatum, 391
Genu valgum, 388, 390–391
Genu varum, 388, 391
Girth measurement, of extremity, 638, 640
Glenohumeral joint
    active range of motion exercises for, 283
    arthrodesis of shoulder, 290–291
    arthrokinematics of, 274
    characteristics of, 274
    faulty mechanics in, 284–285
    hemireplacement of
        indications for, 290
        postoperative management of, 290
        procedures for, 290
    home program for, 284
    joint mobilization techniques for,
        280–282
        anterior glide, 203–205, 204f
        anterior glide progression, 205
        caudal glide, 200f, 201

caudal glide alternate, 201
caudal glide progression, 201–202,
    201f
elevation progression, 202, 202f
posterior glide, 203, 203f
posterior glide progression, 203, 204f
traction, 200–201, 200f
joint problems
    acute, 279
    acute, management of, 280–281
    chronic, 279
    chronic, management of, 281–285
    frozen shoulder, 279–280
    functional limitations/disabilities in,
        280
    impairments/problems in, 280
    related diagnoses and etiology of
        symptoms in, 278–279
    subacute, 279
    subacute, management of, 281–285
    surgical management of, 287–291
    symptoms of, 279–280
manipulation under anesthesia, 285
passive range of motion exercises for,
    280
pendulum (Codman's) exercises for,
    282–283, 282f, 309
replacement of
    indications for, 287
    long-term results of, 289
    postoperative management of,
        288–289
    procedures for, 287–288
    self-assistive range of motion exercises
        for, 283
self-mobilization of, 284, 284–285f
self-stretching exercises for, 284
stability of, 274
stretching exercises for, 283
Glide (joint motion), 188
Gliding, joint, in patient evaluation, 7
Glossopharyngeal breathing, 670–671
Gluteus maximus muscle
    strengthening of, 410–411, 410–411f
    stretching of, 405–406, 406f
    tight, 391
Gluteus medius muscle, strengthening of,
    409–410, 409f
Glycolytic system, anaerobic, 115–116
Goal(s)
    of aerobic exercise program, 135–137
    for expected functional outcome, 11–12
    fitness goals for nation, 112f
    long-term, 11–12
    of resistance exercises, 57–59
    short-term, 12
    of therapeutic exercise, 13–21
        cardiovascular fitness as, 16–18
        coordination, balance, and functional
            skills as, 20–21
        endurance as, 16–18
        mobility and flexibility as, 18–19
        relaxation as, 20
        stability as, 19–20
        strength as, 14–16
"Going for the burn," 721
Golfer's elbow, 343

Golgi tendon organ (GTO), 149–150
Gout, 476
Graded exercise program, in chronic
    arterial insufficiency, 635–636
Graded oscillation technique(s), of joint
    mobilization, 193–196, 194f, 198
Gravity, 13–14
Greater saphenous vein, competence of,
    638
Grip, 356–357
Ground substance, 152
GTO. *See* Golgi tendon organ

Hallux valgus, 391, 476
Hammer toe, 476
Hamstring curl(s), 460–461, 460f
Hamstring muscle(s), 419–421, 532
    hamstring-setting exercises, 459
    overuse of, 391
    range of motion exercises for, 36–38,
        37f
    stretching of, 406–408, 407f, 454
    testing flexibility of, 716
Hand. *See also* Finger(s); Thumb
    arch of, methods to increase, 362
    bones of, 212f, 353
    claw, 382
    control of, 356–357
        unloaded hand, 356–357
    dorsal aspect of, 378, 378f
    extensor mechanism of, 356
    extensor tendons of, 378, 378f
        repair of ruptured tendons, 371–372
    flexor tendons of, 375, 376f
    function of, 355–356
    grips and prehension patterns of,
        356–357
    joint mobilization, 361–362
    joint problems
        acute problems, management of, 360
        functional limitations/disabilities in,
            359–360
        impairments/problems in, 359
        nonoperative management of,
            358–363
        related diagnoses and etiology of
            symptoms in, 358–359
        subacute and chronic problems,
            management of, 360–363
        surgery and postoperative
            management of, 363–372
    joints of, 212f, 354–355
    lacerated extensor tendons of
        indications for surgery in, 378
        postoperative management in,
            379–380
        surgical procedures in, 378
    lacerated flexor tendons of
        delayed primary repair of, 375–376
        direct primary repair of, 375–376
        indications for surgery in, 375
        postoperative management in,
            376–377
    length-tension relationships in, 355–356
    mechanical resistance exercises for,
        383–384

muscles of, 335
nerves of, 357–358
overuse syndromes, 372–374
pinch, 357
precision handling, 356–357
range of motion exercises for
    cupping and flattening arch, 34, 34f
    self-assisted, 43–44, 44f
referred pain in, 358
self-stretching of, 362
sprain of
    etiology of symptoms in, 374–375
    functional limitations/disabilities in,
        375
    impairments/problems in, 375
    nonoperative management of,
        374–375
strengthening muscles of, 381–384
stretching muscles of, 380–381
tendinitis in, 374
tenosynovitis in, 374
traumatic lesions of, 374–375
volar aspect of, 375, 376f
Handicap
    definition of, 4, 10t
    identification of, 11
    tests to document, 9
Head
    dynamic support for, 503–504, 504f
    posture and, 533
Head halter, 585–586
Head lift, 613–614
    with pelvic tilt, 614
Headache, tension, 526
Healing process
    acute (inflammatory reaction) stage of,
        240, 241t, 242f
        clinical considerations in, 243–246
        treatment considerations in, 246–247
    chronic (maturation and remodeling)
        stage of, 241t, 242–243, 242f
        clinical considerations in, 250–252
        treatment considerations in, 252–253
    subacute (repair-healing) stage of,
        240–242, 241t
        clinical considerations in, 247–248
        treatment considerations in, 249–250
Healthy People 2000, 112f
Healthy subject(s), fitness testing of, 120
Heart rate, 114
    at different ages, 137–141
    exercise, 17, 124
    fetal, 608
    maximum, 124
    in pregnancy, 601
    resting, 17
Heart transplantation, 702
Heart-lung bypass pump, 703
Heat production, in soft tissue under
    stress, 152
Heat therapy, for local relaxation, 164–165
Heel-sitting, 550, 550f
Hemarthrosis, 238
Hematocrit, 607
Hemireplacement
    of glenohumeral joint, 290
    of hip, 394, 399

Hemoptysis, 663, 680
    mild, 697
    severe, 697
Hemothorax, 703, 709
Hindfoot, 470
Hip
    active flexion of, 389
    angle of inclination, 388
    bones of, 220f
    closed-chain exercises for, 412, 413f
    in equilibrium and posture control, 392
    flexors, testing flexibility of, 717
    fracture of. *See* Femur, proximal, fracture
        of
    function of, 387–388
    gait and, 390
    hemireplacement of, 394, 399
    increasing strength, stability, and control
        in weight-bearing, 411, 412–414f,
        415
    joint mobilization techniques for
        anterior glide, 221, 222f
        caudal glide, 219–220, 220f
        caudal glide alternate, 221
        posterior glide, 220f, 221
    joint problems
        acute and subacute lesions,
            management of, 393–394
        functional limitations/disabilities in,
            393
        impairments/problems in, 393
        nonoperative management of,
            392–394
        related diagnoses and etiology of
            symptoms in, 392–393
        subacute and chronic lesions,
            management of, 394
        surgery and postoperative
            management of, 394–399
    in kinematic chain, 388–392
    manual resistance exercises for
        abduction and adduction, 80–81, 80f
        extension, 80, 80f
        flexion with knee extension, 79, 80f
        hyperextension, 80, 80f
        internal and external rotation, 81, 81f
    motions and postures of lower
        extremity, 389–390
    muscle imbalances at, 391–392
    nerves in, 392
    overuse syndromes
        acute stage of, management of, 402
        chronic stage of, management of,
            402–403
        functional limitations/disabilities in,
            402
        impairments/problems in, 402
        nonoperative management of,
            401–403
        related diagnoses and etiology of
            symptoms in, 401–402
        subacute stage of, management of,
            402–403
    posture and, 533
    range of motion exercises for
        abduction and adduction, 38, 38f
        extension (hyperextension), 36, 37f

internal (medial) and external (lateral)
rotation, 38–39, 39f
self-assisted, 44, 45f
simultaneous flexion and extension,
35–36, 37f
skate board/powder board, 49
suspension, 52f
referred pain in, 392
rhythmic stabilization exercises for, 412
self-stretching of, 404–408
strengthening muscles of, 408–411
abductors and hip hikers, 409–410,
409f
adductors, 411, 412f
extensors, 410–411, 410–411f
external rotators, 411
stretching for, 404–408
abduction, 176
adduction, 176, 176f
adductor and internal rotator muscles,
407f, 408
extension, 175–176, 175f
external rotation, 177
flexor muscles, 404–405
flexion with knee extended, 174–175,
174f
flexion with knee flexed, 174
hip extension and knee flexion,
175–176, 175f
internal rotation, 177
structure of, 387–388
tight muscles or joints of, 389–390
torsion of, 388
total hip replacement, 394–399
Hip hikers, strengthening of, 409–410,
409f
Hold-relax (HR) procedure(s), 159–160,
163
with agonist contraction, 160, 163–164
contract-relax technique, 159
Homans' sign, 638
Home program, 12–13
for cervical traction, 586, 587f
for glenohumeral joint, 284
for lumbar traction, 590
of postural drainage, 686–687
self-stretching in, 160
HR procedure(s). See Hold-relax
procedure(s)
Huffing
after cesarean childbirth, 622–623
to clear airway, 679
Humeroradial articulation, 333
increasing joint play in, 337–338
joint mobilization techniques for
compression, 210, 211f
dorsal or volar glide of radius,
209–210, 210f
traction, 209, 210f
Humeroulnar articulation, 333
increasing joint play in, 337
joint mobilization techniques for
distal glide, 208f, 209
traction, 208, 208f
traction progression, 209
Humerus
depression of, voluntary, 283–284, 284f

elevation through plane of scapula, 278
external rotation with full elevation
through abduction, 277
humeral head control in shoulder
problems, 310–311, 311–312f
internal rotation with full elevation
through flexion, 277
musculature of, stretching of, 546
replacement of head of, 290
Humidification, 679
Hurdler's stretch, 724
Hydra-Gym, 99
Hypermobility, of joint, 191
Hyperplasia, muscle, 15
Hypertension, pregnancy-related, 624
Hypertrophy, muscle, 15, 57, 130
Hyperventilation, 660

Iliofemoral ligament, 533
Iliopsoas muscle, 533
Iliotibial band
self-stretch insertion of, 433, 434f
tight, 391
Immobilization, 26, 143, 148, 154–155, 244
Impairment
clinical evaluation of, 5–9
definition of, 4, 10t
educating patient about, 13
identification of, 9–11
Inactivity, 155
Incentive respiratory spirometry, 668
Incisional pain, postthoracotomy, 702
Incontinence, pelvic floor awareness
training and strengthening, 616
Inflammation
acute
characteristics of, 240
clinical considerations in, 243–246
clinical signs of, 240, 242f
treatment considerations in, 246–247
chronic, 242
characteristics of, 243
clinical considerations in, 250–252,
254–255
clinical signs of, 243
contributing factors in, 254
general treatment guidelines for,
253–257
mechanisms for, 253–254
treatment considerations in, 252–253,
255–256
contraindication to resistance exercises,
65
of joint, 192
subacute
characteristics of, 240–242
clinical considerations in, 247–249
clinical signs of, 242, 242f
treatment considerations in, 249–250
Infrahyoid muscle, 504, 504f
Infraspinatus muscle, strengthening of,
320, 321f
Infraspinatus tendinitis, 291
Inhibition, active. See Active inhibition
Inspection, in clinical evaluation, 5
Inspiration, muscles of, 650

Inspiratory capacity, 656f, 657
Inspiratory reserve volume, 656, 656f
Inspiratory resistance training, 668
Intensity of exercise, 84
Intercostal muscle(s)
external, 650
internal, 651
stretching of, 545
Intermetacarpal joint, joint mobilization
techniques for
traction, 216, 216f
volar glide, 216
Intermetatarsal joint, joint mobilization
techniques for, 232
Intermittent claudication, 631, 635–636
claudication time, 633
Internal oblique muscle, 501f, 503, 503f,
651
Internal pterygoid muscle, 503
Interossei muscle, self-stretching of, 380
Interphalangeal joint, finger, 212f, 355
flexion of, 383, 383f
increasing mobility of, 362
interphalangeal implant arthroplasty,
proximal
indications for, 368
postoperative management of,
368–370
procedures for, 368
joint mobilization techniques for
glides, 218, 219f
rotations, 218–219, 219f
traction, 217, 219f
manual resistance exercises for, 79, 79f
range of motion exercise for, 34–35, 35f
stretching for, 173–174
Interphalangeal joint, toe, 472–473
arthrodesis of, 481
increasing mobility of, 478
joint mobilization techniques for, 232
range of motion exercises for, 40, 40f
Interpositional arthroplasty, 269–270
Intertarsal joint, 472
increasing mobility of, 478
joint mobilization techniques for
dorsal glide, 231f, 232
plantar glide, 231–232, 231f
Intertransverse ligament(s), 502
Interval training, 128
Intervertebral disk
dynamic support for, 501–503, 501–503f
function of, 497–498
lesions of
acute phase, management of, 512
age and, 507
anterior protrusion, 515–516
axial overload, 507
centralization of symptoms in, 510
effect of fluid stasis and inhibition of,
511
effect of isometric activities on, 511
effect of muscle splinting on, 511
effect of postural changes and
activities on, 510
effect of traction on, 511
effect on spinal mechanics, 507–508
etiology of symptoms in, 508–509

Intervertebral disk (*continued*)
  fatigue loading and traumatic rupture, 506–507
  functional limitations/disabilities in, 511–512
  herniation, 508
  impairments/problems in, 511, 517
  lateral shift correction in, 513–516, 514–515f
  in lumbar spine, 512–516, 513–515f
  mechanical reduction of protrusion or swollen tissues, 512–516, 513–515f
  nonoperative treatment of, 510–511
  objective clinical findings in, 510
  onset and behavior of symptoms in, 509–510
  passive extension in, 513, 513f
  passive flexion in, 516
  patient education in, 514–515, 515f, 517
  peripheralization of symptoms in, 510
  posterior or posterolateral protrusion, 513
  prolapse, 508
  protrusions, 508
  related diagnoses, 508
  signs of improvement in, 516–517
  subacute and chronic phase, management of, 516–517
  symptoms of, 512
  traction in, 516
  mechanical relationships to facet joints, 518
  size of, 500
  structure of, 497–498
Intestinal gas pain, 623
Intra-abdominal pressure, 503, 503f
Intubation, 702
Inverted bicycle, 720–721, 720f
Irreversible contracture, 146
Ischiogluteal bursitis, 402
Isokinetic exercise(s), 68–69
  speed-specific, 86–87
Isokinetic testing, 104–107, 105–106f
Isometric contraction, end-range, 159
Isometric exercise(s), 71–72. *See also* Resistance exercise(s), isometric
  multiple-angle, submaximal, 247
  precautions with, 72
Isotonic contraction, concentric, 159
Isotonic exercise(s), 66–68. *See also* Resistance exercise(s)
Isotonic torque arm unit, 98, 99f

Jaw muscle(s), control of, 527–528
Joint
  ankylosed, 7
  evaluation of stability and mobility of, 7
  functional immobility of, 191
  hypermobile, 7, 191
  hypomobile, 7, 191
  inflammation of, 62, 192
    acute, therapy in, 245
    subacute, therapy in, 248
  laxity in pregnancy, 606

  progressive limitation of, 191
  resting position for, 196
  shape of
    ovoid, 185, 185f
    sellar (saddle), 185, 185f
Joint dysfunction, 238
Joint effusion, 191–192
Joint integrity test, 7
Joint mobility, 19, 143, 191
Joint mobilization, 183–233
  accessory movements in, 184
  for ankle
    subtalar joint, 229–230f, 230–231
    talocrural joint, 227–230, 228–229f
  conditions requiring special precautions, 192
  contraindications to, 191–192
  definition of, 184
  direction of movement in, 196–197, 197f
  for elbow and forearm complex
    humeroradial articulation, 209–210, 210–211f
    humeroulnar articulation, 207–209, 208–209f
    radioulnar articulation, 211–212, 211–212f
  for fingers, 361–362
  for foot
    intertarsal joints, 231–232, 231f
    tarsometatarsal joints, 231–232, 231f
  graded oscillation techniques in, 193–196, 194f, 198
  for hand and fingers, 361–362
    carpometacarpal joints, 216–217, 216f, 218f
    intermetacarpal joints, 216, 216f
    interphalangeal joints, 217–218, 219f
    metacarpophalangeal joints, 217–218, 219f
  for hip, 219–222, 220f, 222f
  indications for, 190–191
  initiation and progression of treatment in, 197–198, 198f
  joint position in, 196
  for knee and leg
    distal tibiofibular joint, 226–227, 227f
    patellofemoral joint, 225–226, 225–226f
    proximal tibiofibular articulation, 226, 226f
    tibiofemoral articulation, 222–225, 222–225f
  limitations of, 191
  mechanical effects of, 190
  neurophysiologic effects of, 190
  passive stretching vs., 188
  patient assessment for, 193
  patient position in, 196
  physiologic movements in, 184
  procedures for applying techniques of, 193–199
  reassessment in, 199
  for shoulder girdle complex
    acromioclavicular joint, 205, 206f
    glenohumeral joint, 199–205, 200–204f, 280–282
    scapulothoracic articulation, 207, 207f

    sternoclavicular joint, 205–207, 206–207f
  speed, rhythm, and duration of, 198–199
  stabilization in, 196
  sustained translatory joint-play techniques in, 194–196, 195f, 198–199
  for temporomandibular joint, 528, 529f
  for toes
    intermetatarsal joints, 232
    interphalangeal joints, 232
    metatarsophalangeal joints, 232
  treatment force in, 196
  treatment soreness in, 199
  for ulnomeniscal-triquetral joint, 361, 361f
  for wrist
    glides for intercarpal joints, 214–215
    glides of carpals in proximal row with radius and ulna, 214, 215f
    to increase extension, 361
    to increase flexion, 360
    to increase radial deviation, 361
    to increase ulnar deviation, 361
    radiocarpal joint, 212–215, 212–216f
Joint motion, 185–190
  combined roll-sliding, 187–188
  compression, 189
  convex-concave rule in, 187, 187f
  effects of, 190
  glide, 188
  rolling, 186, 186f
  sliding, 186–187, 187f
  spinning, 188, 188–189f
  swing, 185
  traction, 189–190, 189f
Joint separation, 190
Joint-play technique(s), 184, 190, 248
  in knee pain, 423
  progressively vigorous, 191
  sustained translatory techniques in, 194–196, 195f, 198–199

Karvonen's formula, 124
Keiser Cam II system, 99
Kilocalorie, 117
KIN/COM system, 105
Knee
  abrasion arthroplasty, 438–439
  balance activities for, 464
  bones of, 222f
  chondroplasty, 438–439
  closed-chain exercises for, 456, 461
    dynamic, 462–464, 463f
    isometric, 461–462
  conditioning activities for, 464
  developing strength, stability, and control in weight-bearing, 461–464
  drills for, 464
  endurance exercises for, 464
  extensor lag, 422, 440
  extensor mechanism, 419–420
    surgery and postoperative management of, 436–440

training and strengthening muscles of, 457–460
extensor mechanism realignment, 436
advancement of quadriceps, 439
distal realignment, 439
indications for, 439
postoperative management of, 440
procedures for, 439
proximal realignment, 439
flexor mechanism, 420
training and strengthening muscles of, 460–461, 460f
function of, 419–421
functional training of, 425
gait and, 420–421
joint mobilization techniques for
distal tibiofibular articulation, 226–227, 227f
patellofemoral joint, 225–226, 225–226f
proximal tibiofibular articulation, 226, 226f
tibiofemoral articulation, 222–225, 222–225f
joint problems and capsular restrictions
acute lesions, management of, 423
functional limitations/disabilities in, 422
after immobilization, 422
impairments/problems in, 422
nonoperative management of, 421–425
related diagnoses and etiology of symptoms in, 421–422
subacute and chronic lesions, management of, 423–425
surgery and postoperative management of, 425–431
joints of, 222f, 417–419
lateral retinacular release, 436–438
ligamentous tears, 441–448
functional limitations/disabilities in, 441
impairments/problems in, 441
nonoperative management of, 441–442
reconstruction of ligaments and postoperative management of, 442–443
locking of, 724
manual resistance exercises for
extension, 82
flexion, 81, 82f
meniscal tears. See Meniscal tear(s)
muscle setting exercises for, 461–462
open-chain exercises for, 456
patellofemoral dysfunction. See Patellofemoral dysfunction
plyometric training for, 464, 465f
posture and, 532
range of motion exercises for, 424
self-assisted, 44, 45f
simultaneous flexion and extension, 35–36, 37f
referred pain in, 421
rhythmic stabilization exercises for, 462

runner's, 431
sprains of, 441–448
functional limitations/disabilities in, 441
impairments/problems in, 441
nonoperative management of, 441–442
strengthening and training muscles of, 424–425, 456–461
stretching for, 454–456
extension at end of range, 178–179, 179f
extension in mid-range, 178–179, 179f
flexion, 177–178, 178f
hip extension and knee flexion, 175–176, 175f
synovectomy of, 426–427
total knee replacement, 427–431
trauma to, 422, 441–448
work-hardening activities for, 465
Kypholordotic posture, 534
Kyphosis, 498
increased, 535f, 536–537

Labor (childbirth)
onset of, 597
premature, 623
relaxation and breathing exercises in pregnancy, 618–619
stage 1 of, 597–598, 619
stage 2 of, 598, 599f, 619
stage 3 of, 598
Lactic acid, in muscle, 63
Larynx, 653
Lateral raphe, 501–503, 501–502f
Latissimus dorsi muscle, 501, 501f, 503
strengthening of, 323
stretching of, 315
Leg
asymmetries causing postural problems, 539–540
bones and joints of, 222f, 228f
unilateral short, 390
Leg lift(s), testing strength of back extensors, 715
Leg sliding, 614, 614f
Leg-lowering exercise, 615
Leg-raising exercise, all-fours, 616–617, 617f
Lengthening, permanent, 157
Levator scapulae muscle, 504, 504f
strengthening of, 324
stretching of, 318–319, 318–319f
Lido system, 105
Ligament
composition of, 153, 153f
inflammation of
acute, therapy in, 245
subacute, therapy in, 248
about spine, 499
strength increases in, 16
Ligamentous injury
to foot or ankle, 484–487
to knee, 441–448
tear of, surgical repair of, 267

Load-resisting exercise(s), 84
Lobectomy, 701
Local muscle fatigue, 60
Locked-back mechanism, 517
Long horn sign, 362
Long jump, as test of leg strength, 715
Lordosis, 498
Lordotic posture, 534–535, 535f
Low-back region
pain in pregnancy, 604
testing flexibility of, 716, 717f
Lower extremity
asymmetries causing postural problems, 539–540
musculature of, stretching of, 549
testing strength of, with vertical or long jump, 715
unilateral short leg, 390
Lower respiratory tract, 653–654, 654–655f
Lumbar pillow, 544
Lumbar region
active range of motion exercises for, 543
increasing range of motion in, 547–549, 547–548f
postural problems in, 534–536
range of motion of, safe range, 557
stabilization exercises for, 557–564, 557–564f
strengthening of abdominal muscles, 557–561, 557–561f
strengthening of lumbar extensors, 562–564, 563–565f
Lumbar spine
balance of, 569–570
disk protrusion in
anterior protrusion, 515–516
lateral shift correction in, 513–516, 514–515f
passive extension in, 513, 513f
passive flexion in, 516
patient education in, 514–515, 515f
posterior or posterolateral protrusion, 513–514
symptoms of, 512
traction in, 516
dynamic support for, 501–503, 501–503f
effect of pelvic motion on, 388–389
muscle and soft tissue lesions
acute phase, management of, 523–525
sites of strains of, 522
subacute and chronic phase, management of, 525
range of motion exercises for
extension, 42
flexion, 41, 42f
rotation, 42, 42f
traction on
home program, 590
manual, 587–588
mechanical, 588–590, 589f
positional, 588, 588f
self-traction, 590
Lumbodorsal fascia. See Thoracolumbar fascia
Lumbopelvic rhythm, 389
Lumbrical muscle, self-stretching of, 380
Lumpectomy, 642–643

Lunate-radius articulation, joint mobilization techniques for, 214, 215f
Lung(s)
  anatomy of, 655–656, 655f
  compliance of, 652
  disease of, 689–709. *See also* Obstructive lung disease; Restrictive lung disorder
Lung capacity(ies), 656, 656f
  in obstructive lung disease, 690, 691f
  in restrictive lung disorders, 700, 700f
Lung volume(s), 656, 656f
  in obstructive lung disease, 690, 691f
  in restrictive lung disorders, 700, 700f
Lunges, 413, 414f
  full, 464
  partial, 464, 567
Lymphatic disorder(s), 640–641
Lymphedema
  background of problem, 640
  brawny, 640
  causes of, 640
  evaluation of, 640
  in mastectomy, 641–647
  pitting, 640
  treatment of, 641

Mandible, 503
Manipulation, 184
  under anesthesia, 185
    of glenohumeral joint, 285
Manual resistance exercise(s). *See* Resistance exercise(s), manual
Marching in place, 412
Massage, 165
  in postural problems, 545
Masseter muscle, 503, 504f
Mastectomy, 641–647
  chest wall adhesions in, 643–644
  lymphedema in, 643
  modified radical, 642
  postoperative pain in, 643
  postural faults in, 644
  psychological considerations in, 644–645
  radical, 642
  segmental, 642–643
  shoulder motion after, 644
  simple, 642
  treatment goals and plan of care in, 645–647
  upper extremity weakness in, 644
Material strength, of soft tissue, 150–152
Maximal oxygen consumption, 113, 125
  estimation of, 113
Maximal oxygen uptake, at different ages, 137–141
MCP joint. *See* Metacarpophalangeal joint
Mechanical resistance exercise(s). *See* Resistance exercise(s), mechanical
Medial collateral ligament, injury to, 441
Medial plica synovitis, 431
Medial pterygoid muscle, 504f
Medial shelf syndrome, 431

Median nerve, 336, 357
  compression of, 372
Median sternotomy, 704
Mediastinum, 661
Mediate percussion, in evaluation for chest physical therapy, 661
Meniscal tear(s)
  arthroscopic repair of, 450–452
    indications for, 450
    postoperative management of, 450–452
    procedures for, 450
  functional limitations/disabilities in, 449
  impairments/problems in, 449
  nonoperative management of, 449, 449f
  partial meniscectomy in, 452–453
  related diagnoses and mechanisms of injury in, 448
  surgical repair of, 449–450
Meniscectomy
  partial, 450
    indications for, 452
    postoperative management of, 452–453
    procedure for, 452
  total, 450
Meniscoid blocking, 581
Meniscus, medial, manipulative reduction of, 449, 449f
Mental imagery, 618
Merac system, 105
MET, definition of, 117
Metabolism, changes with aerobic exercise, 130–131
Metacarpophalangeal extension, 383
Metacarpophalangeal (MCP) joint, 355
  flexion with interphalangeal joint extension, 382, 382f
  increasing mobility of, 362
  joint mobilization techniques for
    glides, 218, 219f
    rotations, 218–219, 219f
    traction, 217, 219f
  metacarpophalangeal implant arthroplasty
    indications for, 366
    postoperative management of, 366–368
    procedures for, 366
  stretching for, 173
  of thumb, range of motion exercise for, 34–35, 35f
Metatarsalgia. *See* Excision arthroplasty, for metatarsalgia
Metatarsophalangeal joint, 472–473
  increasing mobility of, 478
  joint mobilization techniques for, 232
  range of motion exercises for, 40, 40f
  restricted motion of, 476
Microtrauma, 64, 253
Midcarpal joint, 353–354
Midfoot, 470
Military press-up, 321, 322f
Mini-squat, 462–463, 463f
Mobility
  exercises for, 19
  goal of therapeutic exercise, 18–19

guidelines for developing, 19
  of joint, 19, 143
  of soft tissue, 18–19
Monosynaptic stretch reflex, 150
Motivation, 13
Motor unit(s), recruitment of, 15–16, 116
Mucus, of respiratory tract, 676
Multi Exercise Pulley Unit, 97f
Multiple gestation, 624
Multiple sclerosis, 61
Multiple-angle isometric exercise(s), 92–93
Multistage testing, for aerobic exercise, 122, 123f
Muscle
  adaptation to training stimulus, 114
  atrophy of, 14, 148
  contractile elements of, 145, 147, 147f
  contractile unit problem, 7
  extensibility of, 144
  hyperplasia of, 15
  hypertrophy of, 15, 57, 130
  inflammation of
    acute, therapy in, 245
    subacute, therapy in, 248
  length-strength imbalances in, 254
  lesions of, 238
  mass at different ages, 138
  mechanical properties of, 147–148, 148f
  microtrauma to, 64
  mobility of, 18
  neurophysiologic properties of, 148–150
  patient assessment, 7–8
  recruitment of motor units, 15–16, 116
  rupture of, 238
    surgical repair of, 266
  strength of. *See* Strength
  tight weakness of, 143
  tightness of, 146
  vascularization of, 17
Muscle fatigue, 721
  local, 60
Muscle fiber, 147, 147f
Muscle guarding, 6, 239, 244
  as indication for joint mobilization, 190–191
  spinal traction in, 580–581
Muscle setting exercise(s), 71
  for knee, 461–462
  for shoulder, 310
Muscle soreness
  acute, 63
  delayed-onset (DOMS), 63–65
    after eccentric exercise, 71
  exercise-induced, 63–65
Muscle spasm, 6, 20, 63, 239, 239f, 244
  as indication for joint mobilization, 190–191
  about shoulder, 283–284
  spinal traction in, 580–581
Muscle spasticity, 6
Muscle spindle, 148–149, 149f
Muscle splinting, in intervertebral disk lesions, 511
Muscle strain, 721
Muscle tear, 7
Muscle tension, 20
Muscle weakness, 7, 143, 148, 239, 254

Muscular endurance, 16–17, 113
  guidelines for developing, 17–18
  resistance exercises to increase, 58
  suggestions for safe program, 725
  testing of, 717
Musculoskeletal system, in pregnancy, 601
Myocardial infarction, aerobic exercise
        program in, 131–134
Myocardial ischemia, 114
Myocardial oxygen consumption, 114, 130
Myofibril, 147, 147f
Myosin, 147, 147f
Myositis ossificans, 342
Myostatic contracture, 146
Myotomy, 267

Nasal cavity, 653
Nautilus system, 98–99
Neck extensor(s), testing flexibility of, 717
Necking, stress-strain curve, 151, 151f, 154
Needs assessment, 4–11
Neurologic test, in patient evaluation, 8
Neutral spine position. See Resting
        position
N-K Unit, 98, 99f
"No pain, no gain," 721, 723
Nucleus pulposus, 497–498
  herniated, 579

Obstetric patient. See Pregnancy
Obstructive lung disease
  asthma, 695–697
  bronchiectasis, 697
  changes associated with, 690, 691f
  chronic. See Chronic obstructive
        pulmonary disease
  cystic fibrosis, 698–699
  definition of, 690
  impairments/problems in, 690–691
Obturator nerve, 392
Older adult, aerobic exercise in, 139–141
1-Mile Walk, 113
1.5-Mile Run, 113
Open heart surgery, 701–702
Open-chain exercise(s), 67–68, 88–89
  for ankle and foot, 491–492, 492f
  for knee, 456
  for shoulder, 325, 326f
Open-circuit portable spirometry, 117
Orthopnea, 660
Orthotron II system, 105
Oscillation, joint, for local relaxation, 165
Osteoarthritis, 143
  characteristics of, 259
  clinical considerations in, 259–260
  of elbow, 336, 339
  of foot and ankle, 476
  of hip, 392–393
  of knee, 421–423
  of shoulder, 278
  of spine, 519
  treatment considerations in, 260
  of wrist and hand, 358–359
Osteokinematics, 184
Osteoporosis, 14

contraindications to resistance exercises,
        62–63
  definition of, 62
  exercise program in, 63
  fracture of proximal femur in, 399
  risk for, 62–63
Osteotomy, 268, 394
  of tibia, 425
Outcome measures, 4
Overflow, 66
Overhead pulley. See Pulley system(s)
Overload, 84
Overload training, 16, 84
Overpressure, 6
Overstretch, 145
Overtraining, 61–62
Overuse syndrome, 152, 154, 238, 253. See
        also specific joints
Overwork, 61–62
Ovoid joint, 185, 185f
Oxford technique, of isotonic resistance
        exercises, 90
Oxygen consumption
  in aerobic exercise, 120
  maximal, 113, 125
  myocardial, 114, 130

Pacing activity(ies), for controlled
        breathing, 672
Pain. See also specific types
  in arterial disorders, 631
  chronic recurring
    contributing factors in, 254
    general treatment guidelines for,
        253–257
    mechanisms for, 253–254
  contraindication to resistance exercises,
        65
  incisional, postthoracotomy, 702
  as indication for joint mobilization,
        190–191
  spinal traction to reduce, 577–578
Painful arc, 7
Palmaris longus muscle, 335
Palpation
  in clinical evaluation, 8
  in evaluation for chest physical therapy,
        660–661
Paralysis
  in arterial disorders, 631
  flaccid, 14
Paroxysmal cough, 679
Partial squat(s), 414
Passive flexibility, 144
Passive insufficiency, 24
Passive movement, 244
  continuous, 244
Passive positioning, in acute problems of
        spine, 505–506
Passive stretching. See Stretching, passive
Patella
  compression of, 419, 431
  function of, 419–421
  malalignment and tracking problems of,
        419, 431
  medial glide of, 433, 434f

medial tipping with friction massage,
        433, 434f
  subluxation/dislocation of, 431
Patellectomy, 436
Patellofemoral compression syndrome,
        413–414
Patellofemoral dysfunction
  acute stage, management of, 432–433
  chronic stage, management of, 435
  etiology of symptoms in, 431
  functional limitations/disabilities in, 432
  impairments/problems in, 431
  nonoperative management of, 431–433
  related diagnoses in, 431–432
  subacute stage, management of, 433,
        434f
  surgery and postoperative management
        of, 436–440
Patellofemoral joint, 418–419
  joint mobilization techniques for
    distal glide, 225, 225f
    medial-lateral glide, 226, 226f
Pathologic fracture, 62, 400
Patient education, 13–14
  in acute problems of spine, 505–506
  in intervertebral disk lesions, 514–515,
        515f, 517
  in postural problems, 544
  preoperative, 263
Patient evaluation, 4–13, 4f
  assessment in, 9–11
    identifying diagnosis and impairment,
        9–11
    identifying functional
        limitations/disabilities, 11
    identifying handicaps, 11
    for joint mobilization, 193
    preoperative, 263
    referrals in, 11
  case history in, 5
  for chest physical therapy, 657–663
  clinical
    cardiovascular system, 8
    documenting functional limitation,
        disability, or handicap, 9
    inspection in, 5
    neurologic tests in, 8
    palpation in, 8
    provocation-selective tension
        procedures in, 5–8
    respiratory system, 8
  needs assessment in, 4–11
  for passive stretching, 161
Pectoralis major muscle, 651
  strengthening of, 323
  stretching of, 315–317, 316–317f
Pectoralis minor muscle, 651
  stretching of, 317f, 318
Pectoralis muscle, stretching of, 673, 674f
Pectus carinatum, 659
Pectus excavatum, 659
Pelvic clock, 615–616
Pelvic floor
  awareness training and strengthening,
        616
  dysfunction in pregnancy, 605–606, 605f
  elevator exercise for, 616

Pelvic floor (*continued*)
  functions of, 605–606
  isometric exercises for, 616
  relaxation exercises for, 618–619
  strengthening after vaginal delivery, 620
  structure of, 605, 605f
  treatment of dysfunctions of, 606
Pelvic lift, 561, 561f, 615
Pelvic motion training, in pregnancy,
     615–616
Pelvic region
  pain in pregnancy, 604
  postural problems in, 534–536
Pelvic rotation, 389
Pelvic shifting, 388
Pelvic tilt, 557
  anterior, 388
  control of, 569–570
  lateral, 389
  posterior, 388
  quadruped, 614
  resisted posterior, 615
Pelvis
  in kinematic chain, 388–392
  motions of, 387
Pendulum exercise(s), for glenohumeral
     joint, 282–283, 282f, 309
Percussion, for postural drainage,
     680–681, 681f
Percussion test, for varicose veins, 638
Periarthritis. *See* Frozen shoulder
Perineum, in pregnancy, 617–618
Peripheral airway disease, 690–695
Peripheral joint mobilization. *See* Joint
     mobilization
Peripheral vascular disease, 629–647
Permanent lengthening, 157
Peroneus brevis muscle, 474
Peroneus longus muscle, 474
Peroneus tertius muscle, 474
Pes anserinus muscle, 420
Pes cavus, 473
Pes planus, 388, 390–391, 421, 473
Pes valgus, 391, 421
Phalanges, proximal, dorsal dislocation on
     metatarsal heads, 476
Pharynx, 653
Phlebography, 637–638
Phlebothrombosis, 637
Phosphagen, 115
Physical therapy diagnosis, 9–11
Physiologic movement(s), in joint
     mobilization, 184
Pigeon breast, 659
Pinch, 357
Pisiform, 354
Piston action, of thorax, 652
Pitting edema, 640
Placenta
  abruptio placentae, 607
  expulsion of, 598
  placenta previa, 623
Plan of care
  aerobic exercise program in, 135–137
  development of
    establishing goals for expected
       functional outcome, 11–12

factors influencing decisions, 11
  short-term goals in, 12
  evaluation of, 12
  home program in, 12–13
  implementation of, 12
Plantar fascitis, 483
Plantar nerve, 475
Plastic range, 151, 151f
Plasticity, of soft tissue, 147
Pleural effusion, 699
Pleurectomy, 701
Plica syndrome, 432
Plica synovalis, 431
Plyometric training, 70, 91–92
  for knee, 464, 465f
  for shoulder, 328, 328f
Pneumonectomy, 701
Pneumonia, 707–708
  acute lobar, 707–708
  bacterial, 708
  bronchopneumonia, 707
  prevention of, 707
  segmental, 708
  treatment goals and plan of care in,
     708
  viral, 708
Pneumothorax, 703, 709
Polymyositis, 143
Popliteus muscle, 420
Portal(s), in arthroscopic surgery, 266
Posterior cruciate ligament
  injury to, 441
    nonoperative management of,
       441–442
  reconstruction of
    indications for, 447
    postoperative management of,
       447–448
    procedures for, 447
Posterior tibialis muscle, in shin splints,
     483
Postimmobilization arthritis, in shoulder,
     279
Postimmobilization stiffness, of wrist and
     hand, 359
Postoperative care
  goals and guidelines for exercise,
     264–265
  precautions in, 265
Postpartum period
  aerobic exercises in, 620
  after cesarean childbirth, 621–623
  strengthening exercises in, 620
  after vaginal delivery, 620
Postthoracotomy patient, 700–707
  with chest wall incision, 704, 704f
  impairments/problems of, 703
  risk of pulmonary complications in, 702
  treatment goals and plan of care for,
     705–707
Postural control
  endurance for, 551–571
  hip in, 392
  training and strengthening muscles of
     ankle and foot, 490–494, 491–493f
Postural drainage
  contraindications to, 680

definition of, 679
  discontinuation of, 686
  goals of, 679–680
  home program of, 686–687
  manual
    percussion, 680–681, 681f
    shaking, 681–682
    vibration, 681, 682f
  modified, 686
  positions for, 682, 683–684f
  treatment procedures for, 682–686
Postural dysfunction, 534
Postural fault, 534
Postural habit(s), 534
Postural pain syndrome, 534
Postural problem(s), 531–573
  avoiding recurrences of
    adaptations of environment, 573
    body mechanics, 571–573
    preventative exercises, 572
  in cervical region, 535f, 538–539
  chronic rehabilitative stage of, 541
  etiology of, 533
  external postural support in, 544
  functional position in, 551
  impairments/problems in, 540–541
  increasing range of motion in, 545–551
    cervical and thoracic region, 545–547,
       546f
    lateral flexibility in spine, 549–551,
       549–550f
    lumbar region, 547–549, 547–548f
  hip muscle imbalances in, 391
  from lower extremity asymmetries,
     539–540
  modalities and massage in, 545
  movement and balance control in,
     569–571
  pain syndromes related to, 534
  patient awareness of, 568
  patient education in, 544
  in pelvic and lumbar region, 534–536
  proprioceptive awareness and, 568–571
  reinforcement techniques during
     treatment, 568–569
  reinforcing learning, 571
  relationship of faulty posture to pain,
     571
  relaxation techniques in
    active range of motion, 542–543
    general conscious relaxation
       techniques, 543–544
  retraining kinesthetic awareness,
     568–571
  in shoulder, 291
  stabilization exercises for
    cervical and thoracic regions,
       552–557, 553–556f
    frontal plane strengthening in,
       567–568, 568f
    preparation for functional activities,
       564–567, 566f
    thoracic and lumbar regions, 557–564,
       557–564f
  stabilization exercises in, 551–571
    general guidelines for, 551–552
  subacute phase of healing, 541

in thoracic region, 536–538
treatment goals and plan of care in, 542
Postural splint, 571
Postural strain, on spine, 522
Posture
  definition of, 532
  equilibrium of, 532–533
  evaluation of patient for chest physical
      therapy, 659
  flat low-back, 535f, 536
  flat neck, 535f, 539
  flat upper back, 535f, 537
  forward head, 535f, 538–539, 569, 569f
  kypholordotic, 534
  lordotic, 534–535, 535f
  maintenance of, 500–501
  after mastectomy, 644
  in obstructive lung disease, 691
  in pregnancy, 602, 604, 612–613
  relaxed or slouched, 535–536, 535f
  round back, 535f, 536–537
  scoliosis. See Scoliosis
Powder board, range of motion exercises
      for hip, 49
Power
  aerobic, 58
  anaerobic, 58
  resistance exercises to increase, 58–59
Power grip, 356–357
Precision handling, 356–357
Pre-eclampsia, 624
Pregnancy, 595–627
  abdominal muscle exercises in,
      613–615, 613–615f
  aerobic exercise in
    fetal response to, 608
    maternal response to, 606–608
  balance in, 602
  breathing exercises in, 618–619
  cardiovascular system in, 601
  center of gravity in, 602
  changes in
    first trimester, 596
    second trimester, 596
    third trimester, 596
  diastasis recti in, 602–604, 603–604f
  exercise in
    contraindications to, 612
    exercises that are not safe, 619–620
    fitness exercises, 611
    goals and plan for, 609–610
    guidelines for instructions in,
        610–611, 610f
    precautions for, 612
    sequence for exercise class, 612
  high risk
    conditions considered high risk,
        623–624
    definition of, 623
    exercise programs for, 625–627
    goals and plan for treatment in,
        624–625
    guidelines and precautions in, 625
    impairments/problems of bed-bound
        patient, 624–625
  joint laxity in, 606
  low back and pelvic pain in, 604–605

musculoskeletal system in, 601
pelvic floor awareness training and
    strengthening in, 616
pelvic floor dysfunction in, 605–606,
    605f
pelvic motion training in, 615–616
perineum and adductor flexibility
    exercises in, 617–618
posture in, 602, 604, 612–613
posture exercises in, 612–613
potential impairments/problems in,
    608–609
relaxation exercises in, 618–619
reproductive system in, 600
respiratory system in, 600
stabilization exercises in, 615
thermoregulatory system in, 601–602
upper and lower extremity strengthening
    in, 616–617
urinary system in, 600
varicose veins in, 605
weight gain in, 598–600
Preoperative care
  evaluation procedures in, 263
  patient education in, 263
  for thoracotomy, 703
Preterm rupture of membranes, 623
ProFitter, 102, 103f
Progressive arterial occlusive disease,
    630
Progressive limitation, as indication for
    joint mobilization, 191
Progressive relaxation technique(s), 166
Progressive resistance, 251
Progressive resistive exercise(s), 83–84, 89
Pronated foot. See Pes planus
Pronator quadratus muscle, 335
Pronator teres muscle, 335
Provocation test, 5–8
Proximal interphalangeal implant
    arthroplasty, 368–370
Pseudomyostatic contracture, 146
Psoas bursitis, 401
Psoas major muscle, 501f
Pulled elbow, 338
Pulley system(s)
  isotonic resistance exercises, 97–98,
      97–98f, 102, 104
  prolonged mechanical passive
      stretching, 157
  range of motion exercises, 47–48
  resistance exercises for elbow, 346, 346f
Pull-up(s), as test of upper extremity
    strength, 714–715
Pulmonary edema, 700
Pulmonary embolism, 700
Pulmonary fibrosis, 699
Pulmonary surgery, 701. See also
      Postthoracotomy patient
  with chest wall incision, 704, 704f
Pulmonary system. See Respiratory system
Pulse, palpation in arterial disorders, 632
Pump-handle motion, of thorax, 651
Pursed-lip breathing, 671–672
Pushed elbow, 338
Push-up(s)
  standing, 616

as test of upper extremity strength, 714
with trunk stabilization, 566, 566f

Q angle, 419
Quad sets. See Quadriceps setting
Quadratus lumborum muscle, 501f, 502
  strengthening of, 409–410, 409f
Quadrectomy, 642–643
Quadriceps femoris muscle, 419–420, 532
  advancement for realignment of knee
      extensor mechanism, 439
  stretching of, 454–456, 455f
  training and strengthening of, 457–460
Quadriceps lag, 422, 440
Quadriceps setting, 457
  in pain-free positions, 433
  in partial weight bearing, 435
  with straight-leg raising, 433–434
Quadruped exercise(s), 562, 563f
Quadruped pelvic tilt, 614

Radial head
  excision of
    indications for, 339
    postoperative management of, 340
    procedure for, 339–340
  subluxation of
    distal, 338
    proximal, 338
Radial nerve, 335–336, 358
Radiocarpal joint, 212f, 353
  joint mobilization techniques for
    dorsal glide, 213, 213f
    radial glide, 213, 214f
    traction (distraction), 213, 213f
    volar glide, 213, 214f
Radioulnar joint
  distal, 333–334
    increasing joint play in, 338
    joint mobilization techniques for,
        211–213, 212f
  proximal, 334
    increasing joint play in, 338
    joint mobilization techniques for, 211,
        211f
Rales. See Crackles
Range of motion (ROM), 24
  active, in patient evaluation, 6
  loss of, 143
  passive
    end-feel in, 6
    overpressure in, 6
    in patient evaluation, 6–7
  in postural problems, 545–551
Range of motion (ROM) exercise(s)
  active
    definition of, 25
    indications and goals for, 26
    limitations of, 27
    in pain-free range, 247
    in postural problems, 542–543
    precautions and contraindications to,
        27
  active-assistive
    definition of, 25

Range of motion (ROM) exercise(s)
(*continued*)
  indications and goals for, 26
  for ankle, 39, 39f
  assistive, 45–52
  for biceps brachii muscle, 32, 32f
  for cervical spine, 40–41, 41f
  continuous passive motion, 52–53, 54f
  for elbow, 31, 32f
  for extensor digitorum muscle, 35, 36f
  finger ladder, 47, 47f
  for flexor digitorum profundus and
    superficialis muscles, 35, 36f
  for forearm, 33, 33f
  full-arc, 88
  through functional patterns, 54
  for hamstring muscles, 36–38, 37f
  for hand, 34, 34f
  in high-risk pregnancy, 625–626
  for hip, 35–39, 37–39f
  for interphalangeal joint
    of fingers, 34–35, 35f
    of toes, 40, 40f
  for knee, 35–36, 37f, 424
  for lumbar spine, 41–42, 42f
  for metatarsophalangeal joint, 40, 40f
    of thumb, 34–35, 35f
  overhead pulleys, 47–48
    for elbow, 48
    for shoulder, 48, 48f
  passive
    definition of, 25
    indications and goals for, 25–26
    limitations of, 26
    precautions and contraindications to, 27
  procedures for application of, 27–28
  reciprocal exercise unit, 51–52
  for rectus femoris muscle, 38
  for scapula, 30–31, 31f
  self-assisted
    for ankle and toes, 44, 46f
    for arm and forearm, 43, 44f
    for glenohumeral joint, 283
    for hip and knee, 44, 45f
    for wrist and hand, 43–44, 44–45f
  short-arc, 88
  for shoulder, 29–30, 29–30f, 280, 283,
    309–310, 310f, 314–320
  skate board/powder board for hip, 49
  for subtalar joint, 39, 40f
  suspension, 49–51, 50–52f
  for temporomandibular joint, 528
  for thumb and fingers, 34–35, 35f
  for toes, 40, 40f
  for transverse tarsal joint, 39, 40f
  for triceps brachii muscle, 32–33, 33f
  using anatomic planes of motion, 28–42
  using combined patterns of motion
    lower extremity, 43
    upper extremity, 42–43
  wand exercises, 45–47, 46–47f
    for elbow, 46
    for shoulder, 46, 46–47f
  for wrist, 33, 34f
Raynaud's disease, 630–631, 634
Raynaud's phenomenon, 630–631

Reactive hyperemia, test for, 632–633
Reactive neuromuscular training, 91
Reciprocal exercise unit, 51–52
Reciprocal inhibition, 160
Recruitment of motor unit(s), 15–16, 116
Rectus abdominis muscle, 651
Rectus femoris muscle
  overuse of, 391
  range of motion exercises for, 38
  stretching of, 404–405, 405f, 455–456
Referral, 11
Referred pain
  in buttock region, 392
  in foot, 475
  in hand and wrist, 358
  in hip, 392
  in knee, 421
  in shoulder, 278
Reflex muscle guarding, 239
Reflex sympathetic dystrophy, 281
  etiology of symptoms in, 308
  impairments/problems in, 308
  management of, 308–309
  related diagnoses in, 307
Rehabilitation Xercise Tubing, 96
Reinforcement technique(s)
  in postural correction, 568
  tactile, 569
  verbal, 568
  visual, 568
Relaxation
  effects of spinal traction, 577
  general, 166
  goal of therapeutic exercise, 20
  guidelines for promoting, 20
  local
    biofeedback for, 165
    heat therapy for, 164–165
    joint traction or oscillation for, 165
    massage for, 165
  progressive, 166
Relaxation exercise(s)
  for cervical region, 543–544
  in postural problems, 542–543
  in pregnancy, 618–619
  therapeutic basis of, 20
Remodeling, 241t, 242–243, 242f
Repair of injury, 240–242, 241t
Repetition maximum, 85
Repetitive strain injury, 238, 253
Repetitive trauma syndrome. *See* specific
  joints, overuse syndromes
Reproductive system, in pregnancy, 600
Residual volume, 656f, 657
Resilience, 151
Resistance exercise(s), 56–107
  accommodating, 68
  for ankle and foot, 492, 492f
  contraindications to
    inflammation as, 65
    pain as, 65
  eccentric, 69–71
  for elbow, 344–347, 345–346f
    flexion, 348–349, 349f
    pronation and supination, 349
  equipment for, 94–106
    isokinetic, 104–107, 105–106f

    isometric, 104
    isotonic, 95–104
    principles for use of, 95
  goals of
    increase muscular endurance as, 58
    increase power as, 58–59
    increase strength as, 57
  isokinetic, 68–69
    eccentric isokinetic training, 94
    equipment for, 104–107, 105–106f
    velocity spectrum rehabilitation,
      93–94
  isometric, 71–72
    brief repetitive (BRIME), 92
    equipment for, 104
    multiple-angle, 92–93
    muscle-setting exercise, 71
    precautions with, 72
    in rehabilitation and conditioning,
      92–93
    resisted isometric exercise, 71–72
    stabilization exercises, 72
  isotonic
    circuit weight training, 91
    concentric vs. eccentric, 67
    constant vs. variable, 66
    daily adjustable progressive resistance
      technique of, 90
    DeLorme technique of, 89–90
    equipment for, 95–104
    manual vs. mechanical, 66
    open chain vs. closed chain, 67–68
    Oxford technique of, 90
    stretch-shortening drills, 91–92
    variable-resistance exercise, 66–67
  manual
    for ankle, 82–83, 82f
    for cervical region, 555
    definition of, 57, 72–73
    for elbow, 77–78, 78f
    for fingers and thumb, 79, 79f
    for forearm, 78, 78f
    for hip, 79–81, 80–81f
    for knee, 81–82, 82f
    modifications of, 83
    principles of, 73–75, 73–74f
    for scapula, 77, 77–78f
    for shoulder, 75–77, 76–77f
    for toes, 83
    for wrist, 78f, 79
  mechanical
    bouts and frequency of exercise,
      85–86
    definition of, 57, 83–84
    duration of exercise, 86
    for elbow, 346, 346f
    intensity of exercise, 84–85
    mode of exercise, 87–88
    number of repetitions, 84–85
    open chain vs. closed chain, 88–89
    position of patient, 88–89
    repetition load, 85
    short-arc vs. full-arc, 88
    speed of exercise, 86–87
    submaximal exercise, 84
    variables of, 84–89
    for wrist and hand, 383–384

precautions for
  cardiovascular, 59–60
  exercise-induced muscle soreness,
    63–65
  fatigue, 60–61
  osteoporosis, 62–63
  overwork/overtraining, 61–62
  recovery from exercise, 61
  substitute motions, 62
progressive resistance, 251
  for shoulder, 310–312, 311–313f,
    320–327, 321–327f
specificity of training, 65
transfer of training, 66
Resisted test, 7–8
Resistive exercise(s), progressive, 83–84,
  89
Resistive reciprocal exercise unit, 100–101,
  101f
Respiration
  active, 651
  at different ages, 138
  external, 657
  internal, 657
  mechanics of, 651–653
  muscles of, 650–651
    weakness of, 699
Respiratory rate, in aerobic exercise, 607
Respiratory system
  adaptive changes leading to increased
    endurance, 17
  anatomy and function of, 653–655,
    654–655f
  changes with aerobic exercise
    with exercise, 130
    at rest, 130
  chest physical therapy, 649–687
  evaluation of, 8
  during exercise, 17
  in pregnancy, 600
  response to aerobic exercise, 119
  structure and function of, 650–657
Resting position
  of joint, 196
  of spine, 551
Restrictive lung disorder
  atelectasis, 709
  causes of
    extrapulmonary, 699
    pulmonary, 699–700
  changes associated with, 700, 700f
  definition of, 699
  impairments/problems in, 700
  pneumonia, 707–708
  postthoracotomy, 700–707
Reticulin fiber, 152
Retinacular release, lateral
  indications for, 436
  postoperative management of, 436–438
  procedures for, 436
Revascularization surgery, 635
Reversibility principle, 126
Rheumatoid arthritis, 143
  characteristics of, 257
  clinical considerations with, 257
  of elbow, 336, 339
  of foot and ankle, 476

of knee, 421–423
of shoulder, 278
of spine, 519
treatment considerations in
  in active disease, 257–258
  in remission period, 258–259
of wrist and hand, 358–359
  acute stage, management of, 363
  chronic stage, management of, 363
  nonoperative management of, 363
  repair of ruptured extensor tendons,
    371–372
  subacute stage, management of, 363
  surgical management of, 363–372
Rhomboid muscle, strengthening of, 323
Rhonchi. See Wheezes
Rhythmic stabilization exercise(s), 20, 72,
  83
  for ankle and foot, 492, 493f
  for hip, 412
  for knee, 462
  for shoulder, 325, 326f
  for spine, 551
  for trunk, 565–566
Ribs, 500, 650
  movements during respiration, 651–652
Rocker board, 412, 491, 491f, 493, 493f
Rockport Fitness Walking Test, 113
Rolling (joint motion), 186, 186f
ROM. See Range of motion
Rotator cuff
  impingement lesions of, 293
  short rotator muscles, 278
  stabilization of, 283–284
  tears of, 292
    indications for surgery in, 298
    postoperative management of,
      298–300
    surgical procedures in, 298
Round back, 535f, 536–537
Rubor, test for, 632–633
Runner's knee, 431

Sacroiliac back pain, in pregnancy,
  604–605
Salicylate cream, topical, 65
Sandbags, 95
Sarcomere, 147, 147f
  elongation and shortening of, 148, 148f
Sarcomere give, 148, 157
Sartorius muscle, overuse of, 391
Scalene muscle, 504, 504f, 650–651
  stretching of, 545–546, 546f
Scaphoid-radius articulation, joint
  mobilization techniques for, 214,
  215f
Scapula
  elevation of, 324
  manual resistance exercises for
    elevation and depression, 77, 77f
    protraction and retraction, 77, 78f
  manual resistance to motions of, 323
  motions of, 275–276
  protraction of, 324, 327
  range of motion exercises for, 30–31,
    31f

retraction of, 323–324, 324f
  with shoulder abduction and lateral
    rotation, 326–327, 327f
  with shoulder horizontal abduction,
    326, 326f
scapular control in shoulder problems,
  312, 313f
stability of, 276
stretching for, 171, 546
testing flexibility of protractors, 717
upward rotation of, 324
Scapular retraction, 617
  correction of, 569, 569f
Scapulohumeral rhythm, 276–277
Scapulothoracic articulation, 275–276
  joint mobilization techniques for, 207,
    207f
Scar, 18–19
  from cesarean childbirth, 623
  formation of, 243–244
  reinjury of "old scar," 253
  scar tissue adhesions, 146
Sciatic nerve, 392
Scissors, 719
Scleroderma, 143
Scoliosis, 390, 537–538, 538f
  cervical. See Torticollis
  functional (postural), 537, 549
  nonstructural, 537–538
  structural, 537–538, 538f
Segmental breathing, 669–670
  apical expansion, 670, 671f
  lateral costal expansion, 669, 669–670f
  posterior basal expansion, 670
  right middle-lobe or lingula expansion,
    670
Segmental pneumonia, 708
Segmental resection, of lung, 701
Selective stretching, 145
Selective tension procedure(s), 5–8, 618
Self-assisted cough, 677–678, 678f
Self-mobilization, of glenohumeral joint,
  284, 284–285f
Self-stretching, 160
  of adductor pollicis muscle, 380
  of ankle, 489–490, 490f
  of elbow, 345, 345f
  of evertor muscles of ankle and foot,
    490
  of extensor communis muscle, 381
  of extrinsic muscles of toe, 490
  of flexor digitorum profundus muscle,
    381, 381f
  of flexor digitorum superficialis muscle,
    381, 381f
  of foot, 489–490
  of hand and wrist, 362
  of hip, 404–408
  to insertion of iliotibial band, 433, 434f
  of interossei muscles, 380
  of latissimus dorsi muscle, 315
  of levator scapulae muscle, 319, 319f
  of lumbrical muscles, 380
  of pectoralis major muscle, 316–317,
    317f
  of shoulder, 284, 314, 314–316f
  of temporomandibular joint, 528

Self-traction, spinal
  cervical region, 587
  lumbar region, 590
Sellar (saddle) joint, 185, 185f
Semispinalis capitis muscle, 504f
Sensory disturbance, in arterial disorders, 631
Sensory test, 8
Serial cast, 157
Serratus anterior muscle, 651
  strengthening of, 324
Serratus inferior muscle, 501
Serratus posterior muscle, 501
Setting exercise(s). *See* Muscle-setting exercise(s)
Shaking, for postural drainage, 681–682
Shear force, 150
Sherrington's law of reciprocal innervation, 20
Shin splint, 483
Short-arc exercise(s), 88
Short-arc terminal extension exercise, for knee, 458–459, 458f
Shortness of breath
  positions to relieve, 693–694, 694f
  prevention and relieving of, 672
Shoulder
  arthritis in, 278–279
  arthrodesis of, 290–291
  bones and joint of, 200f
  closed-chain exercises for, 324
  correcting flexibility imbalances in, 313–328
  dislocations of
    anterior, 300–303, 302f
    anterior recurrent, 303–304
    closed reduction of, 301, 303
    etiology of symptoms in, 300
    functional limitations/disabilities in, 301
    impairment/problems in, 300
    indications for surgery in, 303, 305
    nonoperative management of, 301–303
    posterior, 300, 303
    posterior recurrent, 305–306
    postoperative management of, 304–306
    recurrent, 300
    related diagnoses in, 300
    surgical procedures in, 303–305
  eccentric training for, 328
  frozen, 279–280
  function of, 274–280
  functional articulations of, 275–276
  gear-shift exercises for, 309–310, 310f
  hemireplacement of, 290
  impingement syndromes
    indications for surgery in, 296
    postoperative management of, 297–298
    surgical procedures in, 296
  increasing endurance of, 328
  instability/subluxations in, 292
  joint mobilization techniques for, 673, 674f
    acromioclavicular joint, 205, 206f

glenohumeral joint, 199–205, 200–204f
    scapulothoracic articulation, 207, 207f
    sternoclavicular joint, 205–207, 206–207f
  joint problems
    acute and subacute problems, management of, 309–313
    co-contraction of shoulder girdle muscles, 312–313
    inhibiting pain and muscle guarding in, 309
    maintaining humeral head control in, 310–311, 311–312f
    maintaining scapular control in, 312, 313f
    maintaining soft tissue integrity and mobility in, 309–310, 310f
    nonoperative management of, 378–387
    subacute and chronic problems, management of, 313–318
    surgical management of, 287–291
  manual resistance exercises for
    abduction and adduction, 76, 76f
    extension, 76
    flexion, 75, 76f
    horizontal abduction and adduction, 76–77
    hyperextension, 76
    internal and external rotation, 76, 77f
  after mastectomy, 644
  muscle spasm about, 283–284
  muscle-setting techniques for, 310
  open-chain exercises for, 325, 326f
  painful shoulder syndromes
    etiology of symptoms in, 292–293
    functional limitations/disabilities in, 294
    impairments/problems in, 293–294
    nonoperative management of, 293–296
    postoperative management of, 296–300
    related diagnoses in, 291–292
  plyometrics for, 328, 328f
  postural imbalance/muscle length-strength imbalance in, 291
  range of motion exercises for, 314–320
    abduction and adduction, 29, 30f
    extension (hyperextension), 29, 29f
    finger ladder, 47, 47f
    flexion and extension, 29, 29f
    horizontal abduction (extension) and adduction (flexion), 30, 31f
    internal (medial) and external (lateral) rotation, 30, 30f
    overhead pulleys, 48, 48f
    rotation, 309, 310f
    self-assisted, 43, 44f, 309–310
    suspension, 51f
    wand exercises, 46, 46–47f
  referred pain in, 278
  reflex sympathetic dystrophy, 307–309
  resistance exercises for, 320–327, 321–327f
    abduction, 310

abduction and scaption, 321–323, 322f
    adduction, 323
    elbow flexion with forearm supinated, 311
    extension, 323
    external rotation, 310, 320, 321f
    flexion, 323
    humeral adduction and scapular depression, 327
    internal rotation, 310, 320–321, 322f
    scaption, 310, 311f
    scapular elevation, 324
    scapular elevation/depression, 312, 313f
    scapular protraction, 312, 324
    scapular protraction and horizontal adduction, 327
    scapular retraction, 312, 323–324, 324f, 326–327, 326–327f
    scapular upward and downward rotation, 312
    scapular upward rotation, 324
    rhythmic stabilization exercises for, 325, 326f
  self-resistance exercises for, 311, 311–312f
  self-stretching of
    abduction and elevation of arm, 314, 315f
    extension, 314, 316f
    external (lateral) rotation, 314, 314–315f
    flexion and elevation of arm, 314, 314f
  stabilization exercises for, 324–325, 325–326f
  strengthening muscles of, 313–318, 320–327
  stretching for
    abduction, 169, 169f
    adduction, 169
    external rotation, 169–170, 170f
    flexion, 168, 168f
    horizontal abduction, 170–171
    hyperextension, 168–169, 168f
    internal rotation, 170, 170f
  structure of, 274–278
  synovial joints of, 274–275
  thoracic outlet syndrome, 306–307
  total shoulder replacement, 287–290
  total-chain exercises for, 325
  weight-bearing exercises for, 312–313
Shoulder girdle
  function of, 276–278
  strengthening muscles that affect posture, 557
Shoulder-hand syndrome. *See* Reflex sympathetic dystrophy
Side-lying abduction, 722
Sit-up(s), as test of abdominal strength, 713
Skate board, range of motion exercises for hip, 49
Skill
  exercises to increase, 725
  testing of, 718

Skin
color and temperature in arterial disorders, 631–632
composition of, 153, 153f
mobility of, 18–19
test for rubor/reactive hyperemia, 632–633
Sliding (joint motion), 186–187, 187f
Sliding board, 102, 103f
Slow-twitch fiber, 116
Soft tissue. *See also* Connective tissue; Muscle; Skin adaptive shortening of. *See* Contracture
clinical conditions resulting from trauma or pathology, 238–239
contracture of. *See* Contracture
elasticity of, 147–148
lesions of, 238
surgical repair of, 266–267
material strength of, 150–152
mobility of, 18–19
noncontractile, mechanical properties of, 150–155
plasticity of, 147
properties that affect elongation of, 146–155
remodeling of, 154
severity of tissue injury
grade 1 (first-degree), 239
grade 2 (second-degree), 240
grade 3 (third-degree), 240
therapeutic methods to elongate, 155–160
Soft tissue release(s), 267
Soleus muscle, 419, 421, 474, 532
Specificity of training, 65, 87, 113, 125
Speed of exercise, 86–87
as indicator of endurance, 717
Spinal nerve root impingement, 579
Spinal stenosis, 518, 579
Spinal traction, 524, 575–590
cervical region, 583–587, 583–587f
contraindications to, 581
dosage of, 582–583
duration of, 582–583
in facet joint lesions, 521
facet joint mobilization in, 576–577
general procedures in, 582–583
home traction
cervical region, 586, 587f
lumbar region, 590
indications for
diskogenic pain, 581
hypomobility of joints, 579–580
meniscoid blocking, 581
muscle spasm or guarding, 580–581
pain from facet joints, 580
postcompression fracture, 581
spinal nerve root impingement, 579
intermittent, 578
in intervertebral disk lesions, 511, 516
limitations of, 581
lumbar region, 587–590, 588–589f
manual, 579, 582
cervical region, 583–584, 583f
lumbar region, 587–588
mechanical, 576, 579, 582

cervical region, 584–586, 585f
lumbar region, 588–590, 589f
safety rules for, 583
for muscle relaxation, 577
for pain reduction, 577–578
position of patient for, 582
positional, 579, 582
cervical region, 584
lumbar region, 588, 588f
precautions in, 582
self-traction
cervical region, 587
lumbar region, 590
static (constant)
continuous or prolonged, 578
sustained, 578
Spine. *See also* Facet joint(s); Intervertebral disk; Postural problem(s)
acute problems of, 496–528
functional position in, 504–505
gravity sensitive, 505
passive positioning in, 505–506
patient education and involvement in care, 505–506
cervical. *See* Cervical spine
chronic problems of, 531–573
contusions of, 521–525
curves of, 498
dynamic stabilization of, 551
functional units of, 497
inert structures influencing movement and stability of, 499–500
joints of, 499
lateral flexibility of, 549–551, 549–551f
ligaments of, 499
lumbar. *See* Lumber spine
muscle and soft tissue lesions, 521–525
acute phase, management of, 522–525
etiology of symptoms in, 521–522
impairments/problems in, 521–522
subacute and chronic phase, management of, 525
muscle function of
eccentric control, 500
limb muscles affecting spinal stability, 501
postural support from trunk muscles, 500–501
postcompression fracture of, 581
range of motion of, 551
resting position of, 551
rhythmic stabilization of, 551
strains of, 521–525
structure of, 497–504
subacute problems of, 531–573
traction procedures for. *See* Spinal traction
transitional stabilization of, 552
Spinning (joint motion), 188, 188–189f
Spirometry
incentive respiratory, 668
open-circuit portable, 117
Splint, postural, 571
Split-traction table, 588–590, 589f
Spondylosis, 519
Sprain, 238
of ankle, 484–485

of hand, 274–275
of knee, 441–448
Sputum evaluation, 663
Squat(s)
mini-squats, 462–463, 463f
modified, in pregnancy, 617
partial, 414, 567
Stability, 72
guidelines for developing, 19–20
Stabilization exercise(s), 19–20, 72, 74f
dynamic, 72
goals of, 19–20
in postural problems, 551–571
in pregnancy, 615
rhythmic. *See* Rhythmic stabilization exercise(s)
for shoulder, 324–325, 325–326f
StairMaster, 102
Standing push-up(s), 616
Standing wall slide, 463–464
Static stretch, 156
Step-down(s), 463
Stepping machine, 102
Step-up(s), 413, 463
Sternoclavicular joint, 275
hypomobility of, 286
joint mobilization techniques for
anterior glide, 206, 207f
inferior glide, 206, 207f
posterior glide, 205–206
superior glide, 206–207, 206f
joint problems
functional limitations/disabilities in, 286
impairments/problems in, 286
nonoperative management of, 286
related diagnoses and etiology of symptoms in, 285–286
surgical management of, 286–287
subluxations or dislocations of, 286
Sternocleidomastoid muscle, 504, 650–651
Sternotomy, median, 703
Straight-leg lowering, 458
bilateral, 561
Straight-leg raising, 423, 433–434, 457–458
bilateral, 561, 619, 718–719
as test of abdominal strength, 713–714
Strain, 238
definition of, 150–152, 151f
of spine, 521–525
Strength
breaking, 151, 151f
at different ages, 138
goal of therapeutic exercise, 14–16
increase in
changes in neuromuscular system, 15–16
guidelines for, 16
physical factors influencing, 14–15
recruitment of motor units, 15–16
normal, 14
resistance exercises to increase, 57
testing of, 712–715
ultimate, 151, 151f, 154
yield, 151, 151f
Strength training, 57

Strengthening exercise(s)
common errors in strengthening
programs
activity is too strenuous, 718–719
fatigue and strain not differentiated,
721
faulty biomechanics, 722–723
original program design is altered,
721–722
overemphasis on exercises
perpetuating faulty posture,
719–721
for gluteus maximus muscle, 410–411,
410–411f
for gluteus medius muscle, 409–410,
409f
for hip
abductors and hip hikers, 409–410,
409f
adductors, 411, 412f
extensors, 410–411, 410–411f
external rotators, 411
in postpartum period, 620
for quadratus lumborum muscles,
409–410, 409f
suggestions for safe program, 723
Stress, definition of, 150
Stress fracture, 152, 154
Stress-strain curve, 150, 151f, 153–154
Stretch receptor, 148–149, 149f
Stretch reflex, monosynaptic, 150
Stretch weakness, 145
Stretching, 143–180. See also Self-
stretching; Spinal traction
active inhibition. See Active
inhibition
of ankle, 179–180
ballistic, 156
of biceps brachii muscle, 319
of cervical spine, 547
contraindications to, 167
cryostretching, 165
cyclic, 158
definition of, 144–145
of deltoid muscle, 319–320
of elbow, 171, 171f
extensors, 348
flexors, 347–348
supinators and pronators, 348
of erector spinae muscles, 547–548, 548f
of fingers, 173–174
flexibility and, 144
of forearm, 171–172
of gastrocnemius muscle, 404
of gastrocsoleus muscle, 724
of gluteus maximus muscle, 405–406,
406f
of hamstring muscles, 406–408, 407f,
454
of hand, 380–381
of hip, 174–177, 174–177f
adductor and internal rotator muscles,
407f, 408
flexor muscles, 404–405
indications and goals of, 161
of intercostal muscles, 545
of knee, 175–179, 175f, 178–179f

of latissimus dorsi muscle, 315
of levator scapulae muscle, 318–319,
318–319f
of lower extremity musculature, 549
overstretch, 145
passive, 19, 25
conditions requiring special
precautions, 192
cyclic mechanical, 158
definition of, 145
joint mobilization vs., 188
maintained vs. ballistic, 156
manual, 155–157
patient evaluation prior to, 161
procedures for applying, 161–162
prolonged mechanical, 157, 158f
of pectoralis major muscle, 315–317,
316–317f
of pectoralis minor muscle, 317f, 318
of pectoralis muscles, 673, 674f
precautions for, 166–167
of quadriceps femoris muscle, 454–456,
455f
of rectus femoris muscle, 404–405, 405f,
455–456
of scalene muscles, 545–546, 546f
of scapular and humeral musculature,
171, 546
selective, 145
of shoulder, 167–170, 168–169f, 283
static, 156
of suboccipital muscles, 546, 546f
techniques using anatomic planes of
motion, 167–180
of tensor fasciae latae, 404, 408, 409f
terms related to, 144–146
of toes, 180
of triceps brachii muscle, 319
of wrist, 172–173, 172f, 381
Stretch-shortening drill(s). See Plyometric
training
Stroke volume, 17, 129
at different ages, 137–141
Structural stiffness, 152
Subacromial bursitis, 291
Subdeltoid bursitis, 291
Sublimis fist, 362
Subluxation, 238
Submaximal exercise, 84
Suboccipital muscle(s), stretching of, 546,
546f
Subscapularis muscle, strengthening of,
320–321, 322f
Substitute motion(s), 62
Subtalar joint, 471–472
arthrodesis, 479
increasing mobility of, 477
joint mobilization techniques for
medial glide or lateral glide, 230–231,
230f
traction (distraction), 229f, 230
range of motion exercises for, inversion
and eversion, 39, 40f
restricted motion of, 476
Suctioning, 679
Supinated foot. See Pes cavus
Supinator muscle, 335

Suprahumeral articulation, 276
Suprahyoid muscle, 504, 504f
Suprapatellar plica synovitis, 431
Supraspinatus muscle
function of, 278
strengthening of, 321–323, 322f
Supraspinatus tendinitis, 291
Surgery. See also Postoperative care;
Preoperative care
common orthopedic procedures,
265–270
complications of, 263
indications for, 262
open vs. arthroscopic, 265–266
Suspension
axial fixation, 50–51, 50–52f
range of motion exercises using, 49–51
vertical fixation, 50, 50f
Swan-neck deformity, 359
Swayback, 535–536, 535f
Swing (joint motion), 185
Sympathetic nervous system, response to
exercise, 119
Sympathetically maintained pain. See
Reflex sympathetic dystrophy
Synovectomy, 268, 364, 425, 478
arthroscopic, 339
of knee
expected results in, 427
indications for, 426
postoperative management of,
426–427
procedures for, 426
Synovitis, 238

Tachypnea, 660
Tactile reinforcement, 569
Talocalcaneal joint. See Subtalar joint
Talocalcaneonavicular joint, 471
Talocrural joint, 471
increasing mobility of, 477
joint mobilization techniques for
dorsal (posterior) glide, 228, 229f
traction (distraction), 227–228, 229f
ventral (anterior) glide, 228–230, 229f
restricted motion of, 476
Talofibular ligament, anterior, tears of,
485–487
Talonavicular joint, 472
Tarsal joint, transverse, 472
range of motion exercises for, supination
and pronation, 39, 40f
restricted motion of, 476
Tarsometatarsal joint, 472
increasing mobility of, 478
joint mobilization techniques for
dorsal glide, 231f, 232
plantar glide, 231–232, 231f
Telemetry, 117
Temporalis muscle, 503, 504f
Temporomandibular joint (TMJ)
dysfunction
causes of, 527
clinical picture in, 526–527
management of, 527–528, 529f

Tendinitis, 238
  bicipital, 291
  in foot or ankle, 482
  in hip, 402
  infraspinatus, 291
  supraspinatus, 291
  in wrist and hand
    acute phase, management of, 374
    etiology of symptoms of, 374
    functional limitations/disabilities in, 374
    impairments/problems in, 374
    subacute and chronic phases, management of, 374
Tendinosis, 238
Tendon
  composition of, 153, 153f
  inflammation of
    acute, therapy in, 245
    subacute, therapy in, 248
  lesions of, 238
  rupture or tear of, 238
    surgical repair of, 266–267
  strength increases in, 16
Tendon anastomosis, in repair of extensor tendons of hand, 371
Tendon graft, in repair of extensor tendons of hand, 371
Tendon transfer, in repair of extensor tendons of hand, 371
Tennis elbow, 343
Tenodesis, 381
Tenosynovectomy, 364
Tenosynovitis, 238
  in foot or ankle, 482
  in wrist and hand
    acute phase, management of, 374
    etiology of symptoms of, 374
    functional limitations/disabilities in, 374
    impairments/problems in, 374
    subacute and chronic phases, management of, 374
Tenotomy, 267
Tenovaginitis, 238
Tension, 150
Tension headache, 526
Tensor fasciae latae
  overuse of, 391
  stretching of, 404, 408, 409f
  tight, 391
Teres major muscle, strengthening of, 323
Teres minor muscle, strengthening of, 320, 321f
Thera-Band, 96
Thermoregulatory system
  in aerobic exercise, 607
  in pregnancy, 601–602
Thompson test, 487
Thoracic outlet syndrome
  etiology of symptoms in, 306
  functional limitations/disabilities in, 307
  impairments/problems in, 307
  nonoperative management of, 307
  related diagnoses in, 306
Thoracic region

active range of motion exercises for, 543
control of, 570–571
increasing range of motion in, 545–547, 546f
postural problems in, 536–538
stabilization exercises for, 552–564, 553–564f
strengthening muscles of extension, 553–554, 553–554f
strengthening of abdominal muscles, 557–561, 557–561f
transitional stabilization of, 555–556, 556f
Thoracic spine, control of, 570–571
Thoracolumbar fascia, 499–500
  anatomy of, 501, 501–503f, 503
Thoracotomy
  postoperative pulmonary conditions, 700–707
  preoperative care in, 703
Thorax
  anterior, mobility of, 545
  bucket-handle motion of, 652
  caliper motion of, 652
  movements during respiration, 651–652
  piston action of, 652
  pump-handle motion of, 651
  structure and function of, 650
3-Min Step Test, 113
Thromboangiitis obliterans, 630, 634
Thromboembolectomy, 634
Thrombophlebitis
  acute, 636–637
    treatment of, 639
  clinical signs and symptoms of, 637
  deep vein, tests for, 638
  prevention of, 638
  risk factors for, 637
Throwing ball, as test of arm strength, 715
Thrust, 185
Thumb
  abduction of, 383
  carpometacarpal joint of, 354–355
    joint mobilization techniques for, 216–217, 218f
    mobilization of, 361–362
    replacement of, 370–371
  manual resistance exercises for, 79, 79f
  opposition of, 383
  range of motion exercise for
    metacarpophalangeal joint, 34–35, 35f
    self-assisted, 44, 45f
Tibial nerve, posterior, 475
Tibial torsion, 391
Tibialis anterior muscle, 474
Tibialis posterior muscle, 474
Tibiofemoral articulation, 418
  joint mobilization techniques for
    anterior glide, 225, 225f
    long-axis traction, 223, 223f
    posterior glide, 223–224, 224f
    posterior glide alternate, 224–225, 224f
Tibiofibular joint, 470–471
  distal
    decreased mobility of, 476

joint mobilization techniques for, anterior or posterior glide, 226–227, 227f
  inferior, 470
  proximal
    decreased mobility of, 476
    joint mobilization techniques for, anterior glide, 226, 226f
  superior, 470
Tibiotalar joint, arthrodesis of, 481
Tidal volume, 656, 656f
Tight weakness, of muscle, 143
Tissue fluid stasis, in spine, 508
TMJ dysfunction. See Temporomandibular joint dysfunction
Toe(s)
  claw, 476
  first, arthrodesis of, 481
  hammer, 476
  joint mobilization techniques for
    intermetatarsal joints, 232
    interphalangeal joints, 232
    metatarsophalangeal joints, 232
  manual resistance exercises for flexion and extension, 83
  range of motion exercises for
    flexion/extension and abduction/adduction, 40, 40f
    self-assisted, 44, 46f
  self-stretching of extrinsic muscles of, 490
  stretching for, flexion and extension, 180
Toe touching, 407–408
  as test of flexibility, 716
Torque arm unit, isotonic, 98, 99f
Torticollis, 525–526
  asymmetric weakness in, 525
  congenital, 525
  hysterical, 526
Total ankle joint replacement, 478
  indications for, 479
  long-term results in, 480
  postoperative management of, 479–480
  procedure for, 479
Total elbow arthroplasty
  constrained metal prostheses in, 341
  indications for, 339–341
  long-term results of, 342
  postoperative management of, 341–342
  procedures for, 341
  semiconstrained or unconstrained replacements in, 341
Total hip replacement, 394–399
  cementless fixation in, 395
  indications for, 395
  postoperative instruction in, 396
  postoperative management of, 396–399
  procedures for, 395–396
Total joint replacement, 270
Total knee replacement, 425
  constrained prosthesis in, 428–429
  expected results in, 431
  fixation in, 429
  indications for, 427
  postoperative management of, 429–431
  procedures for, 427–429

Total knee replacement (*continued*)
  resurfacing (unconstrained) prosthesis
    in, 428
Total lung capacity, 656, 656f
Total shoulder replacement, 287–290
Total wrist arthroplasty
  indications for, 364
  postoperative management of, 365–366
  procedures for, 364–365
Total-chain exercise(s), for shoulder, 325
Toughness, 151
Trachea, 653
  mediastinal shift of, 661
  position of, 661
  tracheal tickle, 679
Tracheobronchial tree
  anatomy of, 653–654, 654–655f
  function of, 654–655
Traction, 189–190, 189f
  for local relaxation, 165
  long-axis, 189
  prolonged mechanical passive
    stretching, 157
  spinal. *See* Spinal traction
Training error, 254
Training stimulus threshold, 114, 124
Transcendental meditation, 20
Transfer of training, 66
Transitional stabilization
  of cervical and thoracic region, 555–556,
    556f
  of spine, 552
  of trunk, 567
Translatoric glide, 188
Transversus abdominis muscle, 501–503,
  501f, 503f, 651
Trapezius muscle, 504f, 650–651
  strengthening of, 323–324
Trauma
  continued reinjury, 253
  returning to activity too soon after, 254
Traumatic arthritis, in shoulder, 279
Treatment goal(s). *See* Goal(s)
Treatment plane, for joint mobilization,
  196, 197f
Triceps brachii muscle, 334–335
  range of motion exercise for, 32–33,
    33f
  stretching of, 319
Triglyceride(s), blood, 131
Triple arthrodesis, of ankle, 479, 481
Trochanteric bursitis, 401
Tropocollagen, 152, 153f
Trunk
  increasing extension of, 548–549, 548f
  increasing flexion of, 547–548, 548f
  posture and, 533
  rhythmic stabilization of, 565–566
  testing flexibility of, 717
  transitional stabilization of, 567
Trunk curl(s), 615
Trunk flexor(s), concentric-eccentric
  resistance to, 561
Tunnel of Guyon, compression in
  etiology of symptoms of, 373
  functional limitations/disabilities in, 373
  impairments/problems in, 373

nonoperative management of, 373
postoperative management of, 374
12-Min Run, 113

UBE. *See* Upper Body Exerciser
Ulnar nerve, 335, 357–358
Ulnomeniscal-triquetral (UMT) joint
  joint mobilization techniques for, 214,
    215f
  self-mobilization of, 361, 361f
  subluxed, unlocking of, 361
Ultimate strength, 151, 151f, 154
Ultrasonography, in arterial disorders, 633
UMT joint. *See* Ulnomeniscal-triquetral
  joint
Universal DVR system, 98–99
Upper Body Exerciser (UBE), 105, 106f
Upper extremity
  testing strength of
    with pull-ups or chin-ups, 714–715
    with push-ups, 714
    throwing ball test, 715
  weakness in mastectomy, 644
Upper respiratory tract, 653
Urinary system, in pregnancy, 600
Uterine cervix
  effacement and dilatation of, 597, 597f
  incompetent, 623
Uterus
  contraction of, 607
  involution in, 598

Valsalva maneuver, 59–60, 610
Variable-resistance equipment, 98–99,
  100f, 102–103
Varicose veins, 605, 637
  percussion test in, 638
  treatment of, 639
Vascular disorder(s) of extremities,
  629–647
  arterial, 630–636
  lymphatic, 640–641
  in mastectomy, 641–647
  venous, 636–639
Vastus medialis muscle, training and
  strengthening of, 457–460
Vastus medialis obliquus (VMO) muscle,
  419
  training and strengthening of, 457–460
    in non–weight bearing, 433–435
    in weight bearing, 435
Velocity spectrum rehabilitation, 87, 92–93
Vena cava compression, 607, 610, 610f
Venous disorder(s)
  acute, treatment of, 639
  chronic, treatment of, 639
  clinical signs and symptoms of, 637
  evaluation of, 637–638
  types of, 636–637
Venous insufficiency, chronic, 637
  clinical signs and symptoms of, 637
  treatment of, 639
Ventilatory muscle training, 667–672

Verbal reinforcement, 568
Vertical jump, as test of leg strength, 715
Vibration, for postural drainage, 681, 682f
Viral pneumonia, 708
Visual reinforcement, 568
Vital capacity, 656f, 657
VMO muscle. *See* Vastus medialis obliquus
  muscle
Vocal fremitus, 660

Walking against resistance, 567
Wall slide, 413–414, 414f, 566–567, 617
  gravity-assisted supine, 455, 455f
  standing, 463–464
Wand exercise(s), 45–47, 46–47f
  for chest mobilization, 674
  for pectoralis major muscle, 317, 317f
Warm-up period, 64, 126–127
Weakness. *See* Muscle weakness
Weight boots, 95
Weight gain, in pregnancy, 598–600
Weight training, circuit, 91
Weight-bearing exercise(s)
  for ankle and foot, 490–494, 491–493f
  for knee, 461–464
  for hip, 411–415, 411–414f
  for shoulder, 312–313
  unilateral, 620
Wheelchair patient, 135, 143
Wheezes, 663
Wobble board, 412
Wolff's law, 13
Work-hardening activity, for knee, 465
Working weight, 90
Wrist
  bones of, 212f, 353
  dorsal aspect of, 378, 378f
  dorsal clearance of extensor tendons of,
    365
  extensor tendons of, 378, 378f
  flexor tendons of, 375, 376f
  joint mobilization
    to increase extension, 361
    to increase flexion, 360
    to increase radial deviation, 361
    to increase ulnar deviation, 361
  joint mobilization techniques for
    glides of carpals in proximal row with
      radius and ulna, 214, 215f
    glides of intercarpal joints, 214–215
    radiocarpal joint, 212–215, 212–216f
  joint problems
    acute, management of, 360
    functional limitations/disabilities in,
      359–360
    impairments/problems in, 359
    nonoperative management of,
      358–363
    related diagnoses and etiology of
      symptoms in, 358–359
    surgery and postoperative
      management of, 363–372
  joints of, 212f, 353–354
  ligaments of, 354
  manual resistance exercises for

flexion and extension, 78f, 79
  radial and ulnar deviation, 79
mechanical resistance exercises for, 383–384
muscles of, 335
nerves of, 357–358
overuse syndromes, 372–374
range of motion exercises for
  flexion and extension, radial and ulnar deviation, 33, 34f

self-assisted, 43–44, 44f
referred pain in, 358
self-stretching of, 362
strengthening muscles of, 381–382
stretching for, 380–381
  extension, 172–173, 172f
  flexion, 172
  radial deviation, 173
  ulnar deviation, 173
tendinitis in, 374

tenosynovitis in, 374
total wrist arthroplasty, 364–366
volar aspect of, 375, 376f
Wryneck. *See* Torticollis

Yield strength, 151, 151f
Young adult, aerobic exercise in, 138–139

Zygapophyseal joint(s). *See* Facet joint(s)